Churchill Livi

Mini Encyclopaedia of Nursing

For Churchill Livingstone:
Senior Commissioning Editor: Sarena Wolfaard
Project Development Manager: Mairi McCubbin
Project Manager: John Ormiston
Designer: Judith Wright
Layout: Judith Campbell

Churchill Livingstone's
Mini Encyclopaedia of Nursing

Edited by
Chris Brooker BSc MSc RGN SCM RNT
Author and Lecturer, Norfolk, UK

Foreword by
Karen Holland BSc MSc CertEd SRN
Associate Head of School, School of Nursing,
University of Salford, Manchester, UK

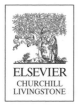

ELSEVIER
CHURCHILL
LIVINGSTONE

Edinburgh London New York Oxford Philadelphia St Louis Sydney Toronto 2005

ELSEVIER
CHURCHILL
LIVINGSTONE

An imprint of Elsevier Limited

First published 2005
ISBN 0 443 07487 9

British Library Cataloguing in Publication Data
A catalogue record for this book is available from the British Library
Library of Congress Cataloging in Publication Data
A catalog record for this book is available from the Library of Congress

Notice
Knowledge and best practice in this field are constantly changing. As new research and experience broaden our knowledge, changes in practice, treatment and drug therapy may become necessary or appropriate. Readers are advised to check the most current information provided (i) on procedures featured or (ii) by the manufacturer of each product to be administered, to verify the recommended dose or formula, the method and duration of administration, and contraindications. It is the responsibility of the practitioner, relying on their own experience and knowledge of the patient, to make diagnoses, to determine dosages and the best treatment for each individual patient, and to take all appropriate safety precautions. To the fullest extent of the law, neither the publisher nor the editor assumes any liability for any injury and/or damage.

The
Publisher's
policy is to use
**paper manufactured
from sustainable forests**

Printed in Spain by GraphyCems

CONTENTS

FOREWORD

When I was approached by Chris Brooker to write the Foreword to this book, I began to consider what it would look like and why nurses might need it.

I recollected using an encyclopaedia during my school days and remembered its value for project work and gaining a superficial understanding of countries and animals that I would probably never have an opportunity to see. It stimulated my interest in certain areas of world life and was a valuable reference resource. It also encouraged me to pursue in more detail those areas that were either necessary for schoolwork or of personal interest.

Reflecting on this prior perception of what an encyclopaedia contained and turning to the *Oxford English Dictionary* definition of 'book giving information on all branches of knowledge or of one subject, usually arranged alphabetically', I began to read *Churchill Livingstone's Mini Encyclopaedia of Nursing*.

My first impression was a sense of wonderment at how much work had been undertaken to develop such a valuable book. In her Preface, Chris explains that it complements the much shorter definitions found in pocket dictionaries. It lives up to this expectation and more.

One of the first areas I explored is that of acid–base balance, an absolute necessity to caring for any patient, and not an easy task to explain succinctly and understandably. The explanation offers not only a brief overview of what it is, but also the possible consequences of any disorders that distort this balance. The approach of providing a brief explanation while still conveying a deeper level of knowledge can be found throughout each alphabetical section. It is not only the physiological that is explained; definitions are also offered for more abstract concepts such as psychosocial theories of ageing and brief overviews of the total care of patients with illnesses such as diabetes.

I find particularly valuable the diagrams that create a link for the student between the written explanation of the human physiology (e.g. the pituitary gland) with a visual representation of the definition. Also invaluable are the sections on practical application, such as the definition of nutritional support, which also offers the reader guidance on how to help people to eat. Such supporting evidence reflects an understanding of the application of theory and practice. Although the book is aimed at nurses, the different sections are also of value to others who work in health and social care services.

I am particularly pleased to see references to the different professional groups a student nurse may meet when working in a multi-professional team. Recent evidence drawn from personal research indicates that lack of awareness on the part of healthcare professionals about their colleagues' roles can hinder the effective delivery of integrated services. Students, in particular, indicate that a better understanding would help them to learn with other professions within the clinical environment. This encyclopaedia gives definitions of the work of many of their colleagues, such as physiotherapists and dieticians.

In conclusion, I believe that, much like the encyclopaedia of my school days, this book will stimulate its readers to further study. It will also prove an invaluable reference resource both for personal use and, most importantly, within the clinical environment in which they learn the art and science of actual nursing practice.

Salford, 2005   Karen Holland

PREFACE

Churchill Livingstone's Mini Encyclopaedia of Nursing provides nurses with in-depth, evidence-based information that covers topics highly relevant to practice in the 21st century, such as accountability, ageing, child protection, communication, consent, disorders of mood, pain, pressure ulcers, reflection, research, stress, etc. The material used has been adapted from a wide range of authoritative sources, to give easy access to expert information in one easy-to-use book. The encyclopaedia expands on and complements the short definitions found in pocket dictionaries of nursing.

The in-depth information provides students with a starting point for planning assignments and essays and forms a quick reference source during clinical placements. It is useful for registered nurses to update knowledge and as a valuable resource when moving to new areas of practice. The inclusion of entries highly relevant to current practice is particularly helpful to nurses returning to practice after a break.

Over 600 main entries are arranged alphabetically and a comprehensive index allows you to locate the sub-headings found within the main entries. For example, the main entry Pressure ulcers has sub-headings that include Risk assessment, Pressure ulcer risk-assessment tools and Classification of pressure damage. Cross-references alert you to related entries and additional information elsewhere in the encyclopaedia. An arrow ⇒, either within or at the end of the entry, is used to indicate cross-references that contain related material.

Churchill Livingstone's Mini Encyclopaedia of Nursing includes practice application boxes, such as 'Helping people to eat', 'Keeping a reflective journal and reflective writing' and 'Sources of evidence for nursing practice', over 185 illustrations, references and many informative tables and text boxes. Many entries also include suggestions for further reading or other learning resources.

I hope that the encyclopaedia will be a valuable addition to the resources already available to nursing students and registered nurses, and that it will provide nurses with an excellent foundation for practice and for professional development.

Norfolk, 2005   Chris Brooker

ACKNOWLEDGMENTS

The editor thanks Roger Watson and Rosie Kneafsey for reviewing the manuscript, Elaine Kwiatek who provided advice about learning disability nursing and all the staff at Elsevier who were involved with the book, in particular Sarena Wolfaard, Mairi McCubbin and John Ormiston for their support and enthusiasm throughout the project.

ABORTION

In the UK, an abortion is defined as the spontaneous expulsion of the fetus or products of conception before 24 weeks of pregnancy. It is defined by the World Health Organization (WHO) as the expulsion of an embryo or fetus that weighs 500 g or less, which equates to a pregnancy of about 22 weeks gestation. In practice it is more common to refer to an abortion as a miscarriage to avoid causing distress, as some women associate the term abortion with a deliberate termination of pregnancy. ⇒ Early pregnancy problems (miscarriage).

TERMINATION OF PREGNANCY

In Great Britain the termination of pregnancy (TOP) is regulated by the Abortion Act 1967, with amendments subsequently made in s.37 Human Fertilization and Embryology Act 1990. The majority of terminations are in the first 12 weeks of pregnancy. The Abortion Act states that a pregnancy can be terminated up to 24 weeks gestation and that two doctors must agree that certain criteria are fulfilled, except in an emergency situation that requires a termination to save the life of the mother.

SURGICAL AND MEDICAL METHODS

The methods include:
* Suction dilatation and curettage (D&C) before the twelfth gestational week. A gemeprost pessary may be inserted before surgery to soften the cervix.
* Mifepristone can be administered for pregnancies up to 63 days of amenorrhoea and also in the second trimester (13–20 weeks gestation). The woman is then admitted 2 days later for the administration of prostaglandin.
* Late terminations of pregnancy (rare) – any surgical procedure that involves the destruction of the fetus and removal of products in parts. Medical termination involves the administration of mifepristone and vaginal prostaglandins, which induce labour.

Practice application – caring for women having TOP
Women who undergo TOP need support and a nonjudgemental attitude from the nurse. Health professionals who do find it difficult through personal or religious beliefs to reconcile this treatment are able to raise their conscientious objection and should not be made to participate in the actual process of termination. However, a nurse could be required to participate in the general care of these women. The decision to have a TOP is extremely distressing and not one made lightly by the woman, so she requires a supportive and professional approach from the nurse. ⇒ Code of Professional Conduct, Family planning, Infections of female reproductive tract, Haemolytic disease of the newborn (anti-D).

ABUSE

Abuse is deliberate injury to another person – either physical, sexual, psychological or through neglect, such as failure to feed or clothe. The term can apply to any group of people, but especially to the most vulnerable in society, such as children, people with learning disabilities, women, refugees and older people.

A

CHILD ABUSE

The physical, sexual or emotional abuse or neglect of children by family and other carers, other children, or health and social care staff. ⇒ Children's rights and protection, Neglect.

SEXUAL ABUSE OF CHILDREN

Sexual abuse involves adults who seek sexual gratification through the use of minors. This may be to have sexual intercourse or anal intercourse, to engage the child in fondling, masturbation or oral sex, and to encourage children to watch sexually explicit behaviour or pornographic material. The most common type of sexual abuse occurs between a father (or father figure) and daughter (incest).

Kempe and Kempe (1984) provide the most common specific definition of sexual abuse in children, "the involvement of dependent, developmentally immature children and adolescents in sexual activities they do not truly comprehend, to which they are unable to give informed consent, or that violate the taboos of family roles."

ELDER ABUSE

The physical (including the excessive use of sedating drugs), sexual, psychological or financial abuse of older people. It may be carried out by those relatives and friends responsible for their care or by health and social care staff.

Resources

Action on Elder Abuse – http://www.elderabuse.org.uk

ACCESS TO HEALTH DATA

ACCESS TO MEDICAL REPORTS ACT (1988)

The Access to Medical Reports Act only applies to reports made for insurance or employment purposes, and does not cover any notes about a patient's condition. A patient has a right to see a medical report compiled by a doctor with responsibility for his or her clinical care if this is then sent to an insurance company or employer.

ACCESS TO HEALTH RECORDS ACT (1990)

The Access to Health Records Act provides a right of access by patients to records kept about them that were created on or after 1st November 1991. A request can be made in writing, enclosing the set fee plus reasonable photocopying charges, and the patient can then receive copies of these notes. This Act applies to manual records only. It means that there is no right to access manually kept information created before 1st November 1991.

It is open to the holder of the manually or electronically stored records to refuse disclosure if, in the opinion of the holder, it is decided that disclosure would cause serious harm to the physical or mental health of the patient. The Act does not require the holder of information to justify such a decision. ⇒ Record keeping and documentation.

ACCIDENTS

⇒ Incident and accident reporting, Moving and handling, Risk assessment and management.

Accountability

Individual professionals are accountable for their own professional practice. They are expected to be able to account for their actions to any enquirer and to justify them on the grounds of best practice and knowledge, informed by good clinical judgement. In addition, each individual has an accountability to their professional peers, their team or department, the organization that employs them and their statutory body (e.g. Nursing and Midwifery Council) and/or their professional organization. There is also a wider accountability to the individual and organizational users of the service, potential users, taxpayers, the government and society as a whole.

These can alternatively be classified as accountability to:

- The public, through criminal law (e.g. murder);
- The patient and/or client, through civil law (e.g. negligence, breach of the duty of care);
- The employer, through contractual law (e.g. breach of confidentiality);
- The profession, through professional 'law' (e.g. inappropriate treatment of a patient or client).

These accountabilities are not necessarily mutually exclusive and a single event may require practitioners, such as nurses, to answer for their actions or omissions in a number of ways. The codes of practice used by the various professions are based upon the concept of accountability. ⇒ Clinical governance, Clinical supervision, Code of Professional Conduct, Evidence-based practice, Negligence, Nursing and Midwifery Council, Professional self-regulation.

Acid–base balance

An acid is a substance that can donate hydrogen ions (H^+). A base, or alkali, is a substance that can accept hydrogen ions. The concentration of H^+ is expressed as $[H^+]$. The acidity or hydrogen ion concentration of a solution is measured using the pH scale that ranges from 1 (strongly acidic) to 14 (strongly alkaline) with a midpoint of 7, which is neutral (*Fig. 1*).

The pH scale is logarithmic, which means that a change of one on the scale represents a tenfold change in the $[H^+]$ (e.g. a solution of pH 7 has ten times more H^+ than a solution of pH 8). This is important when considering the pH of blood, which must lie within a narrow range (pH 7.35–7.45) for homeostasis to be maintained. Outside this range physiological dysfunction occurs rapidly. On a daily basis the amount of H^+ excreted by respiration and in the urine must balance H^+ taken in the diet and produced by metabolic processes.

Effective mechanisms are therefore necessary to prevent accumulation of hydrogen ions and maintain homeostasis. The most important are:

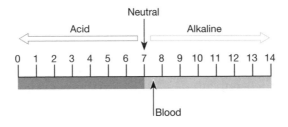

Fig 1 The pH scale

A

- Buffer systems (see below);
- Excretion of carbon dioxide (CO_2) by the lungs, which acts within minutes to adjust the pH;
- Renal excretion of hydrogen ions, which removes excess H^+ over many hours and is also the reason why urine usually has a slightly acidic pH.

pH REGULATION AND BUFFERS

A buffer is a substance that can accept H^+ from an acid solution and donate H^+ to an alkaline solution, and thereby minimize changes in pH by compensating for either a shortage or excess of H^+.

The main human buffering systems are the:
- Bicarbonate system (hydrogen carbonate), the major system, in which the amount of bicarbonate available for buffering is called the *alkaline reserve*;
- Hydrogen phosphate system;
- Plasma proteins, including haemoglobin.

DISORDERS OF ACID–BASE BALANCE

⇒ Electrolyte, Fluid balance and body fluids.
Acidaemia is present when arterial blood pH is less than 7.35 (i.e. closer to the acid part of the range), and the process that leads to the accumulation of excess acid is called *acidosis*. *Alkalaemia* is present when the arterial blood pH exceeds 7.45 (i.e. more alkaline), and the process that leads to the depletion of acid is termed *alkalosis*. When they occur, compensation takes place in an attempt to restore normal blood pH, through either alterations in the amount of CO_2 excreted by the lungs (which is rapid) or changes in the levels of bicarbonate secreted by the kidney tubules (which is slower to take effect). Acid–base disorders are described as either respiratory or metabolic according to their cause:
- *Respiratory acidosis* (e.g. caused by severe impairment of gaseous exchange in the lungs);
- *Respiratory alkalosis* (e.g. caused by overbreathing in panic attacks);
- *Metabolic acidosis* (e.g. caused by a failure to excrete H^+ at a normal rate in acute or chronic renal failure);
- *Metabolic alkalosis* (e.g. caused by excessive loss of hydrogen ions from the gastrointestinal tract through vomiting, aspiration or obstruction).

A mixed disorder may occur in seriously ill patients. The changes that occur in the arterial blood of the four main types in the list above are outlined in *Table 1*.
⇒ Blood gases, Oxygen (oxygen saturation, pulse oximetry).

Further reading

Brooker C and Nicol M (2003). *Nursing Adults. The Practice of Caring*, Ch 8. Edinburgh: Mosby.

ACQUIRED IMMUNE DEFICIENCY SYNDROME

Acquired immune deficiency syndrome (AIDS) is a term used to denote a particular stage of infection with human immunodeficiency virus (HIV). The Centers for Disease Control (CDC) in Atlanta define AIDS as the development of an AIDS-defining illness in a patient with HIV infection. CDC criteria for AIDS in a patient infected with HIV include the presence of candidiasis of the bronchus, trachea, lungs or oesophagus, invasive cervical cancer, Kaposi's sarcoma, pulmonary tuberculosis or other mycobacterial infection, and *Pneumocystis carinii* pneumonia.

A low CD4$^+$ T cell count of less than 200 per μL (or less than 14% of lymphocytes) in an HIV-positive person is also regarded as AIDS-defining, regardless of symptoms or opportunistic infections. ⇒ Human immunodeficiency virus.

Table 1 Acid–base problems: changes in arterial blood [H^+], $PaCO_2$ and HCO_3^-

Disorder	[H^+]	$PaCO_2$	HCO^{3-}
Metabolic acidosis			
Acute	↑	→	↓
Compensated (by ↑ ventilation)	↗ or →	↓	↓
Metabolic alkalosis			
Acute	↓	→	↑
Compensated (by ↓ ventilation)	↘ or →	↑	↑
Respiratory acidosis			
Acute (duration of hours)	↑	↑	→
Compensated (by renal retention of HCO_3^-; duration of days)	↗ or →	↑	↑
Respiratory alkalosis			
Acute	↓	↓	→
Compensated (by ↑ renal excretion of HCO_3^-)	↘ or →	↓	↓

ACTIVITIES OF DAILY LIVING

Under the term activities of daily living (ADL), most nurses include the usual hygiene activities associated with washing and dressing, and maintenance activities such as eating and drinking. Occupational therapists recognize the activities and tasks essential for self-care or home management. They include:
- Personal activities of daily living (PADL), such as washing, dressing, personal hygiene and eating;
- Domestic activities of daily living (DADL), such as cooking, laundry and cleaning;
- Instrumental activities of daily living (IADL), sometimes used synonymously with DADL, but it includes a wider range of activities, such as using means of communication, shopping, maintaining home and garden, etc.

Competence and independence in ADLs is essential for personal survival, health and well-being. Persons who are unable to cope with the necessary range of activities are likely to be at risk and require care services. ADL assessment and training is an occupational therapy technique in which a period of objective appraisal of a person's ability to perform ADLs is followed by a training programme to improve function. Adaptations may be made to the environment to improve an individual's ability to perform ADLs consistently and competently.

ACTIVITIES OF LIVING MODEL

The activities of living (AL) model (Roper *et al.* 1996) is the only model to have been developed in the UK, although it is based on work in the 1960s of the American nursing theorist Virginia Henderson. It stems from the belief that the person is an individual engaged in certain 'activities of living (ALs)' that enable them to live and grow. The individual's ability to be independent in these activities may be affected by illness or disease, but also by their age. For example, newborn babies are dependent on others for most of their ALs, but gradually become independent in these activities as they mature and develop. Illness, an accident or pregnancy may mean that someone who was previously independent in all ALs may become dependent in some and require the assistance of others. Equally, as we become older we may become increasingly dependent on others for certain activities (e.g. mobilizing), but remain completely independent in others, such as communicating. According to this model, the aim of nursing is to assist the patient as necessary to restore independence and meet the goals planned in partnership with the patient or client. Nursing interventions are also needed to implement the medical care plan and health promotion activities that enable the person to prevent or avoid ill health.

ACTIVITIES OF LIVING

The 12 ALs were developed from the 14 ADLs originally identified by Henderson (1966). They are:
- Breathing;
- Maintaining a safe environment;
- Communicating;
- Eating and drinking;
- Elimination;
- Personal cleansing and dressing;
- Controlling body temperature;
- Working and playing;
- Mobilizing;
- Sleeping;
- Expressing sexuality;
- Dying.

Breathing must be considered of prime importance because it is essential for all other activities (Roper *et al.* 1996), but the other ALs are not in any fixed order of priority. The nurse should vary the order according to the needs and priorities of the patient. The model provides a framework or *aide-mémoire* for a holistic assessment, and the nurse works in partnership with the patient (or family and/or significant others where patients cannot participate) to assess the patient's level of independence and any needs or problems in relation to each of the activities.

The model identifies five factors that influence each activity:
- Physical;
- Psychological;
- Sociocultural;
- Environmental;
- Politico-economic factors.

The influencing factors are crucial to the assessment process and ensure that nurses do not simply focus on the physical needs of the patient, but also consider all the other factors during assessment.

Further reading

Holland K, Jenkins J, Solomon J and Whittam S (2003). *Applying the Roper–Logan–Tierney Model in Practice.* Edinburgh: Churchill Livingstone.

ACTIVITY TOLERANCE

Activity tolerance is the amount of physical activity tolerated by a patient. It may be assessed in people with angina or after myocardial infarction. Graded exercise, including walking, cycling and going up stairs, may be used to rebuild confidence during the convalescent phase after any serious illness or injury – an important aspect of any rehabilitation programme. ⇒ Exercise, Rehabilitation.

ADENOSINE

Adenosine is a nucleoside formed from ribose (a pentose sugar) and adenine; with the addition of one, two or three phosphate groups it forms the nucleotides adenosine monophosphate (AMP), adenosine diphosphate (ADP) and adenosine triphosphate (ATP). These molecules are vital in cellular energetic processes. ⇒ Metabolism.

ADENOSINE DIPHOSPHATE

ADP is an important cellular metabolite involved in energy exchange within the cell. Chemical energy is conserved in the cell, by the oxidative phosphorylation of ADP into ATP, primarily in the mitochondrion, as a high-energy phosphate bond.

ADENOSINE MONOPHOSPHATE

AMP is involved in the release of energy for cell use. The form *cyclic adenosine monophosphate* (cAMP) has an important function as a *second messenger* for many hormones (e.g. glucagon) and in biochemical process in which many reactions are catalysed simultaneously (enzyme cascade).

ADENOSINE TRIPHOSPHATE

ATP is a high-energy compound that, on hydrolysis to ADP, releases chemically useful energy. ATP is generated during the catabolism of organic fuel molecules, such as glucose. ATP molecules are generated during glycolysis, in the reactions of Krebs' citric acid cycle, but most are produced during oxidative phosphorylation of ADP in the electron-transfer chain. The energy from ATP is used to drive metabolic processes, such as the active transport of substances across cell membranes, synthesis of molecules and muscle-fibre contraction.

ADRENAL GLANDS

The two triangular adrenal (suprarenal) glands are situated on the upper pole of each kidney. Each adrenal gland has a middle part or medulla, and a cortex around the outside.

The cortex secretes the steroid hormones or corticosteroids. The three types of corticosteroids are glucocorticoids, mineralocorticoids and sex hormones. Together they control metabolism, chemical constitution of body fluids, sustained stress responses and secondary sexual characteristics. Secretion is controlled either by the pituitary hormone corticotrophin, which is also known as adrenocorticotrophic hormone (ACTH), or changes in body chemistry in conjunction with other hormones. ⇒ Corticosteroids.

The adrenal medulla secretes the catecholamines adrenaline (epinephrine) and noradrenaline (norepinephrine). These hormones are involved in the initial response to stress.

DISORDERS OF THE ADRENAL GLANDS

ADRENAL INSUFFICIENCY

Primary adrenal insufficiency is known as Addison's disease. There is deficient secretion of cortisol and aldosterone because of the primary failure of the adrenal cortex, which causes electrolyte imbalance, diminished blood volume, hypotension, weight loss, hypoglycaemia, muscular weakness, gastrointestinal upsets and pigmentation of skin.

Secondary adrenal insufficiency results from pituitary or hypothalamic disease. Causes include trauma after neurosurgery or, less commonly, after infection, radiotherapy or haemorrhage. However, the most common cause is sudden cessation of glucocorticoid treatment.

Management involves the replacement of deficient hormones, correction of fluid and electrolyte imbalances and, where possible, treatment of the cause.

A

CUSHING'S DISEASE (SYNDROME)

Cushing's disease is a rare disorder, mainly of females, characterized principally by a cushingoid appearance, proximal myopathy, hyperglycaemia, hypertension and osteoporosis. It results from excessive cortisol production by hyperplastic adrenal glands because of increased ACTH secretion by a tumour or hyperplasia of the anterior pituitary gland.

Cushing's syndrome is clinically similar to Cushing's disease, but includes all causes, such as adrenocortical hyperplasia and tumour, ectopic ACTH secretion by tumours and glucocorticoid therapy.

HYPERALDOSTERONISM (CONN'S SYNDROME)

Hyperaldosteronism is the excessive production of aldosterone that causes hypertension, hypokalaemic alkalosis, muscle weakness and, rarely, tetany. Primary hyperaldosteronism is called Conn's syndrome and is caused by hyperplasia or adenoma of the adrenal cortex, whereas secondary hyperaldosteronism is caused by another condition, such as heart failure or increased rennin secretion.

PHAEOCHROMOCYTOMA

Phaeochromocytoma is a condition in which there is a tumour of the adrenal medulla, or of the structurally similar tissues associated with the sympathetic chain. It secretes adrenaline (epinephrine) and allied hormones and leads to hypertensive crises, with associated headache, flushing and tachycardia.

ADRENAL SEXUAL DISORDERS – CONGENITAL ADRENAL HYPERPLASIA (ADRENOGENITAL SYNDROME)

Adrenal sexual disorders result from abnormal activity of the adrenal cortex. A female child shows an enlarged clitoris and possibly labial fusion, perhaps being confused with a male. The male child may show pubic hair and an enlarged penis. In both male and female there is rapid growth, muscularity and advanced bone age.

ADVANCE DIRECTIVE

Advance directives are also known as 'living wills'. They are written declarations made by mentally competent persons that set out their wishes regarding life-prolonging medical interventions if they are incapacitated by an irreversible disease or are terminally ill, which prevents them making their wishes known to health professionals at the time. An advance directive is legally binding if it is in the form of an advanced refusal and the maker is competent at the time of declaration.

ADVANCED LIFE SUPPORT

Advanced life support (ALS) covers the advanced resuscitation techniques used during cardiopulmonary arrest, which may result from ventricular fibrillation (VF) and / or ventricular tachycardia (VT), asystole or electromechanical dissociation, and follow-on from basic life support. ALS involves the use of drugs [such as adrenaline (epinephrine) or atropine] appropriate to the type of cardiopulmonary arrest, artificial aids such as defibrillation and advanced skills to save or preserve life (*Fig. 2*). ⇒ Basic life support, Defibrillation.

PAEDIATRIC ADVANCED LIFE SUPPORT

Paediatric advanced life support (PALS) involves the use of the special techniques, drug doses and equipment appropriate to the body weight and surface area of the child being resuscitated. ⇒ Intraosseous.

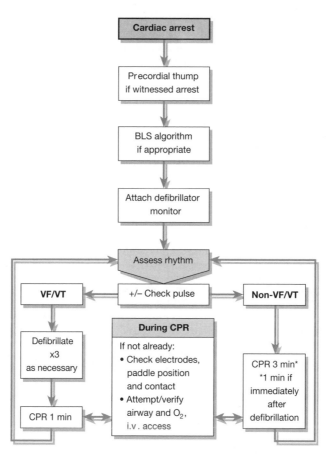

Fig 2 Algorithm – advanced life support (adapted from Resuscitation Council 2000)

BROSELOW PAEDIATRIC RESUSCITATION SYSTEM

The Broselow paediatric resuscitation system is a system designed in the USA for use during paediatric resuscitation. The Broselow tape measure, with its colour segments, is placed alongside the child. This provides the medical team with accurate information, from the colour segment that corresponds to the length of the child, regarding the correct size of equipment and appropriate drug doses to be used for that child. The equipment is stored in colour-coded packaging.

ADVOCACY

Advocacy is the process by which a person supports or argues for the needs of another. Nurses may act as an advocate for their clients and/or patients. Advocacy means speaking up for people who have difficulty doing so for themselves. However, an important variant in health and social care is self-advocacy, which involves teaching and supporting disadvantaged individuals in putting forward their own case. Formal advocacy services tend to be funded most frequently in support of those with learning disabilities or mental health problems. A further variant is class advocacy or collective advocacy, in which a group of people try to win rights or change attitudes on behalf of a cause rather than specific individual clients.

In the UK the work of Help the Aged and other campaigning charities tends to fall into this category. Many healthcare professionals also regard themselves as advocates for their clients or patients, although external advocacy services are frequently critical of the ability of paid staff to be sufficiently independent of the employing organization to act as true advocates

Affect

There is a tendency to use the terms 'affect', 'emotion' and 'mood' interchangeably. However, there are differences. Affect is a subjective interpretation of the feelings that accompany an idea or image. Similar in meaning to mood, it can be defined as a state of emotional tone or feeling that can fluctuate between depression and elation. Affect is the term reserved for the experience of the emotion plus the drive energies presumed to generate the conscious and unconscious feelings associated with it. ⇒ Disorders of mood, Emotion,

Ageing

Old age is difficult to define and several classifications are used. Functionally defined, it may be taken as the age at which a person becomes eligible for a state pension, a group who are commonly referred to as the 'elderly'. However, this used to be 65 years for men and 60 years for women in the UK, but will soon be 65 years for both men and women; it is 55 years in the USA. It should be understood that, at whatever age old age is considered to begin, the age is arbitrary and, largely, socially defined. There is a further classification among those considered to be elderly into the 'old', those aged over 75 years, and the 'very old', those aged over 85 years (Watson 1993). It should be understood that there is a great variety of experiences and ability among all elderly people.

The number of older people is increasing in both absolute and relative terms in the developed and developing countries. A number of factors are conspiring to produce this effect, one of which is the increasing life expectancy at birth. At the other end of the age range it is generally the case in developed countries that fertility is decreasing, which means the number of older people constitutes an ever-increasing proportion of the population.

The projected relative and absolute increase in the number of older people has consequences for individuals who live longer in greater numbers and for the societies in which they live. There is an increased dependency among older people, which arises for reasons of physical and mental disability as well as social dependency. It does not mean that all older people are dependent, in fact the majority are independent, but the dependency does have economic and social consequences. ⇒ Confusion and delirium, Dementia.

PSYCHOSOCIAL THEORIES OF AGEING

It is hard to disentangle the social from the psychological aspects of theories of ageing, so they are usually considered together under the term 'psychosocial'. Moreover, it must be appreciated that, while there are a number of theories of psychosocial ageing, there is little evidence to support any systematic change in the psychology of people as they become older.

DISENGAGEMENT, ACTIVITY AND CONTINUITY THEORIES

Disengagement theory describes a process whereby people gradually disengage from life as they become older. For example, a person may retire from employment and thereby have less involvement with the lives of the people who were also employed in the same company. On the other hand, activity theory describes a process whereby, while people do disengage from certain activities as they become older, they replace these with others that they are able to do physically and economically. For example, an individual who retires from work may take up new hobbies and interests. Of course, the evidence supports both of these theories of ageing, and it is certain that, while there are elements of truth in both theories, neither of these could be described as comprehensive.

Lying somewhere between the above theories is continuity theory, which describes a process whereby people, as they age, struggle to retain as many of the activities of their younger life as possible. Clearly, there is a great variety of experiences among older people in terms of activity, and these are dictated by many factors, such as ability, motivation and financial status.

ERIKSON'S THEORY OF LIFESPAN

One theory that attempts to describe the process of ageing from the cradle to the grave is Erikson's theory of the lifespan in which eight stages of the life process are described (*Box 1*). This is in contrast to the above theories, which really only consider old age and are not developmental. Erikson's theory incorporates adjustment to the process of ageing and further psychological development as people age.

Box 1 Erikson's theory: the eight stages of lifespan development
- Basic trust versus mistrust in infancy.
- Autonomy versus shame and doubt in early childhood.
- Initiative versus guilt in play age.
- Industry versus inferiority in school age.
- Identity versus confusion in adolescence.
- Intimacy versus isolation in young adulthood.
- Generativity versus self-absorption in adulthood.
- Integrity versus despair in old age.

Each stage represents a choice or conflict, and the way that the conflict is resolved affects all subsequent stages. It also affects the development of personality and success in adapting to the world. The internal conflicts in old age are integrity versus despair. The ultimate stage of Erikson's theory sees the older person reflecting on life and evaluating whether or not it has been a worthwhile and positive experience. Erikson's theory is borne out to some extent by the process of life review, whereby older people tend to reminisce more than younger people do in an effort to evaluate the past and their part in it.

The psychosocial theories of ageing presented above are by no means comprehensive, but some conclusions can be drawn. Not one of the theories is comprehensive and none are testable scientifically because it is not possible to measure some of the concepts upon which the theories are based. It is important, however, to be aware of these theories and their influence on practice.

BIOLOGICAL THEORIES OF AGEING

Biological ageing, or senescence, is an indisputable fact with plenty of supporting evidence. There are many classic signs of ageing, some of which become evident even in relatively young people. For example, the loss of hair colour, loss of elasticity of the skin that leads to wrinkling and less joint flexibility are all signs of ageing that are universally displayed, albeit to different extents in people as they age. A congenital condition known as progeria is characterized by premature ageing during childhood. Biological theories of ageing may have hereditary, physiological and cellular components.

A

HEREDITARY THEORIES

The hereditary theories are genetic in nature and propose that we are 'programmed' at birth to age and die. This may be true for individuals in terms of rate of ageing and lifespan. Environmental aspects may play their part by acting on the genetics of individuals. However, no specific ageing genes have yet been identified

PHYSIOLOGICAL THEORIES

There are a number of physiological theories of ageing:
- The notion that 'wear and tear' leads, at different rates between systems and between individuals, to the organs gradually losing their capacity to undertake their physiological functions;
- Another theory is based on a decreased ability to maintain homeostasis as the body ages, which leads to a decreased ability to withstand physiological stresses, such as dehydration, changes in temperature and disturbances to homeostasis caused by disease;
- The cross-linkage theory is based on the accumulation of metabolic waste products with age, which leads to a chemical change in the collagen in the body;
- The immune system has been implicated in ageing because, as we age, it becomes less able to fight infection and may even begin to attack cells of the body – a condition known as autoimmunity.

CELLULAR THEORIES

The remaining theories of biological ageing may be grouped under the heading of cellular theories. These include:
- Cell-doubling theory is based on the notion that the somatic (body) cells are able to double a specified number of times only.
- DNA theories speculate that, with age, the cell is decreasingly able to repair the inevitable errors that take place as DNA is replicated, and such errors lead to malfunctions in cell activity.
- Related to the DNA theories is the speculation that ageing takes place by error catastrophe, whereby errors that accumulate in DNA also accumulate in RNA. The number of errors rises to a critical level beyond which cell function is no longer possible, which results in the death of cells and ageing of the body.
- Free radical theory encapsulates the notion that, with age, the body becomes less able to withstand the effects of oxygen on the DNA and phospholipids, which leads to genetic and cellular damage. Oxygen, despite its crucial role in cell metabolism and survival, is actually a very toxic molecule during the process of metabolism, and in conjunction with certain pollutants, such as cigarette smoke, is potentially very damaging.

Practice application – Clifton Assessment Procedures for the Elderly
One particular instrument, the Clifton Assessment Procedures for the Elderly (CAPE; Pattie and Gilleard 1979) is commonly used in the assessment of older people who appear to be confused. It assesses:
- Psychomotor activity (motor effects of mental activity);
- Cognition (awareness, one of the three aspects of the mind);
- Behaviour.
Psychomotor assessment is carried out using the Gibson Spiral Maze (Gibson 1961). This tests psychomotor ability by asking the person to trace a line from the centre of the spiral outwards, avoiding the obstruction and to complete this as quickly as possible. The time taken to complete the maze and the number of errors form the basis of the score – the lower the score the better.

For the cognitive assessment, the client answers 12 set questions that relate to personal data, orientation and mental ability, to give a possible total score of 12. Clients with depression are expected to score eight or more, while those with dementia are likely to score seven or less (Pattie and Gilleard 1979).

Behavioural assessment is carried out using the Behaviour Rating Scale, which measures the level of dependence or independence based on 18 items, including bathing, dressing, mobility, eliminating and socializing. This scale, in contrast with that of cognitive assessment, identifies dependency level with the highest scores. Therefore, the less the patients can do, the higher their scores.

The CAPE score can be used immediately; however, it is usual to record the scores and repeat the test over a period of time to monitor the person's improvement or deterioration.

Although a helpful instrument, CAPE should be used with caution with some people. Those with mild confusion may be unable to carry out the activities or only partially achieve them. Others may have a limited ability to understand the questions because of a limited knowledge of the language or cultural differences. Others may have sensory deficits and/or failings.

A GEISM

Ageism is stereotyping people according to chronological age, with overemphasis on the negative aspects to the detriment of the positive ones. It is a term that describes a situation in which a discriminatory attitude disadvantages older people on the basis of chronological age. Ageism is also interpreted to be stigmatizing and to demarcate the older person from others who are younger. Further, ageism can affect people of any age. The practice of ageist behaviours is often demonstrated in the choice of words used, for example 'senile' and 'geriatric' are terms that have become derogatory (Behrens 1998). In addition, the media often reinforces this negative stereotyping. An ageist attitude can develop from the process of socialization, parental behaviours, peer influences and teachers' attitudes.

A balanced approach to healthy ageing is adopted by professionals to promote anti-ageist behaviours across boundaries. Healthcare professionals can reduce the impact of ageism by exercising sensitivity in their daily interactions with clients and promoting a positive image of ageing.

A GGRESSION

Nurses may encounter aggressive behaviour in all areas of practice – community settings, emergency departments and in all in-patients areas. The aggressive behaviour may be seen in service users, their family and friends, and also colleagues. Aggressive behaviour does not just mean being assaulted; it also includes making people feel abused or threatened. It is possible to make distinctions between aggression and violence. Aggression refers to a range of behaviours, including verbal, emotional or physical actions, that are intended to produce harm to another. Aggressive acts range on a continuum from verbal or emotional acts to serious physical harm, but, in contrast to violent acts, physical harm is not essential. It is important to stress that the perception of what is an aggressive act may vary. For example, what one person may deem as a verbal 'assault' may be identified by another person as an 'assertion' or a 'defensive' act.

Violence, on the other hand, refers to actual physically destructive acts carried out by one person upon another. This behaviour is intended to produce physical harm. Violent acts are therefore characterized by the use of physical force. They

A

may be directed outwardly to others or inwardly at the individual (deliberate self-harm). ⇒ Anger, Suicide and deliberate self-harm.

> **Practice application – identifying cues that warn of imminent aggression**
> Recognition of anger and impending aggression is essential if measures are to be taken to de-escalate the risk. Some nonverbal cues that may precede aggression include:
> • Body language and other nonverbal cues (e.g. finger pointing, standing close, aggressive posture, fixed eye contact, looking away, etc.);
> • Voice – raised voice and shouting, verbal threats, enlisting assistance from others, etc.

De-escalation is a term that refers to the process of reducing the threat posed by a potential aggressor. Before any action is taken to de-escalate a potentially aggressive incident it is essential that nurses be aware of their own feelings. Fear in this situation is to be expected, and can be used to provide the impetus needed to take the necessary action. Three actions are essential (*Table 2*).

Table 2 Actions to deal with the potential aggressor

Actions	Rationale
Listen to what the aggressive individual is saying	This will provide the information necessary to identify and deal with the source of the individual's anger
Focus on the source of the individual's anger	This will help to prevent the conversion of the focus of aggression to a more physical process
Try not to mirror the aggressive posture	Adopting an aggressive body posture in response to that of the potential aggressor is likely to be interpreted as the nurse's own preparation for aggression (Braithwaite 1992)

A GONIST

An agonist is:
• A muscle that contracts and shortens to perform a movement;
• A drug or other substance that imitates the response of the natural chemical messenger when it binds to molecules on the body cell, such as selective beta$_2$-adrenoceptor agonists (e.g. terbutaline, a bronchodilator) or beta$_1$-adrenoceptor agonists (e.g. dopexamine and dobutamine, positive inotropes).
⇒ Antagonist, Pharmacokinetics and pharmacodynamics.

A IDS TO INDEPENDENCE

Aids to independence is a term to describe any articles that enable a person to retain or regain independence (*Fig. 3*) Such articles include those used:
• To prepare, cook, serve and eat food, as well as to swallow liquids;
• For personal hygiene, dressing and undressing;
• To accomplish walking, ascending stairs and so on;
• For transit.
Their use is explicit in the concept 'aided independence'. ⇒ Mobility (mobility aids).

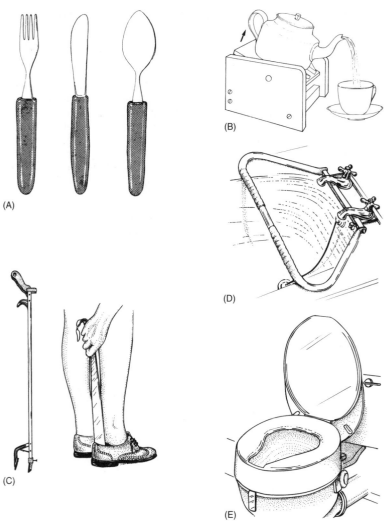

Fig 3 A selection of aids to independence: (A) cutlery with foam-covered handles, (B) tipper for teapot or kettle., (C) easy reacher and shoe horn, (D) bath support rail, (E) raised lavatory seat and lid

AIRWAY

The term airway is used to describe the entry to the larynx from the pharynx.

AIRWAY MAINTENANCE

Any procedure or condition that alters the level of consciousness has the potential to compromise the airway. Altered consciousness may result from cardiac arrest, trauma, drugs overdose, general anaesthetic, etc. In the unconscious person, the airway should be manually supported until the person is able to do so unaided. ⇒ Anaesthesia, Basic life support.

A

AIRWAY MAINTENANCE DURING THE PERIOPERATIVE PERIOD

The process of anaesthesia often requires the use of an airway maintenance device (AMD). A range of these may be used according to the person's airway requirement. They are:

- Oropharyngeal airways, such as the rubber or plastic Guedel, are commonly used for short-term airway maintenance and postoperative airway management (*Fig. 4A*). Oropharyngeal airways prevent the tongue from falling back and obstructing the throat. Nasopharyngeal airways are also available (*Fig. 4B*).
- The laryngeal mask airway (LMA) is used in cases where the person can breathe spontaneously or where assisted ventilation is appropriate and can be maintained. It is inserted relatively easily and, because the inflated cuff sits over and masks the larynx, there is no trauma or damage to the vocal cords or throat (*Fig. 4C*). The LMA is not ideally suitable for procedures in which the LMA can be dislodged. Additionally, emergency surgery or situations with a high risk of regurgitation and aspiration of gastric contents are not ideal scenarios for LMA usage. The trachea is not occluded using this device and aspiration may be a concern.
- An endotracheal tube (ETT) is designed to provide optimal anaesthetic delivery and minimal risk of aspiration. The ETT, which may be cuffed or noncuffed, is inserted nasally or orally and passes through the larynx and

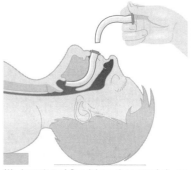

(A)   Insertion of Guedel oropharyngeal airway

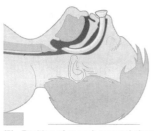

(B)   Position of nasopharyngeal airway

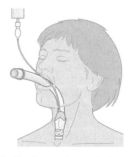

(C)   The laryngeal mask *in situ*

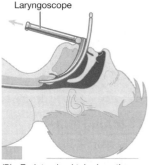

(D)   Endotracheal tube insertion

Fig 4 Airway maintenance devices

vocal cords and down the trachea (*Fig. 4D*). The cuffed tube has a balloon or cuff which, when inflated in the trachea, provides an occlusive seal and thus prevents any fluid draining into the lower airway and lungs. The ETT may cause trauma that leads to sore throats and hoarseness.

Airway obstruction is a major postoperative concern in the unconscious patient and is often caused by the tongue falling back against the posterior pharynx. Placing the person in the recovery position (*Fig. 5*), if his or her condition allows, is often sufficient to re-establish and maintain a patent airway.

Alternatively, where there is danger of the tongue falling back to obstruct the airway and the person cannot be moved safely, the nurse can move the tongue forwards by using the jaw-thrust method (*Fig. 6*).

If the person is unable to maintain his or her own airway, an artificial airway may be inserted, if not already *in situ*, to maintain airway patency. The most commonly used oral airway is the Guedel type, which may be removed easily by the person as consciousness returns.

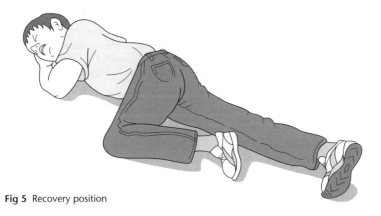

Fig 5 Recovery position

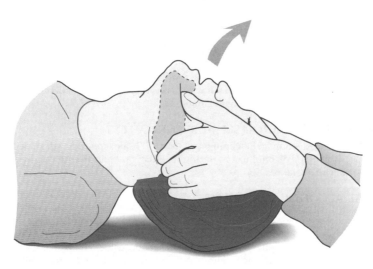

Fig 6 Jaw-thrust

A

> **Practice application – signs of postoperative airway obstruction**
>
> It is essential that the nurse in the recovery unit be able to recognize signs of impaired respiratory function, which may be caused by a partial or total airway obstruction.
>
> Airway obstruction may result directly from the presence of a foreign body. Alternatively it may be an inflammatory or protective response to airway trauma. Signs of airway obstruction might range in severity and may include (from mild to severe):
> * Restlessness;
> * Mouth breathing;
> * Confusion agitation and anxiety;
> * Changes in respiratory rate;
> * Noisy or laboured breathing;
> * Exaggerated use of accessory muscles of the neck and abdomen;
> * Absence of breath sounds and chest movement.

ALCOHOL

Alcohols are a group of organic compounds. Absolute alcohol is occasionally used by injection to relieve trigeminal neuralgia and other intractable pain. Ethyl alcohol (ethanol) is the intoxicating constituent of alcoholic drinks. It potentiates the effects of hypnotics and tranquillizers.

ALCOHOL DEPENDENCE

A syndrome of physical, psychological and behavioural responses related to alcohol misuse. Characteristically, there are withdrawal symptoms and then drinking to relieve these, tolerance to the effects of alcohol, compulsion to drink alcohol, narrowing of repertoire of drinking, etc.

ALCOHOL MISUSE

Long-term alcohol misuse is associated with hepatitis, cirrhosis and portal hypertension, gastritis, iron overload, primary liver cancer, other cancers (e.g. head and neck), pancreatitis, arterial hypertension, ischaemic heart disease and neurological problems caused by alcohol toxicity or B vitamin deficiency. In addition, there are social, emotional and psychological problems, such as relationship difficulties, financial problems and unemployment.

The term *delirium tremens* describes the results of the withdrawal of alcohol after a period of excessive and sustained intake and is represented by a picture of confusion, terror, restlessness and hallucinations.

MICHIGAN ALCOHOLISM SCREENING TEST

The Michigan Alcoholism Screening Test (MAST) is an assessment designed to detect problematic alcohol use by rating its effect on an individual's physical and social circumstances.

FETAL ALCOHOL SYNDROME

Fetal alcohol syndrome (FAS) is defined as stillbirth and fetal abnormality as a result of prenatal growth retardation caused by the maternal consumption of alcohol during pregnancy. It includes both physical and mental abnormalities and is characterized by poor growth, facial, cardiac and limb abnormalities, and learning disabilities.

WERNICKE–KORSAKOFF SYNDROME

Wernicke–Korsakoff syndrome is caused by a deficiency of vitamin B_1 (thiamin). In developed countries, Wernicke–Korsakoff syndrome may result from long-term alcohol misuse that leads to a deficient intake and reduced absorption and metabolism of thiamin. Thiamin deficiency can occur quickly after binge drinking with little food intake.

It is characterized by chronic amnesia (defect of retrieval of recently acquired information) with denial, lack of insight and confabulation. There is a level of impaired consciousness and thinking.

ALLERGY (HYPERSENSITIVITY)

Allergy is a powerful immune response to an allergen (an antigen that produces allergy). The allergen itself is usually harmless (e.g. house dust, food, animal dander and pollen). Upon initial exposure to the allergen the individual becomes sensitized to it, and on second and subsequent exposures the immune system mounts a response entirely out of proportion to the perceived threat. Sometimes the effects are mild, if annoying, such as the running nose and streaming eyes of hay fever (allergic rhinitis). Occasionally, the reaction can be so extreme as to overwhelm body systems and cause death. ⇒ Defence mechanisms, Nose and paranasal sinuses (rhinitis), Respiratory system (asthma).

MECHANISMS OF HYPERSENSITIVITY

There are four mechanisms of hypersensitivity, classified according to what parts of the immune system are involved (*Fig. 7*).

TYPE I, IMMEDIATE-TYPE HYPERSENSITIVITY (ANAPHYLACTIC)

Type I sensitivity occurs in individuals who have inherited very high levels of a type of antibody called immunoglobulin E (IgE). When exposed to an allergen (e.g. nuts), the antibody activates mast cells and basophils, which release their granular contents. The most important substance released is histamine, which constricts some smooth muscle (e.g. airway smooth muscle), causes vasodilatation and increases vascular permeability. Examples of type I reactions include hay fever, nut allergies and the serious situation of anaphylaxis, in which there is profound bronchoconstriction, respiratory distress and shock caused by extensive vasodilatation. The condition can lead to death. ⇒ Shock.

TYPE II, CYTOTOXIC HYPERSENSITIVITY

When an antibody reacts with an antigen on a cell surface, that cell is marked for destruction by a number of mechanisms (e.g. phagocytosis). This is the usual procedure in the elimination of, for example, bacteria, but if the antibodies are directed against self-antigens the result is the destruction of the body's own tissues (autoimmune disease). Type II mechanisms cause other conditions (e.g. transfusion reactions).

TYPE III, IMMUNE COMPLEX MEDIATED HYPERSENSITIVITY

Antibody–antigen complexes (immune complexes) are usually cleared efficiently from the blood by phagocytosis. If not they can be deposited in tissues (e.g. kidneys, skin, joints and the eye), where they cause an inflammatory reaction. Immune complexes, for example, that collect in the kidney lodge in and block the glomeruli, which impairs kidney function (glomerulonephritis).

A

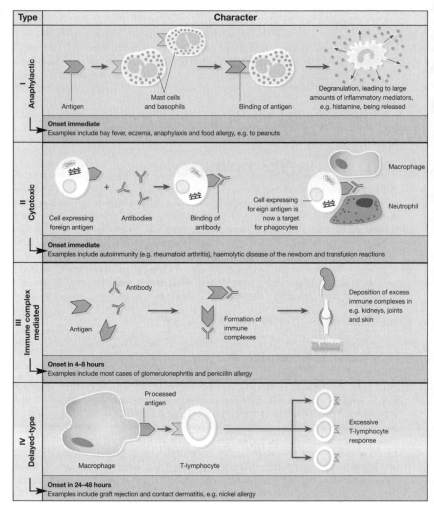

Fig 7 The four types of hypersensitivity

TYPE IV, DELAYED-TYPE HYPERSENSITIVITY

Unlike types I–III, type IV hypersensitivity does not involve antibodies, but is an overreaction of T-cells (T-lymphocytes) to an antigen. Usually this system is controlled and the T-cell response is appropriate. If not, the actively aggressive T-cytotoxic cells damage normal tissues. An example of this is contact dermatitis, such as that caused by an allergy to latex. Graft rejection is also caused by T-cells.

> **Practice application – contact dermatitis**
> Contact dermatitis initially occurs on the site of contact. This may give clues to possible causes (e.g. around the neck where a necklace has been worn). Referral for an allergy patch test is useful and especially supportive for a person who may have an occupational contact dermatitis. The patch consists

of hypoallergenic tape that contains aluminium discs, each with a different allergen. The nursing management involves supporting the person through patch testing, which is quite time-consuming for the person with several appointments in 1 week to read the tests.

If an allergen is identified, then it is important that the person, relative or carer understand how to avoid that substance. This might mean checking the content list of every product they use in the house (e.g. for perfume that is present in foods and shampoos). If they are allergic to latex it is important for all healthcare professionals to know this (e.g. dentists). Sometimes the person will develop Type 1 immediate-type hypersensitivity. This will necessitate the provision of a Medic-alert and the person, relative or others, such as a teacher, are taught how to administer adrenaline (epinephrine). ⇒ Latex sensitivity.

ANTIGEN

A substance that the body recognizes as foreign and that produces a specific immune response.

ATOPIC SYNDROME (ATOPY)

A hereditary predisposition to develop hypersensitivity disorders, such as eczema, asthma, hay fever and allergic rhinitis.

AUTOIMMUNE DISORDERS

Normally, an immune response is mounted only against foreign (nonself) antigens, but occasionally the body fails to recognize its own tissues and attacks itself. The resulting autoimmune disorders, examples of type II hypersensitivity, comprise a number of relatively common conditions that include rheumatoid arthritis, the majority of cases of type 1 diabetes mellitus, pernicious anaemia and Graves' disease.

AMBULATORY TREATMENT

Ambulatory treatment is treatment given on a day-care basis. Interventions, such as blood product transfusion or chemotherapy, and dialysis for chronic renal failure are undertaken. It also includes surgery carried out on the day of admission. ⇒ Day care surgery, Renal failure.

AMINO ACIDS

Amino acids are organic acids in which one or more of the hydrogen atoms is replaced by the amino group NH_2. They are the end product of protein digestion and from them the body synthesizes its own proteins. They are classified as either essential (indispensable) or nonessential (dispensable). Ten (eight in adults and a further two during childhood) cannot be synthesized in sufficient quantities in the body and are therefore essential (indispensable) in the diet – arginine, histidine, isoleucine, leucine, lysine, methionine, phenylalanine, threonine, tryptophan and valine. The remainder, which can be synthesized in the body if the diet contains sufficient amounts of the precursor amino acids, are designated nonessential (dispensable) amino acids. However, some of these are conditionally essential and depend upon adequate amounts of their precursor.

AMNESIA

Amnesia is the complete loss of memory. It can be divided into organic (true) amnesia (e.g. delirium, dementia, trauma, etc.) and psychogenic amnesia (e.g. dissociative states, etc.). The term anterograde amnesia is used when there is impaired continuous recall of events that follow an accident or brain insult, and retrograde amnesia is when the impairment is of events prior to the insult.

AMNESIC SYNDROME

Amnesic syndrome is chronic profound impairment of recent memory with preserved immediate recall, often accompanied by disorientation for time and confabulation (the creation of false memory to fill the gaps in memory). Commonly caused by vitamin B_1 (thiamin) deficiency, which can be secondary to chronic alcohol use, dietary deficiency, gastric cancer, etc. ⇒ Alcohol (Wernicke–Korsakoff syndrome), Memory.

AMPUTATION

Amputation means the removal (surgical or traumatic) of an appending part. However, the term is generally used to describe the removal of a limb, usually the lower limb. The reasons for lower limb amputation include:
- Peripheral vascular (arterial) disease associated with smoking, and as a long-term complication of diabetes;
- To relieve pain and improve mobility (by use of prosthesis), and thereby improve the quality of life;
- Severe trauma;
- Frost bite and burns;
- Bone cancers;
- Severe, intractable bone infection (e.g. osteomyelitis).

Practice application – stump and prosthesis care

On-going skin care issues tend to be related to the contact of the stump with the prosthesis (artificial device) and problems can result from friction, swelling or a moist environment caused by poor hygiene or temperature changes.

As well as being told of the associated health issues, those who wear prostheses must be taught to care for the 'mechanics' of the prosthesis. Generally, the prosthesis should be kept clean, all joints should be fully operational and lubricated, and there should be access to a prosthetist should any problems occur.

Stump bandaging

Following amputation, the earlier the prosthesis is fitted the better it is for the amputee. One of the challenges that faces the amputee and the healthcare team is to control oedema of the stump through the use a rigid dressing.

People are taught the proper technique for bandaging during the time in hospital and are generally expected to be self-caring in this area after discharge home, if functional ability permits.

Elastic shrinker socks are commonly used instead of elastic bandages. Although some may consider these not to be as effective as a properly applied bandage, they are easier for the person to apply and may therefore produce a better outcome than a poorly applied elastic bandage.

Whichever is used, it should be removed at least three times daily and the stump should be massaged vigorously for 10–15 minutes. The bandage or sock must be reapplied immediately after the massage. Applying the correct technique for a stump bandage is extremely important to using a prosthesis successfully. Clearly, the technique differs slightly for below-knee amputations, but the principles remain the same (*Fig. 8*).

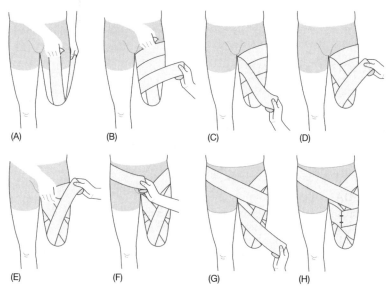

Fig 8 Technique for stump bandaging – above-knee amputation. (A) Begin at the front of the stump, cover the bottom and work upwards towards the top of the back of the stump. (B) Wrap 2–4 diagonal turns around the stump. (C) Take the bandage down towards the bottom of the stump and begin a figure-of-8 pattern from the underside of the stump upwards to cover its sides. (D) Pressure should be directed evenly upwards and outwards from the end of the stump as you wrap. (E) Take the bandage from the front, inside of the thigh and wrap upwards and outwards across the front of the hips. (F) Carry the wrap around behind the hips at the level of the iliac crest. (G) Return the bandage wrap to the stump and finish wrapping with more figure-of-8 turns. (H) Anchor the end of the bandage at the upper front part of the thigh, with safety pins, clips or adhesive tape

ANABOLIC STEROIDS

Anabolic steroids are a group of androgens that have marked anabolic effects (e.g. nandralone, stanozolol, etc.). They increase protein synthesis and increase weight and muscle mass. They are used clinically in the treatment of some breast cancers, and sometimes to increase appetite and a feeling of well-being in patients with terminal cancer. They are subject to considerable misuse by athletes and body builders, who may take many times the therapeutic dose.

ANAESTHESIA

Anaesthesia is defined as loss of sensation. In practice, anaesthesia is more complex and may usefully be described as general, regional or local in nature.

LOCAL ANAESTHESIA

Local anaesthesia (LA) involves the use of agents designed to block nerve impulse transmission in localized sensory nerve endings. The local anaesthetic agents used, such as lidocaine and bupivacaine, are also used for regional blocks. For practical purposes surgery under LA is generally considered to involve topical or well-defined localized tissue infiltration, usually in the conscious patient.

While it is true that the majority of LAs are administered without adverse effect (such as allergic or anaphylactic reaction, and cardiac toxicity), the potential for problems must be recognized and managed.

REGIONAL ANAESTHESIA

Most minor topical procedures utilize a local anaesthetic agent administered directly into those tissues to be incised. On occasions when the amount of the agent required to ensure anaesthesia might be excessive, a regional block may be required. Regional anaesthetics are also designed to provide a pain- and sensation-free environment in a specific region of the body, but provide this over a greater area of tissue than is practicable with local infiltration anaesthesia. They include caudal, Bier's and spinal and epidural blocks.

CAUDAL BLOCK

Caudal anaesthetic may be considered to be a modified epidural injection. For caudal anaesthesia, the local agent is injected into the epidural space through the caudal canal in the sacrum. The anaesthetic is very localized and does not produce the systemic effects of spinal and epidural anaesthetics. Their ease of use means caudal anaesthetics are commonly used for perineal and genital pain relief.

BIER'S BLOCK

Bier's block involves the intravenous injection of local anaesthetic into an extremity, such as a limb that has been exsanguinated using a rubber elasticated (Esmarch) bandage and a double-cuffed pneumatic tourniquet, applied to prevent arterial blood re-entering the vessels. With an upper time limit for the tourniquet of around 90 minutes the surgeon is able to operate on a limb that is both sensation free and presents a bloodless field. It is essential that the technique be undertaken by appropriately trained and experienced practitioners only and with equipment that has had a thorough safety check.

SPINAL AND EPIDURAL BLOCKS

Spinal and epidural injections (*Fig. 9A,B*) are commonly employed in modern anaesthesia and involve the injection of LA and/or analgesic into either the subarachnoid or epidural space (*Fig. 9C,D*). The spinal anaesthetic is injected into the subarachnoid space to mix with the cerebrospinal fluid (CSF). The epidural injection is inserted into the epidural space and has no contact with the meninges. The injection has an anaesthetic effect on tissues distal to the site of injection and is commonly used for abdominal, pelvic and lower limb orthopaedic and perineal surgery.

Local anaesthetic agents, e.g. lidocaine, are commonly used for injection. The sympathetic nerve blockade produced by these agents can promote profound hypotension and patient assessment and preparation for this procedure must take this into account. Prior to injection intravenous (i.v.) access is established and i.v. therapy commenced. In addition, heart rhythm and blood pressure monitoring equipment are sited to ensure constant monitoring of cardiovascular status. Cardiopulmonary resuscitation equipment must be immediately available should any catastrophic hypotensive episode or toxic reaction occur. An i.v. dose of a vasoconstrictive agent, such as methoxamine, must also be available to reverse the vasodilatory effects of the anaesthetic.

The patient may be positioned on their side with the knees drawn up (*Fig. 9A*), or sitting up and leaning forwards. This promotes lumbar spine flexion, vertebral separation and facilitates access for the needle or cannula.

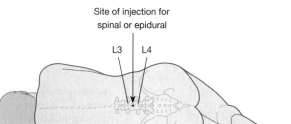

Site of injection for
spinal or epidural

L3 | L4

(A) Position of patient for spinal and epidural injection

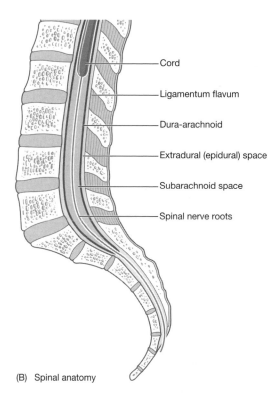

—— Cord

—— Ligamentum flavum

—— Dura-arachnoid

—— Extradural (epidural) space

—— Subarachnoid space

—— Spinal nerve roots

(B) Spinal anatomy

Fig 9 (A), (B) Spinal and epidural injections

To provide the regional anaesthesia, a suitable-sized needle is inserted using strict aseptic principles. For the spinal injection particularly, the introduction of micro-organisms into the CSF may cause life-threatening infection. Epidural anaesthesia may be administered either by a single injection or intermittently via a catheter.

While the use of spinal and epidural anaesthetics is commonly very safe and with minimal risk, the potential for complications must not be underestimated.

A

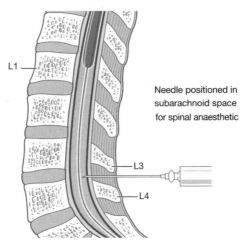

L1

Needle positioned in
subarachnoid space
for spinal anaesthetic

L3

L4

(C)   Position of needle in spinal anaesthesia

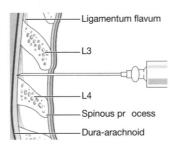

Ligamentum flavum

L3

L4

Spinous pr ocess

Dura-arachnoid

(D)   Position of needle in epidural anaesthesia

Fig 9 (C), (D) Spinal and epidural injections

GENERAL ANAESTHESIA

General anaesthesia (GA) produces loss of sensation with loss of consciousness.
GA is characterized by a medication-induced, reversible state of unconsciousness.
The three key elements ('triad') of anaesthesia are the states of analgesia, sedation
and muscular relaxation. The triad may be achieved through a variety of means,
but a combination of i.v. and inhalational agents is most commonly used. The
process of anaesthesia involves three distinct phases: induction, maintenance and
reversal. For airway maintenance, ⇒ Airway.

Practice application – anaesthetic induction, maintenance and reversal
Critical to the success of any anaesthetic is the preparation of both the patient
and the anaesthetic environment. In the anaesthetic room appropriate cardiovascular and respiratory devices, such as electrocardiograph electrodes, pulse
oximeter, etc., are attached to the person. After induction , specific activities,
such as the fitting of eye protectors prior to laser surgery, are also instigated.

- Induction involves the administration of sleep-inducing drugs to provide sedation during surgery. While inhalational agents may be used (e.g. in needle-shy adults and small children), the i.v. route is most common. Probably the most commonly used induction agent is propofol. This produces a short-acting but very rapid loss of consciousness. There is a high risk of regurgitation and aspiration in emergency anaesthetic-induction situations for which there has been no preoperative fast, or where there is raised intra-abdominal pressure, as in pregnancy. In such cases, a technique that applies pressure to the cricoid cartilage, known as *Sellick's manoeuvre*, may be employed at the time of anaesthetic induction and endotracheal tube intubation.
- Anaesthetic maintenance and reversal – the person is monitored throughout surgery for any signs of physiological disturbance. Assessment and recording of cardiovascular, neurological and respiratory functions, including oxygen saturation and carbon dioxide levels, are maintained throughout the anaesthesia. Throughout surgery, the optimal level of sedation achieved at induction is maintained and may be complemented by the use of analgesics and muscle relaxants. These may be either inhalational or i.v. agents, or more commonly a combination of both. These agents, supplemented by oxygen and usually nitrous oxide, complete the 'triad' and allow the person to be sedated and pain free, and for muscle relaxation to enable adequate surgical access.

As surgery is completed, the effects of anaesthesia, or more usually of muscle relaxation, may need to be reversed and an anticholinesterase, such as neostigmine, may be given. Should reversal of narcotic analgesia be required because of respiratory depression, an antagonist (e.g. naloxone) may be given, though this, of course, reduces the postoperative analgesic effect.

ANATOMICAL TERMS

Anatomy is the study of the structure of the body and the physical relationships between body parts. A set of standard terms, accepted everywhere, is used to describe the position of body structures and their geographical relationships with each other.

THE ANATOMICAL POSITION AND REGIONAL TERMS

The anatomical position of the body is used as a reference point when studying or describing the position of body structures. The person stands in the upright position, faces forwards, the arms at the side with palms facing forwards and the feet together.

Each region of the body can be described using a specific term and many of these regional terms are illustrated in *Fig. 10*.

BODY PLANES

Body structures can be described in relation to three planes (imaginary lines) – median (midsagittal), coronal and transverse – which run through the body (*Fig. 11*).

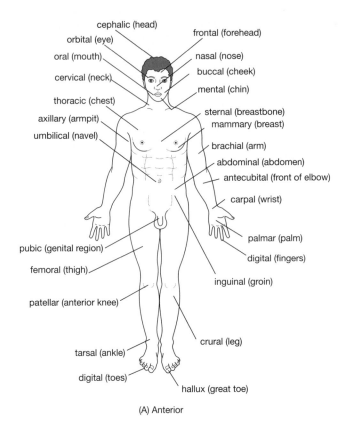

cephalic (head)
frontal (forehead)
orbital (eye)
oral (mouth)
nasal (nose)
cervical (neck)
buccal (cheek)
thoracic (chest)
mental (chin)
axillary (armpit)
sternal (breastbone)
umbilical (navel)
mammary (breast)
brachial (arm)
abdominal (abdomen)
antecubital (front of elbow)
carpal (wrist)
pubic (genital region)
palmar (palm)
femoral (thigh)
digital (fingers)
inguinal (groin)
patellar (anterior knee)
crural (leg)
tarsal (ankle)
digital (toes)
hallux (great toe)

(A) Anterior

Fig 10 (A) The anatomical position and regional terms: anterior

DIRECTIONAL TERMS

Directional terms are used to describe the position of structures relative to each other. They include:
• Superior – above;
• Inferior – below;
• Anterior (ventral) – in front;
• Posterior (dorsal) – at the back (when describing the hands, the terms palmar and dorsal are used, with plantar and dorsal for the feet);
• Efferent – away;
• Afferent – towards;
• Peripheral – at the edges of the body;
• Lateral – away from the median line (middle), on the outer side;
• Medial – towards the median line, on the inner side;
• Distal – furthest away from a given point;
• Proximal – nearest the given point;
• Internal - towards the centre or inside of a cavity;
• External – towards the outside of a cavity;
• Deep – away from the surface of the body;
• Superficial – near or on the surface of the body.
The use of terms that have such a precise meaning helps to avoid mistakes.

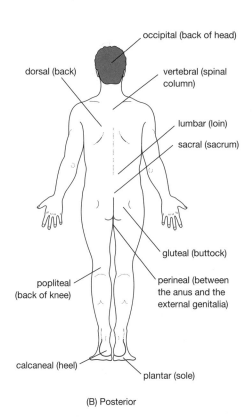

Fig 10 (B) The anatomical position and regional terms: posterior

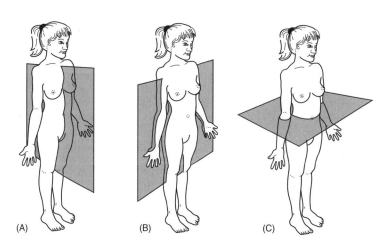

Fig 11 Body planes: (A) median plane, (B) coronal plane, (C) transverse plane

ANGER

Anger can be described as a complex emotion, which can be conceived of in terms of an interplay between environmental events, thoughts and physiological arousal. Chronic anger is associated with a range of psychological and behavioural disorders and medical conditions. ⇒ Aggression.

ANGER MANAGEMENT PROGRAMMES

Anger management programmes have been used successfully with many different types of angry and impulsive people. Programmes are applicable to a variety of situations, for example, work with offenders in the criminal justice system and with people who have certain mental health problems. These programmes typically consist of training in recognition of anger cues, development of self-control and social skills, and role-play practice of these skills.

ANORECTAL PROBLEMS

Anorectal problems are distressing for people because they cause pain and embarrassment, and in some cases people are reluctant to seek professional help. However, many conditions are ultimately treatable, but it is important to eliminate serious pathology, such as cancer. ⇒ Gastrointestinal tract.

FISSURE (FISSURE-IN-ANO)

A fissure-in-ano is a tear in the squamous lining of the lower anal canal, which causes pain on defaecation. Fissures are usually caused by the passage of hard stool, but can also be caused by Crohn's disease, trauma and anal cancer. Dietary changes are helpful; people should be advised to eat a diet high in fibre.

FISTULAE

Fistulae are abnormal communications between two epithelial surfaces, but commonly in this condition a fistula is an opening at the cutaneous surface near the anus. It is common in Crohn's disease. If surgical intervention is considered, the tract is laid open to allow healing by secondary intention.

HAEMORRHOIDS (PILES)

Haemorrhoids are varices in the lower rectum or anus. Internal haemorrhoids originate above the internal anal sphincter. Sometimes they are large enough to protrude from the anus and may become enlarged (i.e. external haemorrhoids), constricted and painful. Haemorrhoids may arise from years of constipation. They result in pain and bleeding on defecation. Management includes advice on a diet high in fibre and bulk-forming laxatives. Haemorrhoids may be treated by injecting the haemorrhoidal veins or they can be ligated or excised during haemorrhoidectomy. Haemorrhoids may rupture or thrombose, whereupon surgery is undertaken immediately.

PERIANAL ABSCESS

Perianal abscess is a cavity that contains pus and occurs when micro-organisms invade the mucosal wall after a tear. The abscess can then track inferiorly to the perianal region or laterally to the ischiorectal fossae. There is a great deal of discomfort with throbbing pain and swelling. Antibiotic therapy is started and the abscess is then incised and drained.

PILONIDAL SINUS

Pilonidal sinus is an abnormal tract that contains a tuft of hair that curls and irritates the skin. It is most frequently situated over or close to the tip of the coccyx. Abscess formation is common after irritation and subsequent infection. Management includes antibiotics and pain relief followed by wide surgical excision, drainage and laying open of the wound. Healing is by secondary intention.

POLYPS

Polyps occur in the mucosa and are small, benign tumour-like projections. They are more common in the sigmoid colon and rectum, and occur more frequently in those over the age of 50 years. A condition known as familial polyposis, when large numbers of polyps occur in the intestine, is considered precancerous, and so the aim of management is surgical removal.

PRURITUS ANI

Pruritus ani is itching felt around the anus. It can be caused by poor hygiene, wearing tight underwear, threadworm infestation or anxiety. Other causes include fissures, incontinence, inflammatory bowel disease, fistulae and skin diseases, such as contact dermatitis.

People should be advised to clean themselves thoroughly after going to the lavatory; moist wipes can be useful. They should be advised to avoid spicy food and to wear loose clothing. If itching persists, anaesthetic cream may be helpful.

Practice application – discharge advice after anorectal surgery
It is important to stress that straining and constipation should be avoided; therefore, people should defecate in response to the initial sensation. They should increase the fibre content of the diet, have sufficient fluids and take exercise and medications to soften the stool.

Frequent perianal hygiene is advised to avoid the risk of infection. Washing the area with warm water is soothing and cleansing, and taking warm baths reduces the pain and keeps the perianal area clean.

The person is advised to observe for any bleeding or signs of inflammation, such as increasing pain. Any problems should be reported to the appropriate health professional. ⇒ Defecation (constipation and faecal impaction).

ANTAGONIST

An antagonist is:
- A muscle that reverses or opposes the action of an agonist muscle;
- A drug or other substance that prevents a biological action when it binds to cell receptor molecules, either on the surface or within the cytoplasm. It blocks the receptor, which cannot then be occupied by any other chemical. Examples are $beta_1$-adrenoceptor antagonists, such as atenolol (beta-blocker), and calcium antagonists (calcium channel blockers), such as nifedipine and verapamil. If the antagonist does not completely block the receptors, it is termed a partial agonist, so the relationship between agonist and antagonist is a competitive one.

⇒ Agonist, Pharmacokinetics and pharmacodynamics.

ANTHROPOMETRY

Anthropometry is the comparative measurement of the human body and its parts to compare and establish norms for sex, age, weight, race and so on. Anthropometric measurements include weight, height, skin-fold thickness, etc. ⇒ Nutrition (methods of assessing nutritional status).

ANTIBIOTICS (ANTIMICROBIALS)

As their name implies, antibiotics act against life – the life in this context being that of micro-organisms. For this reason , these drugs are also known as antimicrobials. Antimicrobial drugs may be antibacterial (e.g. gentamicin), antiviral (e.g. aciclovir), antifungal (e.g. fluconazole), antiprotozoal (e.g. metronidazole) or anthelmintics (e.g. mebendazole).

Antibiotics may act primarily by stopping cell division (bacteriostats), or by killing the micro-organisms directly (bactericides). The cells most susceptible to the effects of bacteriostats and bactericides are those that divide rapidly. ⇒ Infection.

For the antimicrobial drug to be effective, it must be present in sufficient concentration with the person's bloodstream, and therefore in the interstitial fluid.

RANGE OF ANTIBIOTIC ACTIVITY

Antibiotics are classed as *broad spectrum* or *narrow spectrum*. Broad-spectrum antibiotics are effective against a range of different micro-organisms, such as cocci and bacilli. The manner in which different bacteria take the staining substances used by microbiologists for identification causes them to be subdivided into Gram-positive and Gram-negative groups. A broad-spectrum antibiotic may be effective against Gram-positive and Gram-negative groups. Narrow-spectrum antibiotics are highly effective against a specific micro-organism. ⇒ Bacteria.

ANTIBIOTIC RESISTANCE

Over time, antibiotics may become ineffective against a specific micro-organism. This is brought about by a protective change that occurs in the micro-organism. One such change could be that the micro-organism becomes able to produce an enzyme that inactivates the antibiotic. For example, most staphylococci produce beta-lactamases, which inactivate antibiotics, such as penicillin, that contain a beta-lactam ring in their chemical structure (*Fig. 12*).

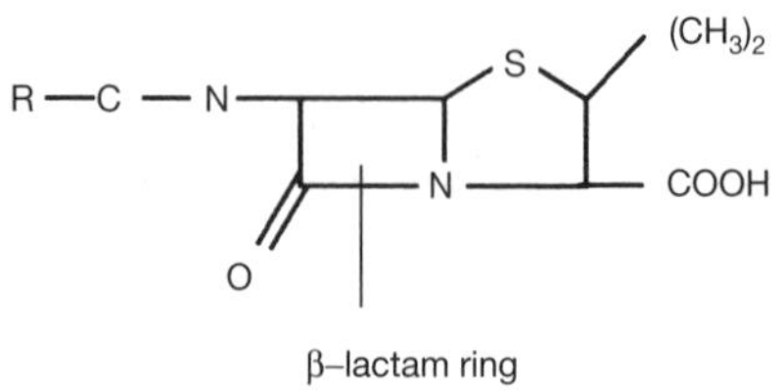

β–lactam ring

Fig 12 The structure of penicillin

Practice application – preventing antibiotic resistance
Prevention of antibiotic resistance is achieved by:
* Avoiding overexposure of micro-organisms to a given antibiotic through unnecessary prescribing;
* Encouraging people to complete the antibiotic course, even though the symptoms have disappeared; and, lastly,
* Avoiding the use of antibiotics 'just in case' an infection develops.

In addition, nurses have an important role in educating the public and junior doctors about the proper use of antibiotics (e.g. antibiotics are unnecessary for minor viral infections). Examples of antibiotic resistance, both in hospital and the community, include methicillin-resistant *Staphylococcus aureus* (MRSA) and vancomycin-resistant enterococci (VRE).

ANTICOAGULANTS

Anticoagulants reduce the propensity of blood to clot. Uses include:
* Obtaining specimens suitable for haematological and chemical analyses for which whole blood or plasma is required instead of serum;
* Collecting blood for transfusion;
* Prophylaxis and treatment of various thromboembolic conditions.
⇒ Deep vein thrombosis, Pulmonary embolism, Thrombosis.

HEPARIN

Heparin must be given parenterally, either by intravenous infusion or by subcutaneous injection. There are two forms of heparin – standard (unfractionated) heparin and low molecular weight heparin (LMWH).

Heparin works quickly and has a short duration of action, although LMWH has a longer action than standard heparin. Heparin is used in the treatment and prophylaxis of deep vein thrombosis (DVT) and pulmonary embolism (PE). It is also used in the treatment of unstable angina, myocardial infarction and to prevent blood coagulation in extracorporeal circuits, such as in haemodialysis. The major side-effect is haemorrhage, and if this occurs the heparin is discontinued. If haemorrhage is severe the antidote protamine sulphate (not fully effective for reversing LMWH) is also administered.

WARFARIN

Warfarin is taken orally. It takes about 48–72 hours to produce anticoagulation and for this reason it is usually started with the heparin. Warfarin is used in the treatment of DVT, PE and to prevent emboli developing in atrial fibrillation and with mechanical prosthetic heart valves. The major side-effect is again haemorrhage, for which the antidote phytomenadione (vitamin K) is given, as well as discontinuing the warfarin.

Practice application – advice during anticoagulant therapy
Nurses should ensure that people know about the many substances that should be avoided while having warfarin. These include alcohol, St John's wort, aspirin, diclofenac and other nonsteroidal anti-inflammatory drugs (NSAIDs), etc. People should be reminded to take their medication as prescribed, and of the importance of taking warfarin at the same time each day. People should know about observing themselves for bruising, swelling, gum bleeding, nosebleeds, haematuria or any evidence of gastrointestinal bleeding, such as black stools.

A

> People should be encouraged to attend the anticoagulation clinic for testing
> – activated partial prothrombin time (APPT), reported as the international
> normalized ratio (INR). It is important that people alter the dose of warfarin
> only as prescribed. Many nurse-led anticoagulation services offer telephone
> helplines and give advice about medication to individuals.

ANTIDEPRESSANTS

Antidepressants are drugs used to manage depression. The three main groups are
monoamine oxidase inhibitors (MAOIs), selective serotonin re-uptake inhibitors
(SSRIs) and tricyclic antidepressants (TCAs). ⇒ Disorders of mood (psychotic
depression).

MONOAMINE OXIDASE INHIBITORS

MAOIs are drugs that inhibit the action of the enzyme monoamine oxidase, and take
3 weeks or longer to become effective. They include phenelzine, but largely have
been superseded by other antidepressants that have fewer side-effects and greater
clinical efficacy. However, newer reversible MAOIs, such as moclobemide, act more
rapidly. Reversible MAOIs are also used in the management of social phobias.

People who receive MAOIs should avoid many other drugs, such as other antidepressants, sympathomimetics (such as amfetamines, dopamine, etc.), pethidine,
anti-epileptics, etc. Alcohol and low-alcohol drinks should also be avoided. Foods
that include cheese, broad bean pods and yeast extract, etc, and stale foods should
be avoided to prevent a serious hypertensive crisis.

SELECTIVE SEROTONIN RE-UPTAKE INHIBITORS

SSRIs are a group of widely prescribed antidepressants that include fluoxetine, parox-
etine and sertraline. They take 2–4 weeks to become effective and act by blocking the
re-uptake of 5-hydroxytryptamine (serotonin) by nerve cells. They have fewer side-
effects than MAOIs and TCAs, but gastrointestinal side-effects are fairly common.
Other side-effects include anorexia, weight loss, insomnia, headache, nervousness
and tremor. More seriously, suicidal ideation has been linked with certain SSRIs.

Many other substances can interact with SSRIs, and these include other antidepressants, alcohol, anaesthetic agents, beta-blockers, etc.

TRICYCLIC ANTIDEPRESSANTS

TCAs are a group of widely prescribed antidepressants (e.g. clomipramine,
amitriptyline, etc.). They act by blocking the uptake of the neurotransmitters 5-
hydroxytryptamine (serotonin) and noradrenaline (norepinephrine). They take
2–4 weeks to be effective and have unpleasant side-effects that include blurred
vision, dry mouth, constipation and urinary retention. They may also be prescribed
for nocturnal enuresis in children and as a prophylactic for migraine. In common
with other antidepressants, TCAs may interact with alcohol and other drugs,
which include sympathomimetics, beta-blockers, etc.

ANTIDISCRIMINATORY PRACTICE

⇒ Fair and antidiscriminatory practice.

ANTIEMBOLIC

Antiembolic (against embolism) is used to describe a drug (e.g. prophylactic heparin) or other measure that helps to prevent the development of deep vein thrombosis (DVT) and an embolus. These measures include:

- Keeping mobile;
- Leg exercises if mobility is limited;
- Correct positioning and intermittent pneumatic external compression system (*Fig. 13A*) in the operating theatre;
- Effective pain relief and early mobilization postoperatively;
- Prophylactic heparin for people having some types of surgery;
- Use of graduated compression stockings (anti-embolic stockings).

⇒ Deep vein thrombosis, Embolism.

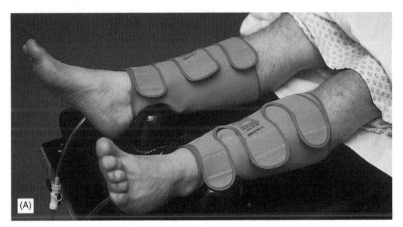

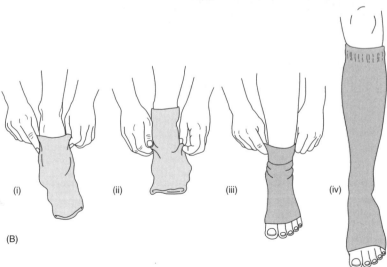

Fig 13 (A) Foltron stockings, (B) fitting antiembolic stockings

A

Practice application – anti-embolic stockings

It is very important that nurses measure patients accurately for anti-embolic stockings, fit these correctly according to the manufacturer's instructions, teach patients and carers about applying stockings and ensure that they are competent to do so (*Fig. 13B*). Thigh-length stockings are reported to be more expensive, more difficult to fit accurately and apply, and less well tolerated by people than are knee-length stockings. Poorly fitting stockings may be constrictive and diminish blood flow, which leads to reports of ischaemia, thrombosis and even gangrene, particularly in people with existing disease, such as diabetes or peripheral vascular disease. Commonly, stockings may fall down or are removed by people who are unaware of their benefits. To help with compliance, it is essential, therefore, that people be fully informed as to the purpose of the stockings.

The circulation should be observed daily for ischaemia and, again, nurses should make sure that people understand how to make these checks.

People with chronic venous insufficiency should be referred to a specialist tissue-viability nurse before graduated compression stockings are used, because there may be situations in which these should be avoided. ⇒ Leg ulcers.

ANTIEMETICS

⇒ Vomiting.

ANTIPSYCHOTICS

Antipsychotics (syn. neuroleptics) are drugs that act on the nervous system. They are used in the immediate management of disturbed patients. People may become disturbed for a variety of reasons, including schizophrenia, affective disorders (e.g. depression) and organic psychoses (e.g. in alcohol misuse). Antipsychotics are often used in the management of people with certain types of schizophrenia. Basically, they all act as antagonists of dopamine receptors, and can be classified as either typical or atypical antipsychotics.

The 'typical antipsychotics' include the phenothiazines (e.g. chlorpromazine, fluphenazine, the butyrophenones (e.g. haloperidol) and the thioxanthenes (e.g. flupentixol). Typical antipsychotics, especially the phenothiazines, give rise to extrapyramidal side-effects, such as akathisia (restlessness), dystonia (abnormal movements), parkinsonian tremor, bradykinesia and rigidity, tardive (late) dyskinesia (see below), antipsychotic malignant syndrome (rare but potentially fatal hyperthermia, etc.), and anticholinergic side-effects, such as dry mouth, constipation, blurred vision, erectile dysfunction, etc.

'Atypical antipsychotics', which include amisulpiride, clozapine, olanzapine, quetiapine, risperidone and zotepine, tend to cause fewer extrapyramidal effects. However, clozapine may cause agranulocytosis and patients must be monitored. Atypical drugs, such as risperidone, are effective against both positive and negative symptoms of schizophrenia. Antipsychotic drugs can be given as a depot injection (e.g. fluphenazine and flupentixol) to ensure that medication is taken regularly when a person is failing to take medication as prescribed. ⇒ Mobility (*Box 23*, disorders of movement).

TARDIVE (LATE) DYSKINESIA

Tardive (late) dyskinesia is characterized by involuntary movement of the orofacial and buccal–lingual muscles, as well as uncoordinated movements of the upper and lower limbs. Tics, abnormal posture, grunting and vocalizations may all occur. It is fairly frequent with prolonged high-dose treatment in older people. The effects may be irreversible, but discontinuation of the antipsychotic by gradual withdrawal provides a better prognosis than continuation. Clozapine is introduced as other neuroleptics are withdrawn.

ANTISEPSIS

Antisepsis is the prevention of infection of tissues or body surfaces by the application of nonantibiotic chemicals (antiseptics). Introduced into surgery in 1880 by Lord Lister, who used carbolic acid. ⇒ Asepsis, Disinfection, Infection.

ANXIETY

Anxiety is the emotional response to distress. It is normal to feel anxious when exposed to stressors, but what differentiates clinical anxiety from everyday anxiety is that the emotional response associated with clinical anxiety is inappropriate to the threat imposed by the stressor and continues after the threat has been removed (Sims and Owens 1993). In reality, it is not always easy to differentiate between normal and abnormal anxiety. Anxiety can be regarded as a continuum from mild anxiety increasing in severity to panic attacks. Clinical anxiety that occurs where there is no apparent danger is called generalized anxiety and the individual complains of feeling anxious all the time.

PANIC ATTACKS

Panic attacks are related to anxiety, and are periods of intense fear, which often occur despite no obvious cause. During a panic attack, the somatic symptoms of the flight-or-fight response are exaggerated, in particular increased heart and respiration rates. The individual experiences palpitations, arrhythmias (such as occasional ectopic beats), hyperventilation and dizziness. Sufferers often think they are having a heart attack and are about to die, which serves to reinforce the panic. ⇒ Obsessive–compulsive disorder, Phobias, Stress.

ANXIOLYTICS

Benzodiazepine anxiolytics (such as diazepam, etc.) provide immediate relief from the unpleasant feelings associated with stress. Their use is a very short-term solution, although in periods of crisis they may be prescribed for a limited period to reduce the anxiety level and facilitate the return of problem-solving thinking. Counselling may be used to aid this process, because if the underlying problems responsible for the anxiety are not addressed, the unpleasant feelings return when the drug is discontinued. The danger is that as the underlying problems remain unresolved, the individual continues to take the drug to avoid the symptoms. This quickly becomes a self-perpetuating cycle and may ultimately lead to dependence upon drugs. Consequently, anxiolytics should only be prescribed for a short period and at the lowest possible dose.

APGAR SCORE

The Agpar score is a measure used to evaluate the general condition of a newborn baby, and was developed by an American anaesthetist, Dr Virginia Apgar. A score of 0, 1 or 2 is given for each of the criteria of heart rate, respiratory effort, skin colour, muscle tone and response to stimulation (*Table 3*). A score of between 8 and 10 indicates a baby in good condition

A

Table 3 Apgar score

Signs and/or criteria	Score 0	1	2
Heart rate	Absent	Slow, below 100/min	Over 100/min
Respiratory effort	Absent	Slow, weak, irregular	Good chest movements or crying
Muscle tone	Limp	Poor tone, some movement	Active resistance, strong movement
Reflex irritability (response to stimulation such as sole flicks)	None	Slight withdrawal	Vigorous movements, cries
Colour (applicable to Caucasian newborns)	Pale or blue	Extremities blue	Completely normal colour

APHERESIS

Apheresis is a technique whereby a single blood component is removed from a patient or donor. During apheresis, the patient's or donor's blood is gradually passed through an automated cell separator. The desired blood component is drawn off and the remainder is returned to the person. The person undergoing apheresis requires two peripheral venous access devices, or a central venous catheter with two lumens, to enable blood to be removed and returned (*Fig. 14*). Apheresis can be used to collect or remove platelets, plasma (plasmapheresis), white cells (leucopheresis) or stem cells.

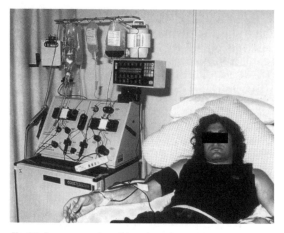

Fig 14 A person undergoing apheresis

Apheresis can have certain advantages over whole blood donation insofar as there is no depletion of red cells and the volunteer can donate more frequently. Apheresis is most commonly used to obtain platelets and plasma from healthy donors. Plasmapheresis is also used to remove plasma from people with disorders that affect plasma proteins and to remove toxic substances from the blood. Fresh plasma can then be transfused (plasma exchange). Leucopheresis can be used to treat patients with very high white cell counts, such as those with chronic leukaemia. Stem cells can be collected for haemopoietic stem-cell transplantation.

APNOEA

Apnoea describes a transitory cessation of breathing from any cause, such as that seen in *Cheyne–Stokes respiration*. It results from a lack of the necessary CO_2 tension in the blood to stimulate the respiratory centre.

Apnoea is a feature of periodic breathing seen in newborn babies. A period of apnoea of 5–10 seconds is followed by a period of hyperventilation at a rate of 50–60 breaths a minute, for a period of 10–15 seconds. The overall respiratory rate remains between 30 and 40 breaths per minute.

APNOEA IN LOW BIRTHWEIGHT BABIES

Apnoea occurs quite frequently in very low birthweight babies, often without definite cause. Attacks are only a problem if they are prolonged and do not respond to simple stimulation.

APNOEA ALARM

An apnoea alarm is a device that gives an auditory alarm signal when a baby has not breathed for a preset time, usually 15–20 seconds. The baby can then be stimulated to breathe before he or she becomes hypoxic. Devices can be used in the community to monitor babies after discharge from hospital, or where there has been a previous sudden infant death in the family. ⇒ Sudden infant death syndrome.

ARTERIAL CANNULA OR LINE

An arterial cannula is one placed in an artery to sample blood for gas analysis and for continuous blood-pressure monitoring. An arterial cannula should always be attached to a pressure transducer and monitor, and have an alarm that indicates any disconnection. ⇒ Blood gases, Blood pressure.

Many high-dependency patients need frequent blood-gas analysis and so an indwelling arterial cannula is inserted to avoid repeated arterial punctures. In addition, the continuous assessment of blood pressure may be required to monitor the effects of vasoactive drug therapy (e.g. inotropes), or to reflect the severity of the illness of the patient. The radial artery is commonly used for continuous blood-pressure monitoring (*Fig. 15*), although others can be used. Although arterial cannulation allows the continuous measurement of blood pressure and observation of waveform, the advantages must be weighed against the potential disadvantages (e.g. haemorrhage from dislodgement or disconnection, infection, peripheral artery damage and embolism).

ARTERIAL DISEASE

Arterial disease is a serious and common cause of morbidity and mortality, especially so in developed countries. ⇒ Coronary heart disease, Hyperlipidaemia, Hypertension, Nervous system (cerebrovascular accident).

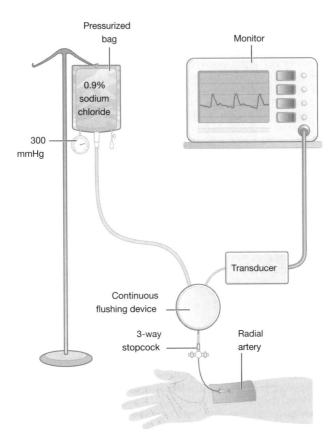

Fig 15 Arterial cannula in the radial artery

ANEURYSM

An aneurysm is a sac formed by localized dilation of a blood vessel, usually an artery, because of a local fault in the wall through defect, disease or injury, which produces a swelling, often pulsating, over which a murmur may be heard. True aneurysms may be saccular, fusiform or dissecting, in which the blood flows between the layers of the arterial wall (*Fig. 16*). An aneurysm may develop in the aorta (e.g. one that affects the abdominal aorta), or in the cerebral blood vessels, in which rupture causes subarachnoid haemorrhage.

ARTERIOSCLEROSIS

Arteriosclerosis is a common degenerative arterial change associated with advancing age. Primarily a thickening of the media (middle) layer and usually associated with some degree of atheroma. It is characterized by hardening of the walls with calcification, narrowing of the lumen and loss of elasticity, which results in decreased blood flow.

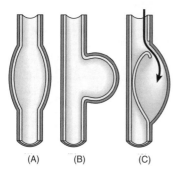

Fig 16 Types of aneurysm: (A) fusiform, (B) sacculated, (C) dissecting

(A)   (B)   (C)

ARTERITIS

Arteritis is an inflammatory disease that affects the walls of the arteries. *Giant cell arteritis* occurs in older people and mainly affects the external carotid artery and its branches, such as the temporal arteries of the scalp. It may also affect the aorta (aortitis). In temporal arteritis there is severe headache, scalp tenderness, pyrexia, anorexia and weight loss. Visual impairment can ensue if there is thrombosis of the ophthalmic artery. Prompt treatment with corticosteroids is effective.

ATHEROMA

Atheroma comprises plaques of fatty (lipid) material that form in the intimal (inner) layer of the arteries (*Fig. 17*). It starts as fatty streaks on the intima, deposition of low-density lipoprotein and plaque formation. Eventually, the lumen of the artery is reduced and ischaemia results. A thrombus may form if a plaque ruptures, which leads to further occlusion of the artery. It is of great importance in the coronary arteries in predisposing to coronary heart disease (angina, coronary thrombosis and myocardial infarction) and heart failure.

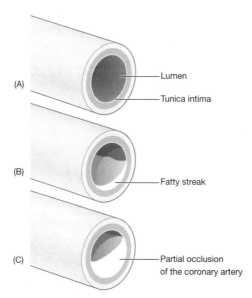

(A)   Lumen

Tunica intima

(B)   Fatty streak

(C)   Partial occlusion of the coronary artery

Fig 17 Atheroma formation: (A) normal artery, (B) early atheroma development, (C) severe atheroma

ATHEROSCLEROSIS

Atherosclerosis is co-existing atheroma and arteriosclerosis.

ARTHRITIS

Arthritis is inflammation of a joint. ⇒ Joint (joint diseases), Rheumatic disorders (rheumatoid arthritis).

ARTIFICIAL FEEDING

⇒ Nutrition (nutritional support).

ASEPSIS

Asepsis is the condition of being free from living pathogenic (disease-producing) micro-organisms. ⇒ Disinfection, Infection.

ASEPTIC TECHNIQUE

Aseptic technique is used to reduce the risk of introducing pathogenic micro-organisms into the body when the integrity and/or effectiveness of the natural body defences are reduced. It includes handwashing, the use of sterile gloves and gowns in theatre, nontouch technique with either sterile gloves (*Fig. 18*) or forceps for the care of wounds, intravenous cannulae and urinary catheterization, and the use of sterilized equipment and lotions. The risk of contamination by air-borne pathogenic micro-organisms is kept to a minimum.

The details of the technique may be modified according to the particular circumstances and the sterile pack used, but the principles are the same (*Fig. 19*).

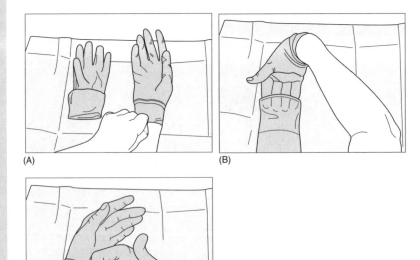

(A)   (B)

(C)

Fig 18 Putting on sterile gloves

A

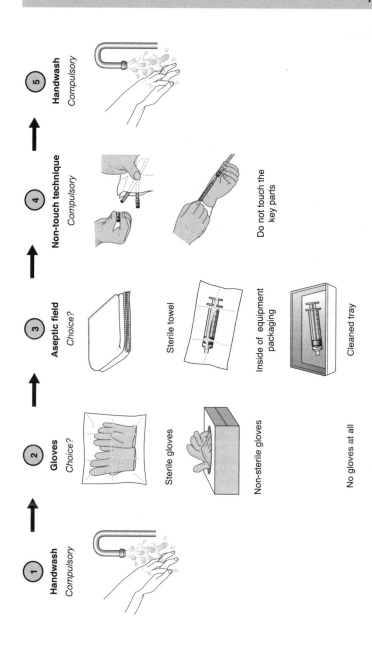

Fig 19 The five core stages of aseptic nontouch technique

Aseptic wound dressing is indicated:
- To remove wound discharge;
- To apply special treatments to a wound (e.g. a venous leg ulcer);
- If signs of wound infection are present;
- Following trauma to the skin (e.g. pressure ulcer);
- During an invasive procedure (e.g. introduction of an intravenous cannula).

A

Further reading

Huband S and Trigg E (2000). *Practices in Children's Nursing. Guidelines for Hospital and Community.* Edinburgh: Churchill Livingstone.

Nicol M, Bavin C, Bedford-Turner S, Cronin P and Rawlings-Anderson K (2004). *Essential Nursing Skills,* Second Edition. Edinburgh: Mosby.

ASPHYXIA

Asphyxia is a lack of oxygen reaching the brain that leads to unconsciousness and, in the absence of effective treatment, eventually death. It may be caused by smoke inhalation, hanging, chest injury, respiratory diseases, drowning, choking, poisoning, electrical injury, etc.

ASSESSMENT

Assessment (evaluation) is the first stage of the nursing process during which client and/or patient problems and needs are identified. ⇒ Nursing process.

ASSESSMENT TOOLS

A variety of validated tools used by nurses to assess many aspects of care, which include:

- Confusion and/or dementia;
- Dependence and/or mobility;
- Depression;
- Moving and handling;
- Nutritional status;
- Oral assessment;
- Pain intensity;
- Pressure ulcer risk;
- Swallowing;
- Wounds.

Further information is provided in the appropriate main entries.

ATTENTION-DEFICIT HYPERACTIVITY DISORDER

Attention-deficit hyperactivity disorder (ADHD) has an onset before the age of 5 years, and is characterized by continuous (pervasive) motor hyperactivity, restlessness, poor attention and concentration, distractibility and impulsivity.

The condition is more common in boys than girls (3:1). Between 30 and 50% of children with hyperactivity also have behavioural problems. No single cause has been found, but there is evidence that biological and neurodevelopmental factors are involved. Family factors, such as parental attitudes, are only involved in the presence of behavioural problems. Treatment includes behavioural modification (to improve concentration and adverse behaviour), school intervention (structured teaching in a small-size class, if possible) and medication (usually centrally acting stimulants, such as methylphenidate, but newer drugs are being developed). Medication may have a positive effect on attention, concentration and activity, but not directly on behavioural problems. However, if a child improves in some of the symptoms, this allows additional interventions to target the comorbid behavioural problems. Hyperactivity, restlessness, attention-deficit and impulsivity improve with age, but other problems, such as poor school performance, impaired social skills and relationships, low self-esteem and behavioural problems, may persist.

AUDIT

Audit is the process of comparing existing practice with an agreed standard.

Clinical audit evolved from medical audit, which entailed physicians examining their practice independently of that of other professionals. It soon became apparent that good patient care resulted from the integrated practice of many professionals and the emphasis shifted to clinical audit. Typically, audits are conducted to evaluate the effectiveness of medicines or treatments. However, almost any aspect of clinical care can be audited. Discharge planning, wound care, nutrition and pain management are other examples of clinical audit topics.

The fundamental first step in effective clinical audit is to identify and agree a standard. This is often the most valuable part of the process because it requires clinicians of all relevant professions to discuss and compare practices, which in itself can improve the consistency and quality of care.

The key stages in the audit process are:
- Deciding on a topic to audit, the reasons for doing the audit, how the care will be measured and which cases should be included;
- Collecting data on practice, from medical records or by observing care;
- Evaluating the findings against the standard and identifying the causes of incompatible performance;
- Acting to improve care;
- Repeating the data collection, evaluation and action steps as often as needed to raise the standard consistently.

Where organizations often fall short is in the action stage. It can be challenging and time consuming to change clinical practice. When faced with the prospect of change, there is often a need for education, persuasion and support to make it happen.

The importance of clinical audit as a tool for improving patient care has re-emerged with the introduction of clinical governance. The setting of clinical standards and the evaluation of practice against those standards are fundamental activities necessary to meet the expectations within clinical governance. The most important role of clinical audit is, however, to assure the best standards of care through a systematic, interactive, peer-supported process. ⇒ Change management, Clinical governance, Quality assurance.

AUTISM (AUTISTIC DISORDERS)

Autism is characterized by onset in the first 3 years of life, delay and deviation in the development of social relationships and communication, and resistance to change. There is an association with learning disability and a range of neurological diseases, particularly epilepsy. The child may show little interest in other people and show preference for his or her own company, be preoccupied with objects, avoid going to parents for comfort and lack empathy. Both comprehension and expression are usually delayed markedly. Children with autism develop no or limited pretend or imaginative play. When behavioural problems occur, these are usually secondary (i.e. a result of impaired communication). The child may have special abilities that involve mechanical tasks (e.g. numbers) and memory, but difficulties in abstract thinking.

Typical autistic disorders occur in 3–4 per 10 000 children. If one includes cases of milder severity, the prevalence rises to 10 per 10 000 children. It is as yet unclear whether there is a spectrum (or continuum) of autistic disorders according to severity, or groups of disorders with different aetiology and presentation.

The diagnosis *Asperger's syndrome* is characterized by the same abnormalities of reciprocal social interaction as autism, together with a restricted and repetitive repertoire of interests and activities, but without the general delay in language

A

or cognitive development of autism. These social difficulties are likely to continue in later life.

The broad diagnostic term *pervasive developmental disorders* is used to describe all autism-like conditions. Autistic disorders are four times more common in boys than in girls. There is a genetic predisposition, with 2–3% of siblings being affected, and a higher proportion has nonspecific language delay. In addition to comorbid neurological conditions, autism is also associated with a number of chromosomal abnormalities, particularly fragile-X syndrome. ⇒ Learning disability.

Management starts with a comprehensive assessment and explanation and/or reassurance to the parents. Support to the family should be long term. Appropriate educational placement is essential, depending on the nature and severity of the problems. Speech and language therapy or a behavioural programme can help to maximize the child's communication skills. Behaviour modification also targets aggression and social difficulties, the latter through graded steps of social stimulation and interaction. The prognosis depends on the number and severity of problems and impairments. In severe disorders, a high proportion of individuals require continuing care and support. In nearly all cases, there is continuing improvement throughout childhood and adolescence, so that each year the child gains some new skills.

Further reading

Glenis LB (2004). *Autism Spectrum Disorders: A Practical Guide to Diagnosis*. Oxford: Butterworth Heinemann.

AUTONOMY

Autonomy (self-determination) is the freedom and ability to act independently and without supervision or control. Autonomy as a quality can exist only insofar as certain conditions are present – to be able to understand one's environment, to make rational choices and to be able to act on the choices made.

Autonomy is a matter of degree. It can be considered on a continuum with 'no control' and 'total control' at the extremes. The greater the degree of autonomy, the more the person is able to do in his or her life. Autonomy is a quality that can be possessed to a greater or lesser degree in different areas, situations and times in our lives. Admission to hospital can result in fear and distress and reduce a person's degree of autonomy, and thus his or her ability to function in that particular situation and at that particular time. Working with patients to produce the conditions necessary for autonomy is a large area of nursing work.

A dilemma exists when it is felt that it is more important to act in the best interests of a person than to respect his or her autonomy. Overriding a person's autonomy is serious, and an action that must be justified. An area of client and/or patient autonomy that nurses work with in practice is to respect and maintain client and/or patient confidentiality.

Bacteria

Bacteria are microscopic unicellular organisms widely distributed in the environment. They may be free-living, saprophytic or parasitic. Bacteria can be *pathogenic* (disease producing) to humans, other animals and plants, or *nonpathogenic*. Pathogens may be *virulent* and always cause infection, whereas others, known as *opportunists*, usually only cause infection when the host defences are impaired, such as during cancer chemotherapy. Nonpathogenic bacteria may become pathogenic if they move from their normal site (e.g. bowel bacteria that cause a wound infection). Many bacteria have developed adaptations that allow them to exploit environments and survive unfriendly conditions (e.g. flagella, pili, waxy outer capsules, spore formation and enzymes, such as beta-lactamases, that destroy some antibiotics). ⇒ Antibiotics, Infection, Micro-organisms.

CLASSIFICATION OF BACTERIA

Bacteria are classified and identified by features that include shape and staining characteristics with Gram stain (positive or negative). Bacteria may be (*Fig. 20*):
- Round – single (cocci), in pairs (diplococci), in bunches (staphylococci) or in chains (streptococci);
- Rod shaped (bacilli);
- Curved or spiral (vibrios, spirilla and spirochaetes).

Gram's stain

A bacteriological stain for the identification and classification of micro-organisms. Those that stain violet are Gram-positive (+ve) and those that stain pink are Gram-negative (–ve).

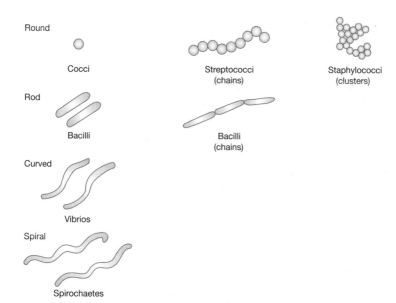

Fig 20 Bacterial classification according to shape

B

Basic Life Support

Basic life support (BLS) is the maintenance of a clear airway, the application of artificial respiration (usually by mouth-to-mouth breathing) and external cardiac massage to save a life without the use of artificial aids or equipment. Artificial respiration and external cardiac massage together comprise cardiopulmonary resuscitation (CPR). The emphasis of BLS is on:

• Assessing and/or checking responsiveness;
• Opening the airway, **A** (*Fig. 21A,B* and also see *Fig. 6*);
• Checking breathing, **B**, by looking for chest movements, and listening and feeling for chest movement. If the person is not breathing the BLS guidelines advice that two effective breaths (mouth-to-mouth) be used before proceeding to check the circulation;
• Confirming the presence of a circulation, **C**, by feeling for the carotid or femoral pulse (as the practice of the pulse check may be a less than reliable technique, especially by lay First Aiders, perhaps the expression 'look for signs of a circulation', which includes a more general assessment of circulation as well as a pulse check, is more appropriate).

When no circulation is present external cardiac massage is commenced at the rate of 100 chest compressions per minute and mouth-to-mouth breathing is continued. The guidelines state that the ratio between chest compressions and mouth-to-mouth breathing is 15:2. If circulation is present, mouth-to-mouth breathing continues and the circulation is checked every minute.

Help is summoned as soon as possible. ⇒ Advanced life support, Airway.

BASIC PAEDIATRIC LIFE SUPPORT

There are major differences between children and adults in both the causes of sudden collapse and also in some of the anatomical features, and these have an impact on the resuscitation techniques used in BLS. The causes of collapse in children and infants are usually respiratory problems and the resulting hypoxia, rather than the cardiac problems that occur in adults. BLS guidelines advise the same stages as for adults and 100 chest compressions per minute. There are, however, many differences, which include artificial respiration, the technique for external cardiac massage in infants and children, and the ratio of chest compressions to mouth-to-mouth or mouth-to-mouth-and-nose (in infants), which is 5:1 for children. Readers are advised to consult Further reading for details of paediatric BLS. ⇒ Advanced life support (Broselow paediatric resuscitation system).

Further reading

Brooker C and Nicol M (2003). *Nursing Adults. The Practice of Caring*, pp. 495–497. Edinburgh: Mosby.
Resuscitation Council (2000). *Basic Life Support. Resuscitation Guidelines*, and *Paediatric Basic Life Support. Resuscitation Guidelines*. Both Online: http://www.resus.org.uk

Bedrest, Complications of

⇒ Mobility (potential complications of immobility).

Behaviour

Behaviour can be defined as the observable general response of a person to internal or external motivating stimuli. The *mediational model* is a way to explain behaviour that takes into account cognitive factors. It was proposed as a result of

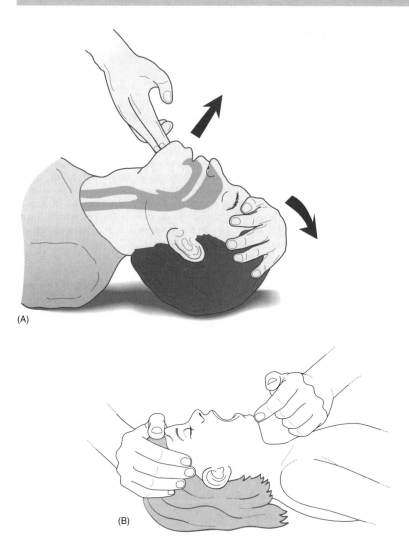

(A)

(B)

Fig 21 Head tilt and chin lift: (A) adult, (B) child

experimental work done by Tolman (1932), who (although a behaviourist) argued for the recognition of mediating factors in the establishment and maintenance of behaviour.

The *stimulus response model* disregards the notion of an intervening variable in the acquisition and display of behaviour. It is the model that is favoured by behaviourists who argue that observable behaviour is the only legitimate object of study and that it can be explained by consideration of the establishment of the links made via association during the learning process (see classical and operant conditioning below). ⇒ Cognition, Illness behaviour.

B

ADAPTIVE BEHAVIOUR

Adaptive behaviour is beneficial or appropriate behaviour in response to a change.

MALADAPTIVE BEHAVIOUR

Maladaptive behaviour is an abnormal or maladaptive response to a situation or change. It may relate to social interactions or to a response to a stressor that results in ill health (e.g. tension headaches, etc.).

BEHAVIOUR THERAPY

Behaviour therapy is a psychotherapeutic approach based on the experimental work that describes classical and operant conditioning. It emphasizes the central role of reinforcement in establishing and maintaining both adaptive and maladaptive behaviour. The focus of the therapy is the observable behaviour. It utilizes a nonmediational model in arriving at a formulation of a problem. ⇒ Cognition (cognitive behavioural therapy).

CLASSICAL CONDITIONING

The early work of Pavlov exemplifies this process of learning, which is the encouragement of new behaviour by modifying the stimulus–response association.

OPERANT CONDITIONING

After the work of Skinner it was recognized that if an organism emits a behaviour and this behaviour is reinforced, the behaviour is likely to be emitted again. The behaviour is seen to have an effect on the environment and, depending on this consequent effect, the behaviour may or may not be reinforced.

BEHAVIOURISM

Behaviourism is a word used in psychology to describe an approach that studies and interprets behaviour by objective observation of that behaviour, without reference to the underlying subjective mental phenomena, such as ideas, emotions and will. Behaviour is seen as a series of conditioned responses. ⇒ Psychology.

BELIEFS

A belief is a personal judgement for which one makes a truth claim, and that one should be prepared to defend by producing sound reason or evidence. While attitudes are generally acquired from others, beliefs comprise the sub-set of attitudes for which we personally make truth claims. To say we believe something to be true does not mean that we know for certain that it is true, so we do not give beliefs unconditional assent. They are formed by culture, family, life experiences and many other factors. ⇒ Culture, Ethics.

BENCHMARKING

Most organizations determine internally what levels of quality and standards to aim for. However, sometimes these levels may be determined using an inappropriate yardstick for guidance and comparison. Benchmarking is the system of comparing an organization's standards against those of an external, but similar, organization chosen especially for excellence in quality. The aim of benchmarking is to strive towards achieving improvements continuously.

Benchmarking in the National Health Service (NHS) is mainly a development of the 1990s. It is seen as another tool in the armoury against poor-quality practice and will help NHS organizations to learn from each other and to contribute to value for money (VFM) initiatives. Benchmarking depends on measurement and audit, and contributes to the cycle of quality improvements in the NHS. ⇒ Quality assurance.

BENZODIAZEPINES

⇒ Anxiety (anxiolytics).

BEREAVEMENT

Bereavement is a response to a life event that involves loss. It includes that which happens to a person after the death of another person who has been important in his or her life. It also occurs in other situations of loss, such as redundancy, loss of home, divorce or loss of a body part (e.g. mastectomy, amputation, etc.). ⇒ Grief.

BIBLIOGRAPHIC DATABASES

⇒ Literature searching and reviews.

BILIARY TRACT

The biliary tract comprises the bile ducts and gall bladder (*Fig. 22*). Bile produced in the liver is transported to the gall bladder for concentration and storage prior to release into the duodenum. ⇒ Gastrointestinal tract, Liver, Pancreas.

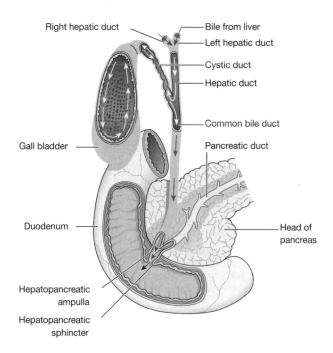

Fig 22 Biliary tract showing direction of the flow of bile from the liver to the duodenum

B

BILE DUCTS AND GALL BLADDER

The right and left hepatic ducts join to form the common hepatic duct just outside the portal fissure of the liver. The hepatic duct passes downwards about 3 cm, where it is joined at an acute angle by the cystic duct from the gall bladder. The cystic and hepatic ducts together form the common bile duct, which passes downwards to be joined by the main pancreatic duct at the hepatopancreatic ampulla. The opening of the combined ducts into the duodenum is controlled by the hepatopancreatic sphincter (sphincter of Oddi). Bile passes through the cystic duct twice, once on its way into the gall bladder and again when it is expelled from the gall bladder to the common bile duct and thence to the duodenum.

The gall bladder is a pear-shaped sac attached to the posterior surface of the liver. It has a fundus or expanded end, a body or main part and a neck, which is continuous with the cystic duct. The functions of the gall bladder include:

- Reservoir for bile;
- Concentration of the bile;
- Release of stored bile.

When the muscle wall of the gall bladder contracts, bile passes through the bile ducts to the duodenum. Contraction is stimulated by the hormone cholecystokinin (CCK), secreted by the duodenum in the presence of fat and the acid chyme in the duodenum.

Relaxation of the hepatopancreatic sphincter (of Oddi) is caused by CCK and is a reflex response to contraction of the gall bladder.

BILIARY AND GALL BLADDER DISORDERS

BILIARY ATRESIA

Biliary atresia is caused by congenital narrowing or absence of a bile duct or other biliary structure. It leads to jaundice and liver damage. Treatment is surgical and includes liver transplant.

CHOLANGITIS

Cholangitis is inflammation of a bile duct usually associated with the impaction of a gallstone, or after surgery.

GALLSTONES (CHOLELITHIASIS)

Gallstones consist of deposits of the constituents of bile, most commonly cholesterol. Many small stones or one large stone may form. The causes are not clear, but pre-disposing factors include:

- Changes in the composition of bile that affect the solubility of its constituents;
- High levels of blood and dietary cholesterol;
- Cholecystitis (see below);
- Diabetes mellitus with high blood cholesterol levels;
- Haemolytic disease;
- Female gender;
- Obesity;
- Long-term use of oral contraceptives;
- Several pregnancies in young women, especially when accompanied by obesity.

Complications of gallstones include:

- Biliary colic if a gallstone becomes stuck in the bile ducts. Strong peristaltic contraction of the smooth muscle in the wall of the duct (spasm) attempts to move the stone onwards. Severe pain is associated with biliary colic.

- Irritation and inflammation of the gall bladder and the bile ducts. There may be superimposed microbial infection.
- Impaction that results in blockage of the cystic duct by a gallstone leads to distension of the gall bladder and cholecystitis. Obstruction of the common bile duct leads to retention of bile, jaundice and cholangitis.

CHOLECYSTITIS

Acute cholecystitis is usually a complication of gallstones or an exacerbation of chronic cholecystitis. Inflammation develops, followed by secondary microbial infection.

The onset of chronic cholecystitis is usually insidious, sometimes after repeated acute attacks. Gallstones are usually present and there may be accompanying biliary colic. There is usually secondary infection with suppuration. Ulceration of the tissues between the gall bladder and the duodenum or colon may occur with fistula formation and, later, fibrous adhesions.

TUMOURS OF THE BILIARY TRACT

Benign tumours are rare. Malignant tumours are relatively rare, but can involve the gall bladder or the bile ducts.

BILIARY SURGERY

Some types of biliary and/or gall bladder surgery are outlined in *Box 2*.

> **Box 2 Biliary and/or gall badder surgery**
> **Cholecystectomy** – removal of the gall bladder, usually laparoscopically via the minimally invasive transperitoneal approach.
> **Cholecystoduodenostomy** – the establishment of an anastomosis between the gall bladder and the duodenum.
> **Cholecystoenterostomy** – the establishment of an artificial opening (anastomosis) between the gall bladder and the small intestine.
> **Cholecystogastrostomy** – rarely performed anastomosis between the gall bladder and the stomach.
> **Cholecystojejunostomy** – an anastomosis between the gall bladder and the jejunum, performed for obstructive jaundice caused by growth in the head of the pancreas.
> **Cholecystotomy** – incision into the gall bladder.
> **Choledochoduodenostomy** – an anastomosis between the common bile duct and the duodenum.
> **Choledocholithotomy** – surgical removal of a gallstone from the common bile duct.
> **Choledochostomy** – drainage of the common bile duct using a T-tube, usually after exploration for a gallstone.
> **Choledochotomy** – incision into the bile duct (see choledocholithotomy).

BIOGRAPHICAL AND HEALTH DATA

Biographical and health data is a term usually applied to information collected at the initial assessment of a person who accesses a healthcare service, whether in hospital or in the community. Most of the biographical data does not change, but it is helpful to the multidisciplinary team of health professionals involved in the care and treatment, enabling them to individualize conversation with the person. The health data, particularly those about dependence or independence for carrying out everyday living activities, may well change during the person's contact with the healthcare service. All data are useful when planning the person's discharge from the service. ⇒ Nursing process.

BIORHYTHM

A biorhythm is any of the cyclical patterns of biological functions unique to each individual, such as variations in body temperature, hormone levels, urine volume, sleep–wake cycles and menstrual cycle.

CIRCADIAN RHYTHM

Circadian rhythm is a term used to describe the daily pattern of life for organisms, including humans. The ultradian rhythm describes a subdivision of time within the circadian rhythm. It has been found that the human body, when deprived of light or other sources of time-keeping (e.g. time-setters such as meal times and live television) adopts a sleep–wake routine that resembles a 24-hour clock. The average circadian rhythm for humans is around 25 hours, although the range of circadian rhythms for different subjects varied from 16 to 48 hours.

Individual circadian rhythms can be considered responsible for the two main personality types, although these are on a continuum and not as polarized as might appear (Borbély 1987). 'Morning types' are those who are alert and bright in the morning, and often do their best work in the morning and by early evening become tired and less efficient. 'Evening types', however, find rising in the morning a chore and do not begin to function at their best until the afternoon. Often they will work late and go to bed late. ⇒ Body temperature, Endocrine (hormones), Menstrual cycle, Sleep.

Practice application – desynchronization: shift work and jet lag
Desynchronization is a phenomenon whereby biological rhythms become disordered because they are no longer synchronized with each other. This can happen during shift work when the working hours change and the sleep–wake cycle has to change suddenly, but hormones and metabolic rhythms take longer to adjust. Thus, the person is sleeping yet the body's hormone secretions are at levels that would be normal for someone who is awake. Compared to the sleeping norm, therefore, the temperature is elevated, there is a higher level of adrenaline (epinephrine) and kidney function is increased, which thus causes disturbances because of the need to void urine; the secretion of the hormone melatonin is decreased (Borbély 1987).

Problems associated with shift work, however, are not just related to desynchronization, but also to the social effect of working 'unsocial hours'.

Nurses need to be aware of the effects of sleep deprivation because shift patterns can seriously affect the standard of care they provide to patients. Sleep-deprived nurses may become less efficient, especially with cognitive tasks (such as drug calculations) or manipulative skills (such as administering intravenous drugs). Nurses may also become irritable, which may affect their relationships with patients, relatives and colleagues.

In recent years there has been a move away from the long rosters of night duty towards shorter internal rotations, as these have been shown to have a less negative effect on individuals through reduced effects of sleep inversion (Brugne 1994).

Jet lag is another example of the body being affected by desynchronization. It can take up to 2 weeks for the effects of jet lag to be overcome and resynchronized by the body when major time zones have been crossed (especially

B

if travel is west to east). Timing of maintenance medication during travelling needs to be considered and managed appropriately, particularly for people with diabetes or asthma, whose medication must reflect their own needs rather than sticking to a strict timetable.

BIPOLAR AFFECTIVE DISORDER (SYN. MANIC-DEPRESSIVE ILLNESS)

⇒ Disorders of mood (bipolar affective disorder, psychotic depression).

BLINDNESS

Blindness is lack of sight or visual impairment. ⇒ Colour vision, Vision (visual impairment).

BLOOD

Blood is a fluid connective tissue that consists of a pale yellow fluid, plasma, in which are suspended the red blood cells or erythrocytes, the white blood cells or leucocytes and the blood platelets (thrombocytes). The plasma contains many substances, including protein clotting factors, nutrients (amino acids, glucose, lipids, minerals and vitamins), enzymes, hormones, gases, drugs and metabolic waste. Blood volume is proportional to size and adults usually have 4–6 L circulating. Cells form around 45% of blood volume, and plasma forms the remaining 55% (*Fig. 23*).

In health the pH of blood remains within the range 7.35–7.45 (see *Box 3* for blood cell counts and other haematological tests. ⇒ Bone (myelodysplasia, multiple myeloma), Bone marrow sampling, Coagulation, Erythrocyte (anaemia), Haemoglobin (haemoglobinopathies), Haemopoiesis, Haemostasis, Leucocytes, Leukaemia, Platelets.

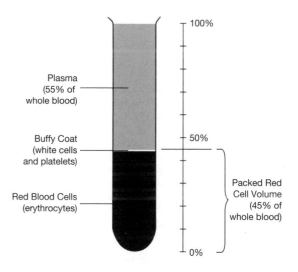

Fig 23 The appearance of anticoagulated whole blood when allowed to settle

Box 3 Haematological tests – reference ranges
Erythrocyte sedimentation rate (ESR), adult
Female, 0–7 mm/h
Male, 0–5 mm/h
NB: Older people may have higher values.
Haemoglobin
Female, 115–165 g/L (11.5–16.5 g/dL)
Male, 130–180 g/L (13–18 g/dL)
Mean cell haemoglobin (MCH)
27–32 pg
Mean cell haemoglobin concentration (MCHC)
30–35 g/dL
Mean cell volume (MCV)
78–94 fL
Packed cell volume (PCV)
Female, 0.35–0.47 (35–47%)
Male, 0.40–0.54 (40–54%)
Platelets
150–400 × 10^9/L
Red cell count
Female, 3.8–5.3 × 10^{12}/L
Male, 4.5–6.5 × 10^{12}/L
Reticulocytes (adults)
25–85 × 10^9/L
White cells
Total: 4.0–11.0 × 10^9/L
Differential:
Neutrophils, 2.0–7.5 × 10^9/L
Eosinophils, 0.04–0.4 × 10^9/L
Basophils, 0.01–0.10 × 10^9/L
Lymphocytes, 1.5-4.0 × 10^9/L
Monocytes, 0.2–0.8 × 10^9/L

BLOOD GROUPS

ABO SYSTEM

There are four groups, A, B, AB and O. The red cells of these groups contain the corresponding antigens (agglutinogens): group A has A, group B has B, group AB has both antigens and group O has neither. In the plasma there are antibodies (agglutinins) that cause agglutination (clumping) of any cell that carries the corresponding antigen. Group A plasma contains anti-B, group B plasma contains anti-A, group O plasma contains both anti-A and anti-B and group AB plasma contains no agglutinins. This grouping is determined by testing a suspension of red cells with anti-A and anti-B serum or by testing serum with known cells. Transfusion with an incompatible ABO group causes a severe haemolytic reaction and death may occur unless the transfusion is stopped promptly. For most transfusion purposes, group A can receive groups A and O, group B can receive groups B and O, group AB can have blood of any group and group O can only have group O (*Fig. 24*). The terms universal donor and universal recipient are outdated and confusing because many other blood groups exist.

	Recipient			
Group	A	B	O	AB
A	+	−	−	+
B	−	+	−	+
AB	−	−	−	+
O	+	+	+	+

(left axis label: Donor)

+ = compatible
− = non-compatible

Fig 24 Blood group compatibility

Rhesus blood group

A further three pairs of antigens coded for by genes designated the letters Cc, Dd and Ee are present on the red cells. When the cells contain only the cde groups, the blood is Rhesus negative (Rh −ve); when the cells contain C, D or E singly or in combination with cde, the blood is Rhesus positive (Rh +ve). For general purposes, only the Dd antigens are of clinical significance. About 85% of the Caucasian population have the D antigen. In contrast to the ABO system, there are no preformed antibodies to the D antigen, but these groups are antigenic and can, under suitable conditions, produce the corresponding antibody in the serum. Antibodies are formed if there is transfusion of Rh +ve blood to a Rh −ve person or immunization during pregnancy by Rh +ve fetal red cells, with the D antigen entering the maternal circulation where the women is Rh −ve. This can cause haemolytic disease of the newborn (erythroblastosis fetalis). ⇒ Haemolytic disease of the newborn (anti-D).

BLOOD AND BLOOD PRODUCTS TRANSFUSION

Transfusion of compatible human blood and blood product is used to replace lost or destroyed blood, and also for severe anaemia with deficient blood production. Fresh blood from a donor may be used, but usually stored blood donated by healthy volunteers is used. It can be given as whole blood, or as plasma-reduced blood (packed-cell). Various components of blood can be transfused as required by the situation, such as platelets, granulocytes (types of white cell), fresh frozen plasma, albumin, cryoprecipitate, factor VIII and factor IX. Before transfusion, the donor red cells are cross-matched against the patient's serum to ensure compatibility and prevent mismatched blood transfusions that result in severe reactions and may be fatal. Autologous blood transfusion may be used where the person's blood is withdrawn and stored prior to elective surgery.

Practice application – principles for safe blood transfusion

A summary based on national guidelines that outline the principles of safe transfusion (British Committee for Standards in Haematology 1999) is as follows:

- Patients do not need to give written consent for a blood transfusion. However, the risks of transfusion should be explained fully and nurses should ensure that patients have all the information they require. The National Blood Service produces a useful patient information sheet.

B

- Before commencing a blood transfusion the nurse should record the patient's temperature, pulse, blood pressure and respiratory rate to establish baseline values.
- To ensure that the correct blood is administered a Registered Nurse or Midwife should check the patient's details against the information on the prescription, the blood bag and the cross-match form. Some hospital policies may stipulate that two nurses participate in this checking procedure. The check should be carried out at the bedside and should include the patient's name, date of birth, hospital number and the blood unit number and expiry date. It should also confirm that the blood group of the donor unit is compatible with that of the patient.
- Blood should not be used after midnight on the expiry date.
- To reduce the risk of bacterial proliferation within blood, transfusions should be initiated within 30 minutes of the blood leaving storage. Blood should not be stored temporarily in drug refrigerators. No drugs should be added to blood.
- Blood should be administered through a blood-giving set, which incorporates a filter above the drip chamber into a peripheral venous cannula or central venous line. A unit of blood is normally transfused over 3–4 hours. The duration of each unit of blood should not exceed 6 hours. Blood that remains in the bag after this period should be discarded in a clinical waste bin.
- Serious transfusion reactions usually become evident within 30 minutes of commencing a unit. The patient's temperature, pulse and respiratory rate should therefore be recorded 15 minutes after the start of each unit. Any significant changes from baseline should be reported to the medical team at once. These checks represent a minimum standard and local policies may require more frequent checks of vital signs. As a general principle, all patients should be observed closely throughout the transfusion.
- Once the transfusion is complete, blood bags can be disposed of in clinical waste bins.

BLOOD CULTURE

If septicaemia is suspected blood cultures should be taken to identify the exact pathogen. Blood must be drawn from a clean venous site using an aseptic technique and placed into special culture bottles (one for an aerobic culture and one for an anaerobic culture). These blood cultures must be taken at specific times and a particular number of days apart, for which local policy should be observed. The blood must be put into the bottle carefully, avoiding any outside contamination that may affect the results of the culture. Preliminary results should be available on the blood culture within 24 hours and appropriate antibiotics commenced if the results are positive. ⇒ Septicaemia, Systemic inflammatory response syndrome.

BLOOD GASES

Blood gases are also known as arterial blood gases (ABGs). The acid–base balance is assessed using ABG analysis. Arterial blood can be analysed to measure the partial pressure of oxygen (PaO_2), carbon dioxide ($PaCO_2$), blood pH and bicarbonate (HCO_3^-) and base excess, which reflect the buffering action of bicarbonate in the blood on hydrogen ions. Normal values are shown in *Box 4*. Arterial blood may be obtained by intermittent arterial puncture or through an arterial cannula.

PaO_2 indicates oxygenation levels of the blood and $PaCO_2$ the effectiveness of ventilation. Hypoxaemia is present when the PaO_2 is lower than normal. When the evaluation of blood gases has been carried out, a pulse oximeter may be used for continuous monitoring of oxygen saturation levels. ⇒ Acid–base balance, Arterial cannula or line, Oxygen (pulse oximetry).

Box 4 Normal values for blood gases
pH, 7.35–7.45
PCO_2, 2.6–6.0 kPa
PO_2, 10.0–13.3 kPa
HCO_3^-, 22–26 mmol/L
Base excess, –2 to +2

BLOOD GLUCOSE PROFILES

Self-monitoring of blood glucose (SMBG) uses capillary blood, usually obtained by a finger prick, for glucose estimation by a hand-held meter. This allows the person to monitor and manage their diabetes. After diagnosis, initially blood glucose tests are usually performed four times a day at most (unless an insulin infusion is running, in which case blood glucose tests are carried out hourly). They should be done just before main meals and at bedtime. When the glucose levels are reasonably well controlled (blood glucose level of 4–9.9 mmol/L), testing frequency may be reduced to twice daily, on one day before breakfast and the evening meal, and on the next before the midday meal and at bedtime, and so on (*Fig. 25A*).

Once the blood glucose levels are well controlled (i.e. blood glucose 4–7 mmol/L before main meals and 4–8 mmol/L at bedtime), testing may be reduced to once daily at various times, with extra tests if there are any concerns (*Fig. 25B*).

Most blood glucose meters are supplied with quality-control solutions. As all blood glucose meters should be subjected to regular quality-control checks in

Date	Before breakfast	Before midday meal	Before evening meal	Bedtime	Notes
	x		x		
		x		x	
	x		x		

(A)

Date	Before breakfast	Before midday meal	Before evening meal	Bedtime	Notes
	x				
		x			
			x		
				x	
	x			x	To gym
		x			
			x		

(B)

Fig 25 Blood glucose monitoring profile: (A) twice daily, (B) four times (various) a day

the clinical setting, so people with diabetes should be shown how to check their own meters on a regular basis, at least once a week, or according to local protocols.

B

Practice application – blood glucose monitoring

- Blood glucose monitoring (BGM) must be performed on clean hands, as any contaminants are likely to affect the result obtained.
- The finger should be pricked on the side (less painful than pricking the pad).
- Blood should be 'milked' out of the finger, rather than squeezed. Squeezing applies pressure and leads to inaccurate results. It is also useful to wait 5 seconds or so prior to 'milking'.
- Washing hands in warm water can also help with blood flow.
- A finger pricker designed for the purpose must always be used. Using lancets alone may cause damage to the fingers and can be extremely painful. To prevent cross-infection the finger pricker must be either single-person use only or specifically designed for multi-person use. Most meters supplied are designed for single-person use only and must *not* be used for another individual.
- The meter (or visually read system) must be used strictly according to the manufacturer's instructions.
- It is essential that sufficient blood be obtained to cover the blood glucose testing strip, as insufficient samples give inaccurate results.
- The results must be recorded. In hospital this is on the appropriate chart, but at home people should also be encouraged to record their results in a blood glucose monitoring diary. Many meters have a memory function, recording the result and the date and time at which the test was performed, but it is not easy to detect patterns in results using this function.

BLOOD PRESSURE

Blood pressure (BP) is the pressure exerted by the blood on the blood vessel walls, and usually refers to the pressure within the arteries as the left ventricle pumps blood into the aorta. The pressure is produced when flow meets resistance, i.e.

blood pressure (BP) = peripheral resistance (PR) × cardiac output (CO)

The factors that contribute to BP include:
- Peripheral resistance;
- Cardiac output;
- Blood volume;
- Venous return;
- Blood viscosity; and
- Elasticity of arterial walls.

Generally, BP is measured indirectly in the brachial artery using a sphygmo-manometer (aneroid or mercury) with a stethoscope, or an electronic device (see *Fig. 26*). Arterial BP may also be recorded directly by the use of an arterial cannula and pressure transducer. The arterial BP has two readings recorded in millimetres of mercury pressure (mmHg):
- *Systolic*, which represents the highest pressure in the left ventricle during systole, when blood is ejected from the heart;
- *Diastolic*, which is the lowest pressure as the ventricles fill during diastole when the aortic and pulmonary valves are closed.

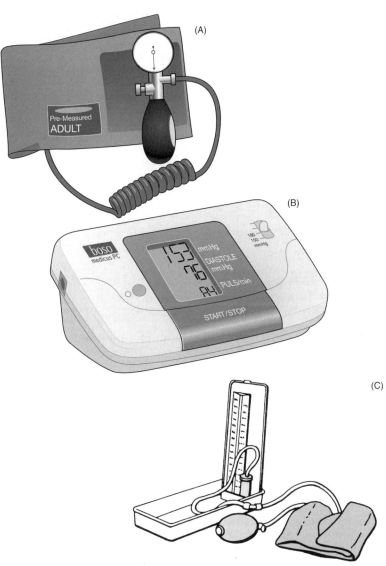

Fig 26 Sphygmomanometers: (A) aneroid, (B) electronic, (C) mercury

Usually values for both systolic and diastolic pressures are recorded, for example 138/88, and BP may be measured with the person lying, sitting or standing. The difference between the systolic and diastolic pressures is termed the *pulse pressure*. ⇒ Arterial cannula or line, Hypertension, Hypotension.

Korotkov or Korotkoff sounds are the sounds heard with a stethoscope while recording noninvasive arterial BP with a sphygmomanometer. The phases are (*Fig. 27*):

B

(1) Sharp, clear sound which represents systolic pressure;
(2) Blowing or swishing sound;
(3) Sharp but softer than in (1);
(4) Muffled, fading;
(5) Silence.

It is unclear whether phase 4 or phase 5 is the best measure of the diastolic pressure. Phase 5 is used for most people and sometimes both phases 4 and 5 are recorded. However, phase 4 should be routinely used in those groups that include pregnant women and children.

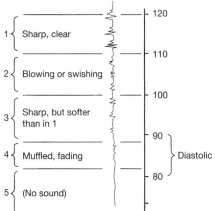

Fig 27 The Korotkov sounds (based on O'Brien and O'Malley 1981)

Practice application – accuracy of blood pressure recording and cuff size
The size of the sphygmomanometer cuff is important in achieving accurate recordings of BP. A bladder that is too large or too small results in a respective under- or overestimation of the blood pressure (O'Brien *et al.* 1995). Different cuffs are available for use on infants, children, adults or a person who is obese, or for taking recordings using the person's thigh. Recommended bladder dimensions are 35 cm length and 12.5 cm wide for adults and grown children, but 18 × 8 cm and 13 × 4 cm cuffs should be available for smaller children and infants. An appropriate-size cuff should be used so that the bladder of the cuff covers at least three-quarters of the circumference of the upper arm, and the middle of the rubber bladder is placed directly over the brachial artery.

Further reading

Nicol M, Bavin C, Bedford-Turner S, Cronin P and Rawlings-Anderson K (2004). *Essential Nursing Skills*, Second Edition. Edinburgh: Mosby.

BODY CAVITIES

The organs that make up the systems of the body are contained in four cavities:
- Cranial;
- Thoracic;
- Abdominal;
- Pelvic.

CRANIAL CAVITY

The cranial cavity contains the brain, and the bones of the skull (cranium and face) form its boundaries (*Fig. 28*).

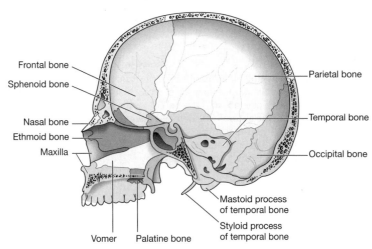

Fig 28 Bones that form the right half of the cranium and the face – viewed from the left

THORACIC CAVITY

The thoracic cavity is situated in the upper part of the trunk. Its boundaries are formed by a bony framework and supporting muscles. The main organs and structures contained in the thoracic cavity are (*Fig. 29*):

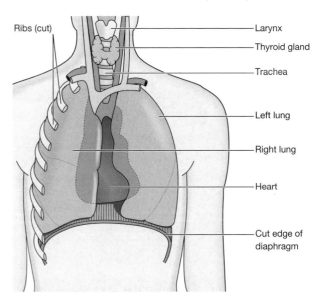

Fig 29 Some of the main structures in the thoracic cavity and root of the neck

B

- Trachea, two bronchi and two lungs;
- Heart, aorta, superior and inferior vena cava, other blood vessels;
- Oesophagus;
- Lymph vessels and lymph nodes;
- Nerves.

The mediastinum is the name given to the space between the lungs. It contains the heart, oesophagus and blood vessels.

ABDOMINAL CAVITY

The largest body cavity, the abdominal cavity is situated in the main part of the trunk. It is bounded by the diaphragm, the muscles that form the abdominal wall, the lumbar vertebrae, lower ribs and the pelvic cavity.

Most of the space in the abdominal cavity is occupied by the organs and glands involved in the digestion and absorption of food (*Fig. 30*):
- Stomach, small intestine and most of the large intestine;
- Liver, gall bladder, bile ducts and pancreas.

Other structures include (*Fig. 31*):
- Spleen;
- Two kidneys and upper ureters;
- Two adrenal glands;
- Blood vessels, lymph vessels and nodes, and nerves.

ABDOMINAL REGIONS

By convention, the surface anatomy of the abdomen is divided into nine regions used to describe the location of organs and structures, or symptoms (*Fig. 32*).

PELVIC CAVITY

The pelvic cavity is roughly funnel shaped and extends from the lower abdominal cavity. Its boundaries are the abdominal cavity, the pubic bones, sacrum and coccyx, the innominate bones and the muscles of the pelvic floor.

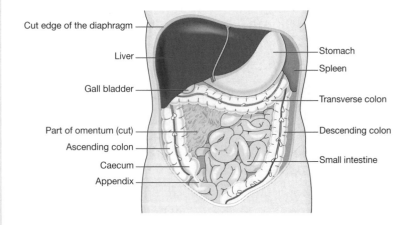

Fig 30 Organs that occupy the anterior part of the abdominal cavity and the diaphragm (cut)

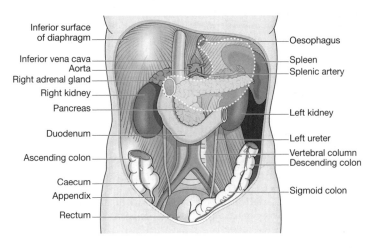

Fig 31 Organs that occupy the posterior part of the abdominal cavity and the diaphragm (cut) – the broken line shows the position of the stomach

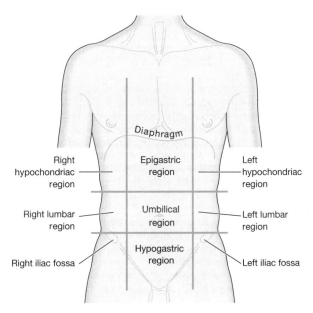

Fig 32 Regions of the abdomen

The pelvic cavity contains the following:
- Sigmoid colon, rectum and anus;
- Some loops of small intestine;
- Urinary bladder, lower ureters and the urethra;
- In the female, the uterus, uterine tubes, ovaries and vagina;
- In the male, some reproductive organs – prostate gland, seminal vesicles, spermatic cord, vas deferens, ejaculatory ducts and the urethra.
⇒ Reproductive systems.

B

BODY IMAGE

Many stigmatizing illnesses have an impact on the way an individual perceives his or her body and therefore his or her body image. Body image is a much-used term that has wide applications in holistic care. Body image affects the social, spiritual, physical and psychological aspects of wellbeing and, as such, an understanding of this subject is vital to the provision of care. Price (1990) suggests that a client's body image has an impact on the process of rehabilitation, having consequences for and affecting the client's wellbeing. He identifies three components to body image (*Box 5*):

• How individuals perceive and feel about their bodies (body reality);
• How the body responds to commands (body presentation);
• How the first two components compare with an internal standard (body ideal).

Box 5 Components of body image (Price 1990)
Reality – as it really is: tall or short, fat or thin, dark or fair. The norm for race and relative to wider social group. It is not a constant state, but dependent upon age and physical changes.
Presentation – dress and fashion. Control of functions, movement and pose. How others perceive us.
Ideal – how a body should look and act (culturally determined and includes contours, size, proportions, odours and smells). Personal norm for personal space. Body reliability, which may be unrealistic. Applied not only to self, but to those around us.

Throughout life there is an attempt to achieve and maintain a balance between the three elements in *Box 5*.

Body image depends not only upon the individual's response to his or her own body, but also upon the appearance, attitude and responses of other. It is important for nurses to remember this when delivering care, as their own responses may have a great impact on how clients perceive themselves.

Body image and self-image are interconnected, self-image being central to an individual's confidence, motivation and sense of achievement. It is a product of an individual's personality, being moulded by socialization, and represents an assessment of self-worth (Price 1990). When the three elements of body image are in a state of equilibrium, meeting both personal and social expectations and therefore enabling a successful presentation of self, there is a corresponding positive self-image. If, however, changes occur that result in an alteration of one or more of the body image components, a negative self-image may follow (*Fig. 33*).

Altered body images can arise from two sources:
• Open (i.e. visible), as with arthritis;
• Hidden (i.e. not readily observable), such as a colostomy.
Personal responses to altered body image arise from the interaction of a variety of factors, which include:
• Visibility;
• Associated guilt or shame;
• Significance for the future – work, social life, personal;
• Support during transition;
• Personal coping strategies;
• Stage of the grieving process.

BODY LANGUAGE

⇒ Communication.

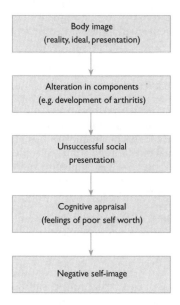

Fig 33 Impact of body image on self-image

BODY MASS INDEX

Body mass index (BMI) is a measurement derived from weight and height: weight in kilograms divided by the square of the height in metres. It is used with other criteria to determine whether an adult is within a healthy weight range and as part of a nutritional assessment. ⇒ Malnutrition, Nutrition (nutritional assessment).

BODY SURFACE AREA

Body surface area (BSA) is calculated from a special nomogram that uses height and weight. It may be used to calculate drug doses in children, especially when the difference between the dose that gives a therapeutic effect and the dose that causes toxicity is small.

BODY TEMPERATURE

Body temperature is the balance between heat production and heat loss in the human body. Core body temperature is maintained at around 37°C throughout the 24 hours, but is subject to a diurnal variation of between 0.2 and 0.3°C over that period. Core body temperature is that which registers in the organs of the central cavities of the body (cranium, thorax and abdomen). Temperature is raised slightly in the late afternoon and/or early evening, during exercise and in women just after ovulation. Shell body temperature is that which registers outwith the trunk (e.g. in the dried axilla or groin). Shell temperature may vary between 36°C at the shoulder and 20°C in the feet. ⇒ Thermoregulation.

DISORDERS OF TEMPERATURE REGULATION

PYREXIA AND HYPERPYREXIA

Pyrexia (temperature 37.6–40°C) and hyperpyrexia (>40°C) are conditions in which the thermoregulatory mechanisms remain intact, but the body temperature is maintained at a high level. Infection is the most common cause of pyrexia.

B

Other causes of pyrexia include dehydration, certain drugs, malignancy, surgery, severe trauma, acute myocardial infarction, blood transfusions reactions, heart failure and hyperthyroidism.

HYPERTHERMIA

Hyperthermia is defined as an increase in core body temperature through the loss of thermoregulatory mechanisms. There is dysfunction of the hypothalamus. This condition is caused by central nervous system (CNS) problems and does not respond to antipyretic therapy. Cerebral metabolism is increased so the brain has great difficulty dealing with the increase in carbon dioxide production. Cerebral vasodilation occurs and may increase intracranial pressure and is thus dangerous to neurologically compromised patients. A temperature of 41–43°C produces nerve damage, coagulation and convulsions. If this dangerous state is not reversed through effective cooling measures the person suffers irreversible brain damage and death.

Conditions that present with hyperthermia include heat cramps, heat exhaustion, heat stroke, malignant hyperthermia and antipsychotic (neuroleptic) malignant hyperthermia. ⇒ Antipsychotics.

HYPOTHERMIA

Hypothermia is defined as a core temperature of less than 35°C. Almost all metabolic processes can be affected by hypothermia. Degrees of hypothermia are classified as mild (body temperature, 32–35°C), moderate (28–31.9°C), severe (20–27°C) and profound (<20°C).

Hypothermia may be accidental or therapeutic. Individuals at the extremes of age and those exposed to adverse environmental conditions are prone to accidental hypothermia. Death usually occurs when core temperature falls below 25°C.

Therapeutic hypothermia may be induced, inadvertent or post-anaesthesia.

FROSTBITE

Frostbite is a localized cold injury to the surface of the body, rather than to its core (as in hypothermia). It results from exposure to sub-freezing temperatures. The fingers, hands, feet, toes and face, especially the nose, ears and cheeks, are at most risk of frostbite.

Practice application – sites for measuring body temperature

For most clinical purposes core temperature can be measured in several ways:

- Under the tongue (close to the sublingual artery) using a single-use, electronic or glass–mercury thermometer. Glass–mercury thermometers have been withdrawn in many countries as there is a risk of cross-infection, and they may break, so exposing people to mercury vapour. Glass thermometers are unsuitable for oral temperature recording in people who have seizures, as well as those who are unconscious or confused, as they may bite on the thermometer causing it to break in their mouth.
- By use of an electronic tympanic membrane thermometer (*Fig. 34*), which correlates well with the pulmonary artery temperature or rectally; however, the rectal site is no longer advocated unless an electronic rectal probe is available.

BOLAM TEST

⇒ Negligence.

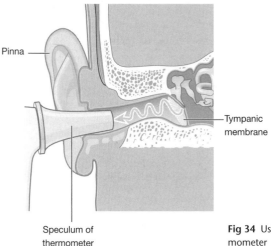

Pinna

Tympanic
membrane

Speculum of
thermometer

Fig 34 Using a tympanic thermometer

Bone

Bone is a connective tissue that has been mineralized to produce an extremely hard substance able to stretch (tensile strength) and withstand considerable compressive forces. Bone consists of:
• Water;
• Organic constituents that include osteoid and bone cells, osteoblasts (bone-forming cells), osteocytes (bone cells) and osteoclasts (bone-resorption cells);
• Inorganic constituents, mainly calcium phosphate.
Bone has the following functions:
• Provides mechanical support and is the site of muscle attachment;
• Protects body organs (e.g. heart, lungs, brain and spinal cord);
• Contains red bone marrow, which is the site for the formation of some blood cells;
• Storage of minerals, notably calcium and phosphorus.
There are two types of bone tissue: hard, dense compact (cortical) bone, and spongy cancellous (trabecular) bone. Several bone types form the skeleton: long (e.g. femur), short (e.g. carpals), flat (e.g. sternum), irregular (e.g. vertebrae) and sesamoid (e.g. patella). The general structure of a long bone is illustrated in *Fig. 35*.

Bone marrow is contained within both the medullary cavity and spaces in cancellous bone. At birth the cavities are filled with blood-forming red marrow, which is gradually replaced by fatty yellow marrow during childhood, until in adults red marrow is confined to the skull, sternum, ribs, pelvis, vertebrae and the ends of long bones. ⇒ Bone marrow sampling, Fracture, Musculoskeletal disorders, Skeleton.

BONE MARROW DISORDERS

Disorders of bone marrow include myelodysplasia, multiple myeloma and aplastic anaemia. ⇒ Erythrocyte (anaemia).

MYELODYSPLASIA

Myelodysplasia, or myelodysplastic syndrome (MDS) describes a group of disorders of the bone marrow characterized by the presence of abnormal stem cells and progressive bone marrow failure. In severe cases, MDS can evolve into acute

B

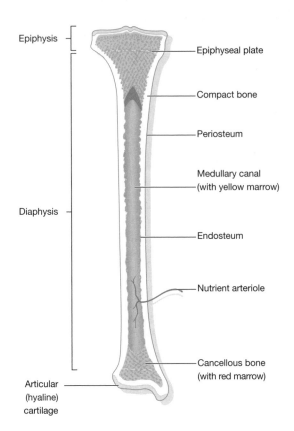

Epiphysis

Epiphyseal plate

Compact bone

Periosteum

Medullary canal
(with yellow marrow)

Diaphysis

Endosteum

Nutrient arteriole

Cancellous bone
(with red marrow)

Articular
(hyaline)
cartilage

Fig 35 Structure of a typical long bone

leukaemia. Treatment may include haemopoietic stem cell transplantation (HSCT), growth factors (e.g. erythropoietin), chemotherapy and supportive measures – regular blood transfusion and chelating drugs to deal with iron overload. ⇒ Leukaemia.

MULTIPLE MYELOMA (MYELOMATOSIS)

Multiple myeloma is a form of bone marrow cancer that affects plasma cells (derived from B-cells). Abnormal immunoglobulins, such as Bence Jones protein, are produced. Bence Jones protein is excreted in the urine of some patients with multiple myeloma. The abnormal immunoglobulins may increase blood viscosity, which can cause renal failure and damage to other organs. There is infiltration of the bone marrow with malignant plasma cells, which leads to anaemia, leucopenia and thrombocytopenia, and bone destruction that can lead to severe bone pain, hypercalcaemia, fractures and spinal cord compression. Treatment includes:

• Cytotoxic chemotherapy and corticosteroids (average survival is about 3 years);
• Cure may be achieved with HSCT;
• High-dose chemotherapy with autologous peripheral blood stem-cell rescue may improve life expectancy for some older adults;
• Bisphosphonates (e.g. pamidronate) to control bone destruction;
• Local radiotherapy for pain control;
• Plasmapheresis to reduce blood viscosity. ⇒ Apheresis.

BONE MARROW SAMPLING

Bone marrow sampling or biopsy is a diagnostic procedure increasingly being carried out by specialist haematology nurses. Sampling of the bone marrow can take two forms, bone marrow aspirate and trephine. Samples are usually taken from the posterior iliac crest.

Practice application – bone marrow sampling

Bone marrow sampling is a very quick procedure, but it can be uncomfortable and some people may prefer to be sedated with short-acting benzodiazepines, such as midazolam, or to inhale nitrous oxide and oxygen.

Prior to sampling, nurses should ensure that people understand and are fully prepared for the procedure. For both types of sampling, the surrounding skin area is cleaned and a local anaesthetic, such as lidocaine, is injected. The bone marrow needle is inserted through the skin into the cortex of the bone, the stylet is removed and a syringe attached to the hub of the needle. Approximately 0.5–1.0 mL of marrow is then aspirated into the syringe, which can cause a sharp pain for a few seconds. A bone marrow trephine uses a similar technique, but a core of bone and marrow is removed.

People sedated with short-acting benzodiazepines should be observed closely until they have recovered fully. Their respiratory rate and oxygen saturation levels should be monitored, as respiratory depression can occur. The puncture site should be observed for bleeding or inflammation, particularly if the person has a low platelet count or white cell count, although bleeding is usually minimal. After a bone marrow test the person may feel some discomfort, which can normally be relieved with a mild analgesic, such as paracetamol.

A variety of tests can be performed on bone marrow. It can be spread on a slide for analysis under a microscope, which enables the number and type of cells present to be assessed. More sophisticated tests can be used to identify specific malignant cells and abnormalities of the chromosomes or DNA.

BONE MARROW TRANSPLANT

⇒ Haemopoietic stem cell transplantation.

BRAIN

⇒ Head injury, Nervous system (neurological disorders).

BREAST

The breasts (mammary glands) are accessory glands of the female reproductive system. At puberty they grow and develop to their mature size under the influence of oestrogen and progesterone. During pregnancy these hormones stimulate further growth. After the baby is born the hormone prolactin from the anterior pituitary stimulates the production of milk, and oxytocin from the posterior pituitary stimulates the release of milk in response to the stimulation of the nipple by the sucking baby, through a positive feedback mechanism.

The mammary glands (*Fig. 36*) consist of glandular tissue, fibrous tissue and fatty tissue. Each breast consists of about 20 lobes of glandular tissue, each lobe being made up of a number of lobules that radiate around the nipple. The lobules consist of a cluster of alveoli that open into small ducts, which unite to form large excretory ducts, called lactiferous ducts. The lactiferous ducts converge towards the centre of the breast where they form dilatations or reservoirs for milk. Leading

B

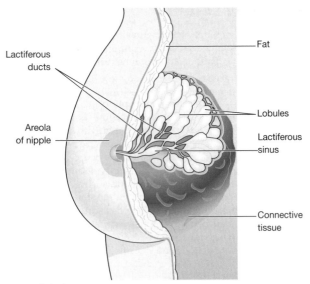

Fig 36 Structure of the breast

from each dilatation, or lactiferous sinus, is a narrow duct that opens on to the surface at the nipple. Fibrous tissue supports the glandular tissue and ducts, and fat covers the surface of the gland and is found between the lobes.

The nipple is a small conical eminence at the centre of the breast surrounded by a pigmented area, the areola. On the surface of the areola are numerous sebaceous glands (Montgomery's tubercles), which lubricate the nipple during lactation.

BREASTFEEDING

The first choice of feed for a healthy baby is breast milk. Breastfeeding secures for the baby the optimum health, growth and development, and immunity against illness (Department of Health 1996). Advantages to the mother include a reduced risk of premenopausal breast cancer, unique contact with her baby, etc.

BREAST MILK

Three types of breast milk are produced. The first is *colostrum*, produced in the 3 days after the baby's birth. This is not as rich as mature breast milk, but it is well suited to the newborn baby's nutritional requirements and contains many maternal antibodies. After about the third day, the mother's milk is 'let down' and mature breast milk is produced. *Foremilk* is the milk released at the beginning of a feed and is high in lactose, but low in fat; later in the feed, *hindmilk* is produced which is four to five times higher in fat, providing more calories and being more satisfying to the baby.

DISORDERS OF THE BREAST

BREAST PAIN

Up to 50% of all women who present at breast clinics do so with either breast pain (mastalgia) and or lumpiness. Breast pain may be cyclical or noncyclical. In cyclical mastalgia, women often report the following in the days before menstruation:

- Discomfort;
- Increased breast size and heaviness;
- Tender lumpiness;
- Increasing pain from mid-cycle that only improves at menstruation.

Management includes reassurance that breast pain is not indicative of cancer. Stopping the oral contraceptive pill can sometimes relieve symptoms. For the remainder, currently three drugs can be prescribed: gamolenic acid, bromocriptine and danzol.

Breast infection

Breast infection is most common in women aged between 18 and 50 years and can be divided into lactation- and several nonlactation-associated infections.

Lactation infection most frequently occurs within the first 6 weeks of breast-feeding. The most commonly isolated micro-organism is *Staphylococcus aureus*, a skin-associated infection.

Management of breast infections includes the appropriate antibiotics, hospital referral if infection does not settle and aspiration of an abscess prior to surgical drainage.

Breast cancer should be excluded in any woman with an inflammatory lesion that is solid on aspiration, or does not settle despite adequate antibiotic treatment.

Benign breast tumours

Benign breast disease accounts for the majority of women who pass through a breast clinic. The most common disorders are fibroadenomas, cysts and papillomas. A definitive diagnosis is made using a combination of clinical examination, fine needle biopsy, ultrasound and mammography. Management depends on the type and size of the benign tumour, and the age and wishes of the woman. Treatment includes aspiration of cysts, excision of fibroadenomas and microductectomy for duct papillomas.

Breast cancer

Breast cancer is a common cancer. In the UK one in 12 women develop breast cancer, and about 1% of all breast cancers occur in men. The majority of breast cancers present as a lump. All lumps should be investigated, though the majority are not malignant. Most breast cancers have painless presentation, but around 20% of women feel some discomfort or altered sensation. A locally invasive breast cancer may cause puckering or dimpling, which is why breast awareness incorporates looking for changes (see Practice application).

Some breast cancers may present with an indrawn nipple or discharge. A small number of breast cancers present with an enlarged axillary lymph node. Inflammatory eczematoid change of the nipple (Paget's disease of the breast) is associated with breast cancer.

Diagnosis involves the triple assessment – clinical examination, imaging (mammography, ultrasound) and fine needle aspiration, and sometimes a biopsy. ⇒ Cancer, Screening and early detection.

Treatment modalities are outlined in *Box 6*.

Practice application – breast awareness

Women should be encouraged to look and feel (with a flat hand) for the following changes and remember that breast tissue extends into the axilla. They also need to consider the hormonal changes that occur through the lifespan, e.g. menstrual cycle, pregnancy and after the menopause when the breasts feel softer:

B

- Any dimpling or puckering on the breasts;
- Skin changes (e.g. 'orange peel' skin, redness or more prominent veins);
- Any change in the shape (the contour) or size in either breast;
- Any lump or thickening in either breast or axilla;
- Any change in either nipple, including any discharge, eczema around the nipple or change in shape or prominence;
- Any changes in sensation, such as an odd or different feeling in the breast or nipple.

Box 6 Treatment modalities for breast cancer

Surgery – wide local excision, lumpectomy or some type of mastectomy (breast reconstruction should be offered to all women after mastectomy).
Chemotherapy – used at all stages of breast cancer: preoperatively (neo-adjuvant), after surgery (adjuvant) or as palliative treatment in advanced breast cancer.
Radiotherapy – used after breast conservation, after mastectomy, for large tumours, palliation of metastases or for local control of fungating lesions.
Hormone therapy – reduction of oestrogen in premenopausal women by removal of the ovaries or use of drugs such as goserelin, or irradiation. In post-menopausal women the sources of oestrogen (adipose tissue and adrenal glands) are blocked by drugs that include tamoxifen and anastrozole (an aromatase inhibitor).

Further reading

Brooker C and Nicol M (2003). *Nursing Adults. The Practice of Caring*, Ch 26. Edinburgh: Mosby.

BRONCHODILATORS

Bronchodilators are any agent that dilates the bronchi (e.g. the drug salbutamol). Bronchodilators may be either selective beta$_2$-adrenoceptor agonists (e.g. terbutaline) or muscarinic antagonists (e.g. ipratropium bromide). ⇒ Drug, Respiratory system (asthma, chronic obstructive pulmonary disease).

BURN INJURIES

Burn injuries have a variety of causes and potentially cause death or lead to injuries that have a lifelong impact on people and their families.

TYPES OF BURNS

Types of burns are:
- Wet heat (scalds) caused by hot water (e.g. kettles or drinks).
- Hot fat burns from cooking fat.
- Burns from bonfires, barbecues and fires caused by smoking in bed.
- Hot objects (e.g. a radiator).
- Radiation (e.g. sunburn).
- Electrical burns from poorly maintained electrical appliances. There may be no obvious skin damage, but usually entry and exit points are present. Electrical burns may cause cardiac arrhythmias and these patients should have cardiac monitoring for at least 24 hours post-injury.
- Chemical burns caused by acids and alkalis often result in extensive skin damage. The antidote for the chemical should be known and used to neutralize its effects.

- Inhalation injury occurs from exposure to hot gases, explosions, head and neck burns, or being confined in a smoke-filled room. Some patients need assisted ventilation.

FIRST AID FOR BURNS

The person should be removed from the source of the burn to a safe place. Regardless of cause the injured part should be bathed in copious amounts of cool water. Time should not be wasted in taking off clothes, as this may cause further injury and pain, the exception being when clothing is contaminated with chemicals. The patient should be kept warm and receive medical attention as soon as possible. If the patient is on fire, roll him or her on the ground to put out the flames. Do not put yourself in danger (e.g. do not enter a house on fire), but always call the fire brigade.

INITIAL MANAGEMENT OF BURNS

Priorities of management include:
- Assessment of depth and percentage of body area involved (see below);
- Fluid replacement and prevention of shock;
- Monitoring;
- Pain control;
- Prevention of hypothermia;
- Emotional support;
- Wound care and preventing infection;
- Maintaining increased nutritional needs, and minimizing scarring and loss of function.

Prognosis depends upon the percentage of body area burnt, age and general condition.

Practice application – assessment of burns

Burns are assessed using both depth and percentage of body surface area affected.

Depth

The patient's skin should be examined to assess the depth and extent of the burn:
- *Superficial burn* (only involves the epidermis) – red, painful and has capillary refill. Heals spontaneously and leaves no scars.
- *Partial thickness/deep dermal burn* (involves epidermis and upper dermis) – red, blistered and has sensation. It blanches under pressure and heals between 14 and 28 days. Some scarring may occur according to genetic disposition. Sometimes partial thickness burns require skin grafting. There is an infection risk.
- *Full-thickness burns* (involves all the layers of the skin and may include subcutaneous fat, muscles and bone). The burn is white, charred and may have a leathery appearance. Thrombosed veins may be visible. There is little sensation as the nerves are damaged and scarring occurs. Skin grafts are required to promote healing. There is an infection risk.

Body surface area

The rule of nines chart can be used initially to assess the percentage body surface area involved (*Fig. 37A*). A more accurate assessment can be made using one of several more-precise charts, such as the Lund and Browder chart (*Fig. 37B*). Adults with 15% or more body surface area involvement should receive fluid resuscitation in a specialized burns unit.

An aid for assessment when the injury is not clearly demarcated is that the patient's palm is considered to be 1%.

B

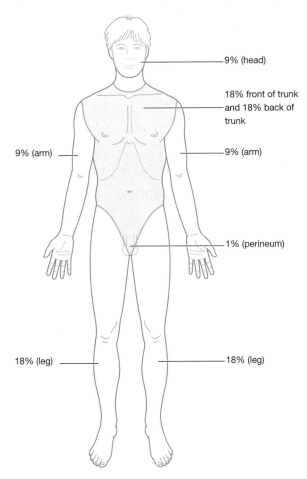

9% (head)

18% front of trunk
and 18% back of
trunk

9% (arm)

9% (arm)

1% (perineum)

18% (leg)

18% (leg)

(A)

Fig 37 Assessment of body surface area affected by burn injury: (A) rule of nines,

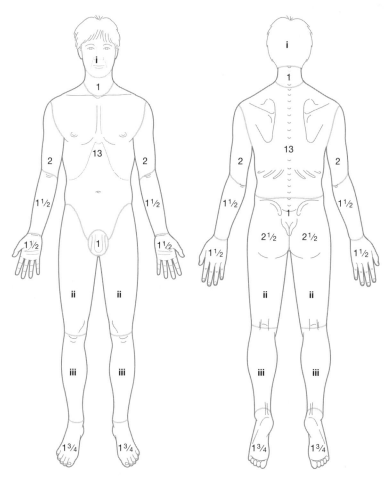

Relative percentage of affected areas by age						
Age (years)	0	1	5	10	15	Adult
i (half the head)	9½	8½	6½	5½	4½	3½
ii (half of thigh)	2¾	3¼	4	4¼	4½	4¾
iii (half of leg)	2½	2½	2¾	3	3¼	3½

The burn is also assessed for depth,
e.g. superficial or deep

(B)

Fig 37 (cont.) (B) Lund and Browder's chart

C

CANCER

Cancer is a disease characterized by cell growth that is purposeless, parasitic and flourishes at the expense of the human host. The terms tumour, growth, lesion, neoplasm and new growth may all be used to describe cancer. Tumour development occurs within an organized multi-step process:

- Genetically altered cell;
- Hyperplasia;
- Dysplasia;
- Cancer-in-situ (a premalignant growth) – surrounding tissue is not compromised and the tumour may be contained locally for an indefinite period of time;
- Invasive cancer – cancer cells invade the blood or lymphatic systems and/or surrounding tissue, the tumour is considered malignant and metastases (secondaries) are likely to be established throughout the body.

⇒ Cell (abnormalities of cell growth).

The individual risk of developing cancer is influenced by genetic factors and exposure to environmental carcinogens (agents that predispose to cancer). Factors known to predispose to cancer include tobacco, a diet low in fibre or high in saturated fat, increased body mass index and lack of physical activity, some drugs (e.g. chemotherapy), alcohol, occupational and environmental exposure to carcinogens (e.g. asbestos), radiation and infection. The age, gender and ethnicity of the person are also important (e.g. cancer is predominately a disease of older adults). Various screening programmes are available for the early detection of cancer (e.g. mammography, faecal occult blood). ⇒ Screening and early detection, Tumour.

COMMON CANCERS

The commonest cancers in the UK include those that affect the lung, breast, bowel (colorectal) and prostate, and these four account for over half of all new cases (Cancer Research UK 2003). Other common cancers are nonmelanoma skin cancer, bladder, pancreas, ovary, uterus, cervix, testis, melanoma, leukaemias, lymphomas, etc.

GRADING AND STAGING OF CANCERS

GRADING

Grading is a method of classifying a tumour based on the histopathological characteristics of the tissue. The aggressiveness or degree of malignancy of the tissue is calculated by comparing the level of cellular abnormality and the rate of cellular division with normal cells in the same tissue. High-grade cancer is aggressive and spreads rapidly, whereas low-grade cancer tends to be latent with slow tumour growth and spread. For selected tumours the grade of the disease is more significant than the stage (1–4) as an indicator of prognosis and treatment.

STAGING

The relationship between the stage of the cancer at the time of diagnosis and the associated mortality and survival underpins the prescription of therapeutic treatment. Tumours are staged according to the TNM (tumour, node, metastasis).

Each disease has its own specific classification criteria. Broadly speaking, the classification system enables clinicians to assess, either by clinical (TNM) or pathological investigation (pTNM), the size of the tumour (T), the absence or presence and extent of regional lymph node metastases (N) and the absence or presence of distant metastases (M). TNM staging may be supported with histopathological grading.

According to the size of the tumour, and based on the extent of disease noted throughout the lymphatic and/or other systems within the body, the clinician determines the disease stage from 0 to 4 (where 0 = no disease and 4 = advanced disease). The classification system is widely used as the criterion for entry into clinical cancer trials, for which it is important to determine response to treatment in people with different stages of a specific cancer. Using the classification as a baseline measurement enables clinicians to evaluate the outcome of treatment.

TREATMENTS FOR CANCER

Surgery and radiotherapy enable localized treatment of cancer, while chemotherapy with cytotoxic drugs and biological therapies (immunotherapy and biological response modifier) have a systemic effect and thus have the potential to treat local and metastatic disease. Side-effects are associated with all treatment modalities, and patients and their families need information and support to make decisions about treatment. ⇒ Cytotoxic chemotherapy, Radiotherapy.

Practice application – identifying warning signs

Perhaps the most important role in the prevention of and screening for cancer is monitoring and surveillance for changes in body structure and function by individuals. Nurses are central in educating the public about body changes that should be reported to a health professional. Specific changes to look out for include (Sarafino 1994):

- Change in bowel or bladder habit;
- A sore that does not heal;
- Unusual bleeding or discharge;
- Thickening of tissue in the breast or testes, or anywhere else in the body;
- Indigestion or difficulty in swallowing;
- Obvious change in a wart or mole;
- Nagging cough or hoarse voice.

CANNULA

A cannula is a hollow tube of plastic or metal used to introduce or withdraw fluid from the body. In some types (e.g. intravenous), to facilitate insertion the lumen is fitted with a sharp-pointed trocar, which is withdrawn when the cannula is *in situ*. The insertion of a cannula, such as into a vein (*Fig. 38*) is termed cannulation. ⇒ Intravenous therapy

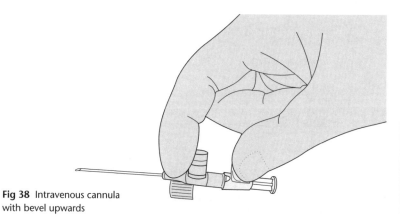

Fig 38 Intravenous cannula with bevel upwards

CARBOHYDRATES

A carbohydrate is an organic compound that contains carbon, hydrogen and oxygen. Formed in nature by photosynthesis in plants, they include starches, sugars and cellulose, and are classified in three groups: monosaccharides, disaccharides and polysaccharides. Carbohydrate is the most important source of body energy (16 kJ or 3.75 kcal/g). ⇒ Gastrointestinal tract (*Table 19*), Glucose, Macronutrients.

GLYCAEMIC INDEX

The glycaemic index is a classification of foods according to their acute effect on blood sugar level. Foods such as simple sugars (e.g. sugar) have a high glycaemic index as they cause an immediate rise in blood sugar. However, low glycaemic index foods, such as complex carbohydrates (high in soluble fibre, e.g. wholegrain cereals, pasta and legumes), are absorbed more slowly and evenly, which avoids sudden swings in blood sugar.

CARDIAC ARREST

Cardiac arrest is the complete cessation of effective output (of blood) from heart activity, so the heart action fails to maintain an adequate circulation. This can be caused by one of three abnormal rhythms:
- Pulseless ventricular tachycardia (VT, *Fig. 39A*) or ventricular fibrillation(VF, *Fig. 39B*);
- Asystole or extreme bradycardia (*Fig. 39C*).
- Electromechanical dissociation (EMD) – the presence of an electrical rhythm compatible with circulation, but with no detectable cardiac output.

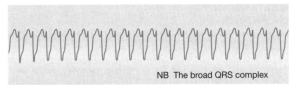

NB The broad QRS complex

(A) Ventricular tachycardia (VT)

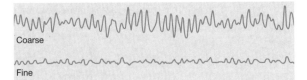

Coarse

Fine

(B) Ventricular fibrillation (VF)

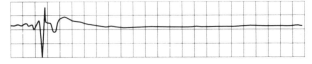

(C) **Asystole**

Fig 39 ECG tracings during cardiac arrest: (A) ventricular tachycardia, (B) ventricular fibrillation, (C) asystole

CARDIOPULMONARY RESUSCITATION

Cardiopulmonary resuscitation (CPR) describes the techniques used to maintain circulation and respiration after cardiopulmonary arrest. It involves:
- Maintenance of a clear airway;
- Artificial respiration using mouth-to-mouth or mouth-to-nose respiration, or with a bag and face mask, or by an endotracheal tube; and
- Maintenance of the circulation by external cardiac massage.

⇒ Advanced life support, Basic life support.

CARDIOTOCOGRAPHY

Cardiotocography (CTG) is a procedure whereby the fetal heart rate is measured either by an external microphone or by the application of an electrode to the fetal scalp, which records the fetal electrocardiogram (ECG) and from it the fetal heart rate. Using an external transducer placed on the mother's abdomen, the uterine contractions are measured.

CARE AND/OR CASE MANAGER

The NHS and Community Care Act 1990 describes the role of the care and/or case manager in the assessment of individual clients to identify and deploy the services to meet their needs.

Care managers are usually staff with assessment skills, such as social workers or home-care organizers who work in Social Service Departments (SSDs). Alternatively, district nurses or nurses who work in SSDs function as care managers. The role involves assessing older or disabled clients who live in their own homes for the amount and type of home care and support they require to live as independently as possible. Each assessment leads to the construction of an individualized 'package of care' for that client, one that may involve intervention by a home carer and/or care worker, social worker, district nurse, other community nurses (e.g. community psychiatric nurse, increasingly known as community mental health nurse), occupational therapist and physiotherapist. ⇒ Social services.

Further reading

Department of Health (1990). *NHS and Community Care Act*. London: DoH.

CARE PATHWAY (PROGRAMME OR PROTOCOL) OR CRITICAL PATHWAY

⇒ Integrated care pathway.

CARE PLAN

The care plan is the document on which nursing information is recorded. In some instances, it is used as a collective term that includes:
- Information from the initial assessment;
- Statement of the person's actual and potential problems with everyday living activities that are amenable to nursing intervention;
- Statement of the goals related to the problems to be achieved by the person;
- Plan of nursing or family interventions and their implementation, together with information from the ongoing assessment;
- Evaluation of whether or not the goals have been, or are being, achieved.

⇒ Nursing process.

C

CARE PROGRAMME APPROACH

The care programme approach (CPA) was developed in the UK because of several high-profile scandals concerning inadequate continuing care in the community of people with severe learning disabilities and mental health problems. The CPA is designed to ensure that these people do not slip through the net by prescribing and monitoring essential requirements for good practice in their care and supervision. These principles are:

- Assessment of health and social care needs;
- Written plan of care agreed with the user and carers;
- Key worker appointed with responsibility for co-ordinating the care programme;
- Regular reviews with multidisciplinary professional and user and/or carer involvement.

CARER

A carer is someone who takes the responsibility for caring for another (child, sick, disabled or older person). The organization Carers UK seeks to restrict the term to cover the 6 million unpaid family, friends and neighbours of vulnerable people in the UK, and not to paid helpers such as care workers, nurses or social workers. They also oppose the term 'informal carer'.

CASTS (ORTHOPAEDIC)

The three varieties of cast (plaster of Paris, resin-reinforced plaster bandages and water-activated polymerizable casts) serve the same purpose, to immobilize the affected part until healing has occurred, so protecting against further damage.

Practice application – care relating to the person in a cast

Plaster of Paris takes a minimum of 24 hours to attain its full strength. The cast should be supported by a soft surface throughout this period (e.g. pillows). A hard surface may result in pressure problems underneath the cast. Artificial heating to facilitate drying should be avoided, as the cast is likely to become brittle.

During this drying period, the extremities of the relevant limb should be inspected on a 2 hourly basis, testing each digit for temperature, colour, sensation and mobility, and where possible palpating a pulse distal to the cast. Acute compartment syndrome may be caused by the application of a cast that is too tight, and so it must be confirmed that the cast impairs neither circulation nor nerve transmission. Any adverse observation should be reported immediately to the appropriate medical staff, plaster technician or nurse. Those people who have been discharged should be instructed to return to the emergency department if there is any evidence of neurovascular impairment. Once the cast has dried, the frequency of such observations may be reduced to a twice-daily basis. ⇒ Compartment syndrome.

Complaints by the wearer of pain beneath a cast should always be acted upon. It may be from the initial injury or the site of surgical intervention. However, pain may also be the result of a developing sore beneath the plaster, as a consequence of swelling of the affected limb or application of a cast that is too tight (potentially highlighting the need for an increased frequency of neurovascular observations in the limb). In any case, such a situation merits immediate consultation with the plaster team or medical staff.

Note that casts on limbs that are paralysed (e.g. in clients with a stroke) should always be bi-valved (split) and kept in place with a crepe bandage wrapped around them. This should be removed on a daily basis to inspect the skin, as the major symptom (pain) of a developing sore or a tight cast will be absent.

C

The cast should be kept dry even during washing. During bathing or any activity that may wet the cast, it may be covered temporarily with a plastic bag.

People should be strongly discouraged from putting items down the side of the cast to relieve itching. The potential resulting trauma to the skin may initiate the development of a sore or crease the lining of the plaster, which results in increased pressure over that area. Note that severe irritation may be an adverse reaction to the material in the cast or lining and, if suspected, should be reported. Pyrexia or offensive odour may also be signs that a sore is developing and should be investigated. A window may be cut in the plaster to facilitate changing of dressings or to check for potential sore development. A cast that has become loose is ineffective and should be renewed.

Exercising the limb should be commenced only after the cast is completely dry.

Clients who are discharged from hospital with a cast should be issued with a set of appropriate and comprehensive instructions that should cover all of the above points. These should always be explained fully and the client's comprehension checked by the nurse. It should not be assumed that the client understands the written instructions.

CATHETERS AND URINARY CATHETERIZATION

A catheter is a hollow tube used to drain urine. Urinary catheterization of both women and men is an established nursing role. While the procedure is relatively simple, it is not without risks.

INTERMITTENT CATHETERIZATION

Intermittent catheterization is used in all areas of nursing when people have problems with residual volumes of urine, such as people with spinal injury, children with spina bifida, older people with hypotonic bladder tendencies and postoperatively. Many people self-catheterize.

INDWELLING CATHETERIZATION

Indwelling (or Foley) urinary catheters may be inserted via the urethra (urethral) or via an abdominal approach above the level of the symphysis pubis (suprapubic). The choice of route is influenced by both the reason for catheterization and, particularly in the case of long-term catheterization, patient needs and physical abilities. An indwelling catheter can be required after surgery, or for the management of incontinence after all alternative methods of management have been unsuccessful or are inappropriate.

Preventing complications of an indwelling catheter, such as infection and encrustation, is achieved by assessing the person to ensure that the correct catheter size and type (see Practice application) with a suitable drainage is used (*Fig. 40*).

CATHETER MANAGEMENT

The natural defences against urinary tract infection include the tightly closed folds of the urethra and the bladder's flushing action caused by regular emptying. The invasive nature of catheterization compromises these defences and, after 30 days, bacteriuria is almost universal. Micro-organisms gain entry to the bladder during catheterization by migrating along the catheter lumen from the collecting bag and via the periurethral route between the mucosa and the catheter.

To prevent this, catheterization must be aseptic, and once *in situ* the drainage system is closed, which allows free drainage but no bacterial entry, unless broken (*Fig. 40*).

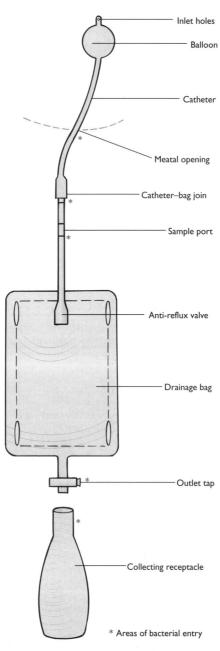

Fig 40 Closed urinary drainage system

Encouraging the catheterized client to increase their fluid intake (unless contraindicated for some reason) has the practical value of maintaining a constant downward flow of urine and reducing bacterial multiplication in the drainage bag. Clients prone to urinary tract infection may benefit from drinking cranberry juice as a preventive measure (Avorn *et al.* 1994). Further complications associated with long-term catheterization and their management are outlined in *Table 4*.

C

Practice application – catheter selection
The factors that influence choice of catheter (size, balloon infill size and material) include the indication for catheterization, client needs and the likely duration of catheterization.

Catheter length and Charriere (Ch) size
Urinary catheters come in two adult lengths: female (23–26 cm) and male or standard (40–44 cm). The longer length must be used on male patients for urethral catheterization because of the length of the male urethra. It may also be used for female patients. The shorter 'female' length can be used only for female patients. Charriere size refers to the external diameter of the catheter. This may also be referred to as French gauge or French units. As a general rule, you should choose the smallest diameter that will provide adequate urine drainage. Using a catheter that is too large can cause bladder irritability, occlude the urethral glands and cause ulceration of the bladder or urethra or strictures (Getliffe 1993). Size 10–12 Ch should be used for females, 12–14 Ch for males and 6–10 Ch for children. A larger diameter catheter is usually required after surgery when haematuria with clots is anticipated.

Balloon infill size
The catheter is held in place by a catheter balloon. Balloon sizes vary from 2.5–5 mL in paediatric catheters, through 10–30 mL in adult size catheters to greater than 50 mL in some specialist urological catheters. Again, the rule is that the smaller the balloon infill the better. The use of a smaller balloon reduces residual urine and ensures that bladder spasms are minimized. For general use, a 10 mL infill is preferable.

Catheter materials
Catheters utilized for short- or medium-term use (up to 4 weeks) are commonly made of latex (after asking about allergies) or Teflon-coated latex. For long-term catheterization, more specialized catheters are used; they may be made of silicone, latex coated with silicone or latex coated with a hydrogel or a hydrated polymer. Those of the last type usually have a lifespan of 12 weeks. Catheters used for intermittent self-catheterization may be composed of either polyvinyl chloride (PVC) or plastic.

Further reading

Getliffe K (1995). Care of urinary catheters. *Nurs Stand.* **10**(1): 25–31.
Robinson J (2001). Urethral catheter selection. *Nurs Stand.* **15**(25): 39–42.

CELL

The cell is the basic structural unit of living organisms. It comprises a mass of protoplasm (cytoplasm), subcellular organelles and usually a membrane-bound nucleus (which contains the genetic material within a nuclear envelope), all within a plasma or cell membrane (*Fig. 41A*). ⇒ Nucleic acids.

C

Table 4 Some complications of catheterization

Problem	Cause	Action
Catheter not draining urine	Kink in tubing	Check tubing and reposition as necessary
	Drainage bag positioned above bladder	Reposition drainage bag below the bladder
	Drainage bag too full	Empty regularly as per procedure
	Inadequate fluid intake	Increase to approximately 10 drinks per day
	Constipation	Clear constipation. ⇒ Defecation (constipation and faecal impaction)
	Encrustation/blocked catheter	
Urine bypassing catheter		
A. While the catheter is still draining	Detrusor spasm caused by:	Recatheterization with smaller catheter
	too large a catheter	Recatheterization with catheter using smaller balloon
	too large a balloon	Increase fluid intake
	concentrated urine	Anticholinergic medication
		Bladder washouts not recommended
B. When there is no drainage from the catheter	Debris	Intermittent bladder washouts
	Encrustation	Change catheter and observe tip for encrustation
		If this is an ongoing problem planned catheter changes should be adopted
Bladder expelling the catheter	Balloon deflation	Replace catheter
	Detrusor spasm	Anticholinergic medication
	Poor support of drainage system	Check tapes, etc., holding the catheter bag
	Self-removal by client	Check for pain and discomfort
	Inflammation around catheter	Remove to allow inflammation to subside; check catheter material
Haematuria	Trauma	Monitor by observation; if bleeding becomes heavy, seek medical advice immediately
	Infection	Urinalysis, urine sample for culture

C

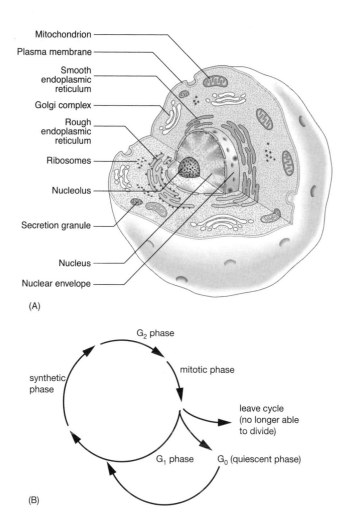

Fig 41 (A) A cell, (B) the cell cycle

The nucleolus is a structure that contains both nucleic acids (DNA and RNA), situated close to the nucleus. There are usually two, involved in nuclear division. Some cells (e.g. the erythrocytes) are non-nucleated, whereas others (such as voluntary muscle) may be multinucleated. The subcellular organelles perform the metabolic processes of the cell (see below).

CELL ORGANELLES

ENDOPLASMIC RETICULUM

The endoplasmic reticulum is a network of channels and membranes concerned with the synthesis and movement of substances within the cell (e.g. proteins and lipids). The rough endoplasmic reticulum found in secretory cells has ribosomes on its surface, whereas the smooth variety has no ribosomes.

C

GOLGI COMPLEX

The Golgi complex comprises membranous sacs involved in the synthesis of glycoproteins and lipoproteins. These are larger and more extensive in secretory cells.

MITOCHONDRIUM (PL. MITOCHONDRIA)

A mitochondrium is membrane-bound organelle situated in the cytoplasm. Mitochondria are the principal sites for energy production, the nucleotide adenosine triphosphate (ATP), from the oxidation of fuel molecules such as carbohydrates. They contain nucleic acids (DNA and RNA) and ribosomes. Mitochondria replicate independently, and synthesize some of their own proteins. They are particularly numerous in metabolically active cells, such as liver and muscle.

RIBOSOMES

Ribosomes are found in the cytoplasm or associated with the rough endoplasmic reticulum. They consist of protein and RNA and are involved in protein synthesis.

CELL CYCLE

The cell cycle describes the sequence of events that occur within a cell from the start of one mitotic division to the start of the next. With the exception of the gametes, all cell replacement in the body occurs by mitotic cell division. The cell cycle involves three major stages, the interphase, nuclear division and cytokinesis (*Fig. 41B*):

INTERPHASE

The interphase is a period of cell growth during which the DNA in the nucleus replicates. There are three distinct phases in interphase, called G_1, S and G_2:
- The G_1 phase occurs immediately after the new cell has been produced. G stands for 'gap' and G_1 is the period between the end of cell division and DNA replication. This is a period of growth in which one centriole pair begins to replicate, as do other cell surface organelles.
- In the S (synthetic) phase DNA replicates precisely, duplicating every chromosome. During this phase the other centriole pair also replicates.
- The G_2 phase is the second gap phase and growth continues. Before mitosis can begin, the parent cell must approximately double its mass and contents. The centriole pairs begin to move apart, the nuclear membrane starts to disintegrate, chromosomes begin to condense and the spindle begins to form as the cell moves into the early prophase of mitosis.

DIVISION OF THE NUCLEUS

The mitotic (M) phase is the period during which the nucleus and its constituent chromosomes divide. $\Rightarrow$ Mitosis.

CYTOKINESIS

Cytokinesis is the division of the cytoplasm.

QUIESCENT PHASE

Some cells enter a 'resting' G_0 (quiescent) phase in which no cell division occurs, but some cells can rejoin the cell cycle when extra cells are needed (e.g. liver cells after surgical resection).

ABNORMALITIES OF CELL GROWTH

As with any complex process the scope for error is ever present. Errors range from a failure of growth through several abnormalities to a breakdown in control mechanisms, which allows the development of cancers.

APLASIA

Aplasia means 'absence of growth' and applies to a situation in which an organ or structure fails to develop during intrauterine life. It affects paired structures, and only one of the pair develops (e.g. kidney). A less severe form is hypoplasia in which incomplete organ development results in a smaller-than-normal structure with possible loss of function.

ATROPHY

Atrophy is an acquired change that occurs when a previously normal structure becomes wasted and smaller. There is normal deterioration, such as ovarian atrophy during the climacteric, and abnormal deterioration, such as when a structure is starved of nutrients, a blood supply, subjected to constant pressure or after long-term disuse (e.g. immobility that leads to muscle loss).

HYPERTROPHY

In hypertrophy individual cells increase in size, which results in an overall enlargement of the organ. This may occur where use is increased (e.g. the leg muscles in a runner). It can happen as part of the compensation mechanisms whereby the body tries to minimize the effects of declining function (e.g. heart failure).

HYPERPLASIA

Hyperplasia is an increase in actual cell numbers, such as bone marrow hyperplasia (which increases erythrocyte production in some types of anaemia) or when an individual lives at high altitude.

METAPLASIA

In metaplasia there is a change in cell type, usually with the cells becoming less specialized. This is a reversal of differentiation, which may be seen in areas such as the cervix. It results from long-standing irritation or infection. If the cause is removed the cells return to normal.

DYSPLASIA

Dysplasia is a change in the size and shape of the cells that form the covering and lining tissues of the body (epithelia). It results from chronic irritation and commonly affects the skin, cervix and oesophagus. These serious changes can lead to cancer. Interestingly, even at this stage a spontaneous reversal to 'normal' can still occur if the chronic irritation ceases.

NEOPLASIA

Neoplasia, which means 'new growth', is characterized by very marked cellular changes. This includes changes in DNA structure and abnormal, unco-ordinated cell division that gives rise to a tumour. They may be:
- Benign localized tumours, which may cause problems from pressure or hormone production;
- Malignant tumours, which are invasive both locally and by their ability to metastasize, that is spread to distant parts of the body via the blood or lymphatics. ⇒ Cancer.

C

CENTRAL STERILE SUPPLIES DEPARTMENT (UNIT)

The Central Sterile Supplies Department (CSSD) is an area in which sterile packs and/or packets are prepared. These contain the equipment and/or swabs and dressings necessary to carry out particular activities that require aseptic technique.

Hospital Sterilization and Disinfection Units (HSDUs) are CSSDs that have extended their work to include disinfection of equipment.

CENTRAL VENOUS CATHETER AND LINE

A central venous catheter is a special catheter inserted into a large central vein via a peripheral vein or by using a skin tunnel. Used in critical care situations to measure pressures, administer drugs and infuse hypertonic fluids, it also allows long-term vascular access for the administration of nutritional support, drugs (chemotherapy, analgesics and antibiotics) and blood products. ⇒ Nutrition.

CENTRAL VENOUS PRESSURE

Central venous pressure (CVP) measures the pressure of blood in the right atrium and is used in the clinical setting to reflect fluid status. A central venous catheter (central catheter and line) is inserted into a large vein, such as the subclavian or internal jugular, and progressed until the catheter tip is in or very near the right atrium of the heart (*Fig. 42*). This is an aseptic procedure and a chest radiograph (X-ray) is performed after insertion to check:
- The correct position of the catheter;
- That during the procedure the pleura had not been punctured accidentally to cause a pneumothorax.

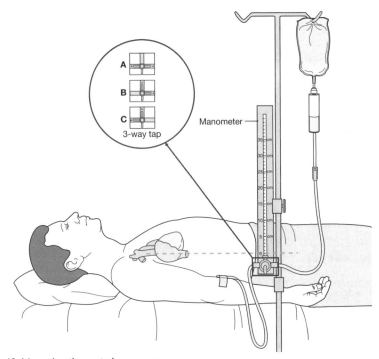

Fig 42 Measuring the central venous pressure

> **Practice application – central venous pressure**
> The CVP can be measured using a water manometer or a pressure transducer attached to a monitor. The normal values are 5–12 cmH$_2$O and 3–9 mmHg, respectively. A number of factors in addition to fluid status can affect the CVP, including pulmonary hypertension, right ventricular failure and peripheral vasodilatation. Therefore, CVP should be interpreted only in conjunction with other observations, such as heart rate and blood pressure. In addition, the trend in CVP is more meaningful than a single, isolated reading.

C

C EREBROSPINAL FLUID

$\Rightarrow$ Nervous system.

C ERVIX

Cervix means a neck, but usually refers to the cervix uteri (uterine cervix) or the neck of the uterus. The cervix is mostly fibrous tissue. The lining of the endocervical canal is columnar epithelium, but changes to stratified squamous epithelium in the part of the cervix (ectocervix) that protrudes into the vagina, which offers some protection from trauma (e.g. during intercourse). During the reproductive years oestrogen stimulates basal cell proliferation in the epithelium of the ectocervix. The change from one type of epithelium to another occurs in an area known as the squamocolumnar junction (SCJ), which is also called the transformation zone. The cervix has two openings – the internal os into the uterine cavity and an external os that opens into the vagina. The protrusion of the cervix into the vagina forms four fornices (deep gutters); the deep posterior fornix receives the semen during coitus.

The type and quantity of mucus produced by the cervical glands change during the menstrual cycle. Examination of this mucus forms the basis of a natural method of family planning. $\Rightarrow$ Family planning.

CANCER OF THE CERVIX

The incidence of cancer of the cervix is falling because of the introduction of the cervical screening programme, as abnormalities are being detected and treated while in a preinvasive state. The modified screening programme being introduced in England recommends that women aged 25–49 years old have cervical screening every 3 years. The frequency may be increased in high-risk women or where early abnormalities have been found. Younger women will not be offered routine screening. Women aged 50–64 years are to have screening every 5 years.

The SCJ is the most common site for cancer. Abnormalities are graded histologically and cytologically to give an indication of the extent of the disease. Preinvasive disease is graded as cervical intraepithelial neoplasia (CIN) I, II or III, which describes the amount and type of abnormality. Preinvasive disease is usually treated in the colposcopy clinic and often does not require hospital admission. $\Rightarrow$ Gynaecological examination (cervical cytology, colposcopy), Human papilloma virus.

FIGO (International Federation of Gynaecology and Obstetrics) provides a classification that stages cancer of the cervix from 0 (preinvasive disease) to IVb (distant metastasis).

The symptoms include postcoital bleeding (bleeding after intercourse), postmenopausal bleeding and an offensive persistent blood-stained vaginal discharge. Advanced tumours may be easily identifiable on inspection of the cervix.

The management options include surgery, radiotherapy and chemotherapy, which may be used alone or in combination, depending on the grade and stage of the cancer. Treatment may be curative or palliative. Unless the disease is advanced, radical surgery is usually recommended. This includes a Wertheim's hysterectomy, whereby the uterus, tubes, ovaries and upper third of the vagina are removed. This may be followed by radiotherapy, depending on the histology results.

CHICKENPOX

⇒ Communicable diseases (varicella).

CHILD AND ADOLESCENT MENTAL HEALTH

At any time, between 15 and 20% of children and adolescents have significant mental health problems and disorders.

The characteristic mental health disorders of young life include anxiety, depression and behavioural problems – broadly divided into *oppositional disorders* (usually of mild severity and in younger children) and the more severe *conduct disorders* (in older children and adolescents, and often associated with delinquency, i.e. committing offences), attention-deficit hyperactivity disorder, somatizing disorders, autism and eating disorders. The aetiology is often multifactorial, and involves interaction between developmental, psychological, biological and social factors.

The management and/or treatment interventions include psychological therapies (psychotherapy and/or behaviour, cognitive and family therapies), and pharmacological and residential therapies.

In the UK, child mental health services are organized using a four-tier model, which includes the full range of services from primary care to specialist settings. Links with primary health, education, social services and hospital child services are essential.

Nurses are involved in the assessment and treatment of child mental health problems across all four tiers. These include specialist community public health nurses (health visitors), school nurses and/or health advisers , community mental health nurses, community paediatric nurses, hospital paediatric and mental health nurses. ⇒ Anxiety, Attention-deficit hyperactivity disorder, Autism, Disorders of mood, Eating disorders, Somatization, Suicide and deliberate self-harm.

CHILDREN'S RIGHTS AND PROTECTION

The rights and protection of children are taken very seriously in the UK. The individual countries of the UK have enacted legislation that allows for the appointment of a Children's Commissioner and changes to the services set up to safeguard children. The Children's Commissioner is a central and influential figure with overall responsibility for improving and ensuring child protection.

CHILDREN ACT 1989

In the UK the Children Act 1989 is an Act of Parliament (became law in 1991) that clearly defines the rights of children, their protection, welfare and care.

CHILDREN'S CHARTER

A Children's Charter was introduced by the UK Government in 1996 to ensure that children and their parents had a better understanding of their rights in terms of healthcare, such as having treatment and care explained, and certain expectations (e.g. being on a ward specifically for children and young people).

CHILD PROTECTION OFFICER AND/OR CO-ORDINATOR

A child protection officer is a suitably qualified and experienced individual (with a nursing, health visiting or social work background) employed by a social services department to oversee and/or co-ordinate the interagency child protection activities to safeguard children in a particular location. In addition, all NHS trusts employ a designated senior nurse with a child protection role.

CHILD PROTECTION REGISTER

In the UK, a register of children deemed to be at risk of neglect, abuse, etc. The register is administered by social services, but is used in interagency child protection work.

EMERGENCY PROTECTION ORDER

An emergency protection order (EPO) replaces a place of safety order. It is an order issued by the court when it believes that a child may suffer significant harm. It transfers parental responsibility rights and allows for the child's removal to a safe place.

GUARDIAN AD LITEM

A guardian ad litem is a person with a social work or childcare background who is appointed to ensure that the court be informed fully of the relevant facts that relate to a child, and that the wishes and feelings of the child be established clearly. The appointment is made from a panel set up by the local authority.

CHIROPODY

⇒ Podiatry.

CHLAMYDIAE

Chlamydiae are micro-organisms of the genus *Chlamydia*. They are intracellular parasites and have features common to both bacteria and viruses. *Chlamydia psittaci* infects birds and causes psittacosis in humans. Subgroups of *C. trachomatis* cause genital tract infection in adults, and are sexually transmitted and/or acquired. The micro-organism also causes trachoma. ⇒ Sexually transmitted/acquired infection, Vision (visual impairment).

CHOLERA

Cholera is an acute enteritis that occurs in Africa and Asia, where it is endemic and epidemic. It is caused by the bacterium *Vibrio cholerae* and is associated with faecal contamination of water, overcrowding and insanitary conditions. There is diarrhoea (rice-water stools) accompanied by agonizing cramp and vomiting, which result in dehydration, electrolyte imbalance and severe collapse.

The chief aim is to maintain the circulation by replacement of water and electrolytes. Three days' treatment with tetracycline or co-trimoxazole reduces the duration of excretion of vibrios and the total volume of fluid needed for replacement. Mortality rates are high for patients who do not have adequate fluid and electrolyte replacement.

CHOLESTEROL

Cholesterol, a fatty substance, is made by the body in the gut and liver and is also found in the diet. It belongs to a large group of molecules called lipids. The synthesis of cholesterol in the body is influenced by dietary saturated fat intake. It is essential to the body for the growth and development of cell membranes and steroid hormones. Cholesterol in the body binds with proteins to create lipoproteins. These lipoproteins can be divided into different groups. The two

C

major groups are high-density lipoproteins (HDLs), which have a protective effect for coronary heart disease (CHD) risk, and low-density lipoproteins (LDLs), which lead to the development of atheroma. High levels of LDL and low levels of HDL are associated with CHD risk. The normal values for blood lipids are outlined in *Box 7*. ⇒ Coronary heart disease.

Box 7 – Normal values for blood lipid profile
Cholesterol (total)
Ideally, <5.2 mmol/L
Mild increase, 5.2–6.5 mmol/L
Moderate increase, 6.5–7.8 mmol/L
Severe increase, >7.8 mmol/L
HDL-cholesterol
Male, 0.5–1.6 mmol/L
Female 0.6–1.9 mmol/L
Triglycerides (fasting)
0.6–1.7 mmol/L

ABNORMAL BLOOD LIPID PROFILES

Hyperlipidaemia is excessive total fat in the blood. An increase in the level of triglycerides is called *hypertriglyceridaemia*. *Hypercholesterolaemia* is high blood cholesterol levels, which can be reduced through diet modification (see Practice application), physical activity or drugs.

A diet low in fat lowers the blood cholesterol level, yet cholesterol is essential to the body, and so it is the ratio of HDL to LDL that is important. To maintain a healthy ratio of LDL to HDL requires more than attention to diet alone. Exercise, considered beneficial in the reduction of CHD, is thought to increase HDL levels, while smoking may reduce them.

Measures that are considered to improve cholesterol levels include stopping smoking, increasing exercise and drinking one unit of alcohol a day (e.g. a small glass of red wine).

DRUG THERAPY

Cholesterol-lowering drugs (resins), which prevent cholesterol absorption from food, are used for some people with familial hypercholesterolaemia. In all other people with CHD and increased cholesterol levels (>5 mmol/L), the HMG-CoA reductase inhibitors (statins), such as simvastatin, are used.

Practice application – diet modification
Individuals can be encouraged to adopt a healthier diet by introducing small changes into their diet and eating habits. Interventions include:
• Using low fat spreads;
• Trimming fat off meat;
• Increasing the intake of oily fish;
• Grilling food instead of frying it;
• Not adding salt to cooked foods or in the cooking of vegetables;
• Using herbs and spices to replace salt;
• Having at least five portions of fruit and vegetables per day;
• Not spreading fat on bread when making sandwiches;
• Choosing thick-sliced instead of thin-sliced bread;
• Eating less processed food (hidden fat, sugar and salt);
• Keeping alcohol intake within safe limits.

CHORIONIC GONADOTROPHIN

Chorionic gonadotrophin or human chorionic gonadotrophin (hCG) is a hormone produced by the trophoblast cells and later the chorion. It maintains the corpus luteum until placental hormone secretion is advanced sufficiently. The presence of hCG in blood or urine is used to confirm pregnancy. High levels may indicate choriocarcinoma (chorionepithelioma). It has been used therapeutically for delayed puberty in the male. Also, hCG acts as a tumour marker for testicular cancer.

CHROMOSOMES

Chromosomes are the genetic material present in the nucleus of the cell. They appear as microscopic threads within the cell nucleus as the cell prepares to divide. Chromosomes consist of strands of deoxyribonucleic acid (DNA) molecules known as genes. Humans have 23 pairs (46) in each somatic (body) cell: 22 pairs of autosomes and one pair of sex chromosomes (females have XX and males have XY; *Fig. 43*). The exceptions are the mature gametes (oocytes and spermatozoa) with half the usual number (haploid number *n*) as a result of reduction division during meiosis. This means that the set of 23 unpaired chromosomes inherited from each parent results in an individual with 46 chromosomes (diploid number 2*n*). The male gamete determines genetic sex of the embryo by whether it contributes a Y chromosome (genetic male) or an X chromosome (genetic female).

Genetic material is also present in the mitochondria, where it codes for metabolic processes and can be responsible for the inheritance of conditions, such as optic nerve atrophy. ⇒ Genes and genetics, Meiosis, Mitosis.

CHROMOSOMAL DEFECTS

Chromosomal disorders can give rise to problems of varying severity, described below.

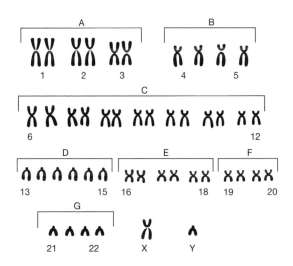

Fig 43 The 46 chromosomes of a human cell arranged in 23 pairs (male)

C

ANEUPLOIDY

Aneuploidy describes a chromosome number that is not a multiple of the normal haploid (n) number of 23. It includes trisomy, such as Down's syndrome in which the individual has 47 chromosomes (three chromosomes, i.e. an extra chromosome 21, where normally they would be paired), and monosomy in which there are 45 chromosomes (e.g. Turner's syndrome).

POLYPLOIDY

In polyploidy there is a multiple of the normal haploid (n) chromosome number of 23, other than the normal diploid ($2n$) number of 46 (e.g. 69). Polyploidy is not compatible with life.

STRUCTURAL CHANGES

Rather than the loss or addition of whole chromosomes, problems can also arise from structural changes to chromosomes. For instance, part of a chromosome can be deleted, as happens in *cri-du-chat* syndrome. Inversion and duplication of small parts of a chromosome can occur, or part of a chromosome becomes attached to another chromosome. This is known as translocation and accounts for some cases of Down's syndrome.

Many of these chromosomal abnormalities arise from mistakes that occur during various stages of meiosis and during recombination and chiasmata (crossing over) formation. The origin of non-disjunction is shown in *Fig. 44*. ⇒ Learning disability.

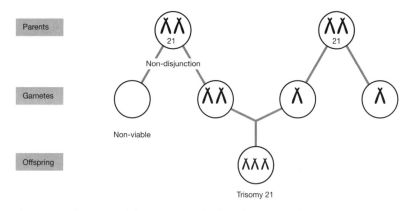

Fig 44 Non-disjunction of chromosome 21 leading to Down's syndrome

CHRONIC (LONG-TERM) ILLNESS

A chronic illness is one that exhibits one or more of the following qualities (*Table 5*). It is permanent, associated with irreversible change in the body's function or structure, and requires extended rehabilitation, long periods of healthcare support or a major adaptation in the person's lifestyle. Most chronic illnesses exhibit more than one of these characteristics.

Nurses have always been active in the care of people with long-term illness and disability, but in the future many of the most advanced nursing roles are likely to be with this client group. Nurses are taking more and more responsibility in both

Table 5 Definitions of chronic illness (Strauss 1976)

Definition	Example of chronic disease
Permanence	Diabetes
	Peripheral vascular disease
Residual disability	Cerebrovascular accident (CVA; stroke)
	Multiple sclerosis
Nonreversible pathology	Arthritis
	Osteoporosis
Requires extended rehabilitation	Serious head injury
	CVA (stroke)
Requires major adaptation in lifestyle	Heart failure
	Epilepsy
Requires long periods of supervision, observation or care	Breast cancer
	Asthma

managing and delivering the care of clients with chronic illness in a range of settings, including hospital wards, outpatient clinics and GP surgeries. People with severe disability increasingly receive almost all their care in settings outside traditional hospitals. Even in long-term care settings, such as nursing homes, care can be far more dynamic and challenging than simply 'care-taking', which was often seen as the main nursing role in the past.

A number of relatively new nursing roles are emerging in the care of people with chronic diseases. Nurse practitioners take on a more complete responsibility for the care of people with a wide range of conditions, including asthma, diabetes, Parkinson's disease and rheumatoid arthritis. They often take full responsibility for managing medication within pre-defined protocols, referring to doctors only when particular new problems emerge. It is believed that a nursing perspective towards care moves the focus from simple disease management to one that enables clients to discuss their wider concerns and issues, which in turn allows for the development of more successful coping strategies. ⇒ Disability, Exercise (exercise tolerance), Rehabilitation.

Practice application – goal setting in chronic illness

With a chronic illness or impairment the goal of 'cure' is not a realistic one. The goals are individual and must be arrived at in negotiation with the client. This is particularly important in chronic conditions, since a client's sense of control and mastery is an important determinant of his or her ability to cope with the condition. Many difficulties can occur when goals are not agreed explicitly between clients and professionals:

- Goals should be set collaboratively between clients and professionals;
- Goal-setting should begin with a clarification of the role of clients and professionals in setting and achieving goals;
- The professionals' role is to advise the clients and help arrive at goals that are neither unrealistically high nor too low;
- Long-term goals should have achievable sub-goals so that both clients and professionals can identify the extent of progress;
- Professionals and clients should identify strategies through which goals are achieved;
- 'Noncompliance' is often a result of clients and professionals working towards different goals;

- Goals must accommodate clients' hopes, expectations and aspirations beyond the management of impairment – their need for 'normality';
- Clients may be more likely to accept goals identified by professionals if professionals show a willingness to work towards the clients' goals.

C

CHRONIC WOUNDS

Chronic wounds are those associated with prolonged healing times, such as large burns, pressure ulcers and leg ulcers. Chronic wounds frequently produce large amounts of exudate. ⇒ Burn injuries, Leg ulcers, Pressure ulcers, Tissue viability, Wounds and wound care.

CIRCADIAN RHYTHM

⇒ Biorhythm.

CIRCULATION

Circulation is a passage of material in a circle. It is usually used to mean circulation of the blood, that is the passage of blood from the heart to arteries to capillaries to veins and back to the heart (*Fig. 45*). ⇒ Extracorporeal (extracorporeal circulation), Fetus (fetal circulation), Heart (coronary circulation), Liver, Lymphatic system, Nervous system (cerebral circulation).

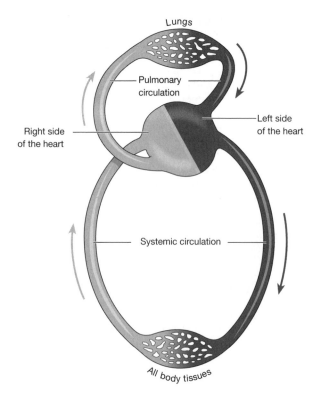

Fig 45 The relationship between the systemic and pulmonary circulations

SYSTEMIC CIRCULATION

Oxygenated blood from the lungs is returned to the left atrium (of the heart) and passes into the left ventricle and is pumped out to the body via the aorta. It moves through smaller arteries to the capillary networks, where nutrients and oxygen diffuse from the blood to cells. Carbon dioxide and other waste diffuse from the cells to the blood. The blood, with high levels of waste, returns via veins that eventually form the venae cavae, which empty into the right atrium.

PULMONARY CIRCULATION

The deoxygenated (low in oxygen) blood leaves the right ventricle (of the heart) via the pulmonary artery, which branches to each lung. The artery branches again within the lung and eventually forms the capillary networks around the alveoli. Gaseous exchange occurs: oxygen diffuses into the blood and carbon dioxide into the alveoli, and oxygenated blood returns to the left atrium via the pulmonary veins.

HEPATIC PORTAL CIRCULATION

Venous blood from the digestive tract, pancreas and spleen, which is rich in nutrients and hormones, passes through the liver, via the hepatic portal vein, prior to its return to the systemic circulation through the hepatic vein to the inferior vena cava.

CIRCUMCISION

⇒ Female genital mutilation, Penis (penile problems).

CLIMACTERIC

The climacteric describes a period of time during which ovarian activity declines and eventually ceases. In most women it occurs between the mid-forties and mid-fifties. The menopause is the ending of menstruation and is a single event that occurs during the climacteric. The average age of the menopause is thought to be 50–51 years, which has remained constant over many centuries and across different parts of the world. Many women use the word menopause to describe the climacteric. Premenopausal women who have their ovaries removed surgically, destroyed with radiotherapy or 'switched off' with drugs experience the menopause.

PHYSIOLOGICAL EVENTS

Ovarian decline results in a failure to ovulate and, consequently, the ovary no longer produces progesterone. This affects the production of other hormones and, for a short time, gonadotrophin levels rise, but then eventually all ovarian activity ceases. The lack of oestrogen causes the internal genitalia, ovaries, uterus and vagina to shrink. Tissue lining these structures becomes very thin, the vaginal acidity decreases, labia shrink and pubic hair disappears.

SYMPTOMS

During the climacteric, women may experience a combination of symptoms, some of which cause them to seek help from a health professional, including:
- Vasomotor symptoms, including hot flushes, night sweats, palpitations, insomnia;
- Psychological symptoms, including irritability, lack of concentration, reduced libido, depression;
- Irregular bleeding, including an increase in interval between periods, diminishing periods or missing periods.

C

The sustained lack of oestrogen can have long-term effects, including:

- Atrophy of vaginal and urethral mucosa that leads to a decrease in vaginal acidity, which increases the risk of infection, vaginal dryness and dyspareunia, and of urinary symptoms, such as urgency, frequency and cystitis.
- Uterovaginal prolapse caused by atrophy and changes in the pelvic floor muscles and supporting ligaments.
- Osteoporosis, a reduction in bone mass makes women more susceptible to fractures.
- Cardiovascular disease, there is a marked increase in the incidence of coronary heart disease and strokes in women after the menopause.
- Changes to the hair and skin, and breast atrophy.

MANAGEMENT

Medical intervention, if required, usually involves hormone replacement therapy (HRT). However, many women feel that the climacteric is a natural progression in their life and may just require advice and information about the current symptoms. For others, it is a significant event and they want help with distressing symptoms, such as hot flushes. For this group HRT can be prescribed in various forms, including tablets, skin patches, implants, gels and nasal sprays. Topical vaginal creams to counter atrophic changes in the vaginal mucosa are appropriate for some women. Unopposed oestrogen with no progesterone therapy can cause hyperplasia of the endometrium. Consequently, women with an intact uterus must be prescribed combined oestrogen–progesterone HRT, but this may result in the woman having a regular bleed, which is not acceptable to all. A woman who has had a hysterectomy only requires oestrogen.

All women should be informed about the risks associated with long-term use of HRT (e.g. the increased incidence of breast cancer associated with both combined HRT and oestrogen-only HRT).

Other drugs used during the climacteric include:

- Selective (o)estrogen receptor modulator (SERM), such as raloxifene, which is used to prevent and treat osteoporosis, and has no effect on vasomotor symptoms;
- Clonidine (antihypertensive drug), which may reduce hot flushes;
- Bisphosphonates, such as etridonate, which are used in the management of osteoporosis.

Practice application – nurse-led initiatives for women experiencing the climacteric

Specialist nurses, both in hospital outpatients and primary care, now run menopause clinics, where they provide advice on how women can deal with their symptoms. Women often find it extremely helpful to talk through their symptoms with a nurse, particularly if the nurse is female. The menopause often occurs at the same time in a woman's life as other significant events, such as children leaving home or older relatives becoming more reliant. There are many different HRT preparations and a woman may have to try several types before she finds one that suits her. She requires considerable support during this time, as she may feel disillusioned if her symptoms persist. The nurse can also monitor any side-effects.

Some women decide to use complementary therapies to alleviate distressing symptoms and nurses should support this decision while being mindful that some herbal medicines may interact with prescription medicines. Self-help groups can also help to increase a woman's control over symptoms and to increase her self-esteem. Women are often receptive to health education at this time and nurses can take the opportunity to stress the importance of exercise, healthy diet (with sufficient calcium), maintaining the correct weight, smoking cessation, maintaining hobbies and interests, and attending for cervical and breast screening.

Women will also need advice about contraception during the perimenopause. Ovulation, and hence conception, may occur after the last period, so women who wish to avoid pregnancy should use contraception for up to 2 years if their last period was before the age of 50 years, or for 1 year if it occurs after 50 years of age.

Further reading

Beral V and Million Woman Study Collaborators (2003). Breast cancer and hormone-replacement therapy in the Million Women Study. *Lancet* **362**(9382): 419–427.

CLINICAL EFFECTIVENESS

⇒ Evidence-based practice, Health economics, Protocols and policies.

CLINICAL GOVERNANCE

Clinical governance is a term for the framework introduced after the English White Paper *The New NHS: Modern, Dependable* (Department of Health 1997), within which all NHS organizations are accountable for their services and are required to have in place an active programme of continuous quality improvement within an overall, coherent framework of cost-effective service delivery. It embraces the process of clinical audit as a quality-improvement tool. Clinical governance requires that:

- Good practice be identified and built upon;
- There is in place in all NHS organizations a programme to manage risk;
- Mistakes are learnt from, free from a culture of blame;
- Lifelong learning is encouraged so that professionals may be supported and developed in their role of delivering quality care.

⇒ Accountability, Audit, Protocols and policies, Quality assurance, Risk assessment and management.

CLINICAL GUIDELINES, PATHWAYS

⇒ Protocols and policies.

CLINICAL SUPERVISION

Most of the healthcare professions have some means of supporting practitioners and students in clinical practice, although the level of support varies from profession to profession. Good clinical supervision should be separated from the managerial role and is designed to support all practising professionals, to offer a safe and supportive environment in which issues that relate to their practice can be discussed.

Clinical supervision works well when the two participants have negotiated a shared and explicit understanding of the purpose of the activity, and have clear boundaries and specific review points. In this way, arrangements can be made that meet the unique needs of the individuals concerned within certain agreed parameters.

Ideally, specific preparation should be given to those who undertake the supervisory role, whether supporting students or supporting registered and/or qualified practitioners. The literature identifies a range of desirable skills and personal attributes for those who undertake the supervisory role effectively. They include

C

a sense of humour, patience, being open minded, approachability, self-awareness, honesty, objectivity, maturity, sincerity, warmth, trustworthiness and understanding. Individuals need to be professional, nonthreatening and nonjudgemental, flexible, self-confident, committed, assertive and prepared to give regular feedback. In addition, supervisors need to be good role models who command peer respect, have demonstrable clinical competence, show good interpersonal skills, be facilitators of learning and the development of initiative and independence and be reflective practitioners (NBS 1999). ⇒ Preceptorship.

CLOSTRIDIUM

Clostridium is a genus of bacteria. These are large Gram-positive, spore-forming anaerobic bacilli found as commensals of the gut of animals and humans and as saprophytes in the soil. Many species are pathogenic because of the production of exotoxins, such as *C. botulinum* (botulism); *C. difficile* (pseudomembranous colitis); *C. perfringens (welchii)* (gas gangrene) and *C. tetani* (tetanus). ⇒ Food problems (food poisoning), Gangrene (gas gangrene).

Practice application – managing *C. difficile* diarrhoea

Pseudomembranous colitis is caused by superinfection with *C. difficile* in people whose normal bowel flora has been destabilized by the use of antibiotic therapy. It is characterized by watery diarrhoea and can be life threatening. Treatment is with oral metronidazole or vancomycin. However, both these antibiotics have been found to cause *C. difficile* diarrhoea in some people, particularly when administered intravenously.

It is important to educate patients and staff about the need for isolation and other infection-control precautions. An adequate fluid balance must be maintained and, if possible, the volume of diarrhoea being passed recorded.

Implement the following stool precautions:

- Wash hands and dry thoroughly after contact with stool and/or before leaving the room;
- Wear gloves and aprons when in contact with stool (masks are *not* necessary);
- Bedpan washer – ensure it is heating to 80°C and holding for 1 minute;
- Bedpan macerator lid must be kept closed for 1 minute after the cycle has finished to minimize aerosol dispersal;
- Disposable crockery and cutlery are *not* required;
- Change *all* bed linen daily, as the linen is infected (use red alginate bags);
- Waste must be discarded into yellow bags;
- Explain to patients the need for handwashing after using the lavatory and before eating;
- Visitors do *not* need protective clothing, but *must* wash and dry their hands thoroughly before leaving the patient area or room;
- Stool specimens, if required for clearance, must *not* be obtained while still on treatment;
- Stool precautions may be discontinued once the patient has had a formed stool for 48 hours;
- Decontaminate nursing and/or medical equipment as appropriate;
- For disinfection of the room after cleaning (*not* the mattress or pillows), the infection control nurse will advise on the appropriate disinfectant;
- Check the terminal cleaning is satisfactory and, once cleaned, the room or area can be used immediately.

COAGULATION (CLOTTING OF BLOOD)

Coagulation (clotting) is the third of four overlapping processes involved in haemostasis. Coagulation occurs through a series of complex reactions that use an enzyme cascade amplification to start the formation of a fibrin clot to stop bleeding. There are two pathways or systems, intrinsic and extrinsic, which converge to follow a common final pathway. Coagulation starts when platelets breakdown, tissue is damaged and thromboplastins are released. Various factors are involved in coagulation: I, fibrinogen; II, prothrombin; III, tissue thromboplastin; IV, calcium ions; V, labile factor (proaccelerin); VII, stable factor (proconvertin); VIII, antihaemophilic factor (AHF); IX, Christmas factor; X, Stuart–Prower factor; XI, plasma thromboplastin antecedent; XII, Hageman factor and XIII, fibrin-stabilizing factor.

During the coagulation cascade, coagulation factors in the blood act sequentially to convert the plasma protein prothrombin into thrombin. Thrombin then converts the plasma protein fibrinogen into fibrin, a durable substance that reinforces the primary platelet plug to form a more stable haemostatic plug (*Fig. 46*). ⇒ Haemostasis.

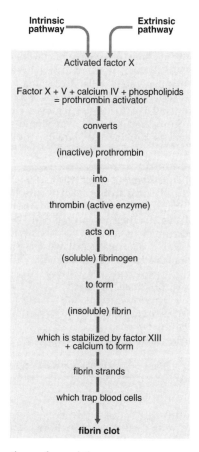

Intrinsic pathway   **Extrinsic pathway**

Activated factor X

Factor X + V + calcium IV + phospholipids = prothrombin activator

converts

(inactive) prothrombin

into

thrombin (active enzyme)

acts on

(soluble) fibrinogen

to form

(insoluble) fibrin

which is stabilized by factor XIII + calcium to form

fibrin strands

which trap blood cells

fibrin clot

Fig 46 Final common pathway of coagulation

C

COAGULATION SCREEN

The coagulation screen measures:
- Prothrombin time (PT) – assesses the extrinsic coagulation pathway;
- Activated partial thromboplastin time (APTT) – assesses the intrinsic coagulation pathway;
- International normalized ratio (INR) – measures PT of the person compared with a standard;
- Plasma levels of fibrinogen and platelet count.

COCAINE

Cocaine is a powerful local anaesthetic obtained from the leaves of the coca plant. In the UK it is a class A controlled drug [Misuse of Drugs Act (1971) and Misuse of Drugs Regulations (1985)]. It is highly addictive and subject to considerable criminal misuse. Toxic, especially to the brain, it may cause agitation, disorientation and convulsions. Crack cocaine is a highly potent and addictive form. ⇒ Controlled drugs, Drug , Substance misuse.

CODE OF PROFESSIONAL CONDUCT

As professionals, all nurses, midwives and health visitors are governed by a code of conduct. The Nursing and Midwifery Council (NMC) published a new *Code of Professional Conduct* in 2002, an overview of which is provided in *Box 8*. The code acts as a guide for nurses. It is not law, but it is a framework for behaviour and a statement about how the profession considers its members should behave (Rumbold 1999). Registered nurses and midwives are accountable to the NMC, which means that they can be called to account for their behaviour and judged against that expected in the *Code of Professional Conduct*. Nurses found guilty of misconduct may have their name removed from the register, which thus prevents them from practising as a registered nurse or midwife. ⇒ Competence/competencies, Nursing and Midwifery Council, Professional self-regulation.

Box 8 *The Code of Professional Conduct* (NMC 2002a)

Each of the clauses listed here is accompanied by sub-clauses that explain the purpose of the code and expand on what they mean. The full document is available from the NMC, in libraries and on the NMC web site, which is at http://www.nmc-uk.org.

The *Code of Professional Conduct* states that registered nurses and midwives are personally accountable for their practice and in caring for their patients and clients must:
- *'respect the patient or client as an individual'*;
- *'obtain consent before you give any treatment or care'*;
- *'protect confidential information'*;
- *'co-operate with others in the team'*;
- *'maintain your professional knowledge and competence'*;
- *'be trustworthy'*;
- *'act to identify and minimise risk to patients and clients'*.

COGNITION

Cognition is a generic term used to describe those mental processes involved within the collection and storage of information. It is also a general term used to describe the mental and internal events that cognitive psychology concerns itself with. It can be used to refer to mental images and symbols that may be reported by individuals as their thoughts about an event. ⇒ Psychology.

COGNITIVE PSYCHOLOGY

Cognitive psychology is an approach in psychology that studies the internal mental processes. Behaviour is explained using a model that takes account of mental events (mediational model). ⇒ Behaviour.

COGNITIVE DISORDER AND DISTORTION

Cognitive disorder is a disorder associated with the way in which an individual perceives and interprets the world. The underlying thought processes are seen as instrumental in determining how people behave and their emotional reactions.

Cognitive distortion is associated with cognitive disorder. Psychological stress is seen as a result of dysfunctional cognitions in which perceptions are interpreted inappropriately in disabling ways.

Therapeutic strategies associated with the above include:
- Cognitive therapy;
- Rational emotive therapy;
- Personal construct therapy;
- Transactional analysis;
- Neurolinguistic programming (NLP).

Cognitive disturbance describes a self-defeating attitude or responses that may become habitual, particularly when directed towards lowered self-esteem.

COGNITIVE BEHAVIOURAL THERAPY

Cognitive behavioural therapy is an approach to therapy that uses techniques from both behavioural and cognitive perspectives in therapy. It emphasizes the importance of using a mediational model in arriving at a formulation of a problem, but highlights the importance of using both aspects of operant and classic conditioning in enabling clients to overcome their difficulties (see Cognitive restructuring below). ⇒ Behaviour.

COGNITIVE RESTRUCTURING

Cognitive restructuring is a technique used in the practice of cognitive therapy that, through a process of challenging an individual's interpretations of an event, attempts to enable the clients to reconsider their construction of the event and to think about it in a different kind of way. This is to encourage a different affective response.

COLOUR VISION

High-definition colour vision depends on the activity of the cones (special photoreceptor cells) present in the retina of the eye. There are three subtypes of cones, which contain one of three visual pigments. These three cone subtypes respond to bright light of the green, blue or red wavelengths. Normal colour vision is inherited as a dominant gene (if present its characteristic is expressed) on the X chromosome.

COLOUR VISION TESTING

Colour vision testing is used to detect defects in the function of the three subtypes (green, blue or red) of cone cells. It is thought that 7% of the male population suffer from colour blindness, many of whom may be unaware that anything is wrong. Colour sensitivity is reduced in some ocular conditions, including optic neuritis and some macular disorders.

C

The usual method of testing is the Ishihara test, which involves people looking at a series of colour plates with numbers or letters embedded within them. They are asked to say what the letter or number is. People with normal colour vision are able to see the number or letter on every plate, whereas those with defective colour vision may see none of them (monochromatic defect), or may only be able to identify some of them, depending on which type of cone is defective.

DISORDERS OF COLOUR VISION (COLOUR BLINDNESS)

Colour blindness results from a dysfunction in or the absence of a photoreceptor subtype (cones) stimulated by red, green or blue light, which leads to difficulty distinguishing between certain colours. Colour blindness caused by deficiency of one of these cone subtypes often affects the red or green cones. Red–green colour blindness is inherited as a recessive gene (its characteristic is only expressed in the absence of a dominant gene on the homologous chromosome) on the X chromosome [males have one X chromosome and one Y chromosome (XY) and females have two X chromosomes (XX)]. It follows that colour blindness is more common in males who only have one X chromosome, and they are affected if they inherit the recessive gene. Females, however, because they have two X chromosomes, only have defective colour vision if they inherit the recessive gene from both parents. Achromatopsia is complete colour blindness in which there is an inability to see colours.

COMMISSION FOR HEALTHCARE AUDIT AND INSPECTION

The Commission for Healthcare Audit and Inspection (CHAI, known as The Healthcare Commission) undertakes the work previously done by the Commission for Health Improvement (CHI), the Mental Health Act Commission, the independent healthcare part of the National Care Standards Commission and the NHS 'value for money' work of the Audit Commission. The functions of CHAI include:

- Encouraging improvement in care (quality and effectiveness) and its provision (economy and efficiency);
- Inspection of healthcare services (management, provision and quality), and monitoring the use of public resources;
- Investigation of serious service failures, and reporting serious concerns to the Secretary of State;
- Production of the annual performance ratings for NHS organizations;
- Act as an independent review for NHS complaints, etc.

COMMISSION FOR HEALTH IMPROVEMENT

⇒ Commission for Healthcare Audit and Inspection.

COMMISSION FOR SOCIAL CARE INSPECTION

The Commission for Social Care Inspection (CSCI) undertakes the work previously done by the Social Services Inspectorate (SSI), the social care work of the National Care Standards Commission and the work of the joint SSI–Audit Commission team. The functions of the CSCI include:

- Inspection of social care organizations (private, public and voluntary) using national standards, publish reports and register those that meet the minimum standards;
- Inspection and publication of the star ratings for local social service authorities;
- Production of an annual report to Parliament;
- Validation of performance assessment statistics on social services.

COMMITTEE ON SAFETY OF MEDICINES

The Committee on Safety of Medicines (CSM) is an independent body that monitors drug safety and advises the UK licensing authority about the quality, efficacy and safety of medicines. The CSM advises the UK licensing authority (Medicines and Healthcare Products Regulatory Agency) on whether new drugs and/or substances should be given marketing authorization. Another function is the on-going safety monitoring of existing medicines to ensure that they reach the required standards of efficacy and safety. ⇒ Drug (adverse drug reactions), Medicines and Healthcare Products Regulatory Agency.

COMMUNICABLE DISEASES

These are infectious (contagious) diseases that can be transmitted directly or indirectly from one person or animal to another. They include diseases that range from the common cold to serious infections such as diphtheria, measles, rabies, typhoid, yellow fever, etc. ⇒ Epidemiology.

COMMUNICABLE DISEASE TERMS

CARRIER

A carrier is a person or animal that harbours an infectious agent without clinical disease and serves as a potential source of infection.

INCUBATION PERIOD

The incubation period is the time interval between infection or exposure to disease and the appearance of the initial symptoms.

PRODROMAL PERIOD

The prodromal period is the interval between the time when early signs of the disease appear to the time when the overt clinical disease is evident.

QUARANTINE

Quarantine is a period of isolation of infected people or suspected cases with the objective of preventing spread to others. For contacts it is usually the same period as the longest incubation period for a particular disease.

COMMUNICABLE AND/OR INFECTIOUS DISEASES OF CHILD-HOOD

Although many of these infectious diseases are associated with childhood, they do occur in adults. In addition, some, such as rubella, can affect the unborn child. ⇒ Defence mechanisms (active artificially acquired immunity – immunization).

MORBILLI, RUBEOLA (SYN. MEASLES)

Morbilli is an acute infectious disease caused by a paramyxovirus. Morbilli is endemic, worldwide in distribution and usually affects children. It is highly contagious and spreads via droplets. The incubation period is about 10 days. The disease has an initial catarrhal stage, with a cold-like illness, fever, sore and watery eyes, cough, photophobia and Koplik's spots (small white spots inside the mouth). After 3–4 days a maculopapular rash appears (*Fig. 47A*). It may be complicated by a secondary bacterial infection, such as otitis media or pneumonia. Other effects include eye damage from corneal ulcers and encephalitis. The mortality rate is very low in previously healthy and well-nourished individuals, but in developing countries the mortality is high. Active immunity is

C

offered as part of the routine immunization programme, in conjunction with protection against mumps and rubella (MMR), and passive immunity is available in special cases.

MUMPS (SYN. INFECTIOUS OR EPIDEMIC PAROTITIS)

Mumps is an acute, specific inflammation of the parotid glands, caused by a paramyxovirus. It is spread by droplets and mainly affects children and young adults. The incubation period is around 18 days. It is characterized by fever, malaise, swelling of the parotid salivary glands and pain. It can be complicated by orchitis, oophoritis, pancreatitis and meningitis. Active immunization is offered as part of the routine programme, in conjunction with protection against measles and rubella (MMR).

RUBELLA (SYN. GERMAN MEASLES)

Rubella is an acute, infectious disease, with an incubation period of 14–21 days. It is caused by a virus and spread by droplet infection. There is mild fever, a pink, maculopapular rash and enlarged occipital and posterior cervical lymph nodes (*Fig. 47B*). Complications are rare, except when contracted in the first trimester of pregnancy, when it may produce fetal abnormalities, such as heart defects, deafness, cataracts and brain damage. Immunization is available as part of the routine programme, in conjunction with protection against measles and mumps (MMR), and subsequently to individuals who did not receive MMR or any nonpregnant woman of childbearing age with insufficient immunity.

SCARLET FEVER (SYN. SCARLATINA)

Scarlet fever is an infectious disease with an incubation period of 2–4 days. It follows infection by a strain of Group A beta-haemolytic streptococcus, and occurs mainly in children. It begins commonly with a throat infection, followed by fever and the outbreak of a punctate erythematous rash on the skin of the trunk, and then by desquamation (*Fig. 47C*). The tongue becomes bright red – 'strawberry tongue'. Characteristically, the area around the mouth is pale (circumoral pallor). It is usually treated with penicillin.

VARICELLA (SYN. CHICKENPOX)

Varicella is an infection caused by the herpesvirus varicella-zoster virus (VZV), which primarily affects children. The virus is airborne, and the incubation period is 12–21 days. There is mild pyrexia and a skin rash (*Fig. 47D*). Successive crops of vesicles appear first on the trunk and develop through various stages to pustules that scab and usually heal without leaving scars, but scarring with pits is possible. The disease is usually mild, but may cause serious infection in neonates, adults and those who are immunocompromised. Varicella acquired during the first 5 months of pregnancy may cause fetal abnormalities. Severe neonatal infection can be caused by the woman having varicella in the days just before delivery. ⇒ Herpesviruses and herpes.

NOTIFIABLE DISEASES

Local authorities have a statutory responsibility to control infectious diseases within their boundaries. To facilitate this some communicable diseases must be notified to the Proper Officer, usually by the doctor who makes the diagnosis. *Table 6* shows the infectious diseases that are notifiable in England and Wales.

Notifications of infectious disease are necessary for several reasons. Firstly, close family or other contacts may have been exposed to the infection and require treatment or monitoring for signs of infection (e.g. tuberculosis, meningococcal

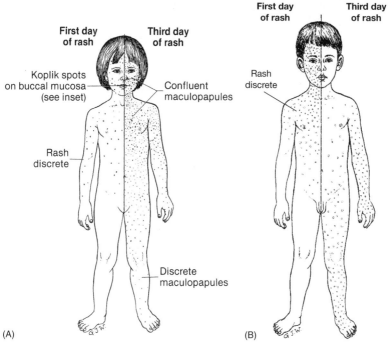

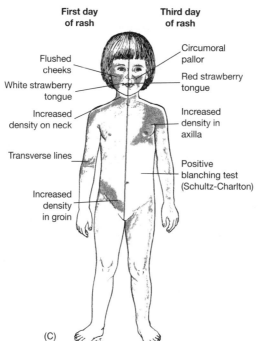

Fig 47 Rash distribution: (A) Morbilli (measles), (B) rubella (German measles), (C) scarlet fever (scarlatina), Rash distribution: (*cont.*)

C

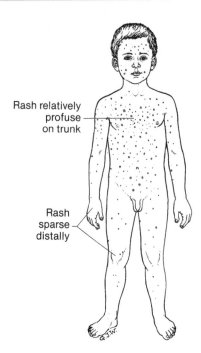

Rash relatively profuse on trunk

Rash sparse distally

Fig 47 *(Cont.)* (D) varicella (chickenpox)

meningitis). Secondly, the infection may have been acquired from contaminated food or water and require investigation to identify the source of infection (e.g. food poisoning). Finally, the information is analysed and used at both local and national level to monitor fluctuations in levels of infection and the effect of vaccination programmes, to detect epidemics at an early stage and to plan preventative programmes.

COMMUNICATION

We communicate much of who we are and our intentions when we approach situations without ever having to say anything. Our capacity as nurses to observe people's demeanours consciously is an essential skill. Alongside this skill of observation, we need to be aware of our own manner, as those around us can readily perceive this whether they are conscious of doing so or not. The process of communication can be described as a cycle that comprises the following (Macmillan 1996):

- History – what both the sender and recipient bring to the encounter, consciously and unconsciously. This includes personal history, society's history and the individual's own history in society.
- Intention – what the sender intends to communicate and what the recipient expects from the encounter. This, too, is both conscious and unconscious.
- Interaction – how the sender gives the message and how the recipient perceives it. This includes the words chosen, the tone used and the body language. Unconscious intentions influence these choices and perceptions.
- Consequences – these are the result of the interventions made and the impact they have on the participants. Senders may not be aware of the consequences they hoped to invoke. Likewise, recipients might respond to a message in ways of which they are unaware.

Table 6 Notifiable diseases, England and Wales

Public health (Control of Diseases) Act 1984

Cholera
Food poisoning
Plague
Relapsing fever
Smallpox
Typhus

Public Health (Infectious Diseases) Regulations 1988

Acute encephalitis
Acute poliomyelitis
Anthrax
Diphtheria
Dysentery
Leprosy
Leptospirosis
Malaria
Measles
Meningitis
Meningococcal septicaemia
Mumps
Ophthalmia neonatorum
Paratyphoid fever
Rabies
Rubella
Scarlet fever
Tetanus
Tuberculosis
Typhoid fever
Viral haemorrhagic fever
Viral hepatitis
Whooping cough
Yellow fever

This model works well for verbal and nonverbal as well as conscious and unconscious processes of communication. We can observe much from other people's body language as well as from the tone of their voices. Likewise, we give away much about ourselves without necessarily intending to do so (i.e. unconsciously). We do this by our posture and the words we choose (e.g. by using words like 'tell' and 'demand' instead of 'ask').

VERBAL COMMUNICATION

Verbal communication can be defined as the language – written and spoken – that we use to convey information to others. The way in which we use language varies according to the situations we are in and with whom we are communicating. Sign language used by people with hearing problems is verbal communication. As with any language, it has its own vernacular, social conventions and dialect.

C

The way we talk or write to people who are intimates in our personal lives is different from the way in which we communicate in a professional or formal relationship. In nursing practice we need to weigh our words – written and spoken – to ensure that they convey the meaning we intend (the 'intention' of the cycle).

When people are anxious or distressed, it is more likely that they will hear our message within a frame that is intimately personal and not necessarily from the perspective that we intend. As nurses we need to choose carefully the language we use, to demonstrate some understanding of how the world may seem to a frightened, angry patient or the person in pain. This is where nonverbal communication – or body language – becomes so important.

NONVERBAL COMMUNICATION

Nonverbal cues express our emotions, sense of occasion, status and sense of who we are and of whom we are relating to. How close (proximal) are we to those with whom we are making a relationship? Do they seem comfortable near us or do they move away? Each of us has a sense of the space around us, such as intimate (body contact to 18 inches) and personal (18 inches to 4 feet), etc. The parameters of this are arguably culturally determined, particularly in relation to gender, age and social status.

Should others around us behave inappropriately within these parameters, our verbal and nonverbal responses will be very evident, although they vary between individuals. For example, if people enter our intimate space uninvited, we back away from them.

The importance of nonverbal cues is very clear in our use of idiom and metaphor. Phrases such as someone's handshake 'was like a wet fish' and 'we jumped for joy' convey sensual as well as linguistic messages. We can feel the handshake and visualize the joy.

How we look at each other, our gestures, facial expressions and frequency of eye contact express much more than words. How we present ourselves (e.g. our posture, dress, the way we move, whether we smile or shake hands on greeting) gives clues to others about who we are and how we might be feeling. The ways in which these cues are interpreted depend on a number of factors. They also vary in place, time and situation. For example, in some cultures it is rude to look your superior in the eye, while in others it is rude not to make eye contact with the person talking to you, regardless of status.

Nurses' uniforms are an integral part of the nursing profession's culture. This nonverbal cue gives a very clear identification of who we are and where we are in the hierarchy of the profession. It is also a mark of our status in wider society.

PARALINGUISTICS

Paralinguistics, the tone and pitch of our voices and the emphasis we put on words or phrases, also convey meanings. The variety of accents and regional phrases also adds richness and colour to our heritage of language, whatever languages we speak. However, this can be confusing to those who are not familiar with them. Conscious and unconscious communication and shared and different psychological defences can be manifest in our paralinguistics as well as in our verbal and nonverbal cues.

Further reading

Ellis RB, Gates B and Kenworthy N (2003). *Interpersonal Communication in Nursing.* Edinburgh: Churchill Livingstone.

COMMUNITY

A community is a social group determined by geographical boundaries and/or common values and interests. Community has also come to imply shared relationships, lifestyles and a greater frequency and intimacy of contact among those who live in a community. For example, the Chinese community in China town and the East End community in London, in which the common interests, values and bonds maintain cohesive networks.

COMMUNITY CARE

Community care is a term applied to the care of people in the community (outside hospital). Such care is delivered by health and social care professionals and unpaid carers, such as family and friends. The community concept hence circumscribes the idea of primary healthcare and nursing practice. The community or primary care setting is increasingly recognized as being at the forefront of the development and delivery of health services. ⇒ Primary healthcare.

COMMUNITY NURSE

Community nurse is a generic term that describes those nurses based in the community and concerned with the health, well-being and care of people in their homes and other community settings. Their role also includes health promotion, health education and the prevention of illness and disability. Community nurses include specialist community public health nurses (health visitors), district nurses, community mental health nurse or learning disability nurses, community children's nurses, practice nurses, family planning nurses and school nurses.

COMMUNITY MENTAL HEALTH TEAMS

Community mental health teams developed in the UK over the final two decades of the 20th century and are to be found in most areas in recognition that most people with mental health needs live in the community. Teams are based according to historical and geographical factors, and generally include a community mental health nurse (also called community psychiatric nurse – CPN), a consultant psychiatrist, a specialist social worker, a clinical psychologist and others. The function of the team is to support people and their carers who live in the community. This may be done directly or by facilitation through generic health and community services.

> **Practice application – community mental health team for the elderly; the role of the nurse**
> The role of the mental health nurse includes:
> • Assessment of nursing needs, provision and evaluation of care plan;
> • Advice to other professional workers in the community;
> • Support for carers and relatives;
> • Specific specialist treatment (e.g. giving injections and different therapies according to the skill and expertise of the individual nurse);
> • Referring agent for different assessments and care;
> • Education of others about mental health disorders in older people.

COMPARTMENT SYNDROME

Acute compartment syndrome may occur in any muscle compartment, but in the context of musculoskeletal conditions it is more commonly associated with limb fractures. ⇒ Casts.

C

The condition is caused by an increase in the tissue pressure, either through bleeding into the soft tissues, or because of oedema and inflammation within the compartment. This leads to decreased perfusion with subsequent ischaemia, and muscle necrosis if treatment is delayed. The affected limb may be pale, painful, pulseless or have altered neurological sensation, and in all cases the patient complains of increased pain on extension of the affected limb. Diagnosis can also be confirmed through measuring intra-compartmental pressures. Treatment involves urgent decompression through fasciotomy [division of the fascia (connective tissue) that surrounds and separates muscles]. Hence the nursing intervention in compartment syndrome involves:

• Monitoring neurovascular status of the affected limb (see Practice application);
• Informing medical staff of any deficits obtained in the neurovascular assessment;
• Postsurgical wound management after fasciotomy.

Practice application – observations to detect compartment syndrome
Observations are referred to as the five Ps:
• Pain – increasing in nature;
• Pallor – of the extremities with swelling;
• Pulse – diminished or absent;
• Paraesthesia – altered sensation, often tingling;
• Power loss – inability to move the associated extremities.

COMPETENCE AND COMPETENCIES

It has arguably been taken for granted that nursing and midwifery are professions that encompass competence within the workforces. However, the issue of competence is a major topic, and is being debated and decided upon through a number of initiatives that include the *Fitness for Practice* (UKCC 1999), *Agenda for Change* (NHS Executive 1999) and *Making a Difference* (Department of Health 1999a).

All of these documents discuss and promote the development of nursing competencies, spanning pre-registration nursing and midwifery programmes, and practitioners who work at higher levels. Reference is also made to the uses of National and Scottish Vocational Qualifications (S/NVQs) for nonprofessional carers.

There are a number of definitions for the word 'competence'. On the whole, the notion is that an individual, a healthcare assistant, a nursing student or a qualified practitioner working at higher level demonstrates competence to an assessor through normal working practices and the compilation and presentation of a portfolio of evidence.

The theme of competence is not restricted to the UK, and members of the European Community are debating similar issues, striving to define the term and to define competencies for nursing that are acceptable to all members of the European Union. ⇒ Professional self-regulation.

COMPLAINTS MANAGEMENT, HEALTH SERVICE COMMISSIONER (OMBUDSMAN)

Used positively, the management of complaints can improve services and be a good learning experience for the professionals involved, as well as resulting in improved patient and client care.

Primary Care Trusts (PCTs), NHS Trusts, Strategic Health Authorities and general practitioners (GPs) must publicise their complaints procedures and must have a designated person to respond to complaints. Access to the Health Service Commissioner (Ombudsman) is available for all those who are not satisfied with the response they have received.

There are two levels at which complaints against the NHS are made and handled – that of local resolution and that of independent review:

- Local resolution – there are a variety of possible stages. Ideally, complaints are dealt with and resolved as close to the source of complaint as possible, by the staff to whom the complaint is made. If that is not possible, then referral must be made to the relevant complaints manager.
- Independent review panels – these are set up where local resolution has failed. The panel is required to produce a confidential report that sets out the results of its investigations, together with its conclusions and recommendations.

At either stage, complainants are informed of the roles and responsibilities of the Health Service Commissioner (Ombudsman), should they wish to pursue matters further.

COMPLEMENTARY MEDICINE AND THERAPY

Complementary medicine refers to a range of therapeutic modalities currently perceived as adjuncts to conventional medicine. More recently, the term *integrated medicine* has been promoted to imply a fusion between allopathic and complementary systems of healthcare. Such therapies present a multidimensional perception of health and well-being. This is broadly based upon a premise that health represents a harmonious state of being, which involves a conscious awareness and balanced interaction between an individual's mind, body, emotional well-being, spirit and the environment in which he or she lives. Care of a person is tailored to meet specific individual needs by recognizing the interaction and impact of each of these dimensions upon health and well-being.

Many therapies share a perception of some form of universal energy that is present in all forms of life. Imbalances in one or more dimensions of an individual's existence may result in an energy imbalance or ill health at some level. Complementary therapies aim to rebalance or reharmonize different energy dimensions in the human body by stimulating the body's own innate predisposition towards health and well-being.

Currently, the evidence base for complementary therapies is very poor.

INDIVIDUAL THERAPIES

ACUPUNCTURE

Acupuncture is a technique that involves the insertion of fine needles into specific parts of the body. There are approximately 365 points along meridians (channels through which energy, known as *Qi*, flows) at which needles can be inserted into the body to alter the energy flow. Sometimes the herb moxa is also used to warm and stimulate certain points. This is known as moxibustion.

ALEXANDER TECHNIQUE

The Alexander technique is a series of techniques used to improve the functioning of mind and body in a movement known as 'psychophysical' re-education. It is based on the belief that poor posture can lead to ill health, injury and chronic pain. The technique aims to promote postural improvement through self-awareness.

AROMATHERAPY

Aromatherapy is a complementary therapy that involves the use of fragrances derived from essential oils. These may be combined with a base oil, inhaled or massaged into intact skin.

C

BIOFEEDBACK

Biofeedback is a treatment based on the presentation of immediate visual or auditory information about usually unconscious body functions, such as blood pressure, heart rate and muscle tension. Either by trial and error or by operant conditioning a person can learn to repeat behaviour that results in a satisfactory level of body functions.

CHIROPRACTIC

Chiropractic specializes in the diagnosis and treatment of mechanical disorders of joints and their effects on the nervous system. The spine is afforded particular attention. Displacement of spinal vertebrae may result in the manifestation of a range of seemingly unrelated symptoms. The aim of chiropractic is not to treat the symptoms, but to identify the subluxation and correct it manually.

GUIDED IMAGERY

Guided imagery is a technique in which the person is asked to imagine a particular situation or state, and can be used with other interventions as a coping strategy in the control of pain and other symptoms.

HEALING

Healing is a therapeutic form of energy exchange that may occur between two or more individuals with the conscious intention to improve health and well-being.

HERBAL MEDICINE

Herbal medicine is the therapeutic use of herbs or mineral remedies by trained practitioners to promote health and recovery from illness.

HOMEOPATHY

Homeopathy is a system of medicine based on the *Law of Similars* (let like be treated with like). Effectivity is obtained by the process of dilution, in which extracts from natural sources, such as plants and minerals, are diluted many times in a water-and-alcohol base. At each dilution the mixture is vigorously shaken, a process known as succussion.

HYPNOSIS

Hypnosis is the deliberate use of a trance state, an altered state of consciousness. This may be initiated by a therapist or by the patient (self-hypnosis) utilizing the mental mechanism of suggestion to bring about a state of relaxation or an improvement in health and well-being. It may also be used to facilitate smoking cessation, and for forms of anaesthesia, as in skin suturing, and pain relief.

MASSAGE

Massage is the conscious use of gentle muscle manipulation, employing stroking or light kneading to promote a sensation of relaxation.

OSTEOPATHY

Osteopathy is a system of manual medicine concerned with mechanical, functional and postural assessment and treatment. This usually involves manipulation of joints and spinal vertebrae directed towards resolving mechanical problems of the body. Thus, abnormal tension in muscles and ligaments can be relieved and self-healing facilitated.

REFLEXOLOGY

Reflexology is a complementary therapy based on the premise that the internal organs of the body are mapped out on the soles of the feet and palms of the hands. It is believed that gentle pressure upon the areas that relate to specific organs can initiate a therapeutic response.

RELAXATION

Relaxation is a state of altered consciousness characterized by the release of muscle tension, anxiety and stress. Relaxation techniques are being incorporated into healthcare and health education programmes. They include progressive muscle relaxation, visual guided imagery, yoga and meditation.

THERAPEUTIC TOUCH

In the context of complementary therapy, therapeutic touch is a nontouch therapy directed towards initiating the body's self-healing mechanisms. It is based upon the idea that healing occurs through an energy field interaction between therapist and client.

More generally, it describes the use of touch as a therapeutic intervention in its own right, rather than as a necessary function of nursing activity. It may involve therapeutic massage or simply appropriate bodily contact, indicating empathy and support.

VISUALIZATION

Visualization is the technique of using the imagination to create any desired changes in an individual's life.

YOGA

Yoga is a discipline that uses breathing techniques, exercises and postures to relax, reduce stress and generally enhance physical, psychological and spiritual well-being.

Further reading

Rankin-Box D (2001). *The Nurse's Handbook of Complementary Therapies*, Second Edition. Edinburgh: Bailliere Tindall.

COMPLIANCE

⇒ Concordance.

CONCEPTION AND FERTILIZATION

Conception and fertilization is the creation of a state of pregnancy – fertilization of an oocyte (ovum) by a spermatozoon. Conception requires that a spermatozoon reaches and penetrates a secondary oocyte to complete meiosis II prior to the fusion of the two nuclei at fertilization (*Fig. 48*).

After spermatozoa are deposited in the vagina during coitus they must make their way through the cervix and uterus and into the uterine tube. Nature has ensured an abundance of spermatozoa, but only a few thousand actually reach the ampulla of the uterine tube. Before spermatozoa can penetrate an oocyte they must undergo the processes of capacitation and acrosome reaction. The spermatozoon carries enzymes that it uses to gain access to the oocyte. Capacitation involves structural changes to the acrosome that make the enzymes available for release. Many spermatozoa must release their enzymes by the acrosome reaction

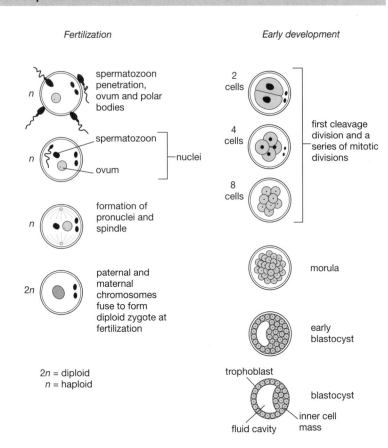

Fertilization   Early development

spermatozoon penetration, ovum and polar bodies

2 cells

spermatozoon

4 cells

nuclei

ovum

8 cells

first cleavage division and a series of mitotic divisions

formation of pronuclei and spindle

morula

paternal and maternal chromosomes fuse to form diploid zygote at fertilization

early blastocyst

trophoblast

2n = diploid
n = haploid

blastocyst

inner cell mass

fluid cavity

Fig 48 Fertilization and early development

to 'break through' the defences around the oocyte, but only one actually latches on to and penetrates the secondary oocyte. These are vital mechanisms that prevent the entry of further spermatozoa (polyspermy).

Once penetration by the spermatozoon head has occurred, the secondary oocyte completes meiosis II to produce the functional ovum and the second polar body. The haploid nuclei of both ovum and spermatozoon enlarge to form the pronuclei. A mitotic spindle forms between the two pronuclei and the maternal and paternal chromosomes combine to form the diploid zygote – fertilization is complete. ⇒ Family planning (types of contraception), Meiosis, Pregnancy.

Practice application – preconception care
Preconception care refers to the physical and mental preparation for childbearing of both parents before pregnancy. Health-promoting activity focuses on measures aimed at reducing the risk of fetal problems and maternal complications during pregnancy and labour. The measures include the importance of an adequate diet, such as the provision of sufficient folic acid in the diet of women of childbearing age, and for the couple to avoid the use of alcohol, drugs (prescribed, over the counter and recreational) and smoking in the months before they decide to have a baby.

CONCORDANCE

Until a few years ago, patients and clients who failed to follow the prescribed treatment regimen, such as taking medicine as directed, were described as being 'non-compliant'. Health professionals thought noncompliance was a problem caused by the behaviour of irrational patients who did not keep to (or perhaps wilfully ignored) the instructions given by their doctors.

Concordance is a fairly new approach to the prescribing and taking of medicines. It is an agreement reached after negotiation between a person and a healthcare professional that respects the beliefs and wishes of the person in determining whether, when and how medicines are to be taken. Although reciprocal, this is an alliance in which the healthcare professionals recognize the primacy of the person's decisions about taking the recommended medications, or following some other treatment regimen, such as dietary restrictions.

Concordance has also been called *partnership in medicine taking*. It includes:
- Sharing beliefs between patient and professional;
- An explicit agreement on whether medicines are the best way forwards;
- Making the best use of medicines and their potential benefits, while accepting the limits to those benefits and respecting those beliefs that the patient does not want to change.

Resource

http://www.concordance.org/uk

CONDITIONING

⇒ Behaviour.

CONFIDENTIALITY

All codes of conduct or ethics for the healthcare professions address the issue of confidentiality in some way, at least in principle. Frequently, additional detailed advice is also available. All practitioners are expected to honour and respect the confidential information that they obtain in the course of their professional practice. Such information should not be disclosed to others without the patient's consent. Those who are being cared for have a right to expect that the information they disclose during the course of their care is kept confidential to those who are involved in their care. This is the basis of trust upon which care is given.

Information obtained during the course of professional practice should only be shared with others in exceptional circumstances. The principle of confidentiality should only be breached when disclosure is required by law or the order of a court, or is necessary in the public interest. The public interest can be interpreted as the interests of an individual, groups of individuals or society as a whole. The decision as to whether to disclose information must lie with the individual practitioner concerned and must be taken as a result of a considered assessment of all the relevant facts. The resultant decision should be recorded meticulously.

CONFUSION AND DELIRIUM

Confusion is marked by poor attention and thinking, which lead to difficulties in comprehension, loss of short-term memory and often irritability alternating with drowsiness. As a term used by nurses, confusion can be difficult to identify with. It is not easily distinguished from other terminologies, such as disorientation or delirium, which are sometimes used synonymously, and it is generally associated with negative mental health status.

C

Confusion is observed as behaviour. It results from adverse physiological, psychological or environmental factors, which in turn interfere with the functioning of the nervous system. Therefore, confusion on its own is not a condition, but is a symptom of underlying pathology. Some of the factors that may lead to confusion are listed in *Table 7*. Although confusion can occur in individuals of all ages, it is, however, far more likely to be observed in older people.

There are two types of confusion – short-term and long-term. Short-term or acute confusion is usually reversible and has a sudden onset. In older people, acute confusion can occur in a variety of serious illnesses. The younger age group can also develop acute confusion; factors that may lead to it include an epileptic seizure, hyperpyrexia, post-electroconvulsive therapy and poisoning. Generally, a confused episode that occurs during an acute physical condition is called delirium. Delirium is always secondary to an underlying medical condition, has a sudden onset, is usually reversible and involves no destruction of brain cells.

In contrast, long-term or chronic confusion occurs following degenerative changes in the brain. This is called dementia. ⇒ Ageing, Dementia.

Table 7 Factors that can lead to confusion

Physical	Psychological	Environmental
Constipation	Anxiety states	Translocation
Diabetes mellitus	Depression	Stressful environment
Drugs or alcohol	Fear	Isolation or loneliness
Fatigue		External or internal stimuli
Hormonal disturbance		
Hypothermia		
Infection		
Neoplasm		
Vascular disorders		
Vitamin deficiencies		
Urinary retention		

Practice application – assessing cognitive function
Many assessment tools are available to assess cognitive function. Some are widely used, such as the Mini-Mental State Examination, which tests ability in ways that include counting backwards in 7 seconds from 100, demonstrating orientation in time and place, identification of objects and writing a simple sentence (Folstein *et al.* 1975). It is a simple tool and is easy and quick to use at the bedside.

CONGENITAL DEFECTS

Congenital defects are abnormal conditions present at birth, and are often genetically determined but can result from environmental factors (e.g. maternal rubella infection). ⇒ Genes and genetics (genetic diseases).

They exist before or at birth, and are usually associated with a defect or disease (e.g. congenital heart disease). Many congenital defects are amenable to corrective surgery.

ATRESIA

Atresia is the imperforation or closure of a normal body opening, duct or canal, such as of the oesophagus, bowel, anus, bile duct, etc.

CLEFT LIP AND/OR PALATE

A cleft lip is a fissure that extends from the margin of the lip to the nostril; it may be single or double, and is often associated with cleft palate. Cleft palate is the failure of fusion between the right and left palatal processes (*Fig. 49*). The cleft may vary, but, when complete, extends through both soft and hard palates into the nasal cavity.

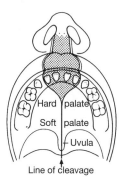

Fig 49 A cleft palate

CONGENITAL HEART DISEASE

Developmental abnormalities in the anatomy of the heart that result, postnatally, in symptoms that include cyanosis, dyspnoea, heart murmurs, etc. These include:
- Atrial septal defect (ASD);
- Ventricular septal defect (VSD);
- Fallot's tetralogy, a cyanotic defect that comprises a ventricular septal defect, subvalvular pulmonary stenosis, right ventricular hypertrophy and malposition of the aorta overriding the ventricular septum;
- Patent or persistent ductus arteriosus;
- Patent foramen ovale;
- Dextrocardia, in which the heart is on right side the thorax.
⇒ Fetus (fetal circulation).

DEVELOPMENTAL DYSPLASIA OF THE HIP

Developmental dysplasia of the hip (DDH) was previously known as congenital dislocation of the hip. However, the term DDH is more useful as it covers the various degrees and causes of the disorder. There is usually poor development of the acetabulum, which allows femoral head dislocation. Early diagnosis is vital (see Practice application). The treatment of DDH depends on the severity and age of the child, but usually involves various types of abduction splinting (using a special harness), skin traction (or a hip spica cast may be required), a closed reduction under general anaesthesia or possibly surgical intervention.

Practice application – early recognition of developmental dysplasia of the hip (Ortolani and Barlow test)

The diagnosis of developmental dysplasia of the hip (DDH) should be made in the newborn period if possible, since treatment initiated before 2 months of age achieves the highest rate of success.

In the newborn dysplasia usually appears as hip-joint laxity rather than as outright dislocation. Subluxation and the tendency to dislocate can be demonstrated by the Barlow or Ortolani test. These tests should only be undertaken by an experienced and competent clinician.

With the infant quiet and relaxed in the supine position on a firm surface and the legs facing the examiner, the hips are flexed (not forced) at right angles and the knees are flexed. The examiner places the middle finger of each hand over the greater trochanter and the thumbs on the inner side of the thigh at a point opposite the lesser trochanter. The knees are carried to mid-abduction, and each hip joint is submitted, one at a time, first to forwards pressure exerted behind the trochanter and then to backwards pressure exerted from the thumbs in front as the opposite joint is held steady. If the femoral head can be felt to slip forwards into the acetabulum on pressure from behind, it is dislocated (*Ortolani's test*; *Fig. 50*). Sometimes an audible 'clunk' can be heard on exit or entry of the femur out or into the acetabulum. If, on pressure from the front, the femoral head is felt to slip out over the posterior lip of the acetabulum and immediately slips back in place when pressure is released, the hip is said to be dislocatable or 'unstable' (*Barlow's test*).

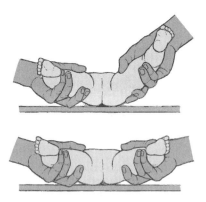

Fig 50 Ortolani click (if infant is under 4 weeks of age)

EXOMPHALOS

Exomphalos results from the failure of the gut to return to the abdominal cavity during fetal development. The intestines protrude through a gap in the abdominal wall, still enclosed in peritoneum.

NEURAL TUBE DEFECTS

Neural tube defects (NTDs) are a range of congenital defects that involve the neural tube. It is recommended that women take folate (folic acid) supplements before and during the first weeks after conception, to reduce the risk of NTDs in the fetus.

ANECEPHALY

Anecephaly is an absence of the brain, a condition is incompatible with life. Raised levels of alphafetoprotein in the amniotic fluid indicate it.

HYDROCEPHALUS

Hydrocephalus ('water on the brain') is an excess of cerebrospinal fluid (CSF) inside the skull caused by a disruption in normal CSF circulation or loss of brain tissue. A valve (e.g. Spitz–Holter type) is used to drain excess CSF and return it to the bloodstream.

MENINGOCELE

Meningocele is a protrusion of the meninges through a bony defect (spina bifida). It forms a cyst filled with CSF.

MENINGOMYELOCELE (MYELOMENINGOCELE)

Meningomyelocele is a protrusion of a portion of the spinal cord and its enclosing membranes through a bony defect in the spinal canal. It differs from a meningocele in being covered with a thin, transparent membrane, which may be granular and moist.

MYELOCELE

Myelocele is an accompaniment of spina bifida wherein development of the spinal cord itself has been arrested, and the central canal of the cord opens onto the skin surface and discharges CSF.

SPINA BIFIDA

Spina bifida is a congenital defect in which there is incomplete closure of the neural canal, usually in the lumbosacral region. In *spina bifida occulta* the defect does not affect the spinal cord or meninges. It is often marked externally by pigmentation, a haemangioma, a tuft of hair or a lipoma, which may extend into the spinal canal. In *spina bifida cystica* there is an externally protruding spinal lesion. It may vary in severity from meningocele to myelomeningocele. The condition can be detected during pregnancy by an increased concentration of alphafetoprotein in the amniotic fluid or by ultrasonography.

TALIPES

Talipes is any of a number of deformities of the foot and ankle. *Talipes calcaneovalgus* is a condition usually caused by intrauterine posture. The foot is fixed in an upturned position with the sole against the uterine wall. Improvement and usually complete recovery occurs with active movement after birth. In *Talipes equinovarus* the heel is drawn up, the foot inverted and the hindfoot adducted (in the equinovarus position). Treatment usually involves manipulation, splinting in a favourable position or surgical intervention in some cases.

TRACHEO-OESOPHAGEAL FISTULA

Tracheo-oesophageal fistula usually occurs in conjunction with an oesophageal atresia. The fistula usually connects the distal oesophagus to the trachea.

CONSCIOUSNESS

Consciousness is a complex concept that implies a person consciously perceives the environment through the five sensory organs, and responds to the perceptions. ⇒ Anaesthesia, Sleep.

ALTERED CONSCIOUSNESS

The level of consciousness is normally changed during sleep. It can also be altered by some drugs, including alcohol, general anaesthesia, metabolic disturbances such as hyper- and hypoglycaemia, head injuries, strokes, etc. ⇒ Confusion and delirium, Glasgow coma scale, Head injury, Nervous system (neurological disorders).

CONSENT, INFORMED CONSENT, INFORMED CHOICE

Consent may be defined as the giving of approval to a particular course of action. However, without an understanding of the implication of that action, any consent remains uninformed.

For consent to be valid, patients must:
• Be competent to make a decision;
• Have received appropriate and sufficient information;
• Not be acting under duress.

The NHS Plan (Department of Health 2000a) identified the need for change in the way patients give consent to treatment, care and research. The Government has introduced new consent-to-treatment forms and a model for consent to treatment (Department of Health 2001). This publication provides explicit guidance on issues of consent and, along with its associated documents that address specific client groups, should be essential reading for all nurses who work in surgical care.

In all areas of healthcare to obtain consent to treatment or procedure is integral to everyday nursing activity. Indeed, without consent, even touching patients might be considered a trespass against them (i.e. battery or assault).

The exact nature of informed consent has developed substantially over the years, although it remains a contentious issue for both medical staff and lawyers. For patient consent to fulfil the requirements of both the law and the professional bodies, it must be informed. In English law, consent can be obtained through implied, verbal or written means, although there is no legal distinction between these forms (Dimond 2001).

Implied consent, while open to misinterpretation, is obtained on the premise that the recipients have agreed to treatment by their actions or behaviour. Patients who roll up their sleeves in the presence of a phlebotomist provide implied consent to the provision of a blood sample. Such an act comprises legally valid evidence of consent, but from a professional perspective is satisfactory only for the more trivial or minimal of interventions. The essence of informed consent is the patient's awareness of the implications of the proposed action. The consent may be a verbal agreement, but for reasons of documentation and the ability to provide evidence of the process, written consent is most desirable.

A consent form signed by both patient and the operative practitioner is evidence of an interaction between the two. As such, it is likely to provide the only acceptable evidence that informed consent was obtained. It also provides a permanent record that implies the patient was made aware of the proposed procedure, its consequence, possible risks and any alternatives. Note that a nurse may well undertake the operation. The increasing number of clinical nurse consultant appointments in colorectal work, for example, has seen them undertake invasive operative procedures. Within the consultation the patient has both legal and moral rights (see Practice application).

AGE AND FACTORS THAT REDUCE THE POTENTIAL FOR INFORMED CONSENT

Patients can sign the consent form if they are of the legal age of 16 years and above and/or have the mental capacity to understand fully all that is involved. ⇒ Gillick competence.

If the patient is unable to sign the form, the parent or legal guardian may do so. Where an adult lacks the mental capacity, either temporarily or permanently, to give or withhold consent no one has the right to give approval for a course of action. However, treatment may be given if it is considered to be in the patient's best interests, provided an explicit refusal to such an action has not been made by the person in advance. The consent form must be signed before any premedication is given and, in signing the form, patients give their consent to the administration of an anaesthetic and performance of surgery. This includes a signed declaration by the medical practitioner that the nature and purpose of the proposed operation has been explained.

> **Practice application – rights in consent**
> Patients have the right to:
> • Quality information;
> • Know alternatives;
> • Ask questions;
> • Consult others and/or obtain a second opinion;
> • Have time to consider the options;
> • Change their mind.

CONSTIPATION

⇒ Defecation

CONTACT LENS

A contact lens is a glass or plastic lens worn under the eyelid in direct contact with the conjunctiva (in place of spectacles) for therapeutic or cosmetic purposes.

> **Practice application – care of contact lens**
> Wearers of hard or soft contact lenses may occasionally contract conjunctivitis. There is a trend for young people to wear nonprescription contact lenses to alter the colour of their eyes, but these people are not always given help and advice on how to care for them. The most frequent cause of conjunctivitis is contamination of the contact lens case itself. Contact lens wearers should wash their hands before and after they insert and remove their lenses to help reduce the risk of infection. In addition, the lens case should be washed in hot soapy water and left to air-dry. Wearers do not always do this because they simply forget or the conditions are less than ideal (e.g. when busy at work or in a nightclub).
> Manufacturers of lens cleaning solutions are continuing to develop one-step cleaning and soaking solutions. Many of them are also providing lens cases with each new bottle of contact lens solution. Many contact lens prescriptions are available as daily disposable, which eliminates the need for cleaning and storage. Some wearers, in an attempt to economize, occasionally reuse disposable lenses. This is clearly a practice that is not recommended and must be discouraged.

CONTINENCE

Continence is the ability to control urination and defecation. The person is able to recognize the requirement to pass urine and/or defecate and is able to delay until they reach a suitable place.

C

LOSS OF CONTINENCE

Loss of continence is termed incontinence. It is the inability to control urination or, less commonly, defecation. Other definitions may incorporate other aspects of the problem, such as time periods. Urinary incontinence is not uncommon in adults, particularly women, and the incidence increases with age (Milsom *et al.* 2001). Milsom *et al.* (2001), using a definition of overactive bladder symptoms (frequency, urgency and nocturia, with or without urge incontinence), estimated the prevalence in the UK as being 5.15 million.

Prevalence studies show faecal incontinence to be more common than healthcare professionals previously realized. A UK study of 15 904 adults over the age of 40 by the Medical Research Council Incontinence Study Team (Perry *et al.* 1988) found that 8% of those of age 65–84 years and 16% of those aged over 85 years reported faecal incontinence. The different types and/or causes of urinary and faecal incontinence are outlined in the entry for incontinence. ⇒ Incontinence.

Practice application – maintaining continence
The studies above illustrate that loss of continence is a major problem affecting many people. Nurses have a central role in providing education and advice to help people to maintain continence. This might include:
• Bladder retraining;
• Teaching pelvic floor awareness and exercises;
• Advice about fluid and fibre intake, and reducing caffeine intake;
• Reviewing medication likely to affect continence;
• Bowel training that establishes a regular schedule for going to the lavatory;
• Advising on adaptations to clothing that overcome problems with dexterity.

Further reading

Brooker C and Nicol M (2003). *Nursing Adults. The Practice of Caring*, Ch 12. Edinburgh: Mosby.
Getliffe K and Dolman P (1997). *Promoting Continence*. London: Bailliere Tindall.
Royal College of Physicians (1995). *Incontinence – Causes, Management and Provision of Services*. London: Royal College of Physicians.

CONTINUING PROFESSIONAL DEVELOPMENT

Continuing professional development (CPD) is also referred to as continuing education (CE), and it can be thought of as lifelong learning, which embraces the acceptance of education occurring at all points in the lifespan. This implies, of course, that the teaching methods appropriate to adult learners must be used, focusing on learning derived from experience, using a student-centred, needs-based approach. This approach allows the learner to set her or his own agenda and assess its success. It stresses active, rather than passive, learning and frequently using peers as a source for knowledge. It also embraces the linkage of education and work – the application of learning to practice and the notion that practice itself is not static. Alongside this is the acceptance that theory not only informs practice, but also that knowledge can be embedded in, and emerge from, practice. Dynamic, changing practice is underpinned by education that is work-focused. The nature of work changes rapidly these days. The education that fits a practitioner for practice now may not be relevant in 5 years, let alone for a whole working life. Practitioners need to be able to access knowledge and skills, and to develop attitudes to upgrade, consciously, systematically and continuously, their existing repertoire. CPD is a way of meeting this need for education 'on the job', and practitioners should be encouraged and supported to undertake professional development additional to the statutory 5 days of study every 3 years currently required for re-registration as a nurse in the UK. ⇒ Postregistration Education and Practice, Profiles and portfolios.

CONTROLLED DRUGS

In the UK The Misuse of Drugs Act 1971 imposes controls on those drugs liable to produce dependence or cause harm if misused. It prohibits certain activities in relation to controlled drugs (CD). Currently, only doctors and dentists can prescribe CDs, but plans exist to add some CDs to the Nurse Prescriber's Extended Formulary.

However, the Misuse of Drugs (Notification of and Supply to Addicts) Regulations 1973 state that medical practitioners may not prescribe, administer or supply CDs to addicted persons as a means of treating their addiction, unless specifically licensed to do so.

The Misuse of Drugs (Supply to Addicts) Regulations 1997 revoked the requirement for prescribers to provide the Home Office with information about drug addicts, but there is an expectation that practitioners will report cases of drug misuse to the local Drug Misuse Database.

CDs are divided into three classes that reflect the level of harm caused by each drug if misused. The three legal classes are:
- Class A (most harm) – alfentanil, cocaine, diamorphine (heroin), dipipanone, lysergide (LSD), methadone, methylenedioxymethamfetamine (MDMA or ecstasy), morphine, opium, pethidine and Class B drugs when they are in injectable form;
- Class B (intermediate) – oral amfetamines, barbiturates, codeine, ethylmorphine, pentazocine;
- Class C (least harm) – certain drugs related to amfetamines (e.g. benzfetamine), cannabis, most benzodiazepines, androgenic and anabolic steroids and growth hormone.

In the UK the reclassification of cannabis from a Class B to a Class C drug occurred in January 2004. However, the production, supply and possession of cannabis are still illegal.

The Misuse of Drugs Regulations 1985 further subdivides drugs into five schedules. Each schedule details the requirements for import, export, production, supply, possession, prescribing and record keeping. They are:
- Schedule 1 – drugs that are often used illegally (e.g. cannabis and hallucinogens, such as lysergide). Possession and supply are only permitted with Home Office authority.
- Schedule 2 – addictive drugs, including amfetamine, cocaine, diamorphine (heroin), morphine, pethidine, secobarbital and glutethimide. The prescription, safe custody and storage of Schedule 2 CDs must fulfil the full CD requirements, which includes maintaining registers.
- Schedule 3 includes barbiturates (except secobarbital), buprenorphine, diethylpropion, flunitrazepam, mazindol, meprobamate, pentazocine, phentermine and temazepam. They are subject to special prescription requirements (except phenobarbital and temazepam), but not to safe custody (with exceptions, e.g. temazepam). Registers do not need to be kept, only invoices for 2 years.
- Schedule 4 CDs are neither subject to CD prescription rules nor to safe custody. Part I includes benzodiazepines (except flunitrazepam and temazepam) and zolpidem. Part II includes anabolic steroids, clenbuterol, chorionic gonadotrophin (HCG), somatropin, etc.
- Schedule 5 includes medicines, such as some cough mixtures, that by virtue of their strength are exempt from most CD regulations except the keeping of invoices for 2 years.

Health professionals should be familiar with those that relate to drugs in Schedules 2 and 3.

Practice application – Controlled drug prescription and storage rules

Prescriptions for CDs are required to fulfil the following conditions:
- Hand written;
- Have the name and the address of the patient clearly written in ink;
- The dosage form must be hand written (e.g. tablets) and the strength must be specific;
- The total quantity of the preparation, or the number of dose units, given in both words and figures;
- The dose stated;
- If for dental treatment, this must be stated clearly.

Pharmacists are not allowed to dispense the drug unless each of the above is correct. General practitioners, dentists and hospital staff must keep accurate records of all purchases, amounts of the drugs issued and dosages given.

The rules for the storage of CDs are:
- The locked cupboard for CDs should be a locked cupboard within a locked cupboard, and attached to the wall;
- In hospital the keys to the cupboard are kept on the person in charge of the ward, or deputy;
- Supplies can be obtained by prescription signed by a medical officer, and the drugs can only be given under written instructions;
- Ward stocks of CDs in frequent use can be ordered in special CDs order books, and the person in charge must sign each order;
- A careful written record of each dose given to a patient must be kept. This record must state the patient's name, the time the drug was administered and the dosage. Both the practitioner (usually a nurse) who gives the drug and another nurse who has checked the source of the drug as well as the dosage against the prescription sign the record.

All containers used for CDs must bear special labels to distinguish them clearly. A hospital pharmacist must check the contents of the CD cupboard at regular intervals against the record books. Any discrepancies must be investigated fully.

CORONARY (ISCHAEMIC) HEART DISEASE

Coronary heart disease (CHD) is caused by atheroma affecting the coronary arteries, which eventually may lead to angina, myocardial infarction (MI) or heart failure. CHD is a leading cause of morbidity and premature death in developed countries. The risks factors for CHD are multifactorial. Important modifiable risk factors for CHD have been identified as hypercholesterolaemia (high cholesterol level in the blood), hypertension (high blood pressure), physical inactivity and smoking. Other modifiable factors include poor nutrition with high fat intake, obesity and diabetes. A multifactorial approach to identifying the risk factors and offering appropriate advice is the cornerstone of prevention and treatment. ⇒ Arterial disease, Cholesterol (abnormal blood lipid profiles).

ANGINA PECTORIS

Angina pectoris is characterized by a severe but temporary attack of cardiac pain that may radiate to the arms, throat, lower jaw or the back. It results from myocardial ischaemia, and often the attack is induced by exercise (angina of effort).

The initial treatment is likely to consist of drug therapy and advice about positive lifestyle changes. The drugs used include:

- Glyceryl trinitrate (GTN), or another nitrate such as isosorbide dinitrate $\Rightarrow$ Nitrates;
- Diltiazem and verapamil (to dilate the coronary arteries);
- Beta-adrenoceptor antagonists, such as atenolol, to decrease the myocardial oxygen demand;
- Low-dose aspirin to reduce the risk of further platelet aggregation and of the atheroma developing further;
- HMG-CoA reductase inhibitor (statin), such as simvastatin for individuals who have high blood cholesterol levels (>5.0 mmol/L).

Unstable angina may occur in a patient with known angina, or may itself be the initial sign of CHD. In unstable angina, chest pain develops without exertion, often while the patient is either resting or sleeping.

For situations in which angina severely affects activity and quality of life, angioplasty and stent insertion, myocardial revascularization or surgical treatment is considered.

CORONARY ARTERY BYPASS GRAFT

Coronary artery bypass graft (CABG) is a surgical procedure used if percutaneous transluminal coronary angioplasty (PTCA, see below) is not possible. The diseased coronary arteries are bypassed with a graft, a portion of the saphenous vein from the leg or alternative vessels, such as the internal mammary artery. For traditional coronary artery bypass surgery, a median sternotomy approach is employed, the heart is stopped and a cardiopulmonary bypass (CPB) is used to maintain the circulation and gaseous exchange.

Minimally invasive cardiac surgery (MICS) avoids the median sternotomy and a CPB, and is used in selected patients. There is a shorter hospital stay and morbidity and mortality may be reduced.

PERCUTANEOUS MYOCARDIAL REVASCULARIZATION

Percutaneous myocardial revascularization is a laser technique used to increase the blood supply to the myocardium by creating channels from the endothelium to the subepicardial surface. A catheter is passed through the femoral artery and into the left ventricle. A laser energy source on the tip of the catheter is placed directly against the myocardium to create the channels that supply blood to the myocardium.

PERCUTANEOUS TRANSLUMINAL CORONARY ANGIOPLASTY

Percutaneous transluminal coronary angioplasty (PTCA) is a technique whereby a catheter, with a small balloon on the end, is inserted into the femoral artery and passed into the coronary arteries. The balloon is inflated, which stretches the stenosed portion of the artery and widens the lumen. An intracoronary stent (wire-mesh tube) is placed in the coronary artery to keep it open. Patients are prescribed glycoprotein IIb/IIIa inhibitors, such as abciximab, to avoid vessel occlusion by thrombus aggregating to the arterial wall or the stent.

MYOCARDIAL INFARCTION

Myocardial infarction (MI) occurs when there is an abrupt cessation to blood flow within the coronary arteries that leads to an area of infarction (muscle death) in the myocardium (e.g. the occlusion of the coronary artery may be caused by a thrombosis). The patient experiences a 'heart attack' with a sudden intense chest pain, which may radiate to the arms and lower jaw.

C

Diagnosis of MI is made from the history and clinical presentation, a 12-lead electrocardiogram (ECG) and blood tests that include cardiac enzyme levels. Cardiac enzymes are released from damaged myocardial cells (and in some cases from other cells). They are also released according to the time since the injury, so it is important to draw blood samples at clearly defined intervals. The enzymes usually measured are creatinine phosphokinase MB fraction (MB-CPK), troponin I, aspartate aminotransferase (AST) and lactate dehydrogenase (LDH).

Management of acute MI includes aspirin, thrombolytic therapy, pain relief, antiemetics, oxygen therapy, bed rest, observations (including continuous ECG) and later mobilization and cardiac rehabilitation (phases 1 to 4, of which phase I usually occurs in hospital). PTCA may be used to open the occluded artery, but for the procedure to be effective it must be performed as quickly as possible.

After MI patients should be cared for in a coronary care unit for the first 12–24 hours because of the risk of life-threatening arrhythmias, such as ventricular fibrillation, and the need for skilled staff to monitor the effects of thrombolyic therapy.

Practice application – discharge home after a myocardial infarction

During phase 1 of cardiac rehabilitation the patients and their family members should be given time to talk to a specialist nurse about CHD and its management. Verbal information, supplemented with written material, is a useful strategy. Discharge planning should include a discussion of when patients should return to work, to driving and to any forms of exercise. This information should be tailored to the needs of the individual patient and so should be given by a specialist nurse who works in cardiac rehabilitation. Successful discharge depends on addressing the following:

- Assessment of physical, psychological and social needs;
- Smoking – advice on smoking cessation, clinics and nicotine replacement patches;
- Dietary advice – to promote healthy eating and reducing obesity (refer to a dietician if necessary);
- Alcohol consumption – limit consumption to 2 units of alcohol/day;
- Employment issues – may need to consider strategies to reduce stress or a change in employment;
- Physical activity – may need to consider strategies to increase physical activity;
- Sexual activity – advice regarding the resumption of sexual activity;
- Education about medication;
- Rehabilitation – referral to a programme of cardiac rehabilitation and details of this;
- Telephone helpline number and nurse-initiated telephone follow-up;
- Information on cardiac support groups.

HEART FAILURE

Heart failure can be categorized as either acute heart failure, such as that caused by cardiogenic shock after MI ($\Rightarrow$ Shock), or chronic heart failure in which deteriorating cardiac function occurs over a longer period of time.

The causes of chronic heart failure include CHD and MI, hypertension, valvular heart disease, cardiomyopathy, congenital heart disease and alcohol or drug misuse.

The heart is unable to maintain a cardiac output sufficient to perfuse the tissues and cells. Blood pressure is low and the pulse rate is likely to be raised and may well be irregular.

Most cases of heart failure result from left-sided failure. If the left side of the heart is not pumping well, the left ventricle starts to dilate to accommodate the increased blood volume. In time, this leads to back pressure in the lungs and fluid accumulates in the alveoli (pulmonary oedema). ⇒ Pulmonary oedema.

Right-sided heart failure existing in isolation is likely to be associated with a chronic lung condition that has placed excessive strain upon the right ventricle, for example cystic fibrosis or chronic obstructive pulmonary disease (COPD). Most forms of congenital heart disease also place a strain on the right side of the heart and may result in right-sided heart failure.

A combination of both right- and left-sided heart failure is termed congestive heart (cardiac) failure.

Medical treatment of heart failure includes:
- Diuretics, such as furosemide or spironolactone ⇒ Diuretics;
- Angiotensin-converting enzyme (ACE) inhibitors, such as captopril;
- Digoxin (positive inotrope) ⇒ Glycosides, Inotropes;
- Beta-blockers (negative inotropes), such as carvedilol;
- Vasodilators, such as nitrates, can be used to improve cardiac output. Arterial dilation may be used to reduce the work of the heart. Hydralazine (vasodilator) and amlodipine (calcium-channel blocker) are the more commonly used drugs for this purpose.

Revascularization of the myocardium through PTCA or CABG may be considered. Additionally, some patients may be offered other treatment options. ⇒ Heart (left ventricular assist device, heart transplantation).

Practice application – reducing salt intake in heart failure

As a high intravascular sodium level leads to water retention, limiting salt (sodium chloride) intake in food or cooking can also reduce oedema. Salt intake should be reduced to about 2–3 g/day and patients with heart failure should be referred to a dietician. Additionally, the nurse can encourage a low-salt diet through advice on how to shop and cook. For example, many convenience and sweet foods contain high levels of salt and are best avoided. Adding salt at the table or during cooking should also be avoided. In situations where partners shop and cook for the household, they should also be given information on how to avoid a high salt intake. Low-salt diets can be very bland, but spices and herbs can be used to flavour food in the absence of salt.

Further reading

Brooker C and Nicol M (2003). *Nursing Adults. The Practice of Caring*, Ch 19. Edinburgh: Mosby.
Department of Health (2000). *National Service Framework for Coronary Heart Disease. Modern Standards and Service Models*. London: Department of Health.

CORTICOSTEROIDS

Corticosteroids are three groups of steroid hormones produced by the adrenal cortex – glucocorticoids, mineralocorticoids and sex hormones. ⇒ Adrenal glands.

Synthetic corticosteroids, such as prednisolone and dexamethasone, are used for their anti-inflammatory and immunosuppressive properties (e.g. in asthma, inflammatory bowel disease, rheumatoid arthritis, some skin conditions or after transplant surgery). The benefits of therapy must always be weighed against the risk of serious side-effects associated with high doses and/or sustained use (*Fig. 51*).

C

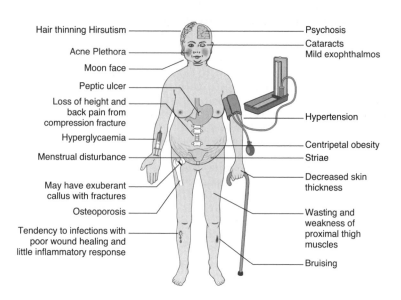

Hair thinning Hirsutism

Acne Plethora

Moon face

Peptic ulcer

Loss of height and back pain from compression fracture

Hyperglycaemia

Menstrual disturbance

May have exuberant callus with fractures

Osteoporosis

Tendency to infections with poor wound healing and little inflammatory response

Psychosis

Cataracts
Mild exophthalmos

Hypertension

Centripetal obesity

Striae

Decreased skin thickness

Wasting and weakness of proximal thigh muscles

Bruising

Fig 51 Adverse effects of corticosteroid therapy

Practice application – information for people taking corticosteroids ('steroids')
To avoid acute adrenal insufficiency individuals who have been taking steroid treatment (for any condition) for 3 weeks must be advised of the following:
- Do not stop taking the medicine suddenly – the dose should be reduced gradually;
- Read the patient information leaflet that comes with the medicine;
- Carry a steroid treatment card at all times, and show it to anyone who treats him or her;
- Wear a Medic-Alert bracelet (or similar);
- Contact the GP urgently if an illness develops or if contact with a person with an infectious illness occurs. If the individual has not had chicken pox, contact with people who have it, or shingles, should be avoided. If contact does occur, the person should contact their doctor immediately.

COUNCIL FOR THE REGULATION OF HEALTHCARE PROFESSIONALS

The Council for the Regulation of Healthcare Professionals (CRHP) is a recently established statutory body in the UK set up to oversee the regulation of health professionals. Its remit includes (CRHP 2003):
- Promoting the interests of the public and patients;
- Reporting to parliament and advising ministers;
- Promoting best practice in regulation, and developing principles of regulation;
- Promoting co-operation and consistency in the regulation of the different professional groups (currently nine regulatory bodies).

The CRHP can refer individual conduct decisions, concerning fitness to practise, to the High Court (England and Wales) or the Court of Session in Scotland if they are considered to be wrong or too lenient.

C

COUNSELLING

Counselling is a professional activity in its own right, and it may be more appropriate in the nursing context to think of nurses as using counselling *skills* rather than being counsellors to their patients. Each person brings his or her internal world and outward behaviour into a common space in which counselling work is carried out. This can happen only if the space is protected from intrusion or distraction and the two people engage with each other in a voluntary way. In the past, for nurses the word 'counselling' has been incorrectly linked to disciplinary procedures, and it is important to extract it from such a context and place it within the general framework of supportive one-to-one contact between people.

The basic aim of counselling is to help individuals help themselves. It is a process of consultation and discussion in which one individual listens and offers guidance or advice to another who is experiencing difficulties. The counsellor does not direct or make decisions for the client.

The goal of counselling is to enable people to be in touch with their own resources so that they can move towards greater freedom, autonomy and independence. It assumes that any conflict or anxiety that arises within the personal world of the individual can only be dealt with using the resources within that person. An individual may ask for help or advice from another person, but until such assistance is actually accepted, it cannot be used for self-help. ⇒ Communication, Empathy.

Further reading

Kenworthy N, Snowley G and Gilling C (2002). *Common Foundation Studies in Nursing*, Third Edition, Ch 9. Edinburgh: Churchill Livingstone.
Rogers C (1974). *On Becoming a Person*, Fourth Edition. London: Constable.

CRANIAL NERVES

⇒ Nervous system.

CREUTZFELDT–JAKOB DISEASE

Creutzfeld–Jakob disease (CJD) is a rare but well-known condition, especially the new form of variant CJD (vCJD). A form of CJD called sporadic CJD has been recognized for many years. Variant CJD shares some clinical features, but has different aetiological patterns.

Sporadic CJD is associated with older people and a rapid deterioration. It is found around the world and does not coexist in the same areas as endemic bovine spongiform encephalopathy (BSE), which is characteristic of vCJD.

Variant CJD is associated with a younger onset and a slower deterioration, although there is an overlap of the two forms. There may be a connection between BSE and vCJD as the two conditions overlap in geographical area, both are caused by a similar prion and the histological pattern is similar. The incidence in Britain is low and the incidence of vCJD is falling. CJD is caused by an abnormal deposition of abnormal prion protein in the brain. Prion proteins can cause other normal proteins to take on the prion form.

Patients with CJD have a variety of symptoms and signs associated with the parts of the brain first affected. Psychiatric symptoms may be present. In the later stages atrophy of the brain leads to dementia, sensory and motor failure and ultimately to death.

CRITICAL APPRAISAL

⇒ Evidence-based practice, Literature searching and review, Research.

CULTURE

The conceptual framework of culture encompasses dimensions such as human behaviour and the influences of knowledge and inheritance: the acquisition of ideas, values, customs, codes, rituals, taboos, language, ceremonies and other related cultural forces, such as spirituality and religion. The evolution of culture is contingent upon the human's innate potential to gain knowledge and to transfer his or her experiential learning to succeeding generations.

Although culture is often defined as a sociological concept, its role in behavioural science is recognized. For example, how a person communicates is influenced not only by social backgrounds and sociocultural beliefs (Béphage 2000), but these influences also determine the expression of psychological needs.

A prerequisite to good healthcare practice is considered to be able to recognize and be sensitive to clients' diverse sociocultural beliefs and practices. ⇒ Personal hygiene, Transcultural nursing.

CURRICULUM VITAE

Curriculum vitae (CV) is literally 'the course of one's life'. It is a summary of personal details, education, professional qualifications and attainment and employment experience.

Further reading

Brooker C (2002). *Churchill Livingstone's Dictionary of Nursing*, Eighteenth Edition, pp. 512–516. Edinburgh: Churchill Livingstone.

CYSTIC FIBROSIS

Cystic fibrosis is an autosomal recessive disorder caused by the mutated cystic fibrosis transmembrane regulator (CFTR) gene that affects the exocrine glands (especially those in the gastrointestinal tract, pancreas, goblet cells in the respiratory mucosa and sweat glands). The condition is particularly common in Caucasian populations, where it has a frequency of around 1 in 2500 live births; diagnosis may be confirmed by high levels of sodium in sweat (see Practice application). Meconium ileus, which causes intestinal obstruction in newborns, may occur. The affected glands have a faulty cell membrane ion (chloride and sodium) transport and produce viscous mucus, which leads to blocked, dilated ducts, stasis, infection and fibrosis. The lungs and pancreas are affected primarily, which gives rise to repeated chest infections, respiratory problems and cardiac failure and digestive problems that lead to malabsorption.

Current management centres upon physiotherapy, antimicrobial drugs and replacement of pancreatic enzymes, but advances in management include identification of the defective mutated gene, gene therapy, heart–lung transplants, antenatal testing and genetic counselling. ⇒ Genes and genetics (genetic diseases).

Practice application – sweat test
The sweat test measures the amount of sodium and chloride in sweat, and is used to confirm a diagnosis of cystic fibrosis. The drug pilocarpine is introduced into the skin by iontophoresis (by means of a constant electrical current) to stimulate the sweat glands and induce sweating. The sweat is collected and tested.

CYTOTOXIC CHEMOTHERAPY

Cytotoxic chemotherapy is used mainly to treat cancer. Cytotoxic drugs ultimately cause cancer cell death by altering DNA and preventing mitosis or by initiating the apoptotic response. They are classified, according to their precise action on the cell cycle, into cell cycle phase specific (CCPS) and cell cycle phase nonspecific (CCPNS) drugs. The CCPS drugs are only active at a particular point in the cell cycle, while CCPNS drugs operate anywhere in the cycle. ⇒ Cell (cell cycle).

Cytotoxic drugs are further classified into five groups according to their biochemical action. The drug groups are:

- Alkylating agents (CCPNS) act to form cross-linkages between the DNA strands (e.g. cyclophosphamide and busulfan);
- Antimetabolites (CCPS – S phase) block enzymes necessary for DNA synthesis (e.g. 5-fluorouracil and fludarabine);
- Anti-tumour antibiotics (CCPNS) primarily interfere with DNA function, but may also alter the cell membrane (e.g. bleomycin and epirubicin);
- Vinca-alkaloids and plant derivatives (CCPNS) interfere with DNA replication (e.g. etoposide and vincristine);
- Miscellaneous agents (CCPNS) work in a variety of ways to alter DNA structure and inhibit replication (e.g. asparaginase and irinotecan).

Cytotoxic drugs are available for administration orally, by injection (intravenous, intramuscular, intra-arterial) and directly into structures such as the bladder (intravesical). Chemotherapy is blood-borne and thus has the potential to treat both primary disease and metastases, which explains its use in a variety of clinical settings from acute to palliative care.

Cytotoxic drugs cause toxicity as a result of their nondiscriminatory action on rapidly dividing tissue. The systemic mode of administration results in widespread toxicity. Side-effects may be acute at the time of treatment, subacute (short term) 3–7 days after treatment or at least 1 week after treatment (long term). Not all patients experience all of the common toxicities (*Fig. 52*), since each drug has different actions and toxicities.

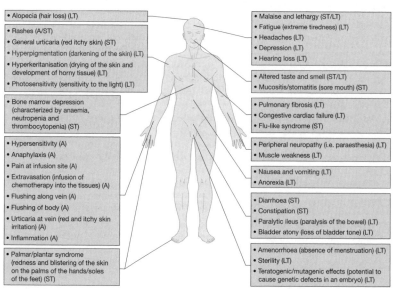

- Alopecia (hair loss) (LT)
- Rashes (A/ST)
- General urticaria (red itchy skin) (ST)
- Hyperpigmentation (darkening of the skin) (LT)
- Hyperkeritanisation (drying of the skin and development of horny tissue) (LT)
- Photosensitivity (sensitivity to the light) (LT)
- Bone marrow depression (characterized by anaemia, neutropenia and thrombocytopenia) (ST)
- Hypersensitivity (A)
- Anaphylaxis (A)
- Pain at infusion site (A)
- Extravasation (infusion of chemotherapy into the tissues) (A)
- Flushing along vein (A)
- Flushing of body (A)
- Urticaria at vein (red and itchy skin irritation) (A)
- Inflammation (A)
- Palmar/plantar syndrome (redness and blistering of the skin on the palms of the hands/soles of the feet) (ST)

- Malaise and lethargy (ST/LT)
- Fatigue (extreme tiredness) (LT)
- Headaches (LT)
- Depression (LT)
- Hearing loss (LT)
- Altered taste and smell (ST/LT)
- Mucositis/stomatitis (sore mouth) (ST)
- Pulmonary fibrosis (LT)
- Congestive cardiac failure (LT)
- Flu-like syndrome (ST)
- Peripheral neuropathy (i.e. paraesthesia) (LT)
- Muscle weakness (LT)
- Nausea and vomiting (LT)
- Anorexia (LT)
- Diarrhoea (ST)
- Constipation (ST)
- Paralytic ileus (paralysis of the bowel) (LT)
- Bladder atony (loss of bladder tone) (LT)
- Amenorrhoea (absence of menstruation) (LT)
- Sterility (LT)
- Teratogenic/mutagenic effects (potential to cause genetic defects in an embryo) (LT)

Fig 52 Effect of chemotherapy-associated toxicity (A, acute; ST, short term; LT, long term)

DATA

Data are pieces of information, usually collected for a specific purpose. In clinical nursing, data requested on the patient assessment form are collected at an initial interview with the patient. Other data are collected by ongoing assessment and evaluation. ⇒ Statistics.

Data collected at the initial interview are analysed, with the patient when possible, to identify the patient problems (actual or potential) being experienced in everyday living that are amenable to nursing intervention. The cause may or may not be the medical diagnosis.

Data can be collected through interviews, during which a structured form, such as a patient assessment form, may be used. In some circumstances an unstructured interview might be appropriate. The data are referred to as subjective or soft data. The nurse, as a skilled interviewer, prompts and reflects so that the patient describes his or her condition as factually as possible. The nurse records the information as factually as possible to decrease bias. Other data are the result of measurement (e.g. the amount of urine passed in 24 hours) and yet others are the result of tests (e.g. urinalysis), and these are called objective or hard data. ⇒ Confidentiality.

DATA PROTECTION ACTS (1994, 1998)

The Data Protection Acts set out the requirements that relate to the accuracy, security and access to information held electronically about individuals. Anyone who undertakes research that uses personal records held on a database is required to register under the Act with a local data protection officer. This measure helps to ensure that the data are being used for the purpose stated, and to maintain confidentiality and security of the system.

These Acts and subsequent Order allow the patient to have access to electronically stored data by giving sufficient notice in a required form. The Acts do not apply to manually kept records. ⇒ Access to health data.

DAY-CARE SURGERY

The criteria used to define the concept of day-care surgery are perhaps best provided by the Royal College of Surgeons (1992) guidelines. These describe day-care surgery as appropriate for the patient who is admitted for an operative procedure, who requires the facility for postoperative recovery and yet who does not require an overnight hospital stay. Also note that the term ambulatory surgery (the patient will walk in and walk out) is often used interchangeably with day-care surgery.

A number of minor operative procedures, however, are commonly performed as day cases. Hernia repair, dental extraction, minor gynaecological surgery and excision of skin lesions and lipoma are regularly carried out in day units, as are many endoscopic procedures, such as cystoscopy, bronchoscopy and gastroscopy.

There have been major technological advances in surgery and the development of minimally invasive techniques. Endoscopic equipment and ever-improving anaesthetic and pharmacological protocols have all provided impetus to the strategy to increase the number of patients who have day-care surgery. Part of the reason for the increase is that patients generally prefer it (see Practice application).

Practice application – benefits of day-care surgery for patients and health-care providers
- Reduced waiting list times;
- Increased numbers treated;
- Patients benefit from being able to go home;
- Reduced disruption to normal lifestyle;
- Fixed date for surgery;
- Greater patient control and improved psychological effects;
- Maintenance of personal privacy through going home.

There are also benefits to the healthcare provider, such as:
- In-patient beds are not required, which allows sicker patients access to care;
- Risk of cancellation because of bed shortages is no longer a direct issue;
- Direct referral from GPs and optometrists is increasingly common, thus avoiding the need for a consultant out-patient appointment.

Clearly, not all surgical procedures, nor indeed patients by virtue of their health status, are either eligible or suitable for day surgery. Most NHS trusts have local policies and protocols that determine patient suitability and access to day-care surgery.

All patients should be assessed for suitability using nonageist criteria. Both surgeon and anaesthetist must be in agreement on the choice of day care as a safe and appropriate environment for the patient. The American Society of Anesthesiologists (ASA, 1963) provides a framework that has been accepted as the most convenient, and consequently most commonly used, classification of physical health status. The classification is used in conjunction with broader considerations (*Box 9*), and a decision about suitability for day-care surgery is made.

Box 9 Issues likely to influence suitability and acceptance for day-care surgery
- Relatively fit and healthy (fulfils appropriate ASA criteria);
- Benefits the patient more than in-patient treatment would;
- No evidence of chronic health problem likely to affect recovery adversely, such as chronic obstructive pulmonary disease (COPD), cardiovascular disease and unstable diabetes;
- Length of procedure and amounts of anaesthetic required;
- The presence of appropriate social and home support;
- Patient acceptance;
- Surgical procedure unlikely to cause excessive bleeding, or postoperative pain, nausea and vomiting.

DEATH

Biological death is the irreversible cessation of vital functions usually assessed by the absence of heart beat and breathing. Mechanical ventilation may maintain vital functions even though the brainstem is fatally and irreversibly damaged. Consequently, stringent tests are necessary to diagnose death.

A death certificate is the official document issued by the registrar of deaths to relatives or other authorized person to allow disposal of the body. It is issued after a notification of probable cause of death is completed by the doctor in attendance upon the deceased or the appropriate documentation from the Coroner (England and Wales) or Procurator Fiscal (Scotland). ⇒ Gangrene, Mortality, Necrosis, Persistent vegetative state, Postmortem, Sudden infant death syndrome.

D

> **Practice application – end of life; meeting spiritual, religious and cultural needs**
>
> It is vitally important that health professionals be sensitive to the spiritual, cultural and any religious needs, and that these are discussed sensitively with the patient and family. Nurses may be asked to arrange visits from local religious leaders, provide privacy and opportunity for religious observance and create an environment conducive to the individual patient's spiritual needs.
>
> The importance that health professionals have an understanding, albeit superficial, of the religious beliefs and cultural traditions of their patients cannot be overstated. Nurses must also have a basic knowledge of the customs and taboos that surround death. The final thing nurses normally do for patients is to prepare the body for removal, but for some faiths to have a nurse of a different faith or gender perform the last offices causes great offence and distress to the family. It is essential to ascertain from the patient, family or wider religious community what they require during the final stages and beyond death.

Further reading

Neuberger J (1994). *Caring for Dying People of Different Faiths*, Second Edition. London: Mosby.

DECOMPRESSION SICKNESS

Decompression sickness results from sudden reduction in atmospheric pressure, as experienced by divers on return to the surface and aircrew who ascend to great heights. It is caused by bubbles of nitrogen released from solution in the blood, and the symptoms vary according to the site of these. The condition is largely preventable by the use of a proper and gradual decompression technique. It is variously described as the 'bends, chokes and creeps', depending on the symptomatology, but was originally called caisson disease when identified as a hazard for drivers. It was later recognized as a complication of high altitude.

DEEP VEIN THROMBOSIS

Deep vein thrombosis (DVT) is a thrombus that has formed in a deep vein, usually in the legs or pelvis. It is often a precursor of pulmonary embolism (PE), a potentially fatal condition.

The predisposing factors that cause DVT are venous stasis (slow blood flow), changes to blood coagulation and trauma affecting the veins. These three factors are known as Virchow's triad, but any factor may act in isolation to cause DVT, or they may act together.

Several other factors are associated with DVT, and certain groups of people are at high risk, including:

* Increasing age (>40 years);
* Obesity;
* Pregnancy and during the puerperium;
* Smoking;
* Previous DVT;
* Venous insufficiency and/or varicose veins.

Making a diagnosis from physical signs and symptoms is not always easy, as many patients have only minimal changes or no physical changes can be detected.

The signs and symptoms of DVT include:

- Localized pain or tenderness in the leg or calf (Homans' sign is positive when calf pain is experienced with the foot dorsiflexed);
- Swelling of the ankle, calf or thigh;
- Warmth and redness around the affected area;
- Pallor of the leg;
- Dilated distal veins.

The immediate treatment for DVT is anticoagulation using heparin. Some form of heparin is likely to be prescribed for 5–7 days and an oral anticoagulant, such as warfarin (or more rarely phenindione) is commenced at the same time. The activated partial prothrombin time (APPT) is used to monitor the level of anticoagulation when standard heparin is used and to make adjustments to the dose of warfarin., the aim being to maintain the international normalized ratio (INR) at 2.5 when warfarin is prescribed for DVT; the target INR is increased to 3.5 for recurrent DVT. Warfarin is continued for 3–6 months to dissolve the clot and help prevent recurrence. ⇒ Anticoagulants, Pulmonary embolism.

D

Practice application – prophylaxis for deep vein thrombosis

Prophylaxis for DVT is indicated for patients who are assessed as being at increased risk by virtue of having one of the three predisposing factors, or other factors (see above). This usually involves the use of graduated compression stockings (antiembolic stockings) and subcutaneous heparin, but the benefits of physiotherapy and early mobilization should be stressed. ⇒ Antiembolic.

Nurses have an important preventive role by assessing patients at risk of DVT and implementing the measures discussed above. Several risk scales are available, such as the Autar DVT risk assessment scale (Autar 1996).

Evidence is growing for a link between DVT risk and long-haul flights. The associated immobility, venous stasis, dehydration and reduced air pressure all contribute to the formation of a DVT. People who contemplate long flights should consider these risks and those with a history of thromboembolic conditions should be encouraged to seek medical advice. Passengers who undertake long flights should be advised to avoid dehydration by drinking plenty of nonalcoholic fluids, take regular exercise around the plane and perform foot and ankle exercises while sitting. Some experts suggest that compression stockings should be worn during long flights, but this has yet to be tested through large-scale randomized controlled trials.

Further reading

Wallis M and Autar R (2001). Deep vein thrombosis: clinical nursing management. *Nurs Stand*. **15**(18): 47–54.

DEFECATION

Defecation is the intermittent voiding per anus of faeces previously stored in the rectum. The large intestine propels the waste towards the rectum by strong peristaltic movements called mass movements, which are linked to the gastrocolic reflex and occur after meals. The rectum fills with faeces, which in turn initiates an urge to defecate.

As the rectum is distended by faeces (normally empty), the defecation reflex is initiated through the sacral part of the spinal cord. Impulses also travel to the cerebral cortex, which can inhibit the reflex until defecation is appropriate. As well as this inhibition we have voluntary control through the pudendal nerve and can keep the external anal sphincter closed. When defecation is appropriate the spinal reflex can proceed. Parasympathetic nerve activity causes the sigmoid colon and rectum to contract and relaxes the internal sphincter, and there is voluntary relaxation of the external sphincter (*Fig. 53*).

Defecation is aided by voluntary straining, which involves Valsalva's manoeuvre. The amount of straining required depends on faecal consistency – it is much easier to pass a soft bulky stool than one that is hard and constipated.

In infants defecation occurs as a reflex response to faeces in the rectum – voluntary control of the external anal sphincter is not achieved until the child is 18 months or older. Reflex defecation also occurs with sacral spinal cord lesions, after cerebrovascular accident or when the pudendal nerve is damaged.

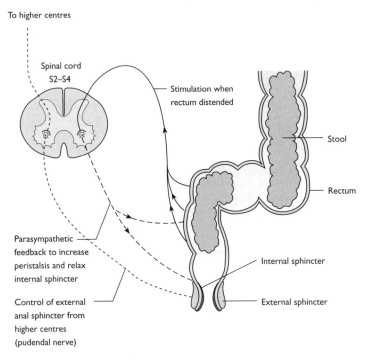

Fig 53 Mechanism of defecation

COMPOSITION OF FAECES

Faeces contain mainly water with some epithelial cells, mucus, bacteria, fibre or nonstarch polysaccharide (NSP), such as undigested cellulose residue, electrolytes, stercobilin, which colours normal stools, and various chemicals, which account for the characteristic odour.

ASSESSMENT OF FAECES

The assessment of faeces should include the type of stool and frequency. This can be aided by pictorial charts, such the Bristol Stool Chart, which grades stools on a scale from 1 to 7 with type 1 for separated hard lumps, like nuts (hard to pass), and type 7 for watery, no solid pieces, entirely liquid.

CONSTIPATION AND FAECAL IMPACTION

Constipation is common and is particularly so in people over the 65 years of age. The common definition of constipation is defecation less frequently than every third day (Wald 1994). However, some people believe daily defecation is normal and important to maintain health and for them any other pattern represents constipation. The diagnosis of constipation should be based on the criteria known as the 'Rome' criteria (Thompson *et al.* 1992):

- Straining for at least a quarter of the time;
- Lumpy and/or hard stools for at least a quarter of the time;
- A sensation of incomplete evacuation for at least a quarter of the time;
- Two or fewer bowel movements per week.

The causes of constipation are outlined in *Table 8*.

Table 8 Causes of constipation

Mechanism	Causes
Insufficient material in the bowel	Lack of fibre in the diet Poor fluid intake
Abnormal neurological control	Spinal nerve injury that affects the autonomic nervous system Hirschsprung's disease (a condition in which there is an absence of nerves in the wall of the bowel) Psychological factors, by an inhibitory effect on the autonomic innervation
Obstruction	Tumours Diverticular disease Haemorrhoids Congenital abnormalities
Pregnancy	High progesterone levels that cause a decrease in motility of the gastrointestinal tract
Metabolic	Diabetes mellitus Hypothyroidism Dehydration
Drugs	Aluminium (antacids) Anticholinergics Diuretics Iron Analgesia opioids Verapamil
Laxative misuse	Over-use of laxatives can cause damage to the nerves in the colon, which results in atonic bowel
Environmental	Anything that prevents defecation (e.g. lack of privacy, dirty toilets, insufficient toilets)
Immobility	Lack of exercise means the bowel itself is less active The client may have difficult reaching the toilet

Leakage of liquid faeces around an impacted mass of hard, constipated faeces may be mistaken for diarrhoea. Acute constipation may indicate obstruction or paralysis of the gut of sudden onset. ⇒ Incontinence (faecal incontinence).

LAXATIVES

Laxatives (also known as aperients) are drugs used to prevent or treat constipation. They may be given orally, or rectally as suppositories or an enema. They may be classified as:

- Bulking agents (e.g. methylcellulose) that retain water and form a soft bulky stool;
- Softeners (e.g. arachis oil enema) that lubricate or soften the faeces;
- Stimulants [e.g. docusate (also a softener), senna, sodium picosulfate, bisacodyl and gylcerin suppositories] that cause peristalsis by stimulating local nerves;
- Osmotic laxatives (e.g. lactulose, phosphate enemas) that increase fluid in the bowel lumen through osmosis;
- Combined softeners and stimulants (e.g. co-danthramer).

⇒ Enemas and suppositories.

DIARRHOEA

Diarrhoea is frequent loose stools that may, if prolonged or excessive, lead to dehydration, perianal soreness, hypokalaemia, acidosis (metabolic) and malabsorption. The causes include:

- Infection;
- Dietary change or indiscretion;
- Food sensitivity;
- Drugs (e.g. antibiotics);
- Laxative misuse;
- Anxiety;
- Irritable bowel syndrome;
- Inflammatory bowel disease;
- Colorectal cancer (alternating with constipation);
- Systemic diseases (e.g. hyperthyroidism).

ANTIDIARRHOEALS

Antidiarrhoeals are agents that relieve diarrhoea, such as loperamide and codeine phosphate, which are antimotility drugs. Bulking agents, such as methylcellulose (see above), may be used to treat diarrhoea in diverticular disease and to control the stool consistency in people with a stoma.

DEFENCE MECHANISMS

An individual is under constant attack from an enormous range of potentially harmful invaders, which include such diverse entities as bacteria, viruses, cancer cells, parasites and foreign (nonself) cells (e.g. in tissue transplant). The body therefore has developed a wide selection of protective measures, which can be divided into two categories:

- Nonspecific defence mechanisms that protect against any of an enormous range of possible dangers;
- Specific defence mechanisms, which are grouped together under the term *immunity*, and that direct the resistance against only one particular invader.

It is worth noting that normal defence mechanisms can become abnormally exaggerated, or fail to function. ⇒ Allergy, Immunocompromised (immunosuppressed) patient, Immunodeficiency.

NONSPECIFIC DEFENCE MECHANISMS

Nonspecific defence mechanisms are the first lines of general defence; they prevent entry and minimize further passage of microbes and other foreign material into the body.

DEFENCE AT BODY SURFACES

When skin and mucous membrane are intact and healthy they provide an efficient physical barrier to invading microbes. Intact skin also provides chemical and biological protection. The normally acid secretions form a chemical barrier ('acid mantle') that protects against some microbes. Both sebum and sweat contain antimicrobial substances. Biological protection is afforded by the normal bacterial flora of the skin and immune cells in the skin, which deal with microbes that penetrate the frontline defences.

Hairs in the nose act as a coarse filter and the sweeping action of cilia in the respiratory tract moves mucus and inhaled foreign materials towards the throat. It is then expectorated or swallowed.

The one-way flow of urine from the bladder minimizes the risk of microbes ascending through the urethra into the bladder.

PHAGOCYTOSIS

Phagocytic defence cells, such as macrophages and neutrophils, are attracted to sites of inflammation and infection by chemotaxis, in which chemicals are released by injured cells and invading microbes. Phagocytes are nonselective and trap, engulf and digest foreign cells or particles (*Fig. 54*). Macrophages have an important role as a link between the nonspecific and specific defence mechanisms. After dealing with an antigen, they act as *antigen-presenting cells* (APCs), by displaying the antigen to stimulate T-cells and activate the immune response (see below). ⇒ Leucocytes (monocytes).

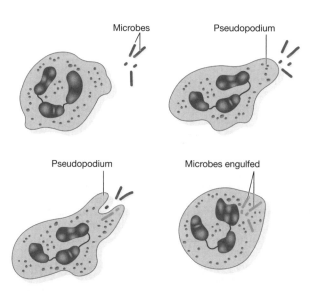

Fig 54 Phagocytic action of neutrophils

D

NATURAL ANTIMICROBIAL SUBSTANCES

Hydrochloric acid is present in high concentrations in gastric juice, and kills the majority of ingested microbes.

Lysozyme is an antibacterial chemical present in some leucocytes, tears and other body secretions. It is not present in sweat, urine and cerebrospinal fluid.

Antibodies are present in nasal secretions and saliva and are able to inactivate some microbes (see below).

Saliva washes away food debris that may serve as a culture medium for microbes. Its slightly acid reaction inhibits the growth of some microbes.

Interferons are substances produced by T-lymphocytes and by virus-infected cells. They prevent viral replication within cells and the spread of viruses to other cells.

Complement is a system of about 20 proteins found in the blood and tissues. It is activated by the presence of *immune complexes* (an antigen and antibody bound together) and by foreign sugars on bacterial cell walls. Complement:

- Helps to destroy microbes;
- Stimulates phagocytosis;
- Attracts phagocytic cells, such as neutrophils, into an area of infection.

INFLAMMATORY RESPONSE

The inflammatory response is the physiological response to tissue damage. Its purpose is protective, and it isolates, inactivates and removes both the causative agent and damaged tissue so that healing can take place.

The numerous causes of inflammation include:
- Micro-organisms;
- Physical agents, such as extremes of temperature, mechanical injury, ultraviolet and ionizing radiation;
- Chemical agents (e.g. acids, alkalis);
- Antigens that stimulate immunological responses.

The cardinal signs of inflammation are redness, heat, pain, swelling and loss of function.

The acute inflammatory response is described in the series of overlapping stages of increased blood flow, increased formation of tissue fluid and migration of leucocytes. A summary of events includes:
- Immediate, but short-lived, vasoconstriction.
- The release of inflammatory chemicals or mediators (e.g. histamine, etc.) by damaged tissue, mast cells and basophils, cytokines and complement activation. This leads to vasodilation and local hyperaemia as blood flow increases to the area.
- The release of inflammatory chemicals also increases capillary permeability with the exudation of fluid and proteins that leak from the blood to the tissues. The exudate brings extra supplies of oxygen, fuel and leucocytes, which helps to dilute any microbial toxins.
- Extra leucocytes – neutrophils initially, monocytes (which become macrophages) later and lymphocytes (where pathogens are involved) migrate to the inflamed area attracted by inflammatory chemicals and chemicals released by micro-organisms in a process called *positive chemotaxis*. Meanwhile, slower blood flow allows the leucocytes to marginate (move to the sides of the capillaries).
- The leucocytes stick to the capillary endothelium and move through the capillary wall to the damage zone by a process called *diapedesis*.

- Once the neutrophils, and later the macrophages, reach the damage zone they start to remove micro-organisms and damaged tissue by phagocytosis. Pus, if formed, is a mixture of dead leucocytes, tissue debris, micro-organisms and exudate. Phagocytosis is enhanced by the presence of antibodies (immunoglobulins) and complement.
- The last stage of the inflammatory response is for the macrophages to clear the debris, so that the processes of healing can proceed. ⇒ Wounds and wound care (wound healing).

SPECIFIC DEFENCES

The cell type involved in immunity is the lymphocyte. Once released into the bloodstream from the bone marrow, lymphocytes are divided into two functionally distinct cell types (T and B):
- T-cells mature in the thymus gland, where they are programmed to recognize only one type of antigen (anything that stimulates an immune response). Mature T-cells provide *cell-mediated immunity* (see below).
- B-cells mature in the bone marrow. Some B-cells differentiate into *plasma cells* that produce *antibodies* (immunoglobulins), which are proteins designed to bind to, and cause the destruction of, an antigen. As with T-cells, each B-cell targets one specific antigen; the antibody released reacts with one type of antigen and no other. B-cells provide *humoral immunity* (see below).

Although the two parts of the immune system are covered separately, it is important to stress their interdependence.

CELL-MEDIATED IMMUNITY

T-cells are released into the circulation. When they encounter their antigen for the first time, they become sensitized to it. If the antigen has come from outside the body, it needs to be 'presented' to the T-cell by an APC, for example, macrophages. Macrophages are part of the nonspecific defences, because they engulf and digest antigens indiscriminately, but they also participate in immune responses. If the antigen is an abnormal body cell, such as a cancer cell, it too displays foreign (non-self) material on its cell membrane that stimulates the T-cell. Whichever way the antigen is presented to the T-cell, it stimulates the division and proliferation (*clonal expansion*) of the T-cells. Several types of specialized T-cells are produced, each of which is still directed against the original antigen, but which will tackle it in different ways (*Table 9*).

HUMORAL (ANTIBODY-MEDIATED) IMMUNITY

B-cells, unlike T-cells (which are free to circulate around the body), are fixed in lymphoid tissue (e.g. the spleen and lymph nodes). B-cells, unlike T-cells, recognize and bind antigen particles without having to be presented with them by an APC. Once its antigen has been detected and bound, and with the help of a T-helper cell, the B-cell enlarges and begins to divide (clonal expansion). It produces two functionally distinct types of cell, *plasma cells* and *memory B-cells*.

Plasma cells secrete antibodies [immunoglobulins (Ig) of five classes (IgG, IgA, IgD, IgM and IgE)] into the blood. Plasma cells produce only one type of antibody, which targets the specific antigen that originally bound to the B-cell.

Antibodies:
- Bind to antigens, which labels them as targets for other defence cells, such as T-cytotoxic cells and macrophages;
- Neutralize bacterial toxins;
- Activate complement.

D

Memory B-cells remain in the body long after the initial episode has been dealt with, and rapidly respond to another encounter with the same antigen by stimulating the production of antibody-secreting plasma cells.

Table 9 T-cells

Type of T-cell	Mode of action	Role in cell-mediated immunity
Memory T-cells	These provide cell-mediated immunity by responding rapidly to another encounter with the same antigen	Provides immunological memory for cell-mediated immunity
T-cytotoxic or killer cells (CD8 cells)	These are activated by T-helper cells. These directly inactivate any cells that carry antigens. They attach themselves to the target cell and release powerful toxins, which are very effective because the two cells are so close together	The main role is in the destruction of abnormal body cells (e.g. virus-infected cells and cancer cells)
T-helper cells (CD4 cells)	These are essential for correct functioning of not only cell-mediated immunity, but also antibody-mediated immunity	Their central role in immunity is emphasized in situations in which they are destroyed, as by HIV. When T-helper numbers fall significantly, the whole immune system is compromised. T-helper cells are the most common of the T-cells; their main functions include:

1. production of special chemicals called *cytokines* (e.g. interleukins and interferons), which support and promote T-cytotoxic cells and macrophages

2. activate B-cells to produce antibodies, although B-lymphocytes are responsible for antibody manufacture, they need to be stimulated by T-helper cells first |

T-delayed hypersensitivity cell (CD4 cells)
Involved with macrophages and other T-cells in chronic inflammation and cell-mediated delayed hypersensitivity.

T-suppressor cells (CD8 cells)
Stop or slow the activity of B-cells and other T-cells once the immune response has dealt with the antigen. Normally keep the immune response within appropriate limits

ACQUIRED IMMUNITY

When antigens (e.g. microbes) are encountered for the first time there is a *primary response* in which a low level of antibodies can be detected in the blood after about 2 weeks. Although the response may be sufficient to combat the antigen, the antibody levels then fall, unless there is another encounter with the same antigen within a short period of time (2–4 weeks). The second encounter produces a *secondary response* in which there is a rapid response by memory B-cells, which results in a marked increase in antibody production. Further increases can be achieved by later encounters, but eventually a maximum is reached. This principle is used in active immunization against infectious diseases.

Immunity may be acquired *naturally* or *artificially* and both forms may be *active* or *passive* (*Fig. 55*). Active immunity means that the individual has responded to an antigen and produced antibodies, the lymphocytes are activated and the memory cells that form provide long-lasting resistance. In passive immunity the individual is given antibodies produced by someone else. The antibodies are then destroyed and, unless lymphocytes are stimulated, passive immunity is short-lived.

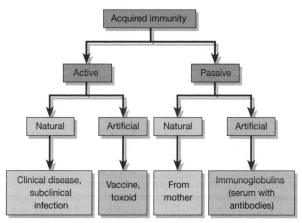

Fig 55 Summary of the types of acquired immunity

ACTIVE NATURALLY ACQUIRED IMMUNITY

Active naturally acquired immunity occurs when the body is stimulated to produce its own antibodies by having the disease or a subclinical (subliminal) infection.

ACTIVE ARTIFICIALLY ACQUIRED IMMUNITY – IMMUNIZATION

Active artificially acquired immunity develops in response to the administration of dead or live artificially weakened (attenuated) microbes (*vaccines*) or deactivated microbial toxins (*toxoids*). The vaccines and toxoids retain the antigenic properties that stimulate the development of immunity, but they cannot cause the disease. Many microbial diseases can be prevented by artificial immunization, such as measles, tetanus, poliomyelitis, etc. Active immunization against some infectious disorders confers lifelong immunity (e.g. diphtheria, whooping cough or mumps). In other infections the immunity may last for a number of years or for only a few weeks before revaccination is necessary. Apparent loss of immunity may result from infection with a different strain of the same microbe, which has different antigenic properties, but causes the same clinical illness (e.g. influenza virus).

Passive naturally acquired immunity

Passive immunity is acquired by the passage of maternal antibodies across the placenta to the fetus and to the baby in colostrum and breast milk. The variety of different antibodies provided depends on the mother's active immunity. The immunity is short-lived, but offers some protection until the infant's immune system matures and immunocompetence is achieved.

Passive artificially acquired immunity

In passive artificially acquired immunity, ready-made human antibodies are injected into the recipient. The source of the antibodies may be an individual who has recovered from the infection. Specific immunoglobulins may be administered *prophylactically* to prevent the development of disease in people who have been exposed to the infection, or *therapeutically* after the disease has developed.

Defibrillation

Defibrillation is the application of a direct current (DC) electric shock to the heart to restore normal cardiac rhythm using a defibrillator. Defibrillation is used to treat pulseless ventricular tachycardia (VT) or ventricular fibrillation (VF) during cardiac arrest.

Two paddles are placed on the chest wall, one on each side of the heart – one in the right upper sternum, mid-clavicular region, and the other at the fifth intercostal space, mid-axilla region. An electrical current of between 200 and 360 joules is delivered through the paddles. This causes all the myocardial cells to contract so that the sinus node can fire and the heart return to a sinus rhythm. As an electrical current is being used, strict safety measures are necessary. The paddles should only be charged once they are in position on the chest wall and all personnel should stand well clear of the patient or bed when the electric shock is delivered. Clearly, it is also important to ensure that there is no spillage of water, which could conduct the electric current, in the vicinity. ⇒ Advanced life support, Heart (Synchronized DC cardioversion).

IMPLANTABLE DEFIBRILLATOR

For people who have recurrent VT or VF, artificial implantable defibrillators (AICD) are used. The implantable defibrillator (also known as an internal cardioverter) can sense the heartbeat. If VT or VF is detected, the device fires a small electric shock to restore the rhythm to normal.

Deliberate self-harm

⇒ Suicide and deliberate self-harm

Delusions

A delusion is a belief that is held with absolute and compelling conviction, is not amenable to modification by experience or argument, is largely idiosyncratic, impossible, incredible or false and described clearly by the sufferer and not simply assented to after a leading question. The idiosyncratic nature of delusion beliefs helps to distinguish delusions from eccentric beliefs that are part of belonging to a particular religious, political or other social group (e.g. accounts of alien abduction).

Delusions are generally subclassified according to their basis in abnormal mood (e.g. delusions that concern sinfulness, catastrophe, guilt in severe depression and grandeur in mania). Such delusions are said to be 'mood congruent', in contrast to 'incongruent' delusions that have no such basis and are thought to be more typical of schizophrenia.

Some commonly encountered delusions include:

- Delusions of *reference*, in which sufferers are convinced that people are saying things with a double meaning, or that items in newspapers, on TV or in advertisements refer to themselves and that people are tracking them, spying on them or checking up on them in some way;
- In delusions of *misidentification*, innocent bystanders seem to be members of the Mafia or the secret police, doctors and nurses are impostors, and even family or friends have been replaced by lookalikes (*Capgras syndrome*);
- Perhaps the most commonly encountered are delusions of *persecution* that involve someone or some organization on a campaign to harm, defame or destroy the sufferer.

Other fairly common delusions include *grandiose identity* (beliefs that the sufferer is of royal blood, Christ, etc.) or *grandiose ability* (e.g. chosen for a special mission in life, a genius, etc.), as well as *guilt, catastrophe, depersonalization* and *hypochondriacal* delusions.

Some delusions appear as primary experiences in themselves. Their content cannot be explained by other delusions and seem to arise from some very ordinary perception. For example, it has been known for a patient to have a sudden insight that he was God when a traffic light turned from amber to green. These experiences are called 'primary delusions' and are thought to be strongly suggestive of schizophrenia. They sometimes occur after a period of perplexity in which the sufferer is vaguely aware that something strange is going on – familiar surroundings seem changed in some way, and there is an ominous or threatening atmosphere (*delusional mood*). ⇒ Hallucinations.

DEMENTIA

The word dementia, which means 'madness' or 'insanity', is a label applied to a number of diseases that lead, not to madness, but to progressive loss of cognitive function (Watson 1993). Such diseases include Alzheimer's disease (see below), Lewy body disease, Pick's disease and cerebrovascular (multi-infarct) dementia. While dementia is certainly not an inevitable consequence of ageing, there is an association between ageing and dementia such that it is more common in older age groups.

Being progressive, dementia is mild in its early stages, with small lapses of memory being ascribed by the individual sufferer and significant others (friends and family) to the effects of ageing. However, the memory loss eventually begins to have a significant negative impact on sufferers and those close to them. Subtle personality changes may take place, as well as noticeable changes in behaviour.

A most distressing aspect for family members is that dementia sufferers may forget who they are and may become hostile or aggressive towards people who were once familiar. Other aspects of this middle stage of dementia may include loss of social (including sexual) inhibition, which leads to embarrassing situations for those around the sufferers. Wandering may be a feature of dementia while the sufferers are still active, which may result in dangerous situations, becoming lost, 'turning night into day' by being up all night wandering around the house and engaging in repetitive behaviour. Clearly, this is exhausting and anxiety provoking for those who live with them, and other aspects (e.g. excessive eating and incontinence) may have significant adverse economic and social implications.

Following on from the early and middle stages of dementia described above, there is a late-stage dementia that leads to a very high level of physical dependency and may require the individual to be taken into institutional care. ⇒ Ageing (Practice Application – Clifton Assessment Procedures for the Elderly), Confusion and delirium, Memory (age-associated memory impairment).

D

ALZHEIMER'S DISEASE

Alzheimer's disease is seen mainly in older people, but it can affect younger adults as well. It is characterized by memory loss, behavioural changes (such as aggression) or wandering. Mood changes and depression may occur and eventually loss of control over voluntary movement. Dementia occurs in later stages.

Histological changes in the brain include plaques that consist of damaged cells and abnormal proteins, such as amyloid precursor protein, which gives rise to beta-amyloid fragments. The beta-amyloid fragments appear to cause most of the loss of neuronal function. Alzheimer's disease is also characterized by neurofibrillary tangles in the neurons. Later, a marked atrophy of brain tissue occurs.

The aetiology is unknown, although genetic links or a history of brain injury may be implicated in some cases. Environmental factors and viruses have all been suggested as causes, but no evidence has been found to corroborate these suggestions.

Drugs that may help to maintain function in the earlier stages of Alzheimer's disease include donepezil hydrochloride, rivastigmine and galantamine. They inhibit acetylcholinesterase, the enzyme that breaks down the neurotransmitter acetylcholine (which is depleted in Alzheimer's disease), and in addition galantamine is a nicotinic receptor agonist. They may also increase the amount of acetylcholine in the brain. These drugs are not suitable for all patients with Alzheimer's disease and the National Institute for Clinical Excellence (NICE) recommends that they normally be used for patients with a Mini-Mental State Examination score above 12 points and that certain other conditions are met, such as that the diagnosis of Alzheimer's is made in a specialist clinic and the views of the carers are sought (NICE 2001).

Practice application – caring for people with Alzheimer's disease and their families

The care of people with Alzheimer's disease depends on the stage of the illness. In the early stages, people are aware of the changes, which can be very frustrating and frightening. In the later stages, they may become dependent on carers for every aspect of care.

Key points are as follows:

* Support the sufferers and family members with information and practical help;
* Try to maintain active participation of both sufferers and carers;
* Stimulating activities, such as games and creative pastimes, or reminiscence increase sufferer confidence and may help to preserve some functions;
* Carers frequently find the behavioural changes very difficult to cope with – support, contact with self-help groups and respite care may help;
* Plan care to minimize confrontation in behavioural challenges – do not argue with or reprimand sufferers, but find a distracting activity instead;
* Maintain sufferers' dignity by treating them as adults;
* Plan care to help sufferers with activities that can no longer be performed, but maximize self-care where possible.

Resource

Alzheimer's Society – http://www.alzheimers.org.uk

DEMOGRAPHY

Demography is the study of population. Demographic indices include age distribution, birth and mortality rates, occupation and geographical distribution. They are used to obtain a profile of a given population, compare different areas and to plan services. For example, knowing that there are more people over retirement age in a particular geographical area allows the relevant NHS Trusts and Social Services Departments to plan appropriate interventions and services for an ageing population.

DENTITION

The natural teeth collectively in an individual. ⇒ Teeth.

DEOXYRIBONUCLEIC ACID (DNA)

⇒ Nucleic acids.

DEPERSONALIZATION AND DEREALIZATION

Depersonalization and derealization are sensory distortions that occur where anxiety, depressed mood, schizophrenia or temporal lobe epilepsy are featured, as well as in individuals who do not have mental health problems. Depersonalization is the term utilized to describe the individual's feelings of lost personal identity, of being 'different', changed or strange and unreal. Depressed individuals may describe the feeling as 'if in a dream' or 'like an automaton'. Mild depersonalization can occur in states of physical and mental fatigue.

Derealization relates to similar feelings about one's environment, and the two may be seen to coexist frequently. ⇒ Delusions, Hallucinations.

DEPRESSION

⇒ Disorders of mood.

DIABETES MELLITUS

Diabetes mellitus (hereafter referred to as diabetes) is the general term used to describe a group of diseases characterized by hyperglycaemia (a high blood glucose level). Diabetes results from defects in insulin secretion or insulin action, or both, which affect the metabolism of carbohydrates, proteins and fats. ⇒ Pancreas.

The diagnosis of diabetes is based on the symptoms and venous plasma glucose results. In the symptomatic individual a random venous plasma glucose result >11.1 mmol/L is indicative of diabetes. In those without symptoms two fasting venous plasma glucose samples must be taken, on different days; results >7 mmol/L indicate diabetes. ⇒ Blood glucose profiles.

An oral glucose tolerance test (OGTT) may be performed instead. ⇒ Glucose (Practice application – oral glucose tolerance test).

Diabetes may be classified as *Type 1* or *Type 2*. *Type 1* is caused by autoimmune destruction of insulin-producing cells in the pancreatic islets, and if uncontrolled leads to ketoacidosis. *Type 2* results from varying degrees of insulin resistance, often caused by obesity and impaired insulin secretion, and if uncontrolled leads to hyperosmolar nonketotic hyperglycaemia (HONKH). Type 2 may also be *secondary* to other diseases (e.g. pancreatitis, Cushing's syndrome, haemochromatosis), *genetic* [e.g. maturity onset diabetes of the young (MODY), mitochondrial diabetes] or *gestational diabetes* diagnosed in pregnancy, which usually resolves afterwards, when it reflects the increased burden placed on the pancreatic beta cells by hormone changes in later pregnancy.

D

PRESENTATION AND MANAGEMENT OF DIABETES

TYPE 1

The onset is usually very rapid, occurring over days or weeks. Individuals usually present with a history of polyuria, polydipsia, lethargy and weight loss. They may have minor infections, such as oral candidiasis (thrush), pruritus vulvae, balanitis or boils. Some individuals present with diabetic ketoacidosis (DKA). The medical management of Type 1 diabetes is always treatment with dietary therapy and insulin (see below).

TYPE 2

The symptoms of Type 2 diabetes are the same as those in Type 1 diabetes, although the onset is slow in comparison. However, people with Type 2 diabetes are resistant to ketosis. Weight loss can be a feature of Type 2 diabetes, but it is not extreme and, indeed, may go unnoticed.

Most people with newly diagnosed Type 2 diabetes are overweight. They may be aware of symptoms of hyperglycaemia (lethargy, polyuria and polydipsia), but may deny these or have attributed them in the past to increasing age. Many are identified via opportunistic screening. Very occasionally people with newly diagnosed Type 2 diabetes may present with HONKH.

People with Type 2 diabetes may be treated with:

- Diet alone;
- Diet and oral hypoglycaemic agents (OHAs, see below);
- Diet and insulin;
- A combination of all three regimens, although this is not very common.

INSULIN THERAPY

Insulin can be extracted for commercial use from the pancreases of cattle (bovine) and pigs (porcine). Human insulin is bioengineered, some by modifying porcine insulin, but most is produced by recombinant DNA technology.

Types of insulin:

- Short-acting insulins – soluble insulins that are clear in appearance and have a short duration; they start to be absorbed 20–30 minutes after injection and peak between 1.5 and 4 hours after injection. The duration of these insulins is approximately 6–8 hours post-injection.
- Analogue insulins ('designer') – alterations to the structure enable immediate absorption after injection. This allows people to have a flexible regimen as it enables them to inject immediately before eating or, indeed, up to 15 minutes afterwards. The peak absorption is 0.5–2 hours post-injection and the duration is about 5 hours.
- Intermediate insulins – isophane insulins are insoluble suspensions of insulin combined with protamine, which delays the absorption of the insulin. Isophane insulins start to be absorbed about 1 hour after injection; their peak is between approximately 2 and 12 hours, depending on the specific insulin used, and the duration is between 18 and 24 hours, again depending on the specific insulin. Lente insulins (with added zinc ions) tend to start being absorbed later than the isophane insulins, at about 2 hours after injection, but peak at similar times and have approximately the same duration.
- Long-acting insulins – ultralente insulins are very long acting; they start to be absorbed 2–4 hours after injection, their peak is between 4 and 24 hours and they last up to 28 hours after injection.
- Biphasic or 'mixed' insulins are a combination of soluble and isophane insulins in varying proportions.

All types of insulin are supplied in one strength, 100 units/mL. Insulin may be administered using an insulin syringe and needle, a preloaded insulin device, a reusable insulin pen or an insulin doser (*Fig. 56*).

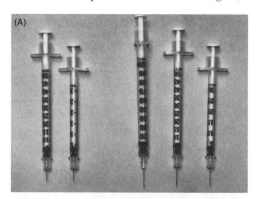

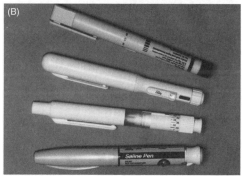

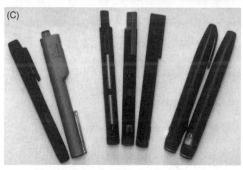

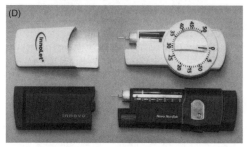

Fig 56 Insulin administration equipment: (A) insulin syringes; (B) insulin devices (preloaded); (C) reusable insulin pens, (D) insulin dosers

Insulin is injected subcutaneously and may be injected into the upper outer arms, the abdomen, the upper outer thighs or the buttocks (*Fig. 57*).

All subcutaneous injections of insulin should be delivered at 90° to the skin surface, whatever the length of the needle (8 mm, 12.7 mm). To ensure that it is delivered into the subcutaneous tissue, rather than muscle, raising a skin fold is necessary for most individuals at most injection sites (apart from the buttocks). In the past subcutaneous injections were delivered at 45° to the skin; this practice should not occur when using modern insulin needles.

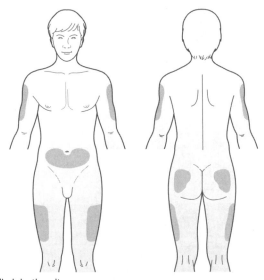

Fig 57 Insulin injection sites

ORAL HYPOGLYCAEMIC AGENTS

As many as 50% of people with Type 2 diabetes need to take oral therapy to help control their blood glucose levels. Types of OHA are:

- Sulphonylureas (e.g. glibenclamide, gliclazide);
- Biguanides – metformin is the only biguanide available in the UK;
- Alpha glucosidase inhibitors – acarbose is the only example currently available in the UK;
- Meglitinides – the only meglitinide currently available is repaglinide;
- Amino acid derivatives – nateglinide is the only available amino acid derivative.

ACUTE COMPLICATIONS OF DIABETES

HYPOGLYCAEMIA

Hypoglycaemia (a low blood glucose level) occurs in people with diabetes treated with insulin or sulphonylureas. It is not, however, a feature of Type 2 diabetes treated with diet alone. The underlying causes of hypoglycaemia are usually:

- Unexpected activity, e.g. gardening;
- Missed or delayed meals;
- Excessive alcohol intake;
- Excess insulin;
- Long duration of diabetes.

Those having a mild hypoglycaemic episode (hypo) most commonly appear pale and sweaty and may have a fine tremor. There is commonly a 'glassy-eyed' appearance also. Each individual is likely to experience the same symptoms with each episode of hypoglycaemia, although these may change over a period of years.

Individuals experiencing a moderate hypo may appear as if they are drunk. They often have slurred speech, an uncoordinated gait and may be verbally and physically aggressive. Those experiencing a severe hypo will be unconscious and may be having a seizure.

D

Practice application – dealing with 'hypos'
- Mild hypos should be treated initially with 10 g of oral glucose (e.g. dextrosol). If glucose is not available, anything that contains sucrose may be used as an alternative.
- Moderately severe hypos may be treated in the same way if the individual is able to swallow. Many people carry Hypostop, a clear gel that contains glucose; it is packaged in a tube, which is easily transportable and opened.
- Oral glucose of any kind must not be given to people with severe hypoglycaemia until they have regained consciousness. This is vital to protect the airway and prevent fluids and/or food entering the respiratory tract. Glucagon may be given. It must be given by injection, which can be subcutaneous, intramuscular or even intravenous (not frequently given i.v.).
- Individuals must always be given a meal after glucagon administration, as the hormone stimulates the release of all the glycogen stored in the liver.
- Severe hypoglycaemia may also be treated with intravenous glucose.

DIABETIC KETOACIDOSIS

Diabetic ketoacidosis (DKA) is an uncommon acute complication of diabetes, which usually involves people with Type 1 diabetes. It occasionally affects people with Type 2 diabetes at times of acute physiological stress and during serious intercurrent illnesses, such as myocardial infarction or cerebrovascular events.

It is caused by an absolute or relative insulin deficiency. The result is:
- Hyperglycaemia, which can be extreme (>13 mmol/L);
- Polyuria and glycosuria, polydipsia;
- Dehydration and loss of the electrolytes sodium and potassium;
- Electrolyte imbalance;
- Hypovolaemia and shock;
- Metabolic acidosis (as ketones are weak acids).

The priority in managing DKA is to rectify the fluid and electrolyte losses and to treat the insulin deficiency. Local protocols may differ slightly and so should always be checked.

LONG-TERM COMPLICATIONS OF DIABETES

In general the long-term, or chronic, complications of diabetes are categorized into micro- and macrovascular categories. Microvascular complications, as the name suggests, affect small blood vessels and nerves. Retinopathy, which affects the retina in the eye, and nephropathy, which affects renal function and neuropathy (sensory, motor or autonomic nerve damage) are included in this category. Macrovascular complications affect large blood vessels and include ischaemic heart disease, cerebrovascular events and peripheral vascular disease. ⇒ Eye (diabetic retinopathy), Coronary heart disease, Nervous system (cerebrovascular accident), Peripheral vascular disease, Urinary system (diabetic nephropathy).

Further reading

Brooker C and Nicol M (2003). *Nursing Adults The Practice of Caring*, pp. 403–428. Edinburgh: Mosby.

Resources

Diabetes UK – http://www.diabetes.org.uk

DIALYSIS

Dialysis is a process by which solutes are removed from solution by diffusion across a porous membrane; it requires the presence of a favourable solute gradient. ⇒ Renal failure (renal replacement therapies), Urinary system.

DIETETICS

Dietetics is the study, interpretation and application of the scientific principles of nutrition to maintain health and manage illness.

DIETICIAN

A dietician is a person qualified in the principles of nutrition and dietetics. Dieticians work in a variety of settings, including the community, hospitals, schools, institutions (e.g. residential homes), retail food outlets (e.g. shops), restaurants and hotels, large employers (e.g. local authorities) and in the food processing industry. ⇒ Malnutrition, Nutrition.

DIETARY REFERENCE VALUES

Nutritional requirement is the amount of a specific nutrient (macro- and micronutrient) required by an individual to reduce the risk of diet-related disease and maintain health. These differ for different individuals depending on age, gender, activity and physiological status. In the UK nutritional requirements have been estimated for different groups of the population and have been published as tables of *Dietary Reference Values* (DRV; Department of Health 1991a).

Three different values (see below) are usually given for populations of healthy individuals with no metabolic abnormalities. When referring to these values it is important to ensure they are applied to the correct population group. The use of these values replaces the recommended daily allowances (RDAs).

ESTIMATED AVERAGE REQUIREMENT

Estimated average requirement (EAR) is an estimate of the average requirement of a group of people. This means that 50% of the group actually requires more and 50% actually requires less. The EAR is usually used to estimate energy requirement.

REFERENCE NUTRIENT INTAKE

Reference nutrient intake (RNI) is the amount of nutrient required to ensure that the needs of most of the group (97.5%) are met. RNI is commonly used as an estimate of the micronutrient requirement of a population.

LOWER REFERENCE NUTRIENT INTAKE

Lower reference nutrient intake (LRNI) is the amount of nutrient sufficient for that small group of the population (2.5%) who have a low requirement.

Disability

Disability is frequently associated with chronic illness. Disability is an emotive and controversial term. For many years WHO's International Classification of Disease Impairment and Handicap (ICDIH) system provided a standard definition of disability as an inability to function at the level an individual might reasonably expect (WHO 1980). Disability is contrasted with impairment, which is a pathophysiological condition, and handicap, the social disadvantages that occur consequent to the impairment or disability.

However, the ICDIH classification has been criticized widely as focusing too much on impairment as the sole cause of disability and handicap at the neglect of the role society plays in causing disability and handicap (Oliver 1998). An alternative classification is offered by disabled people themselves, who have formulated the 'social model' of disability. The 'social model' is based on a simple dichotomy between impairment and disability (Oliver 1998). According to this approach, impairment neither directly causes nor justifies disability. Disability is regarded as a form of discrimination against the impaired. *Fig. 58* shows the contrast between these two definitions.

An example of the social causation of disability and handicap is the failure of many organizations to provide adequate access to places of work for those with sight or mobility problems. Even where impairment presents the individual with minimal obstacles, the stigma attached to many chronic diseases and disabilities can cause significant handicap. An obvious example is human immunodeficiency virus (HIV) infection whereby the individual can suffer significant handicap because of discrimination despite being physically unaffected by the virus. Stigma is attached to many other chronic diseases, including cancer and, in many cultures, tuberculosis.

A new classification, the *International Classification of Functioning Disability and Health* (ICF; WHO 2001), was devised recently, and takes into account some of the criticisms levelled by the social model. The separate classification of handicap is dispensed with. Disability is defined as a loss of function at the level of the individual that is caused by an interaction between personal factors (including impairment) and environmental factors (including discrimination; WHO 2001).

The value of this view of disability is that it draws attention away from 'cure' of the impairment as the only remedy for disability. This is as relevant to those whose disability is caused by chronic illness as to those whose disability has been caused by accident or congenital conditions. For example, chronic illnesses that lead to mobility impairment would be far less disabling if wheelchair access to public transport and buildings were universal. The nurse who cares for those with disability must be mindful that disability is not simply caused by the person's impairment. Cure of the impairment is frequently impossible and not necessarily the most desirable strategy. However, this does not mean that disability is inevitable or not subject to improvement through nursing care. ⇒ Chronic (long-term) illness, Rehabilitation.

Resources

Disabled Living Foundation – http://www.dlf.org.uk
Equal Opportunities Commission – http://www.eoc.org.uk
Royal Association for Disability and Rehabilitation (RADAR) – http://www.radar.org.uk

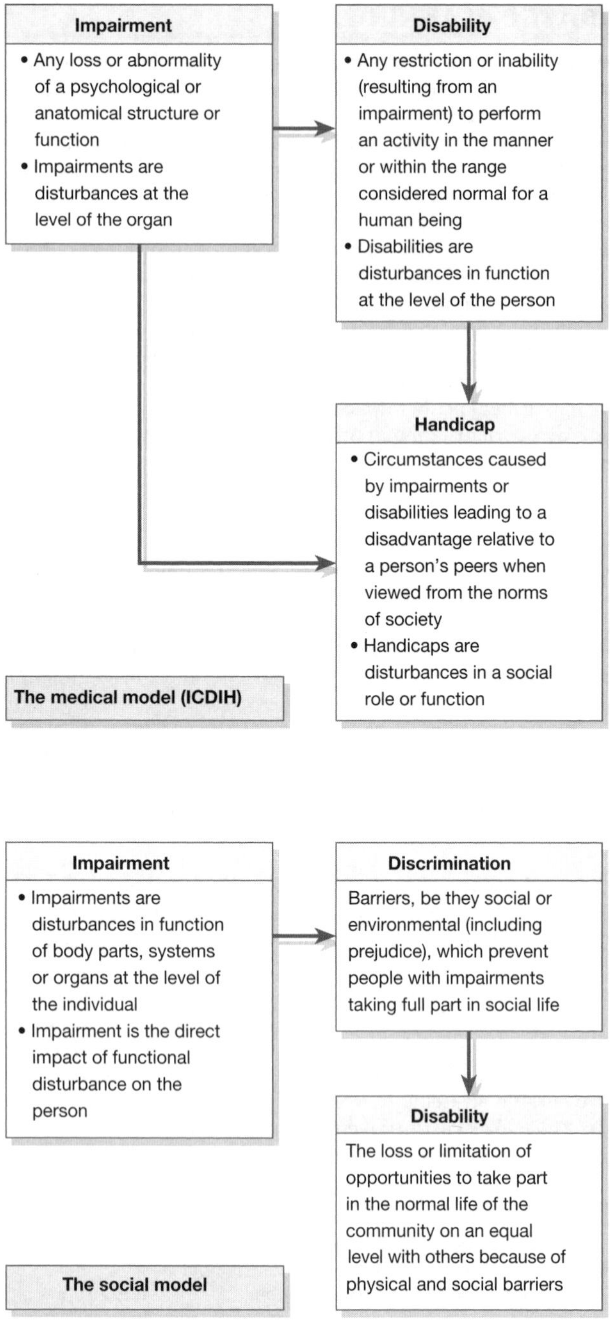

D

(A)

(B)

Fig 58 Contrasting definitions of disability (A) medical model (ICDIH), (B) social model

DISCHARGE PLANNING

A successful outcome for patients depends on high-quality, multidisciplinary discharge planning, particularly so with the increasing use of day-care surgery and planned early discharge from acute healthcare settings. The aim of successful discharge is to provide a seamless transition of care between the day-care or hospital unit and the community (Department of Health 2000a).

All hospitals have a discharge policy that is developed by, and agreed with, the appropriate stakeholders, including primary care and social services. In many cases, this may include a telephone follow-up or support service through which patients may seek clarification or advice on aspects of their care or concerns regarding postoperative discomforts.

The aims of quality discharge planning are to:
- Maximize self-care ability;
- Prepare patients (and family members and/or carers) physically and emotionally for discharge to a suitable environment;
- Provide appropriate verbal and written information to patients and family members;
- Ensure appropriate resources and facilities are in place to meet the individual requirements of patients;
- Promote a co-ordinated and seamless discharge through quality communication between the hospital unit and community to ensure continuity of care;
- Maintain quality record-keeping and documentation for professional accountability.

Practice application – preparation for discharge after surgery

Successful discharge planning should begin as soon as individuals enter the healthcare system. An early appreciation of patients' perceptions of their problem, the support systems available to them and their coping abilities is pivotal to identifying the resource requirements for discharge. Regardless of whether patients are undergoing a minor procedure in a day-care setting or the most complex of operations, early planning can significantly and positively influence successful recovery.

Inappropriate discharge has been highlighted as a major reason for patient readmission. Poor- and noncompliance with health information and medication are strongly linked to the quality of the discharge process.

Key educational aspects of a discharge plan
- General effects of surgery and/or anaesthesia (e.g. driving, etc., may be restricted, need for rest and sleep, etc.);
- Procedure-specific advice (e.g. wearing of antiembolic stockings, etc.);
- Specific exercise activity (e.g. pelvic floor strengthening, walking and leg exercises, etc.);
- Dietary and nutritional advice (e.g. fruit, vegetable and fluid consumption to prevent constipation, etc);
- Medication (e.g. dosage, action, side-effects, and special instruction verbally and in written form), such as for pain relief ⇒ Concordance;
- Postoperative complication potential (e.g. advice on the recognition of bleeding, infection, persistent pain, limb swelling, etc., and understanding of when to seek help is confirmed);
- Nurse- and self-administered treatment (e.g. information on dressing changes, care of operation site and suture/clip/staple removal, etc.);
- Continuing and follow-up care (e.g. contact details and documentation for community nurses, out-patient and follow-up appointment, etc.);

- Social support (e.g. confirm arrangements for transport home and home-based social support).

DISCRIMINATION

Discrimination describes the attitude to, and treatment of, a person solely on the grounds of prejudice towards a characteristic of the group to which the person belongs (e.g. gender, religious beliefs, age, sexual preference or skin colour). ⇒ Fair and antidiscriminatory practice.

DISEASE

Disease is any deviation from or interruption of the normal structure and function of any part of the body or mind. It is manifested by a characteristic set of signs and symptoms and in most instances the aetiology, pathology and prognosis are known. It can be acute or chronic. Loss of function that results from direct trauma, such as a fracture, is not generally considered to be a disease, although such an injury may lead to disease (e.g. secondary osteoarthritis).

DISEASE CLASSIFICATION

The *International Classification of Disease* (ICD) is a list of diseases compiled by the World Health Organization (Tenth Revision, ICD-10). For example, ICD-10 Chapter II is Neoplasms and Chapter V is Mental disorders. The chapters are further subdivided into several categories, so Chapter V has 11 categories, such as Mood (affective) disorders, etc.

In the mental health field there is a second classification system, the American Psychiatric Association's *Diagnostic and Statistical Manual* (Fourth Edition 1994), usually abbreviated to DSM-IV. The ICD-10 (WHO 1992) is the main system used in the UK. The DSM-IV is referred to frequently in psychiatric literature, although is not commonly used in clinical practice in the UK. Both classification systems use slightly different terms to describe broadly similar concepts.

DISEASE PREVENTION

Disease prevention reduces the risk of a disease process, illness, injury or disability. It includes preventive services (e.g. immunization and screening), preventive health education (e.g. advice about sensible drinking) and preventive health protection (e.g. taxing tobacco and fluoridating water). Preventive activities are classified as primary, secondary or tertiary prevention:
- Primary prevention (1°) includes all activities to eradicate the cause of disease or decrease the susceptibility of the individual to the causative agent (examples include smoking cessation advice and immunization programmes);
- Secondary prevention (2°) is the detection and treatment of disease before symptoms or disordered function develops (i.e. before irreversible damage occurs), generally achieved through screening (examples include cervical cytology screening and hypertension screening);
- Tertiary prevention (3°) is the monitoring and management of established disease to prevent the complications of the disease process, disability or handicap (e.g. monitoring of patients with diabetes to detect and treat early complications).

⇒ Communicable diseases, Health education, Health promotion.

DISINFECTION

Disinfection is the removal or destruction of harmful micro-organisms, but not usually bacterial spores. Disinfection is commonly achieved by using heat (e.g. pasteurization) or chemical disinfectants (e.g. hypochlorites).

Many disinfectants are too toxic or corrosive to use on living tissue and are only used for previously cleaned equipment (e.g. isopropanol 70% for trolleys and phenolics for environmental use).

Chemicals that can be applied safely to living tissues are used in hand decontamination and to prepare the skin prior to invasive procedures and surgery (e.g. 4% chlorhexidine, isopropanol, povidone iodine). ⇒ Antibiotics, Infection (handwashing).

DISORDERS OF MOOD

The concept of affective disorder owes its origins to Kraeplin, who introduced the category of 'manic-depressive psychosis'. More recently, a separation was proposed into a 'bipolar group' (depressed patients with a history of manic episodes) and a 'unipolar group' (patients with depressive episodes only). Cassano *et al.* (1994) noted that approximately 15–20% of individuals who suffered from psychotic depression fall within the bipolar disorder group and the remaining 80–85% within the unipolar group. There are therefore good reasons to distinguish between 'bipolar' disorder and severe depressive or psychotic disorder. It might be helpful to differentiate *severe* mood disorders from less severe and 'mixed' affective disorders and neurotic depression (*Table 10*). ⇒ Anxiety, Electroconvulsive therapy, Suicide and deliberate self-harm.

BIPOLAR AFFECTIVE DISORDER

Bipolar disorder is a recurrent, episodic, long-term illness that tends to have a number of negative effects for the sufferer, family members and society as a whole (Lish *et al.* 1994). The disorder can be divided into two distinct types, bipolar I and bipolar II. Manic episodes interspersed with depressive episodes are referred to as bipolar I, and depressive disorder with hypomania as bipolar II (Vieta *et al.* 1997).

The clinical features of mania are:
- Euphoria and/or irritability;
- Overactivity;
- Distractibility;
- Socially inappropriate behaviour;
- Reduced sleep;
- Increased appetite and libido;
- Flight of ideas;
- Expansive ideas;
- Grandiose delusions;
- Hallucinations; and
- Impaired insight.

PSYCHOTIC DEPRESSION

Psychotic depression (sometimes called severe depressive disorder) shares many features with neurotic depression, although obviously to a more severe degree. However, people with psychotic depression exhibit other features, including delusions. The main themes of such delusions are usually worthlessness, guilt, ill-health, poverty, nihilism and persecution. Sometimes auditory hallucinations (and rarely visual) also occur. It is possible to differentiate the nature of the delusional thinking as either mood congruent (delusion based on thoughts of guilt, ruin,

D

Table 10 The continuum of mood disorders

	'Mixed' anxiety and depressive disorder	'Mild to moderate' depression	Psychotic depression /bipolar disorders
Main presenting symptoms	Mixed anxiety and depression Good social functioning Often transient (<6 months) May be 'masked' by physical symptoms Onset often linked to ongoing social stress or 'loss' life event	Persistent lowered mood Sleep disturbance (usually initial insomnia) Reduced energy Impaired concentration Recurrent intrusive thoughts Reduced libido Social functioning may be affected Onset often linked to ongoing social stress or 'loss' life event	Persistent lowered (and/or periodically elevated) mood Sleep disturbance (usually early morning waking) Impaired concentration Reduced appetite (may be life threatening) Depressive delusional thinking Reduced libido Social functioning profoundly affected Relationship between onset and life events
Where likely to present	Primary health care	Specialist psychiatric out-patients	In-patient
Pharmacological treatments	Nothing Antidepressants (particularly SSRIs)	Antidepressants (preferably combined with CBT)	Antidepressants Antipsychotics ECT
Psychological treatments	Brief, focused counselling (providing a psychological model for distress) Self-help Education and/or information	CBT (combined with medication to prevent relapse) Relationship interventions (IPT- or EE-based) to improve quality of social support Self-help Education and/or information	Self-help Education and/or information 'Early signs' monitoring Self-management

CBT, cognitive behaviour therapy; ECT, electroconvulsive therapy; EE, expressed emotion; IPT, interpersonal therapy; SSRI, selective serotonin reuptake inhibitor.

misery and repentance) or incongruent (delusion based on ideas of persecution, influence from external forces and poisoning). Cassano *et al.* (1994) point out that many patients may be unaware of being ill. Loss of interest in eating (and sometimes drinking) can be a considerable problem and may be life-threatening, which requires early recognition and prompt action. ⇒ Delusions.

Diuretics

D

Diuretics are substances that increase the production of urine by the kidney (e.g. caffeine in tea, coffee, 'cola' and other drinks).

DIURETIC DRUGS

Carbonic anhydrase inhibitors

Carbonic anhydrase inhibitors are drugs used to reduce intraocular pressure in glaucoma by limiting the production of aqueous humour, rather than as diuretics (e.g. acetazolamide). They act at the proximal tubule (of the nephron) by preventing the reabsorption of bicarbonate (hydrogen carbonate), sodium, potassium and water, all of which increases urine production.

Loop diuretics

Loop diuretics act by preventing reabsorption of sodium, chloride and potassium in the thick segment of the ascending limb of the loop of Henle (of the nephron) by chloride-carrier inhibition. They include furosemide and bumetanide, and are used for hypertension, oedema and oliguria caused by renal failure. Concurrent therapy with potassium is required.

Osmotic diuretics

Osmotic diuretics are pharmacologically inert substances, such as mannitol (a sugar). They are given intravenously to reduce cerebral oedema or raised intraocular pressure in glaucoma or produce a diuresis after drug overdose. The diuresis occurs through the osmotic 'pull' created by the inert sugar (which is filtered by the kidney, but not reabsorbed) during its excretion.

Potassium-sparing diuretics

Potassium-sparing diuretics cause a diuresis without loss of potassium in the urine. They include spironolactone, which is an aldosterone antagonist and competes with its tubular receptor sites in the nephron, resulting in retention of potassium and increased excretion of water and sodium. It also potentiates the action of thiazide and loop diuretics. Other potassium-sparing diuretics include amiloride, which acts on the collecting ducts to reduce sodium reabsorption and potassium excretion by blocking the sodium channels through which aldosterone operates. They are used with potassium-losing diuretics and to treat the oedema of liver cirrhosis.

Thiazide diuretics

Thiazide diuretics, such as bendroflumethiazide, act upon the first part of the distal tubule (of the nephron). They reduce sodium and chloride reabsorption, which increases the excretion of water, sodium and chloride, and, in addition, potassium is lost and calcium conserved. They are used in hypertension, mild heart failure, oedema and in nephrogenic diabetes insipidus.

D

DOPPLER TECHNIQUE

Doppler technique can be used to measure the velocity of blood flow through a vessel to determine the degree of occlusion or stenosis. *Doppler ultrasound technique* is used in the assessment of leg ulcers. It is a noninvasive technique using a hand-held ultrasound probe that determines the volume of blood flow reaching the lower limbs (*Fig. 59*) ⇒ Leg ulcers (ankle brachial pressure index).

Doppler ultrasound technique can also be used to calculate cardiac output and stroke volume by measuring blood flow in the aorta via a probe passed into the oesophagus. It is used to monitor haemodynamic status and response to treatment in critical care situations. *Doppler scanning* combines ultrasonography with pulse echo.

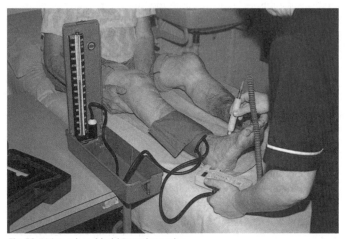

Fig 59 Using a hand-held Doppler probe

DRUG

Drug is the common name for any substance used for symptom control, or the prevention, diagnosis and treatment of disease. The word medicine is usually preferred for therapeutic drugs to distinguish them from the addictive drugs that are misused illegally.

A drug used to alleviate unpleasant symptoms of self-limiting illnesses that does not require a prescription is termed an 'over-the-counter' (OTC) medicine. In the UK these are drugs on the *general sales list* (GSL), such as mild analgesics, on sale to the public through a variety of retail outlets (e.g. supermarkets). There are controls in place regarding the number of tablets that may be purchased (e.g. packs that contain greater quantities may be sold by a pharmacy). *Pharmacy-only medicines* (P) are those drugs that may be purchased by the public from a pharmacy, but only when a qualified pharmacist is present.

Prescription-only medicines (POM) are those medicines that require a written prescription from a doctor or prescribing nurse, except in an emergency when it may be dispensed by a pharmacist, providing certain criteria are met. ⇒ Controlled drugs, Pharmacokinetics and pharmacodynamics, Polypharmacy.

ADVERSE DRUG REACTIONS

Adverse drug reactions (ADRs) are any unwanted drug effects. They range from minor side-effects through to harmful or seriously unpleasant effects. They can be classified into five groups:

- Type A, or augmented effects, are adverse effects that occur as a result of the drug's pharmacology (e.g. constipation caused by morphine);
- Type B, or bizarre effects, are unpredictable adverse effects that are not dose-related (e.g. hypersensitivity reactions to penicillin);
- Type C, or chronic effects, occur after prolonged drug usage (e.g. parkinsonism that occurs with phenothiazine antipsychotics);
- Type D, or delayed effects, occur years after the original drug therapy (e.g. cancers caused by the use of cytotoxic drugs);
- Type E, or ending-of-use effects, are adverse effects that occur when the drug is stopped suddenly (e.g. withdrawal effects, illustrated by delirium tremens that occurs when a person stops misusing alcohol).

YELLOW CARD REPORTING SCHEME

In the UK, there is a system whereby prescribers, and others, report suspected ADRs to the Committee on Safety of Medicines (CSM). The scheme has been operating for over 40 years, and recently has introduced electronic reporting alongside the original yellow cards. Pharmaceutical companies are obliged to report ADRs, whereas prescribers, nonprescribing nurses and pharmacists report on a voluntary basis. Patients are also encouraged to use the scheme to report any ADRs.

DRUG DEPENDENCE

Drug dependence is a state of physical or psychological dependence on a particular drug that arises from repeated administration of a drug on a periodic or continuous basis. It is also called drug addiction. ⇒ Substance misuse.

DRUG ERRORS

See Practice application – drug errors.

DRUG INTERACTION

Drug interaction occurs when the pharmacological action of one drug is affected by another drug, food or beverage taken previously or simultaneously.

DRUG REACTION

Drug reaction is an adverse or unexpected effect associated with the administration of a drug, such as a rash (see Adverse drug reactions above).

DRUG RESISTANCE

⇒ Antibiotics (antibiotic resistance).

DRUG TOLERANCE

In drug tolerance the therapeutic effects of a drug reduce over time, and so an increased dose is required.

D

Practice application – drug errors

Drug errors are preventable prescribing, dispensing or administration mistakes. As human error is inevitable, no matter how knowledgeable and careful healthcare workers are, a technique developed in industry known as 'failure mode and effects analysis' should be used to reduce errors (Cohen *et al*. 1994). This involves identifying mistakes that will happen before they happen, and determining whether the consequences of those mistakes are tolerable or intolerable. Where potential effects are unacceptable actions are taken to eliminate the possibility of error, trap error before it reaches a patient or minimize the consequences of the error when potential errors cannot be eliminated. For example, potassium chloride for injection in vials of 20 mmol per 20 mL has been involved in more fatal medication errors than any other drug (Davis 1995). Failure mode and effects analysis identifies the answer to this problem as removal of the possibility of error (i.e. remove potassium chloride for injection concentrate from ward environments and stock mini-bags of potassium chloride injection 20 mmol per 100 mL instead).

DUTY OF CARE

Duty of care is the legal obligation in the law of negligence that a person must take reasonable care to avoid causing harm. ⇒ Malpractice, Negligence.

DYSENTERY

Dysentery is inflammation of the bowel with evacuation of blood and mucus. accompanied by tenesmus and colic. ⇒ Communicable diseases (notifiable diseases).

AMOEBIC DYSENTERY (AMOEBIASIS)

Amoebic dysentery is an infestation of the large intestine by the protozoon *Entamoeba histolytica*, where it causes mucosal ulceration that leads to pain, diarrhoea alternating with constipation and blood and mucus passed rectally, hence the term 'amoebic dysentery'. If the amoebae enter the hepatic portal circulation they may cause a liver abscess. Diagnosis is by isolating the amoeba in the stools. Metronidazole is the usual treatment, but tinidazole is also used. Diloxanide furoate is used to treat chronic infections.

BACILLARY DYSENTERY

Bacillary dysentery is caused by Shigella, a genus of Gram-negative bacilli. Several species cause dysentery – *Sh. boydii*, *Sh. dysenteriae* and *Sh. flexneri* in tropical or subtropical areas. *Sh. sonnei* causes dysentery in temperate regions and is the most common type in the UK. The organism is excreted by cases and carriers in their faeces, and contaminates hands, food and water, from which new hosts become infected. It commonly affects young children and is spread by the faecal–oral route. Prevention of spread is through meticulous attention to personal hygiene. Treatment, where necessary, is with ciprofloxacin or trimethoprim. Mild cases may not require drug therapy.

DYSLEXIA

Dyslexia is a disorder that affects the ability to read. There are a number of different types of dyslexia, such as *surface dyslexia* and *deep dyslexia*, Many individuals with dyslexia may also exhibit dysgraphia, an acquired problem of written language caused by brain damage. The affected person's ability to spell familiar and/or unfamiliar words is altered in one or many modalities (handwriting, word-processing, etc.). A number of different types of dysgraphia are described.

DYSPHAGIA

Dysphagia is difficulty in swallowing. ⇒ Swallowing and problems with swallowing.

EAR

The ear is the sensory organ concerned with hearing and balance. It has three parts, the outer (external), middle (tympanic cavity) and inner (internal) ear. The outer ear comprises the auricle (pinna) and the external auditory canal (EAC), along which sound waves pass to vibrate the tympanic membrane (ear drum) that separates it from the middle ear. The middle ear cavity is air-filled and contains three tiny bones or ossicles (malleus, incus and stapes). The ossicles transmit the sound waves to the inner ear via the oval window. The middle ear communicates with the nasopharynx via the eustachian tube (pharyngotympanic tube). The fluid-filled inner ear comprises the cochlea (organ of hearing) and the semicircular canals, which are concerned with balance. The cochlea and semicircular canals contain the nerve endings of the cochlear and vestibular branches of the vestibulocochlear or auditory nerve (VIIIth cranial; *Fig. 60*).

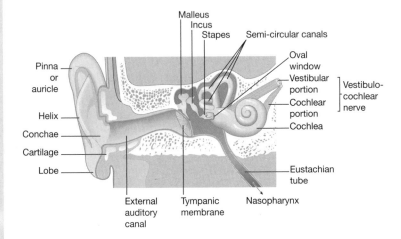

Fig 60 Anatomy of the ear

Practice application – examination of the ear using an otoscope

Ear examination should only be carried out by practitioners who have been appropriately taught and assessed as competent and who can document their findings.

The rule to follow is to begin the examination with the better hearing ear. It is essential to be able to distinguish the different areas of the drum and to be able to draw the features that are visible when examining a patient's ear. It is important to sit at the same level as the patient to ensure that all of the drum is visualized and the patient's safety maintained. A headlight is used during the ear examination (*Fig. 61*), and the tympanic membrane is examined using an otoscope (auriscope; *Fig. 62*). The otoscope has a white light and allows for magnification of the area being viewed.

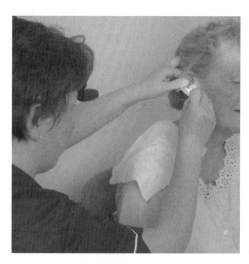

Fig 61 Carrying out an ear examination using a headlight

E

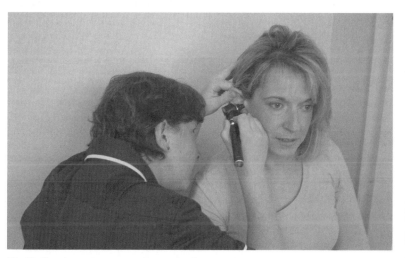

Fig 62 Carrying out an otoscopic examination

EAR DISORDERS

Some ear disorders are outlined below. ⇒ Hearing (hearing assessment, hearing impairment).

ACUTE LABYRINTHITIS

Acute labyrinthitis is an inflammatory and/or infective process that affects the labyrinth of the inner ear. It leads to vertigo.

ACUTE SUPPURATIVE OTITIS MEDIA

Acute suppurative otitis media (ASOM) is an acute infection of the middle ear.

E

CHRONIC SUPPURATIVE OTITIS MEDIA

Chronic suppurative otitis media (CSOM) is a chronic inflammatory process in the middle ear. It may be *tubotympanic*, which is generally referred to as a 'safe' condition, because there is a decreased risk of significant intracranial complications, and it involves a perforation with a margin of the tympanic membrane remaining in the pars tensa. Most of the perforations arise as a consequence of ASOM. In CSOM it may be *atticoantral*, which is associated with a cholesteatoma (squamous debris in the middle ear). Atticoantral CSOM is generally referred to as an 'unsafe' ear because it can be associated with significant intracranial complications.

EXCESS EAR WAX

Excess ear wax is associated with anxiety and repeated ear irrigation. The ageing process results in drier ear wax, which is more likely to become impacted. Excess ear wax may cause inflammation, irritation, conductive hearing loss, brownish smelly discharge, tinnitus and otitis externa.

GLUE EAR

Glue ear is an accumulation of thick mucoid fluid in the middle ear. It is a cause of conductive deafness.

MÉNIÈRE'S DISEASE

Ménière's disease is characterized by episodic vertigo, tinnitus and deafness.

OTITIS EXTERNA

Otitis externa is inflammation of the EAC. It is extremely common and is often associated with infection.

OTORRHOEA

Otorrhoea is discharge from the ear (NB: clear fluid discharge may be leakage of cerebrospinal fluid associated with basal skull fracture).

OTOSCLEROSIS

Otosclerosis is a hereditary condition that affects the middle ear ossicles, most notably the stapes. Bony changes lead to fixation of the ossicles and conductive hearing loss.

TINNITUS

Tinnitus is a sensation of sound that does not come from an external source. Sufferers complain of buzzing, thumping or ringing sounds.

COMMONLY PERFORMED EAR OPERATIONS

Some commonly performed ear operations are outlined in *Table 11*.

Further reading and resources

Brooker C and Nicol M (2003). *Nursing Adults. The Practice of Caring*, Ch16. Edinburgh: Mosby.
Royal National Institute for the Deaf (RNID) – http://www.rnid.org.uk

EARLY PREGNANCY PROBLEMS

The problems of early pregnancy include nausea and vomiting, miscarriage, hydatidiform mole, choriocarcinoma and ectopic pregnancy. ⇒ Abortion.

Table 11 Commonly performed ear operations

Operation	Condition for which performed	Brief explanation of the surgery involved
Myringoplasty	Perforation (hole) in the tympanic membrane structure	A graft of temporalis fascia is most often used and placed under the perforation to seal the hole that exists. With time this should be maintained and the perforation cease to exist
Tympanoplasty	Ossicular or tympanic membrane damage secondary to middle ear disease	The aim of a number of these procedures is to improve the transmission of sound via the tympanic membrane and ossicular chain. There are various degrees of ossicular damage with ear disease, all of which are treated by different types of tympanoplasty
Mastoidectomy	Cholesteatoma	An operation that involves drilling of the mastoid bone, which would normally be filled with air cells. The drilling out of the bone allows for the removal of the disease (cholesteatoma) in the bone
Cochlear implant	Profound hearing loss	This is an electronic device that is implanted with a wire insertion into the cochlea and secured to the skull. Approximately 2 weeks after the insertion an external aid is fitted. This causes stimulation of the electrodes within the cochlea and hopefully stimulates any residual tissue within the cochlea

E

NAUSEA AND VOMITING

Nausea and vomiting are very common in the first trimester of pregnancy and probably affect over half of pregnancies. The exact cause has not been determined, but is thought to result from hormonal changes. Although the vomiting is unpleasant and, in some cases, disrupts daily life, it generally improves by the 16th week of gestation.

HYPEREMESIS GRAVIDARUM

Excessive nausea and vomiting that start between 4 and 10 weeks gestation, resolve before 20 weeks, and require intervention are known as hyperemesis gravidarum. This can lead to serious metabolic problems, including dehydration, electrolyte imbalance, ketosis and weight loss. Hyperemesis gravidarum occurs more often with women who have multiple pregnancies or a hydatidiform mole, both of which are associated with high levels of human chorionic gonadotrophin (hCG; see below).

The management includes admission to hospital, where hypovolaemia and electrolyte imbalance are corrected intravenously. Vitamins may be given parenterally. Fluids and diet are gradually reintroduced.

MISCARRIAGE

It is known that at least one-fifth of all pregnancies end in miscarriage, although this figure is likely to be much higher as many early miscarriages occur before pregnancy has been confirmed and the miscarriage may be considered as a delayed period. The majority of miscarriages occur during the first 12 weeks of pregnancy (the first trimester), when the embryo is undergoing major development into the fetal state. The nurse has a vital role to play in the psychological support of the woman and her partner during this extremely stressful time, as it is now recognized how important this aspect of care is in helping a couple come to terms with the loss of their baby. Most gynaecology units now have specialist 'early pregnancy assessment units', in which specialist nurses can provide both assessment and supportive skills in the diagnosis and treatment of women who suffer a miscarriage.

The different types of miscarriage and their presentation are outlined in *Table 12* (note that early fetal demise is also known as a missed miscarriage). Recurrent miscarriage is defined as three or more consecutive spontaneous miscarriages.

HYDATIDIFORM MOLE

Hydatidiform mole (molar pregnancy or trophoblastic disease) can lead to malignant changes so it merits further consideration. It occurs when the trophoblastic tissue develops abnormally.

Women with hydatidiform mole have a positive pregnancy test and may suffer excessive vomiting in pregnancy (hyperemesis gravidarum) because of the excessive amounts of hCG being secreted by the abnormal trophoblastic tissue. There may be slight vaginal bleeding (*Table 12*). On ultrasound scan, no fetal heart is seen, but instead there is an enlarged placental site, often described as looking like a bunch of grapes. A blood test reveals beta-hCG levels much higher than would be expected for the dates of the pregnancy.

Once diagnosed, the molar pregnancy must be surgically removed as, in a small proportion of cases, the mole can progress to a cancer known as choriocarcinoma. Once a definite diagnosis has been made on histology, the women need to be followed up regularly to ensure choriocarcinoma (chorionepithelioma) does not develop. Choriocarcinoma, should it occur, is usually sensitive to chemotherapy and curable. ⇒ Chorionic gonadotrophin.

ECTOPIC PREGNANCY

In an ectopic pregnancy, the fetus develops outside the uterine cavity. The most common site for an ectopic pregnancy to implant is in the uterine tube, but occasionally it can occur in the abdominal cavity or the uterine cervix.

Once an ectopic pregnancy has been diagnosed, it must be removed because of the devastating effect it will have on the mother's health – the pregnancy cannot be saved. Recent developments in the medical management of ectopic pregnancy include the introduction of drugs [e.g. methotrexate (cytotoxic drug), potassium chloride] directly into the gestation sac, which is left inside the uterine tube for absorption. Medical treatment is only undertaken if the woman is haemodynamically stable and has an unruptured ectopic pregnancy.

Surgery (laparoscopic or sometimes open laparotomy) for ectopic pregnancy is always undertaken as an urgent operation, depending on the condition of the woman; if the tube ruptures it is a surgical emergency that requires immediate intervention. This can be alarming for both patients and their relatives, as the condition can deteriorate rapidly, causing a life-threatening situation. The nurse's role is vital in monitoring patients to assess any changes in condition that may be caused by internal bleeding. Vaginal loss and level of pain must also be assessed closely and any changes reported immediately to medical staff. Nurses must

Table 12 Presentation of different types of miscarriage

Type	Bleeding	Pain	Cervix	Uterus
Threatened	Slight, intermittent	None or mild	Closed	Enlarged Equal to dates
Inevitable	Heavy, often with clots	Cramping, intermittent period-like pains (uterine contractions)	Open	Enlarged
Incomplete	Heavy with clots and possible products of conception	As above	Open	May be smaller than gestational age
Complete	Previous heavy bleeding, patient presents with little bleeding or slight discharge	None, although will complain of severe cabdominal cramps	Closed	Returned to nonpregnant size
Blighted ovum (an embryonic pregnancy)	Slight brownish loss	None	Closed	Smaller than gestational dates
Early fetal demise	Brownish discharge	Nonspecific	Closed	Smaller than gestational dates
Hydatidiform mole	Brownish discharge	Nonspecific	Closed	Larger than gestational dates, may palpate soft as no fetal parts
Septic	Heavy	Abdominal pain with pyrexia	Open or closed	Very tender on examination

also be sensitive to patients' psychological needs. Along with their partners, they will be extremely anxious about their physical condition, which may become life-threatening at any time, but they will also have lost their baby. It is important that patients are not treated as just another surgical case; they must be given the support required by someone who has suffered a pregnancy loss.

Further reading

Brooker C and Nicol M (2003). *Nursing Adults. The Practice of Caring*, pp. 725–730. Edinburgh: Mosby.

EATING DISORDERS

Eating disorders include anorexia nervosa, bulimia nervosa and binge-eating. Eating disorders are more prevalent among females than males.

ANOREXIA NERVOSA

Anorexia nervosa remains a rather rare disorder with an incidence of new cases of 7 per 100 000 population (Turnbull *et al.* 1996). Approximately 4000 cases arise in the UK per year. Anorexia nervosa involves a problem in the definition of self that is triggered by stress in the context of a genetic vulnerability. Family and wider cultural factors are important in maintenance (*Box 10*). The classification is outlined in *Table 13*.

In-patient treatment is necessary for the most severe cases. Psychotherapy that involves motivational aspects, and which addresses the core schemata, is also necessary.

E

Box 10 Essential facets of treatment for anorexia nervosa
- Engender motivation;
- Find out what the patient's beliefs are about the illness;
- Develop a good therapeutic alliance;
- Formulation – links between behaviour and core schemata;
- Match therapeutic processes to stage of change;
- Balance move to change against degree of resistance.

Table 13 Criteria for the classification of anorexia nervosa

DSM-IV	ICD-10 F50
Refusal to maintain body weight over a minimal norm, leading to a body weight 15% below expected	Significant weight loss (BMI <17.5 kg/m^2) or failure of weight gain or growth. Weight loss self-induced by avoiding fattening foods and one or more of the following: vomiting purging excessive exercise appetite suppressants diuretics
Intense fear of gaining weight or becoming fat	A dread of fatness as an intrusive, overvalued idea and the patient imposes a low weigh threshold on her- or himself
Disturbance in the way in which one's body weight, size or shape is experienced, e.g. 'feeling fat' {denial of seriousness of underweight or undue influence of body weight and shape on self-evaluation}	
Absence of three consecutive menstrual cycles	Widespread endocrine disorder: amenorrhoea raised growth hormone raised cortisol reduced tri-iodothyronine (T3)
{Restricting type: Binge–purging type; binge-eating or vomiting/ misuse of laxatives or diuretics}	

{}, proposed addition to DSM-IV; BMI, body mass index

BULIMIA NERVOSA

Bulimia nervosa is increasing rapidly in incidence and prevalence. The disorder is now two to three times more common than anorexia nervosa – an incidence of 14 per 100 000 (Turnbull *et al.* 1996). The aetiology involves developmental stress in the context of a culture that endorses dieting. The classification is outlined in *Table 14*.

Cognitive behaviour therapy is effective in 50% of cases (*Box 11*). In a proportion of cases, these skills can be given in a self-help format. Antidepressants, especially selective serotonin reuptake inhibitors (SSRIs), are also widely used in the treatment of bulimia nervosa disorders.

E

Table 14 Criteria for the classification of bulimia nervosa

DSM-III-R Bulimia nervosa (307.51)	ICD-10 Bulimia nervosa (F50.1)	DSM-IV Binge-eating disorder
Recurrent episodes of binge eating {(1) large amount of food, (2) loss of control} *Feeling of lack of control of eating during binge*	Episodes of overeating	{Recurrent episodes of binge eating (1) large, (2) no control} *Binge-eating associated with at least three of the following:* *rapid eating* *uncomfortably full* *eating without hunger* *shameful, solitary eating* *disgust, guilt, depression after overeating*
Regular use of methods of weight control: vomiting laxatives diuretics fasting and/or strict diet vigorous exercise {DSM-IV Purging (vomiting,laxatives, diuretics), Nonpurging}	Methods used to counteract weight gain: vomiting laxatives fasting appetite suppressants metabolic stimulants diuretics	Marked distress after binge eating
Minimum average of two binges a week in 3 months		Binge eating on average at least 2 days a week for 6 months
Persistent overconcern with shape or weight {Self-evaluation is unduly influenced by body weight or shape}	Morbid fear of fatness with a sharply defined weight threshold	
{The disturbance does not occur exclusively during episodes of anorexia nervosa}	Often a history of anorexia nervosa	Disturbance not always present with anorexia nervosa or bulimia nervosa

Italics, proposed deletion in DSM-IV; {} proposed addition to DSM-IV

Box 11 Essential facets for treatment of bulimia nervosa
- Engender motivation;
- Develop good motivation;
- Formulation – are there links between behaviour and core schemata? Is there a biological disposition to poor weight control?
- Education and/or skills of nutritional balance;
- Education and/or skills of emotional balance.

E

Further reading and resources

Eating Disorders Association – http://www.edauk.com/
Newell R and Gournay K (2000). *Mental Health Nursing: An Evidence-Based Approach*, Ch 14. Edinburgh: Churchill Livingstone.

ELECTROCARDIOGRAM

The electrocardiogram (ECG) depicts the electrical activity of the heart muscle during the cardiac cycle monitored by an electrocardiograph. The normal heart produces a typical waveform, sinus rhythm, which consists of five deflection waves, known universally as the P-QRS-T complex (*Fig. 63*). Each part of the complex represents electrical activity at a different part of the heart:
- P wave – usually a rounded dome-shaped deflection. It occurs as the wave of depolarization passes through the atria to the AV node. Following the P wave is the atria contract (atrial systole). The interval between the P wave and ventricular contraction is termed the PR interval and is measured from the beginning of the P wave to the beginning of the QRS complex.
- QRS complex – represents ventricular depolarization. Initial depolarization of the ventricles is from left to right through the septum (seen in some leads as a negative deflection, termed the Q wave). The next part of the complex is the upright deflection, termed the R wave, which represents depolarization of the ventricular muscle mass, and the S wave occurs as the cells return to their resting electrical state. The whole QRS complex describes the period of time for electrical activity to depolarize the ventricular cells.

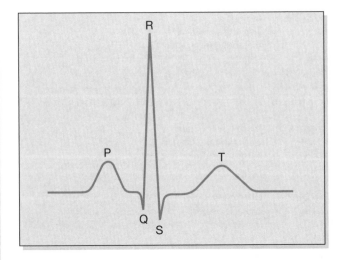

Fig 63 P-QRS-T complex

- ST segment – follows the QRS complex and represents the end of ventricular depolarization and the start of repolarization. It is during this period that coronary artery perfusion takes place. This segment should be an isoelectric line where the ECG complex returns to the baseline and forms a straight line.
- T wave – represents repolarization or the ventricular resting stage. This should be a gently rounded deflection.

THE 12-LEAD ECG

A 12-lead ECG may be used to provide information on the heart activity from 12 different angles (in the same way that 12 people sitting in different parts of a football ground have 12 different views of a goal). For example, through analysing a 12-lead ECG it is possible to identify the exact region of the heart that has been affected in a myocardial infarction. The ECG is recorded using 12 leads – six standard limb leads and six precordial or chest leads. The precordial leads are termed V_1–V_6 and are positioned around the chest wall, while the six standard limb leads (I, II, III and aVR, aVL and aVF) are obtained by placing electrodes on the right and left arms and on the left leg (*Fig. 64*).

BEDSIDE MONITORING

At times it is important to obtain a continuous tracing of the heart rhythm, such as in the coronary care unit where the prompt identification of arrhythmias enables rapid treatment. Three leads are positioned on the right and left upper chest wall and one on the left lower chest wall. Frequently, the lead II position is chosen for bedside monitoring as it records a positive R wave and a clear view of the P wave.

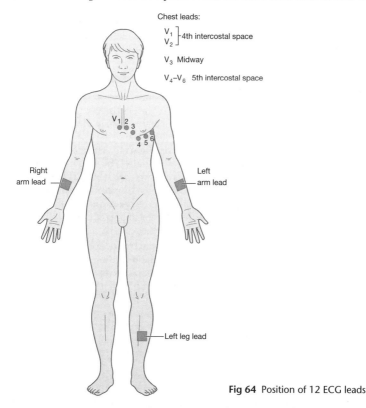

Chest leads:

V_1
V_2 4th intercostal space

V_3 Midway

V_4–V_6 5th intercostal space

Right arm lead

Left arm lead

Left leg lead

Fig 64 Position of 12 ECG leads

HOLTER MONITORING (AMBULATORY) ECG

Holter monitoring records the heart rhythm and rate over a 24 hour period to detect transient ischaemia or arrhythmias. The person continues with their normal activities and keeps a record of times and activities.

EXERCISE TEST TREADMILL (STRESS) ECG

A stress ECG is performed during increasing levels of exertion, such as on a treadmill, to detect arrhythmias or ischaemic changes caused by physical stress. This may induce angina and so must be performed under supervised conditions. Both the ECG and blood pressure are recorded frequently throughout. It is so often used for the diagnosis or prognosis of heart disease or to guide cardiac rehabilitation.

Further reading

Hampton J (1997). *The ECG Made Easy*, Fifth Edition. Edinburgh: Churchill Livingstone.

ELECTROCONVULSIVE THERAPY

Electroconvulsive therapy (ECT) is a physical treatment used for patients with either bipolar disorder or psychotic depression. A device is used that delivers a definite electrical voltage for a precise fraction of a second to electrodes placed on the head to produce a convulsion. The convulsion is modified by use of an intravenous anaesthetic and a muscle relaxant prior to treatment. *Unilateral* ECT avoids the sequela of amnesia for recent events. The mechanism for memory of recent events is probably in the dominant cerebral hemisphere. ECT is therefore applied to the right hemisphere to reduce memory disturbance.

ECT remains a controversial treatment, mainly because of the unwanted effects after treatment, including short-term memory loss, which means that (despite its proved efficacy) it may not be acceptable to some individuals. ⇒ Disorders of mood.

ELECTROENCEPHALOGRAPHY

An electroencephalogram (EEG) is a recording of the electrical activity of the brain. This is especially useful in the diagnosis of epilepsy and sleep disorders, but other conditions, such as tumours, can also produce abnormal patterns. People have electrodes (up to 22) applied to specific locations on the scalp. The readings are taken and recorded onto folding paper, videotape or digitally. The reading is often done for about half an hour, but sometimes a continuous record over a 24 hour period is needed. In this case, people use an attached portable transmitter and the information is gathered at a central point. This continuous technique is called EEG telemetry or just telemetry for short (but beware the other meanings of the word telemetry).

Practice application – preparing people for electroencephalography

An EEG requires people to be relaxed during the recording, as tension in the scalp muscles can affect it. This is helped when people are given complete information about the procedure (e.g. that it is not painful or invasive). They should have clean hair without any gels, spray or oil applied. This information needs to be given in a culturally sensitive manner, as, for some groups, the dressing of hair is part of their culture. Sometimes the person is asked to perform tasks, or lights are shone into the eyes to observe the response of the brain.

ELECTROLYTE

The term 'electrolyte' describes a compound that dissociates into charged particles, called ions, in solution. Ions carry an electrical charge – cations are positively charged and anions negatively charged. For example, sodium chloride (table salt) is described in chemical notation as NaCl, but when in solution it dissolves to form an equal number of Na^+ ions and Cl^- ions. The main electrolytes are the cations sodium, potassium, calcium and magnesium, and the anions are chloride, bicarbonate and phosphate. While water can move freely between the fluid compartments, electrolytes cannot. Sodium is found mainly within the extracellular fluid (ECF), while potassium is nearly all in the intracellular fluid (ICF). Electrolytes constitute the major solutes in body fluids and contribute to their osmotic pressure. They are essential for the transmission of nerve impulses and many metabolic activities in the body. The normal serum levels of the common electrolytes and disorders are summarized in *Table 15*. ⇒ Acid–base balance, Fluid balance and body fluids, Intravenous therapy and/or fusion.

Table 15 Common electrolytes and disorders

Electrolyte	Normal range (mmol/L)	High level in the serum	Low level in the serum
Sodium (Na^+)	135–143	Hypernatraemia	Hyponatraemia
Potassium (K^+)	3.3–4.7	Hyperkalaemia	Hypokalaemia
Calcium (Ca^{2+})	2.1–2.6	Hypercalcaemia	Hypocalcaemia
Magnesium (Mg^{2+})	0.75–1.0	Hypermagnesaemia	Hypomagnesaemia
Chloride (Cl^-)	97–106	Hyperchloraemia	Hypochloraemia
Phosphate (PO_4^{2-})	0.8–1.4	Hyperphosphataemia	Hypophosphataemia

Bicarbonate (HCO_3^-; hydrogen carbonate) 22–28 mmol/L. ⇒ Acid–base balance (disorders of acid–base balance) *Table 1*; Blood gases.

Further reading

Brooker C and Nicol M (2003). *Nursing Adults. The Practice of Caring*, Ch 8. Edinburgh: Mosby.

EMBOLISM

Embolism is the obstruction of a blood vessel by a body of undissolved material. It is usually caused by a thrombus (clot), but other causes include cancer cells, fat, amniotic fluid, gases, bacteria and parasites. Rarer emboli, such as fat, may follow long bone fractures, air may enter the circulation via a penetrating chest wound or during surgery, and amniotic fluid during labour. *Arterial embolism* originates from the left side of the heart or from arterial disease and may travel to various sites, including the brain, bowel or limb; the effects are dependent on the size of vessel affected and the site (e.g. gangrene of a limb or a portion of bowel). ⇒ Deep vein thrombosis, Nervous system (cerebrovascular accident), Pulmonary embolism, Thrombosis.

EMBRYO

An embryo is the human developmental stage that starts 2 weeks after fertilization until the end of week eight of gestation. It is an important stage during which organ development occurs. ⇒ Fetus.

EMOTION

Emotion is an amalgamation of consciously perceived feelings and the objective manifestations that accompany such feelings, such as changes in physiological parameters (e.g. an increase in heart rate). For example, a person may say:

I feel anxious and apprehensive. My mouth is dry and my heart races uncontrollably.
Psychologists view the concept of emotion as consisting of two states: a cognitive mechanism and a state of arousal. The former determines what emotions the individual experiences. An appraisal of the emotion-generating stimuli, based on experience, therefore shows the causes the person responds to. Sometimes the individual may be aroused physiologically and subsequently searches for an explanation (cognitively aroused) for the feelings (e.g. fear, anxiety, depression) experienced.

Supportive contact from a nurse may help to reduce the fears and anxieties felt by clients and their families. Further, using strategies (e.g. catharsis, counselling, biofeedback) to help the person reassess and evaluate the situation that is causing the emotional reactions can improve personal control over subjective experiences, and develop understanding.

In the field of mental health, it is argued that emotional dysfunction is often attributed to biological problems – a common feature in psychopathy (Butler 2000). Furthermore, in chronically depressed individuals, psychosurgical interventions (destruction of specific fibres in the frontal lobes of the brain matter) have been known to improve emotional functioning, with a 50–60% recovery rate from depression (Butler 2000). Intense sufferings caused by some illnesses and diseases can elicit intense emotions. ⇒ Affect, Disorders of mood.

EMPATHY

Empathy is identifying with another person or the actions of another person. Empathy is related to a demonstration of insightful awareness of another person's biopsychosocial experiences. In contrast with sympathy, the empathetic person shows objectivity during interpersonal communication. Losing the ability to remain objective in a situation can be detrimental to effective interventions, and causes professionals to become exhausted emotionally.

The empathetic person is, however, not detached from all emotions, but is able to recognize when personal feelings that could block the therapeutic encounter are aroused in the process.

The skilled practitioner can show empathy by listening and reflecting the sufferer's cathartic response, using silence appropriately while being a supportive presence, and tactfully guiding and directing the client to manage his or her emotions effectively.

EMPOWERMENT

To empower means to enable and is a popular term used by many disciplines, including healthcare, to explain the process of granting power to oneself and others.

EMPOWERMENT AS IT RELATES TO THE INDIVIDUAL

According to Gibson (1991), empowerment is a social process of recognizing, promoting and enhancing individuals' abilities to meet their own needs, solve their own problems and mobilize the necessary resources. This leads to a feeling of being in control of one's own life.

This approach implies that individuals take control of their own lives and accept responsibility for their own action and behaviours. However, a considerable number of people do not believe that they have the necessary control over their lives. They often work and live in environments that by design or by accident leave them with little power. Disempowerment is the result of believing that nothing can be done to change the situation and so rendering oneself dependent on others.

Individual empowerment needs an environment in which there is trust, open and honest communication, mutual respect, courtesy, acceptance of people and valuing of others. ⇒ Health education, Health promotion, Locus of control.

ENDOCRINE

Endocrine means secreting internally. *Endocrine glands* are the ductless glands that produce one or more hormones, which pass directly into the blood or lymph. They include the hypothalamus, pineal body, pituitary, thyroid, parathyroids, adrenals, ovaries, testes and pancreas. Other structures also produce hormones, such as the placenta, gastrointestinal tract, kidneys, thymus and heart (*Fig. 65*). ⇒ Adrenal glands, Ovaries, Pancreas, Parathyroid glands, Pituitary gland, Testes, Thyroid gland.

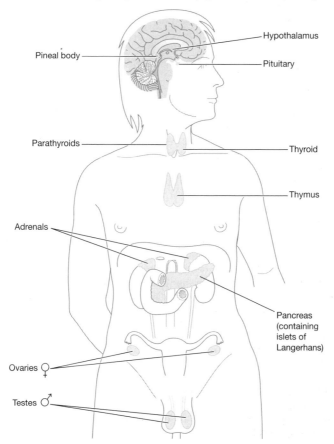

Fig 65 Location of major endocrine structures (both female and male structures are illustrated)

E

HORMONES

A hormone is formed in one organ or gland and carried in the blood to another organ, probably quite distant, where it influences cellular activity, especially growth and metabolism. The majority of hormones are either peptide or steroid in nature. Whereas peptide hormones (e.g. insulin) are water-soluble, steroids such as cortisol are lipid-soluble.

When a hormone arrives at its target cell, it binds to a specific area, the *receptor*, where it acts as a switch that influences chemical or metabolic reactions inside the cell. The receptors for water-soluble hormones are situated on the cell membrane and those for lipid-soluble hormones are inside the cell.

The level of a hormone in the blood is variable and self-regulating within its normal range. A hormone is released in response to a specific stimulus and usually its action reverses or negates the stimulus through a *negative feedback mechanism*. This may be controlled either indirectly, through the release of hormones by the hypothalamus and the anterior pituitary gland, or directly by blood levels of the stimulus.

The effect of a *positive feedback mechanism* is amplification of the stimulus and increasing release of the hormone until a particular process is complete and the stimulus ceases. ⇒ Homeostasis.

LOCAL HORMONES

A number of body tissues not normally described as endocrine glands secrete substances that act locally, which include:
- Prostaglandins (PGs) – lipid substances that act as local hormones and have wide-ranging physiological effects (e.g. inflammatory response, blood coagulation, etc.). Other chemically similar compounds include *leukotrienes* and *thromboxanes*. ⇒ Lipids.
- Erythropoietin (EPO) – a growth factor synthesized by the kidneys. ⇒ Erythrocyte (erythropoietin and the control of erythropoiesis).
- Gastrointestinal (GI) hormones – several local hormones, including gastrin, secretin and cholecystokinin (CCK), regulate digestion. Some GI peptides, such as vasoactive intestinal polypeptide (VIP), are secreted by nerves. Some GI peptides may be classified as hormones in one situation and as neurotransmitters in another, depending on where they come from and what they do.
- Atrial natriuretic peptide (ANP) – secreted by atrial muscle cells in the heart.

ENDOSCOPY

The use of an endoscope (lighted instrument) to visualize body cavities or organs. The older endoscopes were rigid, tubular and made of metal (sometimes still used in certain situations). Those in general use are of the fibreoptic variety, in which light is transmitted by means of very fine glass fibres along a flexible tube (*Fig. 66*). Endoscopes are used for examination by direct view, video imaging or photography, biopsy and treatment (e.g. the introduction of stents to keep the bile duct open, etc.). Endoscopy may be undertaken on a relaxed (sedated) conscious person. Some examinations, however, require a general anaesthetic. ⇒ Day-care surgery.

The endoscopic examinations used for particular body structures are outlined in *Box 12*.

Box 12 Endoscopic examinations
- Arthroscopy – joints;
- Bronchoscopy – tracheobronchial tree (see Practice application);
- Colonoscopy – colon;
- Colposcopy – uterine cervix;

- Cystoscopy – interior of the urinary bladder;
- Hysteroscopy – uterine cavity;
- Laparoscopy (peritoneoscopy) – internal organs of the abdominal and pelvic cavities;
- Laryngoscopy (direct) – interior of the larynx;
- Mediastinoscopy – mediastinum;
- Nasendoscopy – nasal passages and postnasal space;
- Oesophagogastroduodenoscopy (OGD) – oesophagus, stomach and duodenum;
- Pharyngoscopy – pharynx;
- Proctoscopy – anal canal and rectum;
- Sigmoidoscopy – sigmoid colon;
- Thoracoscopy – pleural surfaces.

E

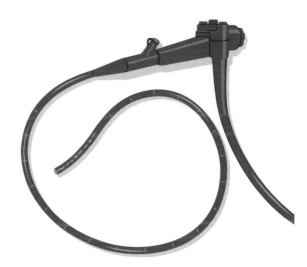

Fig 66 A flexible fibreoptic endoscope

Practice application – fibreoptic bronchoscopy

Bronchoscopy and related procedures (lung biopsy, brushing and lavage) are usually performed under sedation and local anaesthetic to the throat. Sedatives, such as midazolam, may cause respiratory depression, hypoventilation and hypotension, and local anaesthetics applied to the throat may lead to laryngospasm and bronchospasm. Therefore, patients need careful monitoring during the procedure and for 6–8 hours afterwards, as bronchoscopy can cause bronchospasm, hypoxaemia, fever, pneumonia, pneumothorax and haemorrhage.

Fasting is required after local anaesthesia until the effects have worn off. The gag reflex can be tested with sips of water, which should precede free drinking and eating. On discharge, patients should be given information (usually a leaflet) that explains how they should feel during the first 12 hours and details what to do if the prevailing symptoms worsen or new symptoms develop.

E

ENDOTRACHEAL

Endotracheal means within the trachea. An *endotracheal tube* is a plastic tube introduced via the nose or mouth into the trachea to maintain an airway during general anaesthesia and intermittent positive pressure ventilation (*Fig. 67*). ⇒ Airway, Anaesthesia, Intubation.

> **Practice application – care of an endotracheal tube in the critically ill patient**
> The endotracheal tube (*Fig. 67*) must be secured to maintain its position and to avoid accidental extubation. The most common method is to use lengths of material tape attached to the tube and secured around the patient's neck. The tapes must be tight enough to maintain stability of the tube, yet not so tight as to restrict blood flow or cause pressure ulcers.
> Bronchial hygiene, by passing a suction catheter down the endotracheal tube, is required regularly to prevent obstruction of the tube and to remove secretions. Endotracheal suction is an aseptic procedure to avoid the introduction of pathogens into the respiratory tract. Gloves are worn and a technique used that ensures that the part of the suction catheter that enters the endotracheal tube remains untouched and sterile. The nurse should wear protective clothing (gloves and an apron) and ensure effective handwashing and the correct disposal of equipment. The procedure has potential complications in the critically ill patient, including trauma to the trachea and bronchi, infection, hypoxaemia (caused by the interruption of ventilation during suctioning) and cardiovascular instability.

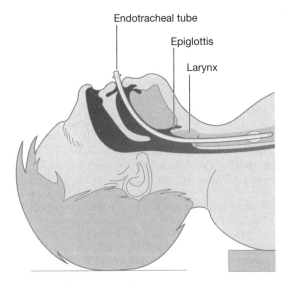

Endotracheal tube

Epiglottis

Larynx

Fig 67 Endotracheal tube: (A) In position

ENEMAS AND SUPPOSITORIES

⇒ Defecation (laxatives).

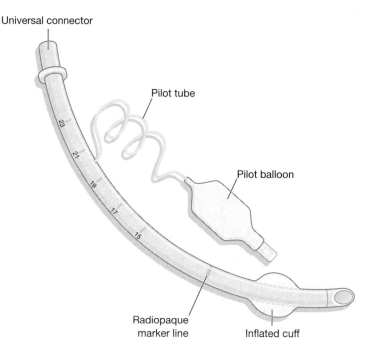

Fig 67 (B) Endotracheal tube

ENEMAS

An enema is the introduction of liquid into the rectum by means of a tube. There are three main kinds (*Fig. 68*):
• Medication – contains medication (e.g. corticosteroids) that should be given slowly and retained as long as possible (prescribed, checked and documented according to local protocols);

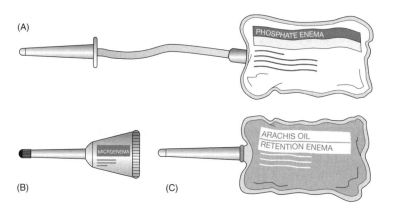

Fig 68 Types of enema: (A) phosphate enema, (B) microenema, (C) arachis oil

- Evacuant – stimulant enemas usually returned, with faecal matter and flatus, within a few minutes (a solution that contains phosphates or sodium citrate is commonly used);
- Retention – enemas that soften and lubricate the faeces and should be retained for a specified time; they usually contain arachis oil (from peanuts) or olive oil.

Microenemas are increasingly being used in both the community and hospital as they cause less discomfort to patients when administered. The other pre-prepared enemas can be obtained with long delivery tubes to facilitate self-administration by patients.

E

> **Practice application – enema administration – maintaining a safe environment**
> - Prior to administration, check that the patient is not allergic to latex, phosphates or peanuts or groundnuts (arachis oil enemas contain oil expressed from peanuts);
> - Although an aseptic technique is not required, all the equipment used should be clean or disposable, and nurses should wash their hands before and on completion of the practice (gloves and aprons are worn for protection);
> - Some enemas require to be warmed prior to administration to reduce the risk of bowel spasm and shock (Addison 2000);
> - Care should be taken to avoid damaging the rectal mucosa or causing pain (particularly if the person has an anal condition, such as a fissure) when inserting the tube of the enema into the rectum. If the tube meets with resistance, it should be withdrawn slightly and no force used.

SUPPOSITORIES

A suppository is a cone or cylinder of a medicinal substance that can be introduced into the rectum, eventually dissolves and may be absorbed through the rectal mucosa. Suppositories may be used to:
- Relieve constipation;
- Evacuate the bowel prior to surgery or certain investigations;
- Treat haemorrhoids or anal pruritus;
- Administer medication, such as antibiotics, bronchodilators or analgesics (prescribed, checked and documented according to local protocols).

Glycerine suppositories lubricate dry, hard stools and have a mild stimulant effect on the rectum. Stimulant suppositories include bisacodyl.

Medication is absorbed well through the rectal mucosa. This route has for many years been a common way to administer medication in continental Europe, but only recently has it become acceptable to people in the UK.

> **Practice application – blunt end first for suppository insertion**
> Moppett (2000) discusses the latest guidance on the insertion of suppositories, suggesting that, for physiological reason, the suppository should be inserted blunt end first into the anus. It is proposed that this aids retention of the suppository, as the anal sphincter muscles close tightly around the apex of the suppository, propelling it inwards. If it is inserted apex first, as was traditional, the sphincter closes over the blunt end, and the muscles are stimulated to expel the suppository. The introduction of the blunt end of the suppository also reduces the need to insert the full length of a finger.

ENTERIC FEVERS

⇒ *Salmonella* (enteric fevers).

ENTEROCOCCUS

A genus of Gram-positive cocci commensal in the bowel (e.g. *Enterococcus faecalis* and *E. faecium*). These cocci cause wound infection and urinary tract infection and occasionally neonatal meningitis. They are increasingly common as a cause of hospital-acquired infection, and many strains are developing antibiotic resistance.

VANCOMYCIN-RESISTANT *ENTEROCOCCUS*

The emergence of vancomycin-resistant *Enterococcus* (VRE) has been causing much difficulty. New resistant strains are reported increasingly, which has lead to some severe untreatable infections.

ENZYME

An enzyme is a protein that acts as a biological catalyst (a catalyst controls or speeds up the rate of a reaction without itself being altered permanently). Enzymes are produced by living cells to catalyse specific biochemical reactions that involve specific substrates. Many reactions in biological systems would proceed too slowly without an enzyme (e.g. carbon dioxide would not be cleared from the tissues without the enzyme carbonic anhydrase). The names of enzymes often reflect their function, so aminotransferases catalyse the transfer of amine groups (NH_2) between amino acids.

Enzyme cascade amplification allows complex physiological processes to proceed more rapidly. Amplification occurs as the product of one reaction triggers the next reaction and so on, such as in blood coagulation.

ENZYME INDUCTION

Enzyme induction is the property of substances, such as some environmental chemicals, alcohol and some drugs (e.g. rifampicin and barbiturates) to increase the production of liver (microsomal) enzymes. This can have the effect of increasing the rate at which the 'inducer' and sometimes other drugs are metabolized and excreted with loss of drug effects (e.g. rifampicin causes inactivation of oral contraceptives), or sometimes it increases drug effects, such as the toxic metabolites produced in a paracetamol overdose.

ENZYME INHIBITORS

Agents, including many drugs, act by inhibiting a specific enzyme either reversibly or irreversibly. Some drugs are substrate analogues (very similar to the usual substrate of the enzyme) and act as competitive inhibitors (e.g. the cytotoxic drug methotrexate inhibits an enzyme needed for folic acid use by cancer cells). Some drugs inhibit liver (microsomal) enzymes and increase the effects of other drugs (e.g. aspirin can prevent the metabolism of oral anticoagulants, such as warfarin, which leads to an increased anticoagulant effect).

EPIDEMIOLOGY

Epidemiology deals with the incidence, distribution and control of disease. The elements of epidemiology are statistical in nature, as diagnosis, treatment and prognosis are uncertain in individual cases, and it is only by looking at larger samples that data can be interpreted more meaningfully. Epidemiology is a quantitative discipline that considers health outcomes, such as death or disease, and attempts to establish relationships between these outcomes and other factors.

Samples of subjects from a population are analysed with respect to the occurrence of the outcome, and the presence of various purported risk factors. A classic case of epidemiological work is the link between smoking and lung cancer. An individual who smokes may or may not develop lung cancer, and nonsmokers can also develop lung cancer. However, the incidence of lung cancer is far higher among smokers than nonsmokers.

ENDEMIC

Endemic describes a disease that recurs in an area. It is applied to a disease that is always present in an area, such as a particular communicable disease.

EPIDEMIC

An epidemic is a particular disease, such as influenza, that simultaneously affects many people (more than normally expected) in an area.

INCIDENCE

Incidence is the number of new cases of a disease that occur in a population over a defined time period.

PANDEMIC

A pandemic is an epidemic that spreads over a wide area, such as a whole country or the world.

PREVALENCE

Prevalence is the total number of cases of a disease that exist in a population at a single point in time. *Prevalence ratio* is the number of cases of a disease that exist in a population at a single point in time, expressed as a ratio of population size. ⇒ Communicable diseases.

EPISTAXIS

Epistaxis (nosebleed) is a common emergency and generally can be controlled fairly easily. Some bleeding, however, is extremely difficult to control and can result in significant morbidity and distress for the patient and may be life-threatening. The causes of epistaxis are varied and may be local (e.g. trauma) or general (e.g. hypertension or anticoagulant drugs, etc.). ⇒ Nose and paranasal sinuses.

Depending on the amount of bleeding, first aid (see Practice application) and stabilization with intravenous fluids or plasma may be needed. Methods of haemostasis include:
• Nasal cautery – if a bleeding point can be located;
• Nasal packing and balloons – where the bleeding point cannot be identified, or is inaccessible (*Fig. 69*).
The complications of nasal packing are outlined in *Table 16*. Should cautery or packing fail to control bleeding, other methods are available, including septal surgery, arterial ligation and arterial embolization.

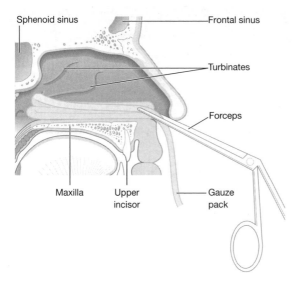

Fig 69 Nasal packing: gauze pack is introduced into the nose in horizontal layers from the floor of the nose upwards.

Practice application – epistaxis; initial care (first aid)
When a patient initially presents with an epistaxis, first aid measures are employed, regardless of their location. These measures are as follows:
• Maintain a calm atmosphere and reassure by explaining all the procedures and care;
• Sit the patient down;
• Provide a receptacle to catch the blood, and also in case of vomiting;
• Encourage the patient to lean forwards over the receptacle;
• Encourage the patient to breathe gently through the mouth and to spit out blood, rather than to swallow it;
• Apply pressure to the soft part of the nose (Little's area) for approximately 10 minutes;
• Apply ice packs to the nose and forehead to ease bleeding through reflex vasoconstriction of the blood vessels;
• Evaluate the extent of blood loss and record the amount.
In a healthcare setting, ensure that oxygen and suction equipment are accessible. Monitor blood pressure and pulse as required (every 15–30 minutes initially) to observe for hypotension and tachycardia that result from blood loss, or hypertension that could be contributing to the epistaxis. Ensure that intravenous access is patent and administer intravenous fluids as prescribed.

Further reading

Phillips S (1997). Epistaxis. *Prof Nurs*. **12**(4): 292–295.

E

Table 16 Complications of nasal packing (adapted from von Schoenberg *et al.* 1993 and Murthy and McKerrow 1995)

Associated with pack insertion	Associated with maintenance of the pack	Associated with pack removal	Late complica- tions
Pain	Hypoxia and hypoxaemia – may lead to myocardial infarction and stroke	Pain or discomfort	Secondary haemorrhage
Vasovagal attack	Obstructive sleep apnoea	Trauma	Adhesions
Cardiovascular collapse (caused by hypovolaemic shock, vasovagal reflex, reactions to local anaesthesia and/or vasoconstricting drugs)	Infection – local (e.g. sinusitis) or general (e.g. bacteraemia or toxic shock syndrome) Fever Abscess	Haemorrhage	Septal perfusion
Trauma to soft palate, nares, mucosa	Pharyingotympanic tube obstruction – may lead to otitis media with effusion, acute otitis media, haemotympanum Bleeding or haematoma		Nasal infection
			Pharyngeal incompetence and stenosis
	Accidental pack displacement that compromises the airway		Paraffin granulomata (rare)
	Unusual chronic inflammatory response induced by petrolatum and lanolin-based ointments used in postoperative packs		

EQUALITY

Equality is for all to be in an equal position relative to one another.

EQUALITY OF OPPORTUNITY

Equality of opportunity is to have equal access to opportunities for healthcare, decent housing, employment, redress in the courts, etc., regardless of class, age, race or gender. ⇒ Inequalities in health.

EQUAL OPPORTUNITIES COMMISSION

In the UK, the Equal Opportunities Commission (EOC) exists to challenge discrimination, champion equality and act as a catalyst for change. Their vision is a society that enables women and men to fulfil their potential and have their contributions to work and home life equally valued and respected, and free from assumption based on their sex.

SOCIAL EXCLUSION

Social exclusion refers to the multiple deprivation experienced by certain population groups who can become socially isolated in their neighbourhood and unable to participate in mainstream activities, such as work or education. Refugees, rough sleepers, teenage mothers and many young people can be excluded socially.

SOCIAL EXCLUSION UNIT

In the UK the government set up the Social Exclusion Unit to study and report on social exclusion and measures aimed at reducing the problem, such as new ways to decrease the number of teenage pregnancies.

Resources

Commission for Racial Equality – http://www.cre.org.uk
Equal Opportunities Commission – http://www.eoc.org.uk

ERYTHROCYTE

Erythrocytes are non-nucleated red blood cells, the most numerous of the blood cells (female, $3.8–5.3 \times 10^{12}$/L; male, $4.5–6.5 \times 10^{12}$/L). Erythrocytes carry oxygen and some carbon dioxide, and buffer pH changes in the blood. The erythrocyte is highly specialized for its purpose of transporting oxygen from the lungs to the peripheral tissues. It has no nucleus and becomes packed with haemoglobin. The erythrocyte lacks mitochondria (and other organelles) and relies only on anaerobic glycolysis for the production of adenosine triphosphate (ATP), which means it does not consume the oxygen it transports. Mature circulating erythrocytes are biconcave discs with a mean diameter of 7.2 μm and a thickness of 2.2 μm, which gives them the optimal surface area to volume ratio to facilitate the transport of oxygen and carbon dioxide in to and out of the cell (*Fig. 70*). ⇒ Blood (*Box 3*).

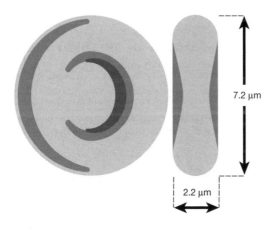

7.2 μm

2.2 μm

Fig 70 Diagrams of a mature erythrocyte

E

In the erythrocyte, haemoglobin binds oxygen at high oxygen levels, such as in the lungs, and releases it at relatively low levels of oxygen, such as in the peripheral tissues. The surface of the erythrocyte carries antigens that are genetically determined, such as the antigens that confer the A, B or O blood types. ⇒ Blood, Haemoglobin.

ERYTHROPOIESIS

Erythropoiesis is the production of red blood cells in the red bone marrow as a result of stimulation by the growth factor erythropoietin (EPO). Other hormones, such as androgens and thyroid hormones, also stimulate the bone marrow. The development of erythrocytes from pluripotent cells takes about 7 days to complete and consists of two main features (*Fig. 71*):
- Maturation of the cell;
- Formation of haemoglobin within the cell.
⇒ Haemopoiesis.

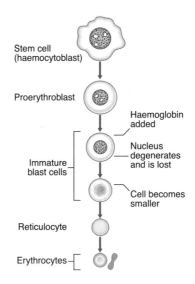

Fig 71 Erythropoiesis

ERYTHROPOIETIN AND THE CONTROL OF ERYTHROPOIESIS

Erythropoietin (EPO) is a growth factor secreted by certain cells in the kidney in response to hypoxia (*Fig. 72*). Active EPO is formed from the renal erythropoietic factor and some is also produced in the liver. It acts on the bone marrow, stimulating erythropoiesis. Recombinant forms of EPO (rhuEPO) are now available to treat patients with chronic anaemia secondary to bone marrow dysfunction or cytotoxic therapy. It is also used for patients with chronic renal failure. ⇒ Renal failure.

DESTRUCTION OF ERYTHROCYTES

The life span of erythrocytes is about 120 days and their breakdown, or haemolysis, is carried out by phagocytic cells found in the spleen, bone marrow and liver.

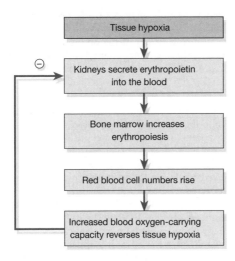

Fig 72 Control of erythropoiesis: the role of erythropoietin

Iron released by haemolysis is retained in the body and reused in the bone marrow to form haemoglobin. Biliverdin is formed from the protein part of the erythrocytes, and is reduced to bilirubin before it is bound to plasma globulin and transported to the liver. In the liver it is changed from a fat-soluble to a water-soluble form before being excreted as a constituent of bile.

ERYTHROCYTE DISORDERS

ANAEMIA

Anaemia is a term used to describe the insufficient oxygen-carrying capacity of blood. Anaemia is said to be present if the haemoglobin concentration of blood falls below 13.5 g/dL in males or 11.5 g/dL in females (normal ranges are 13.5–18.0 g/dL in males, 11.5–16.5 g/dL in females).

The many potential causes of anaemia include traumatic haemorrhage, surgery, disease or its treatment, chronic blood loss, nutritional deficiencies, bone marrow failure (aplastic anaemia), premature destruction of red blood cells and hereditary factors.

General signs and symptoms of anaemia are related to a reduced oxygen delivery to body tissues and impaired metabolism, as well as to the increased demands placed upon body systems. They include:

- Weakness and fatigue;
- Breathlessness, particularly evident on exertion;
- Dizziness;
- Tachycardia and palpitations;
- Angina pectoris and congestive heart failure, particularly in older adults;
- Pallor of the skin and mucosa, particularly the conjunctival membranes. Skin pallor is evident in people with light skins, but in individuals with darker skins it may be detected in the mucosa only.

Other general effects and signs and symptoms are associated with specific types of anaemia. For example, 'spoon-shaped' nails in a person with severe iron deficiency anaemia.

The treatment of anaemia depends on the cause and severity. Mild iron-deficiency anaemia may respond to oral iron and dietary advice, whereas severe haemorrhagic anaemia may require blood transfusion. Some types of haemolytic anaemia are usually treated with corticosteroids and possibly splenectomy (removal of the spleen) to stop the premature destruction of red blood cells. ⇒ Blood.

POLYCYTHAEMIA

Polycythaemia may be primary or secondary and can be defined as a rise in haemoglobin levels beyond the normal. The haematocrit (packed cell volume) is also elevated. In primary proliferative polycythaemia (PPP), the amount of urate in the blood is increased and there is often an increase in the number of neutrophils and platelets. PPP is a disorder that most commonly arises in people over the age of 50 years. It is caused by the mutation of a stem cell that produces excessive numbers of red cells. ⇒ Myeloproliferative disorders.

Secondary polycythaemia can result from hypoxia, such as in lung disease or at high altitude, increased secretion of EPO by the kidneys or tumours, or the misuse of the drug EPO to enhance athletic performance.

People with polycythaemia often have a ruddy appearance and splenomegaly (enlargement of spleen). Symptoms of polycythaemia tend to be related to an increase in blood volume and blood viscosity, and include headaches, fatigue, dizziness, breathlessness, visual disturbances, sweating, pruritus and gout. However, the most serious complication is thrombosis. Thrombi can lead to vascular occlusion, peripheral gangrene, deep vein thrombosis (DVT), embolus formation, stroke and heart attack.

The management of primary polycythaemia includes:
- Measures to maintain the haematocrit within normal limits – venesection, or drugs such as hydroxycarbamide or interferon to suppress bone marrow function;
- Aspirin may be prescribed to reduce platelet activity and inhibit clot formation;
- In older people, radioactive phosphorus may be used to reduce marrow activity, but unfortunately this form of treatment can cause acute leukaemia after some years.

ESCHERICHIA

Escherichia is a genus of motile, Gram-negative bacilli belonging to the family Enterobacteriaceae. Escherichia coli is part of the normal bowel flora. Some strains are pathogenic to humans, causing urinary tract infection, gastroenteritis, meningitis, peritonitis and wound infections. The serotypes that cause gastroenteritis are classified into four groups:
- Enterohaemorrhagic E. coli (EHEC), such as E. coli 0157, a virulent organism that produces a toxin (verocytotoxin) and causes a range of disease from mild diarrhoea to severe haemorrhagic bowel inflammation. Some of the people affected may develop life-threatening haemolytic uraemic syndrome (HUS), which is characterized by intravascular haemolysis and acute renal failure. Affected individuals (mainly children) may require renal replacement therapy. Most make a full recovery, but some will have residual renal problems. Outbreaks of infection have been associated with eating meat and meat products, such as undercooked burgers, unpasteurized milk and vegetables washed in water contaminated with faeces.
- Enteropathic E. coli (EPEC) causes serious diarrhoea in babies, especially in developing countries. Infection occurs through food handlers or faecal contamination of water supplies.

- Enterotoxigenic *E. coli* (ETEC) affects people travelling to areas in which hygiene standards are poor and causes outbreaks of gastroenteritis in developing countries. It results in watery diarrhoea, which can cause fluid and electrolyte imbalance.
- Enterovasive *E. coli* (EIEC) infection is usually via food handlers or water contaminated with faeces. It causes bloodstained diarrhoea.

⇒ Electrolyte, Fluid balance and body fluids, Infection, Renal failure.

ETHICS

Ethics is the study of codes of moral principles derived from systems of values and beliefs and concerned with rights and obligations. The study of nursing ethics as a discipline distinct from bioethics and medical ethics has developed strongly in recent years. The many areas in healthcare that involve ethical issues include abortion, confidentiality, consent, euthanasia, equity of service provision, research, etc. ⇒ Code of Professional Conduct, Research.

BENEFICENCE

Beneficence is the principle that we should do good to others (Latin: *beneficio*) rather than harm (Latin: *maleficio*), and means responsible care or having a duty of care. ⇒ Duty of care, Negligence.

EQUITY

Equity is fairness of the distribution of resources, such that all have access to resources according to need and ability to benefit.

JUSTICE

Justice is an ethical principle based on the assumption of universal human rights. It involves concepts of fairness and justness. It may be described as acting within a set of moral laws, respecting the views and rights of others, or equity in the distribution of resources.

NONMALEFICENCE

Nonmaleficence is the ethical principle of doing no harm.

ETHICAL THEORIES

Three types of ethical theory are:
- Deontological theory – a general approach to the justification of ethical behaviour, in which priority is given to fundamental principles, rights and duties (Greek: *deon* = duty);
- Utilitarianism – the theory advocated in particular by Bentham and Mill that the guiding principle for all conduct should be to achieve the greatest happiness for the greatest number, and that the criterion of the rightness or wrongness of an action is whether it is useful in furthering this goal (the utility principle);
- Virtue ethics – an ethical theory that focuses attention on the possession of sound moral qualities by the moral agent as necessary for consistent moral behaviour, it rejects the apparent dichotomy between deontological (duty based) and utilitarian (consequentialist) theories in favour of emphasis on the agent as having primary responsibility for implementing principles in action.

ETHNICITY

Ethnicity describes the feeling of belonging to a particular group who share common cultural customs and traditions. Sociologists and psychologists often link the term 'ethnicity' with the study of race. Although the two concepts are inter-connected, their meanings are markedly different. Race applies to biological char-acteristics (e.g. skin colour, height, hair types, facial features, etc.), whereas ethnicity denotes cultural lifestyles based on values, beliefs and practices shared by the ethnic groups.

Ethnicity may be recognized by the language used, religion, dress, dietary habits and spiritual practices, for example. Ethnic groups however, may still represent racial groups and their identities.

Race and ethnicity are two of the many variables that help create individuality and, as such, must be acknowledged.

In clinical practice healthcare practitioners must respond positively to ethnic groups' different health beliefs and needs. These needs have not always been met, as demonstrated by minority groups who underutilize healthcare services. The implications for transcultural healthcare practice are numerous.

EUTHANASIA

Euthanasia, when translated literally, means 'good death'. It is only recently that it has come to mean 'the deliberate killing of someone by a fatal intervention'. Euthanasia may be voluntary, involuntary, nonvoluntary, active (e.g. by drug administration) or passive (where treatment is withdrawn or not commenced).

The topic of euthanasia is a matter for world-wide debate. Some countries allow euthanasia under strict control. For example, in 1993 the Dutch government approved euthanasia guidelines that, if followed by a doctor, allow immunity from prosecu-tion. In 1995 the Northern Territory of Australia became the first place in the world to legalize euthanasia, but this was subsequently challenged and overturned. Debate continues in the UK, where euthanasia remains illegal. ⇒ Advance directive.

EVALUATION

Evaluation is commonly accepted as the fourth phase of the nursing process. Care is evaluated to assess whether the stated patient and/or client goals have been or are being achieved. Although it is the final step in the nursing process, it should occur continuously from the first assessment to the person's discharge from the healthcare system. ⇒ Nursing process.

EVIDENCE-BASED PRACTICE

Evidence-based practice (EBP) describes the delivery of healthcare interventions based on the systematic analysis of information available about the effectiveness of the interventions in relation to cost-effective health outcomes. At present, sys-tematic research-based evidence is not available for all areas of healthcare, and some types of care do not lend themselves to scientific research methods. Thus, some of the evidence-based protocols may be developed from the collection of best expert practice in the field. ⇒ Literature searching and review (Practice appli-cation), Research.

Categories of causal evidence are shown below. The strength of the recom-mendation reflects the robustness of the methodological processes, not the value of the findings to practice.

CATEGORIES OF EVIDENCE FOR CAUSAL RELATIONSHIPS AND TREATMENT

Ia Evidence from meta-analysis of randomized controlled trials (RCTs).
Ib Evidence from at least one RCT.
IIa Evidence from at least one controlled study without randomization.
IIb Evidence from at least one other type of quasi-experimental study.
III Evidence from nonexperimental descriptive studies and case-control studies.
IV Evidence from expert committee reports or opinions and/or clinical experience of respected authorities.

STRENGTH OF RECOMMENDATION

A Directly based on category I evidence.
B Directly based on category II evidence or extrapolated recommendation from category I evidence.
C Directly based on category III evidence or extrapolated recommendation from category I or II evidence.
D Directly based on category IV evidence or extrapolated recommendation from category I, II or III evidence.
(Adapted from Shekelle *et al.* 1999.)

CRITICAL APPRAISAL OF EVIDENCE

Not all nurses will be actively engaged in research, but they do need to read research to keep up to date, to answer specific clinical questions or in connection with a course of study or project. Nurses need to be able to evaluate evidence about the effectiveness of interventions. Critical appraisal means being able to weigh up the evidence and make a judgement. Critical appraisal is not about criticizing; it involves assessing the quality of a piece of research and considering its usefulness and effectiveness in the nurse's area of practice (McCaughan 1999). The best evidence is that which has been synthesized from several sources of data, each confirming the same findings. For example, clinical guidance issued by the National Institute for Clinical Excellence (NICE; http://www.nice.org.uk) is based on the best available evidence.

When reading research studies, it is important to consider whether the population under investigation is similar to the patients in your area of practice. The findings for a different population may be very different. The environment in which the study took place is also important. The findings from research conducted in a nursing home cannot be assumed to be applicable to patients in an intensive care unit, and vice versa.

All research studies have weak areas or limitations and a reliable study highlights these. Critical appraisal entails deciding whether the limitations are likely to affect the reliability of the study.

Practice application – sources of evidence for nursing practice
Nurses do not have to do everything themselves. There are now several sources of evidence that have already been appraised critically and put together in a 'user-friendly' form to help the busy professional. There are many and varied sources of evidence available to nurses, who just need to look. Sources include:
• *Evidence-based Nursing* – now also available online (ebn.bmjjournals.com/);
• *Evidence-based Medicine* – published by the BMJ;

E

- National Institute for Clinical Excellence (NICE) –
  http://www.nice.org.uk;
- NHS Centre for Reviews and Dissemination (York) –
  http://www1.york.ac.uk/inst/crd;
- The Cochrane Library (http://www.cochrane.co.uk), which includes
  the Cochrane database of systematic reviews (CDSR) – reviews of controlled trials and a meta-analysis of those studies that meet their strict
  inclusion criteria (that this is regarded as the highest level of evidence);
  a database of abstract reviews of effectiveness (DARE), which is a database of research reviews of the effectiveness of healthcare interventions;
  the Cochrane controlled trials register (CCTR), which is a bibliography
  of controlled trials;
- The Scottish Intercollegiate Guidelines Network (SIGN) –
  http://www.sign.ac.uk;
- UK Department of Health Research and Development –
  http://www.dh.gov.uk/research/index/htm.

Further reading

Chambers R (1998). *Clinical Effectiveness Made Easy: First Thoughts on Clinical Governance.*
  Oxford: Radcliffe.
Crombie I (1996). *The Pocket Guide to Critical Reviews.* London: The BMJ Publishing Group.

EXERCISE

Exercise is the undertaking of physical exertion with the main aim of improving
fitness and health. Exercise and activity are fundamental to mobility and there are
many different types of exercise. ⇒ Activity tolerance, Mobility.
   These include:

- Active – these are exercises undertaken by the person without any assistance, whereas exercises performed by the person, but with assistance from
  the physiotherapist or nurse, are termed active assisted;
- Isometric or static exercises – those carried out without movement (i.e. muscles are alternately contracted and relaxed while the body part remains in a
  fixed position) and used to maintain muscle tone;
- Isotonic exercises – those carried out with movement in which the isotonic
  muscle contraction results in a change in muscle length (shortens or lengthens)
  and movement of its attachments, to increase muscle strength and endurance;
- Passive – exercises that are usually carried out by the physiotherapist or the
  nurse without the assistance of the patient.

AEROBIC AND ANAEROBIC EXERCISE

Aerobic exercise is physical activity that requires the heart and lungs to work
harder to obtain and supply increased oxygen to strenuously contracting skeletal muscles. The long-term physical changes, or adaptations, that result from
aerobic exercise increase the body's ability to deal with endurance exercise.
   Anaerobic exercise is vigorous short-duration exercise in which the skeletal muscle
oxygen supply is inadequate. Metabolic fuel molecules are broken down anaerobi-
cally to produce adenosine triphosphate (ATP) with the conversion of pyruvic acid
into lactic acid. The *anaerobic threshold* describes the point at which aerobic energy
processes alone can no longer meet the musculoskeletal requirements for ATP.
Anaerobic adaptations are long-term physical changes that result from anaerobic
exercise. They increase the body's ability to deal with powerful dynamic exercise.

EXERCISE TOLERANCE

Exercise tolerance describes exercise accomplished without pain or marked breathlessness. The American Heart Association's classification of functional capacity:

Class I   No symptoms on ordinary effort;

Class II   Slight disability on ordinary effort (in the UK it is usual to subdivide this class into Class IIa – able to carry on with normal housework under difficulty – and Class IIb – cannot manage shopping or bed-making except very slowly);

Class III Marked disability on ordinary effort that prevents any attempt at housework;

Class IV   Symptoms at rest or heart failure.

EXPRESSED EMOTION

Expressed emotion (EE) is a research concept that uses a semi-structured interview, known as the Camberwell family interview, to ascertain the effects of certain environments upon the course of schizophrenia. Relatives of clients with schizophrenia were interviewed, and investigations found that when clients returned to live in hostile, critical or overprotective high EE environments they relapsed more frequently than those who took regular medication and returned to live in low EE accepting, supportive environments. These studies have been replicated throughout the world and the measurement of EE is now recognized to be a reliable predictor of relapse. Indeed, the characteristics of EE are not found exclusively in relatives as professional carers share similar attributes (Oliver and Kuipers 1996) and neither are they specific to schizophrenia. The measurement of high EE can also predict relapse in other psychiatric and medical disorders, such as depression.

The characteristics of low and high EE are outlined in *Table 17*. ⇒ Schizophrenia.

Table 17 Response characteristics of low and high EE (adapted from Leff and Vaughn 1985)

	Low EE	High EE
Cognitive	Recognize illness as genuine Lower expectations of the individual	Legitimacy of illness in doubt Expectations unchanged
Emotional	Other-focused Empathetic Calm Objective	Self-focused – 'my goals and needs are more important' Intense anger and/or stress
Behavioural	Adaptive Problem-solving approach Nonintrusive Nonconfrontational	Inflexible Intrusive Confrontational

E

EXTERNAL FIXATORS

External fixators are used in orthopaedic conditions, such as fractures, as an alternative to the use of traction or internal fixation (*Fig. 73*).

Patients should be assisted with proper positioning, utilizing pillows as required for elevation and support. Neurovascular assessment of the affected limb must be performed on a regular basis according to local policy – as a rule of thumb, hourly for 2 hours, then 2 hourly for 12 hours, reducing to 6 hourly, should be sufficient. It is often advisable to administer an analgesic prior to adjustment of pin torque and wound care to facilitate patient comfort in what can be very painful procedures.

The patient should be educated regarding all of the above to enable self-care after discharge.

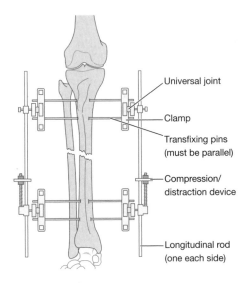

Universal joint

Clamp

Transfixing pins
(must be parallel)

Compression/
distraction device

Longitudinal rod
(one each side)

Fig 73 External fixator – universal day frame

EXTRACORPOREAL

Extracorporeal is outside the body.

EXTRACORPOREAL CIRCULATION

Any situation in which blood is taken from the body, directed through a machine ('heart–lung' or 'artificial kidney') and returned to the body, such as during some types of cardiac surgery or during haemodialysis.

EXTRACORPOREAL MEMBRANE OXYGENATION (ECMO)

The extracorporeal membrane oxygenation (ECMO) circuit is a cardiopulmonary bypass device that uses a membrane oxygenator or 'artificial lung' to support gas exchange. It is used in extreme situations for profound cardiac or respiratory failure. Several methods of perfusion are available, the most common being the venoarterial approach in which, after cannulation, venous blood is drained from the right atrium through the right internal jugular vein and oxygenated blood is returned through the right common carotid artery to the aortic arch.

EXTRACORPOREAL SHOCK-WAVE LITHOTRIPSY

Extracorporeal shock-wave lithotripsy (ESWL) is the use of high-energy shock waves applied externally to break up stones in the kidney or ureter, and sometimes for the treatment of gallstones. The waves break the stones into small pieces that may then be passed in the urine or retrieved endoscopically. Cardiac monitoring is required in ESWL for two reasons – firstly, to synchronize the shock-wave pulse with the R wave of the P-QRS-T complex and, secondly, to monitor for cardiac arrthymias. A double J stent may be inserted into the collecting system as part of this procedure to allow for the passage of stone fragments greater than 5 mm.

E

> **Practice application – patient education after ESWL for kidney stones**
> - Pain – some pain may be experienced as the stone fragments are passed down the ureter. Analgesics are prescribed for the patient to take home.
> - Infection – prophylactic antibiotics are given, as most stones are infected and shattering these can spread infection. The importance of completing the course of antibiotics is stressed. The GP should be consulted if pyrexia develops and increased pain is experienced.
> - Elimination – the patient is advised to drink 2–3 L in 24 hours to help flush out the stone fragments and clear any blood in the urine.
> - Activity – normal activity can be resumed the next day, with a return to work within a few days.

E YE

The eye is the organ of vision situated within the bony orbit. It has three layers: sclera (outer fibrous layer), a middle layer (the uvea, which forms the pigmented choroid, ciliary body and iris) and the light-sensitive retina that contains photoreceptors (cones and rods) and pigment cells (*Fig. 74*). Light that enters the eye is focused on the retina by the lens. Nerve endings in the retina convert the images and transmit them to the brain, in fibres of the optic nerve, for interpretation. ⇒ Colour vision, Vision.

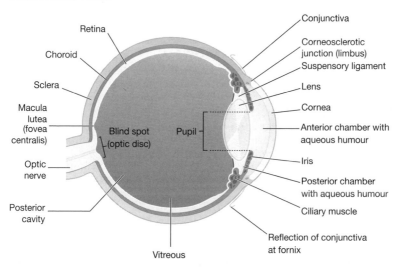

Fig 74 Section through the eyeball

E

The view through the pupil of the structures at the back of the eye using an ophthalmoscope is termed the fundus (*Fig. 75*). This view includes the retina with the optic disc, macula lutea, fovea centralis and the retinal blood vessels. The optic disc can bulge when intracranial pressure is raised, a condition called papilloedema.

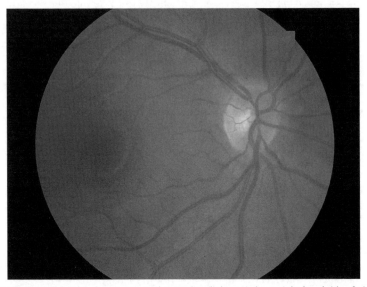

Fig 75 Normal fundus showing normal optic disc (lighter circle on right-hand side of picture) – originally taken from Kanski JJ (1999). *Clinical Ophthalmology*, Fourth Edition. Oxford: Butterworth–Heinemann

ACCESSORY STRUCTURES

The orbit and the eyelids provide protection for the eyeball and orbital contents (muscles, blood vessels and nerves, including the optic nerve, and fat).

EYELIDS, LASHES AND EYEBROWS

The eyelids protect the eyeball from trauma and excess light. The eyebrows protect the eyes from sweat, foreign bodies and intense sunlight.

LACRIMAL SYSTEM

The lacrimal glands produce tears that flow through ducts into the upper conjunctival fornix. Blinking helps to disperse the tear film over the front of the eye and so helps to keep the cornea and conjunctiva moist.

The tear film comprises three distinct layers:
• Outer oily layer – prevents evaporation and spillage of tears;
• Middle aqueous layer;
• Inner mucin layer.
Tears drain into the back of the throat via the nasolacrimal drainage system.

CONJUNCTIVA

The conjunctiva is the thin mucous membrane that lines the eyelids, forms the upper and lower fornices (see Practice application) and is reflected to cover the anterior surface of the eyeball. It is continuous with the cornea.

EXTRAOCULAR (EXTRINSIC) MUSCLES

Six extraocular (extrinsic) muscles move each eyeball. The muscles are innervated autonomically by cranial nerves that give the degree of control of eyeball position and movement needed to focus on distant and near objects. The eyes can also be moved voluntarily. There are four rectus muscles (medial, lateral, superior and inferior) and two oblique muscles (superior and inferior).

PAINLESS VISUAL IMPAIRMENT

CATARACT

Cataract is an opacity of the crystalline lens. It is a very common condition and can affect people of all ages.

DIABETIC RETINOPATHY

Diabetic retinopathy (DR) is a retinal disease caused by diabetes. It occurs more frequently in Type 1 diabetes, but it is also seen in people with Type 2 diabetes. Depending on the disease stage there may be microaneurysms (dots), haemorrhages (blots), exudates and retinal ischaemia (cotton wool spots) and new blood vessels. Later there may be fibrosis that leads to vitreous haemorrhage and retinal detachment. ⇒ Diabetes mellitus.

AGE-RELATED MACULAR DEGENERATION

Age-related macular degeneration (AMD) is a leading cause of blindness in people over 50 years of age. It takes two forms, dry (the most common) and wet. AMD affects the macula lutea, an area necessary for reading and seeing fine features, such as faces.

RETINAL DETACHMENT

Retinal detachment occurs when the neural retina becomes separated from the retinal pigment epithelium. There are two major classifications – with a hole and without. The causes include myopia, after cataract extraction, trauma, age-related degeneration of the retina, diabetes, tumours and inflammation.

PRIMARY OPEN-ANGLE GLAUCOMA

There are many types of glaucoma (raised intraocular pressure, IOP), including primary open-angle glaucoma (POAG) and primary closed-angle glaucoma. POAG is a chronic condition with insidious onset. Often it is only diagnosed when the person attends for routine eye tests. It is known that African Caribbean individuals and people with a close relative who has glaucoma are at a higher risk of developing the condition.

PAINFUL OCULAR CONDITIONS AND TRAUMA

PRIMARY CLOSED-ANGLE GLAUCOMA

Primary closed-angle glaucoma (PCAG) is an acute condition characterized by an elevated IOP. The normal outflow for aqueous humour is blocked because of partial or complete closure of the drainage angle. The condition affects people of middle-age and older. Patients present with severe pain around one eye. The eye is typically red and the pupil is oval and semi-dilated. Visual acuity is reduced and patients are intolerant of light (photophobic). They may also complain of seeing halos around lights. They feel unwell and occasionally experience nausea and vomiting. PCAG is a medical emergency, as the raised IOP can cause permanent damage and loss of vision.

E

ENUCLEATION

Enucleation is the removal of an eyeball, such as for severe damage to the eyeball, a painful blind eye, etc.

CORNEAL DISORDERS

The outer epithelial layer of the cornea can heal without scarring, but damage to the deeper layers can result in permanent scarring. Damage to the inner lining leads to corneal oedema. Disorders of the cornea include injury, infection, degeneration, congenital and nutritional. Any corneal disorder has the capacity to cause corneal oedema, ulcers, opacities or perforation. When the cornea becomes traumatized or diseased, it can result in the following signs and symptoms: pain, photophobia, excess lacrimation (tearing), blepharospasm (eyelid spasm), ciliary injection (blood vessels at the corneal margin become inflamed), miosis (small and/or constricted pupils), reduced vision and discharge of pus.

CONJUNCTIVAL CONDITIONS

CONJUNCTIVITIS

Conjunctivitis is inflammation of the conjunctiva, the main causes of which are bacterial infection, viral infection or *Chlamydia* (e.g. *Chlamydia trachomatis*), which causes trachoma; this is a major cause of blindness world-wide, especially in hot dry climates, where it is widespread. Conjunctivitis may also result from allergies to, for example, drops or eye makeup. Overuse of contact lenses can also cause conjunctivitis. It can be spread to others, especially where face cloths and towels are shared. It is characterized by a minor gritty (foreign body) sensation, photophobia, hyperaemia (red and slightly engorged conjunctiva), purulent discharge with bacterial infection or a watery discharge associated with viral and allergic conjunctivitis.

CONDITIONS OF THE UVEAL TRACT

UVEITIS

Uveitis is inflammation of the uveal tract. It is classified according to the anatomical structures involved:
- Anterior uveitis involves the iris or the ciliary body and occasionally both;
- Posterior uveitis affects the choroid;
- Panuveitis is inflammation that affects the whole uveal tract.

Frequently the cause is unknown, but it may be associated with: trauma, HIV disease or systemic inflammatory disease, such as inflammatory bowel disease.

It is characterized by pain, photophobia, ciliary injection, red eye, tearing, blurred vision, pus in the anterior chamber (hypopyon, *Fig. 76*), the pupil is usually constricted (miosed) and may be irregular and the IOP is raised occasionally.

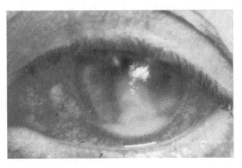

Fig 76 Hypopyon

CONDITIONS THAT AFFECT THE EYELIDS

BLEPHARITIS

Blepharitis is a chronic inflammation of the eyelids and is relatively common. Occasionally, it is associated with conjunctivitis. It is usually bilateral and affects people of any age.

CHALAZION

Chalazion is a swelling in a meibomian gland (secretory glands in the lid).

STYE OR EXTERNAL HORDEOLUM

A stye is an acute infection (usually *Staphylococcus aureus*) of the sebaceous gland at the base of an eyelash follicle.

E

DRY EYES

A deficiency associated with any aspect of the tear film results in dry eye, causing discomfort, but if untreated it may lead to loss of vision. Dry eye can occur at any age. There is (occasionally) red eye, gritty, itchy eye, burning sensation, poor tear production, ache round the eye and (occasionally) sticky eye, usually in the morning.

The treatment is aimed at relieving symptoms, although people may take some convincing that they have dry eye, particularly when they may be complaining that their eyes are watering. This is because the deficient oil film causes tears to spill over into the cheek. Artificial tears are prescribed and should be instilled as often as they are needed.

AGE-RELATED PROBLEMS – ENTROPION AND ECTROPION

Entropion is where the eyelid turns inwards. The eyelashes irritate the eye, which causes marked discomfort as well as tearing (watering) of the eye. If the condition is allowed to go untreated, the cornea is likely to ulcerate and could become permanently scarred. Some temporary relief from the discomfort can be obtained by applying tape to the lower lid. Over-correction causes ectropion (see below). In addition, offending lashes rubbing against the cornea can be removed. Treatment is normally by corrective surgery to evert the eyelid. An alternative to surgery is the use of local injections of botulinum toxin.

Ectropion is where the eyelid turns outwards, away from the eyeball. The eyelids do not close properly, which leaves the eyeball exposed, and the tear film is not distributed evenly. This has an adverse effect on the cornea and conjunctiva. The eye waters because the tears cannot drain into the punctum, and the cheek becomes sore owing to the frequent wiping away of tears. Treatment depends on the cause, but it is usually surgical. However, the quality of the person's lifestyle can be improved by the use of artificial tears and lubricating ointment to the eye and barrier cream to the cheek to protect the skin.

DRUGS USED IN OPHTHALMOLOGY

A list of the common drugs used in ophthalmology is provided in *Table 18*.

E

Table 18 Drugs used in ophthalmology (adapted from Brooker and Nicol 2003)

Drug group and example	Uses
Mydriatics: a: Cycloplegics (antimuscarinics), e.g. atropine sulphate, cyclopentolate hydrochloride b: Noncycloplegics (sympatho-mimetics), e.g. phenylephrine hydrochloride	Dilate the pupil, such as for examination
Miotics, e.g. pilocarpine	Constrict the pupil; improves the drainage of aqueous humour and is used in the treatment of raised intraocular pressure (IOP)
Beta blockers, e.g. levobunolol, timolol maleate	Used to lower IOP in some types of glaucoma; reduces aqueous humour production.
Carbonic anhydrase inhibitors, e.g. acetazolamide, brinzolamide	Inhibit the production of aqueous humour and so reduce IOP
Antiprostaglandin analogues, e.g. bimatoprost, latanoprost	Increase uveoscleral drainage of aqueous humour, used to reduce IOP in some types of glaucoma
Antibacterials: a: Broad spectrum, e.g. chloram-phenicol, gentamicin, ciprofloxacin b: Specific range of action, e.g. fusidic acid	Ocular infection; usually administered topically; may be administered systemically or by subconjunctival or intraocular injection for some infections
Antivirals, e.g. aciclovir, fomivirsen	Used to treat viral infections that affect the eye
Anti-inflammatory: a: Corticosteroids, e.g. hydrocortisone hydrochloride b: Other inflammatory drugs, e.g. levocabastine (antihistamine), sodium cromoglicate	Inhibits inflammation, oedema and allergy Used for allergic conjunctivitis.
Local anaesthetics, e.g. ametho-caine, lidocaine	Short-acting local anaesthesia to surface of the eye
Diagnostic agents, e.g. fluorescein	Highlights damaged tissue; also used when fitting contact lenses, testing for leaking corneal wounds and intravenously for fundal photography (fluorescein angiography)
Lubricants and artificial tears, e.g. liquid paraffin, cabomers	Used to treat 'dry eye' conditions or when normal protective mechanisms are compromised, such as loss of blink reflex in altered consciousness

Practice application – instilling eye medication (adapted from Nicol et al. 2000)

To instil eye medications effectively and safely, patients need information about the procedure from the nurse as well as sufficient opportunities to practise and ask questions. Nurses should reinforce the importance of following eye medication regimens, and the correct care and storage of drops, ointment and any equipment used. Patients should be advised about checking expiry dates on the drugs and reminded that the drug is prescribed for them only. Explain to patients that with some eye drops they may taste the drug as it drains from the eye through the nasolacrimal system. Normally, separate containers for drops or ointment should be used if both eyes are being treated.

Administering eye medication – guidelines for patients

- Check that you are about to instil the correct medications into the correct eye at the correct time.
- Wash your hands.
- Remember that the medication may sting and cause blurred vision for a short time, so do not move about or drive until your vision is back to normal.
- Remove the cap from the medication.
- Gently pull down the lower eyelid to form the small pocket (inferior conjunctival fornix). Both eye drops and ointment are instilled into this pocket (*Fig. 77*).
- Instil the drops or ointment as per prescription (i.e. the number of drops and the order if the treatment involves more than one drug). If you have both drops and ointment, use the drops first, as the greasy ointment may stop the drops working properly. Make sure that the dropper or ointment tube does not touch any part of the eye.
- If you are using ointment, start at the inner part by your nose and squeeze a ribbon of ointment about 1–2 cm in length along the inside edge of the eyelid.
- Shut your eyes gently and count slowly to 60 after instilling your eye medication so that the drug is not absorbed systemically.
- If you need more than one drop per eye, blink normally between drops to disperse the drug.
- Wash your hands.
- Store the medications correctly.
- Check that you have sufficient medications, particularly over weekends and holiday periods.

Seek professional advice if anything unusual happens, such as your eye feeling different after the medication, or if you have any questions about your condition and treatment.

Further reading

Brooker C and Nicol M (2003). *Nursing Adults. The Practice of Caring*, Ch 15. Edinburgh: Mosby.

E

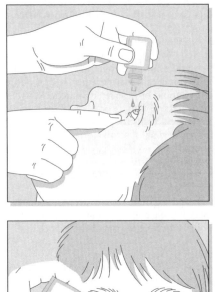

(A)

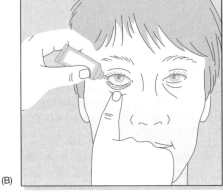

(B)

Fig 77 Instillation of eye medication: (A) drops, (B) ointment

FAIR AND ANTIDISCRIMINATORY PRACTICE

Fair and antidiscriminatory nursing practice, which recognizes and respects alternative cultures and beliefs, is constructed around valuing the individual as a person with rights (Clause 2.1, NMC 2002a). It includes a positive acceptance, promotion and protection of the interests and dignity of people, irrespective of age, gender, race, ability, economic status, sexuality, health problems, culture and political or religious beliefs (Clause 2.2, Nursing and Midwifery Council 2002a).

The UK health service (Department of Health 1998a, 1999a) is underpinned by values of equity and fairness and holds that health services should strive to provide carebased on the best possible evidence and guided by patient's needs and expectations. All patients, without exception, should have equal access to a high standard of care, regardless of where they live or any of the factors discussed above.

The moral principle of justice is highly complex in terms of its meaning and application in practice. Taking the notion of justice according to rights, an understanding of what constitutes an individual's rights is a vital goal for nurses if they are to strive to promote and uphold the rights of patients and/or clients to fair and equitable care.

Violating the rights of patients and/or clients in their care is one of the worst offences that nurses or other health professionals can be guilty of.

FAMILY

The family is assuming a higher profile in modern westernized societies as political leaders, policymakers and social scientists argue for the institution of marriage to be maintained.

The family as a social organization has undergone many changes. Nowadays it is more common to use the term 'families', since there are many family types. For example, in addition to the conventional family types, such as the nuclear family, the extended family, the step family and the compound family (as in some African societies), one must also include lone parent families, cohabitation and gay and lesbian families. Perspectives on the family abound. Functionalists emphasize the role of the family in stress management and in its reproductive and economic activities for society's benefit. Feminists, however, argue that women in families are being oppressed in a patriarchal society. Marxist theorists take the view that the family participates in reproducing a workforce for the benefit of a capitalist society.

The *World Health Report* (WHO 1998a) stipulates that the family forms the basis of the healthcare system, together with personal responsibility and the community. Furthermore, the role of the family in the maintenance of mental well-being and in helping those with mental health problems is emphasized (Department of Health 1999b).

FAMILY-CENTRED CARE

A philosophy of nursing, usually applied to children, that takes into account the needs and circumstances of the whole family, not just the child. In family-centred care the parents and other family members do what were previously considered 'nursing duties', while nurses take responsibility for teaching families, providing support and helping families to make decisions in the best interests of their sick child. These activities may often present nurses with situations in which they have to make some difficult decisions. Such circumstances, therefore, suggest that nurses have to feel competent about the delivery of their practical skills in addition to thinking in a clear and rational manner about the emotional and social care they provide.

Further reading

Béphage G (2000). *Social and Behavioural Sciences for Nurses: An Integrated Approach.* Edinburgh: Churchill Livingstone.

FAMILY PLANNING

Family planning covers the methods used to space or limit the number of children, or to enhance conception.

BIRTH CONTROL

TYPES OF CONTRACEPTION

Types of contraception can be classified by the way they act. The objective is to prevent fertilization or implantation of a fertilized egg, which can be achieved by the following:
- Barrier methods – prevent fertilization by keeping the sperm and oocyte apart, they include the condom, female condom, diaphragm and cervical cap;

- Hormonal methods – prevent ovulation or implantation if an oocyte is fertilized, they include oral contraceptives, either combined oestrogen–progesterone or progesterone only (mini-pill), local progestogens by injection or subdermal implants, intrauterine progesterone-only device (dual function – reduces menorrhagia and provides contraception), transdermal patches and vaginal rings that release oestrogen and progesterone, and levonorgestrel is used for emergency hormonal contraception within 3 days (72 hours) of unprotected intercourse;
- Intrauterine contraceptive devices (IUCDs or IUDs) – prevent implantation, for which various devices are available and may be inert or release progestogen (see above) – a copper-containing IUCD can be used as an emergency contraception if inserted within 5 days of unprotected intercourse;
- Spermicides, such as nonoxinol, in the form of foams, pessaries and sponges – may be used with barrier methods;
- Permanent method – e.g. female sterilization or male vasectomy.

NATURAL FAMILY PLANNING

Natural methods of family planning are those that do not use drugs or appliances. They may use one or a combination of urinary hormone levels, temperature, cervical mucus and menstrual cycle calendar (see Practice application – natural family planning). *Coitus interruptus,* or the withdrawal method, in which the man withdraws the penis from the vagina before ejaculation is used by some couples, but is considered to be very unreliable. ⇒ Infertility (see *Table 24*), Menstrual cycle, Reproductive systems.

Practice application – natural family planning

A commercially produced system that comprises urine dipsticks and a monitoring device that measures hormone levels in early morning urine samples is used to predict the days in the menstrual cycle when conception is possible. Alternatively, the basal body temperature can be recorded daily (i.e. taken each morning on waking before any activity or refreshments are taken) to indicate ovarian progesterone production and thus, by observing the timing of the rise, give an *approximate* guide to the timing of ovulation (*Fig. 78*). This method is used to time ovulation retrospectively by women who want to conceive and by those who do not (as it can be incorporated with the rhythm method of birth control, enabling sexual intercourse to be avoided until 3–4 days after ovulation). This 'typical' pattern of change in temperature during the menstrual cycle is not seen in all women, even with ovulatory cycles.

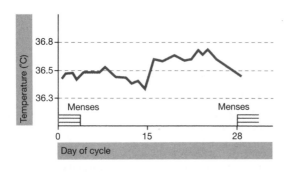

Fig 78 Temperature chart showing typical rise in basal body temperature during the luteal phase of the menstrual cycle

FAT

The main dietary fat is triacylglycerol (also known as triglyceride). Other fats such as phospholipids and cholesterol are important, but can be synthesized in the body. All these fats, as well as others, belong to a large group of molecules called lipids.

SATURATED AND UNSATURATED FATS

Animal fats are generally sources of saturated fats, while oily fish and vegetables are sources of unsaturated fats. The building blocks of triacylglycerols are a glycerol backbone and three fatty acids (*Fig. 79*).

The fatty acids are normally different, thus creating a wide diversity of triacylglycerols. It is these fatty acids that are saturated or unsaturated. In a saturated fatty acid, the carbon atoms are attached to as many hydrogen atoms as possible, whereas in unsaturated fatty acids there are one or more double bonds between carbon atoms, which cannot attach to hydrogen; those with one double bond are monounsaturated and those with two or more double bonds are polyunsaturated (*Fig. 80*).

Heating or hydrogenating unsaturated fatty acid changes the structure. It can become the *trans* form in which the fatty acid molecules pack tightly together to form a solid fat. *Trans* fatty acids are associated with health problems.

Triacylglycerols are a source of the *essential fatty acids* (EFAs) and of the fat-soluble vitamins A, D, E and K. The EFAs are n-6 polyunsaturated fatty acid (PUFA; linoleic acid) and n-3 PUFA (α-linolenic acid). Arachidonic acid is synthesized in the body from linoleic acid.

Although more energy-dense than carbohydrate, fats are not generally used as an immediate energy source [1 g produces 37 kJ (9 kcal)]. It is important that sufficient fat is consumed to provide adequate stores of fuel. Triacylglycerols provide a major reserve of metabolic fuel stored in fat cells (adipocytes).

Lipolysis is the chemical breakdown of fat – stored triacylglycerols are released for energy, stimulated by glucocorticoid hormones. Amino acids and glucose can be converted into triacylglycerols in a metabolic process known as *lipogenesis*, a process stimulated by insulin. ⇒ Gastrointestinal tract (*Table 19*), Lipids, Macronutrients.

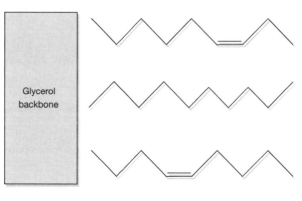

Glycerol backbone

Fatty acids attached to glycerol backbone

Fig 79 Basic structure of a triacylglycerol (triglyceride)

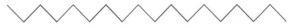

Saturated Fatty Acid
Found in coconut oil, palm oil, dairy products and meat

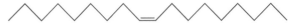

Monounsaturated Fatty Acid with one double bond
Found in olive oil, rapeseed oil, peanut oil, cow's milk and beef

F

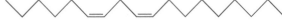

Polyunsaturated Fatty Acid n–6 PUFA Linoleic Acid
Found in corn oil, soybean oil, sunflower oil, poultry and meat

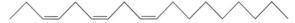

Polyunsaturated Fatty Acid n–3 PUFA αLinolenic Acid
Found in flaxseed oil, cod liver oil and oily fish such as herrings

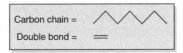

Carbon chain =

Double bond =

Fig 80 Fatty acids – basic structure and sources

FEBRILE

Febrile means feverish, or accompanied by fever.

FEBRILE SEIZURES (PREVIOUSLY CALLED FEBRILE CONVULSIONS)

Febrile seizures occur in children who have an increased body temperature They do not usually result in permanent brain damage and are most common between the ages of 6 months and 5 years. The fever is usually above 38°C and mostly over 38.8°C to precipitate a seizure. A febrile seizure is of short duration and having a febrile seizure does not mean that the child has developed epilepsy. The vast majority of children have a complete recovery. However, a small number of children develop epilepsy after febrile seizures. The children most at risk of developing problems are those who experience more prolonged seizures of over 20 minutes duration with focal features of the seizure. ⇒ Body temperature, Nervous system (epilepsy), Seizure.

FEMALE GENITAL MUTILATION

Female genital mutilation (female circumcision) is excision of the clitoris, labia minora and labia majora. The extent of cutting varies from country to country. The simplest form is clitoridectomy; the next form entails excision of the prepuce, clitoris and all or part of the labia minora. The most extensive form, *infibulation*, involves excision of the clitoris, labia minora and labia majora. The vulval lips are sutured together, but total obliteration of the vaginal introitus is prevented by inserting a piece of wood or reed to preserve a small passage for urine and menstrual fluid. These procedures are illegal in many countries.

FERTILITY

Fertility is the state of being able to produce young. ⇒ Conception and fertilization, Family planning (types of contraception, natural family planning), Infertility.

FERTILITY RATE

Fertility rate is the number of live births that occur per 1000 women of age 15–44 years (e.g. 60 per 1000 women). It can also be described in terms of the total fertile period, that is the average number of live births that would occur per woman if the woman experienced the current age-specific fertility rate throughout her reproductive years (e.g. 1.9 per woman).

FETUS

The developmental stage from the eighth week of gestation until birth. ⇒ Alcohol (fetal alcohol syndrome).

FETOPLACENTAL UNIT

Fetoplacental unit is a term used to describe the interdependence of fetal (adrenal glands and liver) and placental tissues in hormone production during pregnancy. The hormones produced include oestrogen (particularly oestriol), progesterone and human placental lactogen (hPL), also known as human chorionic somatomammotrophin (hCS).

FETAL ASSESSMENT AND SCREENING

Various methods are used to assess fetal well-being and screen for abnormalities.

AMNIOCENTESIS

Amniocentesis is a diagnostic procedure to detect chromosomal (e.g. Down's syndrome), neural tube defects, metabolic and haematological abnormalities of the fetus. It involves inserting a needle under ultrasound guidance through the abdominal wall into the amniotic sac to obtain a sample of amniotic fluid. It is usually performed around the 15th week of pregnancy. There is a risk of complications and some pregnancies are lost through miscarriage.

BLOOD TESTS (MATERNAL BLOOD)

Blood tests include the triple test offered to pregnant women. This measures alpha-fetoprotein (AFP), unconjugated oestriol and total hCG in maternal serum and is used early in pregnancy to predict the estimated risk of conditions such as Down's syndrome.

CHORIONIC VILLUS SAMPLING

Chorionic villus sampling (CVS) is also known as chorion or chorionic villus biopsy. It is a prenatal screening test for chromosomal and other inherited disorders. Samples of fetal tissue are obtained via the cervix to detect genetic abnormalities during early pregnancy (around 11 weeks).

FETOPLACENTAL UNIT FUNCTION TESTS

Fetoplacental unit function tests include 24 hour oestriol levels in maternal urine.

KICK CHARTS

Kick charts are a record of kicks felt by the woman. They are a guide to the amount of fetal movement and hence well-being.

ULTRASOUND SCAN

Ultrasound scans (USSs) are routinely offered during pregnancy to monitor progress and detect fetal and placental abnormalities. An USS is usually performed in the first trimester to show whether the pregnancy is intrauterine, whether there is more than one fetus and whether ovarian cysts or fibroids are present. Scanning at 16–18 weeks shows the presence of fetal abnormalities such as spina bifida and heart defects. More specialized ultrasound equipment is available for nuchal (nape of the neck) scanning used in the diagnosis of Down's syndrome.

FETAL CIRCULATION

The fetal circulation is adapted for intrauterine life. Extra vessels and shunts (ductus arteriosus, ductus venosus, foramen ovale and umbilical vein) allow most blood to bypass the lungs, liver and gastrointestinal tract, as their functions are dealt with by maternal systems and the placenta (*Fig. 81*).

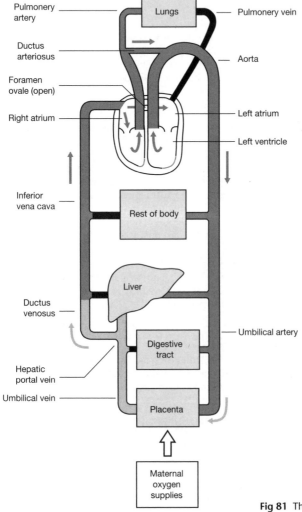

Fig 81 The fetal circulation

FIBRINOLYSIS

Fibrinolysis is the final stage of haemostasis. ⇒ Haemostasis.

FITNESS FOR PRACTICE (THE PEACH REPORT)

Fitness for Practice is a report prepared by the Commission for Education established by the UKCC to look at preregistration nursing and midwifery education and propose education that 'enabled fitness for practice based on healthcare need' (UKCC 1999). ⇒ Competence and competencies, Nursing and Midwifery Council, Professional self-regulation.

FLUID BALANCE AND BODY FLUIDS

Water makes up about 60% of human body weight in the average man, accounting for some 40 L in a 70 kg male adult. Fat (adipose tissue) contains little water and therefore the proportion of body water is lower in obesity and also in females, who have a higher proportion of body fat than males. This is found mainly in the breasts and around the hips. The proportion of body water decreases with age. Age and gender differences in the proportions of body water are shown in *Fig. 82.*

Body water is found in two compartments: the intracellular fluid (ICF) accounts for two-thirds of the total body water and the extracellular fluid (ECF) for the remaining one-third. ICF consists of the watery cytosol within all body cells. ECF includes the plasma in the circulatory system and fluid in the spaces between tissue cells, known as tissue or interstitial fluid. *Fig. 83* shows the water distribution within the two compartments. Homeostasis of many factors, including water and electrolytes in the fluid compartments, is essential for life and health. Although body fluids are discussed here in isolation it is important to remember that fluid, electrolyte and acid–base balance are all interdependent. ⇒ Acid–base balance, Electrolytes.

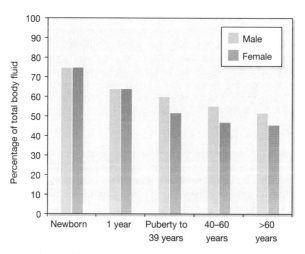

Fig 82 Percentage of total body fluid in relation to age and gender (based on Metheny 1996)

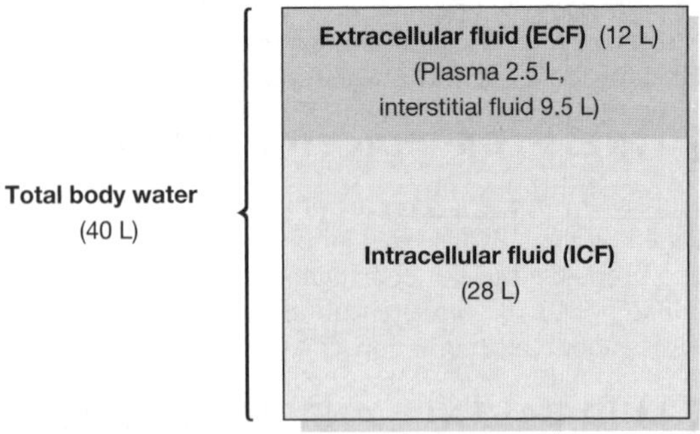

Extracellular fluid (ECF) (12 L)
(Plasma 2.5 L,
interstitial fluid 9.5 L)

Total body water
(40 L)

Intracellular fluid (ICF)
(28 L)

Fig 83 Distribution of body
fluid in a 70 kg adult male

F

MOVEMENT OF WATER AND ELECTROLYTES

Water and other small molecular substances can normally pass freely across the membranes that surround body cells and separate them from capillary membranes. A number of processes are involved.

DIFFUSION

Diffusion takes place when a difference in concentration of substances, known as a concentration gradient, exists. Gases and solutes move from an area of high concentration to one of low concentration until equilibrium is reached (the concentration is the same). No chemical energy is required and therefore transport is described as passive. Diffusion also occurs across a semi-permeable membrane, such as the plasma membrane, and some solutes can also cross it. Water can move freely, while large molecules such as proteins are too large to cross membranes.

OSMOSIS

Osmosis is the movement of water across a semi-permeable membrane down its concentration gradient from an area of high water concentration to one of low water concentration. It occurs when equilibrium cannot be achieved by the movement of solute molecules (e.g. salt or sugar) across the semi-permeable membrane. The pressure needed to oppose this movement of water across membranes is called osmotic pressure and is related to the size of the concentration gradient. The concentration of osmotically active particles in a litre of fluid is known as the osmolality of the solution. Osmosis continues until equilibrium is reached and the concentrations on each side of the semi-permeable membrane are the same. The solutions are then said to be *isotonic*. In the body, isotonic means having the same osmolality as plasma. Solutions with higher concentrations of solutes than those in plasma are *hypertonic* and those with solute concentrations lower than those in plasma are *hypotonic*.

ACTIVE TRANSPORT

Active transport is the transport of substances against their concentration gradient and is described as active because chemical energy, in the form of adenosine triphosphate (ATP), is needed to drive the process. The sodium–potassium pump is an active transport mechanism and is present in cell membranes to maintain homeostasis of sodium and potassium.

FILTRATION

The filtration mechanism is also important in the movement of fluids in the body, but it relies on pressure differences rather than the concentration differences

F

described above. When a pressure gradient exists, the higher (hydrostatic) pressure causes water and other small molecules to be pushed through membrane pores to an area of lower pressure. This process is important in the formation of tissue fluid and in filtration of the blood by nephrons in the kidney.

Practice application – assessment of fluid and electrolyte status
The assessment of fluid and electrolyte status requires a review of the patient's history, together with nursing observations. During the assessment interview, a history of the patient's normal eating and drinking patterns is sought together with any recent changes in habits. This includes approximate daily volumes and preferred types of drinks. The following should be assessed:
• Oral cavity – the oral cavity and the structures within it are normally moist and shiny.
• Thirst – the sensation of thirst is an important indicator of fluid depletion.
• Skin turgor – when pinched up, the skin of a healthy person returns immediately to its normal position when released because of the recoil of elastic tissue (referred to as turgor). When turgor is reduced, the skin remains elevated for some seconds after release (e.g. when a patient has a fluid-volume deficit). Turgor is reduced in older people, and it may be difficult to assess turgor in people who have recently lost weight because the skin can be loose. In infants the fontanelles are also assessed for bulging or depression.
• Oedema – this is present when there is retention of excess interstitial fluid and is especially apparent in dependent areas. The feet and ankles commonly swell when sitting, and the sacrum swells if the patient is in bed. After lying flat overnight, the eyes may be puffy (*periorbital oedema*). *Pitting oedema* is when the oedematous tissue remains indented after firm digital pressure is applied.
• Sunken eyes – a sign of moderate or severe fluid-volume deficit and occurs as a result of loss of interstitial fluid around the orbit.
• Confusion, lethargy and anxiety – these nonspecific symptoms often accompany fluid loss and acid–base disorders. In older people, the presence of confusion is an indicator that all is not well and a more detailed inquiry is required to identify the underlying cause.
• Respiratory status – rate, depth and effort are assessed and recorded, providing baseline information. Abnormalities or trends may indicate an underlying disorder of fluid, electrolyte or acid–base balance. Fluid-volume excess and cardiac failure may lead to pulmonary oedema.
• Pulse – tachycardia is usually the first sign of decreased intravascular volume, but this is not always present in older adults.
• Blood pressure – when the blood pressure is recorded with the patient lying down and then when standing up, a sustained decrease when standing is known as postural hypotension. This often accompanies fluid-volume deficit. In more severe cases, hypotension occurs even when lying flat because of reduced blood volume. Rising blood pressure may indicate fluid overload.
• Jugular venous pressure (JVP) – the jugular veins in the neck provide an indicator of central venous pressure (CVP) as the blood volume determines the level of filling and distension of these veins.
• Central venous pressure – CVP measurements are interpreted together with pulse, blood pressure, respiratory rate, fluid intake and urine output. A trend in any or all of these values is often of significance. Low CVP occurs when blood volume is decreased. Raised CVP occurs when there is increased blood volume. ⇒ Central venous pressure.

- Urinary output – volume, colour and specific gravity. Ongoing monitoring of fluid intake and output is recorded on a fluid balance chart (*Fig. 84*).
- Weight – sudden reduction may indicate fluid deficit. An increase in weight may result from water retention.
- Bowel habit – constipation and diarrhoea.

F

Fluid balance chart

Hospital/Ward:						Date:		

Hospital number:

Last Name:

Forenames:

Date of birth:

Sex:

	Fluid intake			Fluid output				
Time	Oral	IV	Other (specify route)	Urine	Vomit	Other (specify)		
01.00								
02.00								
03.00								
04.00								
05.00								
06.00								
07.00								
08.00								
09.00								
10.00								
11.00								
12.00								
13.00								
14.00								
15.00								
16.00								
17.00								
18.00								
19.00								
20.00								
21.00								
22.00								
23.00								
24.00								
TOTAL								

Fig 84 Fluid balance chart

DISORDERS OF FLUID BALANCE

Disorders of fluid balance may be isotonic or osmolar. Isotonic imbalances occur when water and electrolyte levels are increased or decreased in proportion to their levels in the ECF. In osmolar imbalances a loss or gain of water affects only the concentration of electrolytes, mainly sodium, and therefore the serum osmolality. The principal differences are shown in *Fig. 85*. Although described separately, the disorders below often occur in combination. Details of the signs and symptoms of individual disorders can be found in the Further reading suggestion.

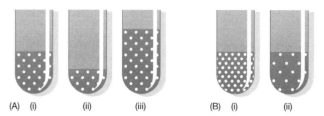

Fig 85 Water imbalance: (A) isotonic imbalance – (i) normal, (ii) fluid-volume deficit, (iii) fluid-volume excess; (B) osmolar imbalance – (i) hypernatraemic, (ii) hyponatraemic

ISOTONIC IMBALANCES
Fluid-volume deficit

In fluid-volume deficit there is loss of electrolytes and water in proportion to their levels in the ECF and therefore serum levels remain normal [*Fig. 85A(ii)*]. This should not be confused with dehydration, which correctly describes an osmolar imbalance (see below). It is usually the result of loss of fluid from the gastrointestinal tract through vomiting, diarrhoea, fistulae or nasogastric or other drainage tubes. Other causes include pyrexia, sweating, increased urine volume and third space events.

Third space events occur when fluid is effectively lost from the circulation (ECF) because of a pathological condition. Susceptible patients include those with major trauma, burns or surgery, intestinal obstruction, sepsis and pancreatitis. The effective fluid loss can amount to several litres and may accumulate in the pleural, peritoneal or pericardial cavities.

Fluid-volume exces

Fluid-volume excess arises when there is retention of electrolytes and water in proportion to the levels in the ECF [*Fig. 85A (iii)*]. It is usually the result of sodium retention accompanied by the retention of water. Fluid moves into the interstitial spaces and accumulation leads to oedema (excess tissue fluid). The causes include congestive cardiac failure, renal failure, cirrhosis of the liver, excessive corticosteroid levels and over-transfusion with i.v. fluids that contain sodium.

OSMOLAR IMBALANCES
Hyperosmolar imbalance

Dehydration, or water depletion, is one form of this condition and occurs when there is water loss without significant loss of electrolytes [*Fig. 85B(i)*].

There is an increase in the serum sodium level and osmolality. This results in movement of fluid out of cells and into the circulation to maintain blood volume.

As the cells become dehydrated, their function is impaired. The kidneys respond by secreting less urine in an attempt to conserve body fluid. Thirst is the natural response to fluid depletion and occurs as the osmolality of the blood increases. This abnormality may occur with a nearly normal ECF volume or may be accompanied by a fluid-volume deficit or excess.

Hypo-osmolar imbalance

Hypo-osmolar imbalance is also known as water excess and it effectively dilutes the ECF [*Fig. 85B(ii)*]. Movement of fluid is from the ECF into the ICF. It is caused by excessive water intake – 'water intoxication', a severe mental health problem also called psychogenic polydipsia – or abnormally high levels of antidiuretic hormone. ⇒ Pituitary gland (diabetes insipidus).

FLUID REPLACEMENT

Fluids and electrolytes may be replaced in several ways:
- Oral – the oral route is used for fluid replacement whenever possible as it is 'normal', noninvasive and free of the discomforts and complications of other routes – electrolyte replacement in the form of oral rehydration salts and/or solution (ORS) may be used;
- Enteral – a nasogastric, nasoenteric or gastrostomy tube may be used to replace fluids;
- Subcutaneous infusion (hypodermoclysis);
- Rectal infusion (proctoclysis);
- Intravenous ⇒ Intravenous therapy and/or infusion;
- Intraosseous ⇒ Intraosseous.

Further reading

Brooker C and Nicol M (2003). *Nursing Adults. The Practice of Caring*, Ch 8. Edinburgh: Mosby.

FOOD PROBLEMS

FOOD ALLERGY AND INTOLERANCE

Food allergy is an abnormal immunological response to foods (such as peanuts, strawberries and shellfish) that can be severe and life-threatening. Signs and symptoms include swelling of the mouth and throat, breathing difficulties, skin rashes and gastrointestinal disturbances. The term is often used erroneously to describe any adverse reactions to food, whether or not the underlying mechanism has been identified. ⇒ Allergy.

Food intolerance or sensitivity is an abnormal reaction to a food that is not immunological in origin, such as lactase deficiency or coeliac disease (see below). Symptoms can be chronic or acute, identification of the food can be difficult and may require an exclusion diet.

COELIAC DISEASE

Coeliac disease (gluten-sensitive enteropathy) is an unpleasant reaction to gluten (cereal protein) that may damage the intestinal villi. Symptoms may be mild or more severe with abdominal bloating and progressive weight loss. Management involves avoiding products that contain gluten, which is found, for example, in wheat-, rye- and barley-based foods.

LACTOSE INTOLERANCE

Individuals who are lactose intolerant lack the enzyme (lactase) to digest milk sugar (lactose). Undigested lactose then passes into the colon, where it can cause diarrhoea and cramping pain. Sufferers may be able to tolerate fermented milk products such as yoghurt and cheese.

FOOD POISONING

Food poisoning is a notifiable disease characterized by vomiting, with or without diarrhoea. ⇒ Communicable diseases (notifiable diseases), *Escherichia*, Gastroenteritis.

FOOD STANDARDS AGENCY

The Food Standards Agency (FSA) is a UK body set up by the Government to oversee food standards and safety.

FORENSIC

Forensic means pertaining to or applied in legal proceedings.

FORENSIC MEDICINE

Forensic medicine encompasses the branches of medicine concerned with the law and that have a bearing on legal problems. It includes the investigation of unexplained death or injury.

The term forensic is also be applied to secure psychiatric hospitals or units.

FORMULARY

A formulary is a collection of formulas. For example, the *British National Formulary* (BNF) describes licensed pharmaceutical products available in the UK, and is produced by the Joint Formulary Committee (British Medical Association and the Pharmaceutical Society).

NURSE PRESCRIBERS' FORMULARY

In the UK, the *Nurse Prescribers' Formulary* (*NPF*) is a limited formulary available to suitably qualified nurses who have completed an approved course and demonstrated prescribing competence. ⇒ Nurse prescribing.

FRACTURE

A fracture is a break in the continuity of a bone. Fractures may be classified into two types:
- Open (compound) – a fracture in which a wound communicates with the fracture haematoma, and thus provides a route for bacteria;
- Closed (simple).

There are essentially three causes of fracture:
- Trauma – direct or indirect;
- Stress or fatigue fractures;
- Pathological fractures – occur in an abnormal or diseased bone and result in a fracture caused by limited force (e.g. osteoporosis, tumour).

Fractures may also be classified according to the pattern of the fracture as it presents on a radiograph (X-ray; *Box 13* and *Fig. 86*).

F

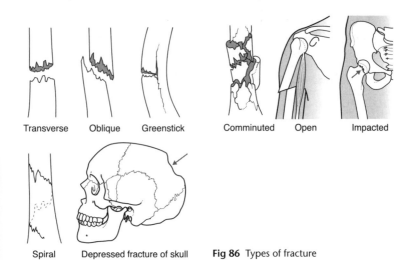

Transverse Oblique Greenstick   Comminuted Open Impacted

Spiral Depressed fracture of skull   **Fig 86** Types of fracture

---

Box 13 Fracture pattern
Comminuted – at least three fragments present.
Greenstick – occur in children. The bone is only fractured halfway through on the convex side of the bend.
Transverse – runs at right angles to the long axis of bone (often direct trauma).
Oblique – fracture line is less than 90° to the long axis of bone (often indirect trauma).
Spiral – fracture curves in spiral fashion (usually indirect trauma).
Complicated – surrounding organs or structures are damaged.
Avulsion – may be produced by a sudden muscle contraction or ligamentous attachment pulling off the portion of bone to which it is attached.
Depressed (commonly to the skull) – as a result of a sharp localized blow.
Compression (crush) – commonly applied to vertebral bodies or ankle (usually indirect trauma).
Segmental (double fracture) – fractured at two distinct levels.
Impacted – one fragment is driven into another (e.g. femur or humerus).

Practice application – recognizing the signs and symptoms of a fracture
These include:
• Local pain and tenderness;
• Swelling;
• Bruising;
• Crepitus (grating noise heard when the broken bone moves);
• Deformity, including shortening;
• Abnormal mobility of the affected part;
• Loss of functional ability to perform daily living tasks;
• Soft tissue damage.

FRACTURE HEALING

The process of fracture healing is summarized in *Fig. 87*.

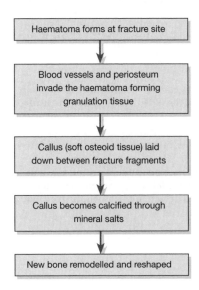

Fig 87 Fracture healing

OVERVIEW OF THE MANAGEMENT OF FRACTURES

Six common treatment modalities are used in fracture management:
• Nonrigid methods of support (e.g. slings, bandages, strapping);
• Continuous traction – skin or skeletal types;
• Plaster fixation;
• Internal surgical fixation;
• External surgical fixation;
• Casts and/or bracing.
⇒ Casts, External fixators, Skeleton, Traction.

COMPLICATIONS OF FRACTURES

Complications of fractures may be classified as immediate (at the time of injury), early (within hours or days) and late (within weeks or months).
    Immediate complications include:
• Haemorrhage – blood loss (1.0–2.5 L) from the bone itself combined with loss from damage to surrounding tissues (e.g. femur);
• Damage to arteries and nerves (e.g. in supracondylar fracture of the humerus; see Practice application);
• Damage to surrounding tissues (e.g. pneumothorax in rib fractures, spinal cord damage in vertebral fractures, brain injury in skull fractures).
Early complications include:
• Wound infection;
• Fat embolism, which occurs particularly with multiple fractures of long bones;
• Generalized problems of immobilization (e.g. pressure ulcer, deep vein thrombosis, chest infection);
• Compartment syndrome ⇒ Compartment syndrome.
Late complications include:
• Delayed union – when the fracture does not unite within the expected time;
• Malunion – when the bone has united soundly but in the wrong position, and surgery may be required depending on the potential disability and outcome;

- Non-union – may not be a serious problem in nonweight-bearing bones (a painless, false joint may occur), but internal fixation or bone grafting may be required;
- Deformity;
- Secondary osteoarthritis ⇒ Joint;
- Aseptic and/or avascular necrosis may occur, particularly after fractures to the femoral head, scaphoid and talus – it results from disruption to the blood supply to the bone after the fracture.

Practice application – neurovascular assessment after supracondylar fracture of the humerus

The jagged end of the proximal fragment may poke into the soft tissue anteriorly and thereby compromise the brachial artery or median nerve. Neurovascular assessment is important to detect problems at an early stage. The following observations are performed:
- The radial pulse on the affected side;
- The skin colour and warmth of the limb distal to the injury;
- Sensation distal to the injury;
- Movement of the fingers;
- Degree of pain.

The medical staff are informed at once if the radial pulse is absent or increasingly difficult to palpate, the limb becomes pale, blue or cold, sensation is altered, pain increases or if the person is unable to move his or her fingers.

Further reading

Brooker C and Nicol M (2003). *Nursing Adults. The Practice of Caring*, Ch 27. Edinburgh: Mosby.

FREE RADICAL

Free radicals are activated oxygen species, such as the superoxide ion and hydroxyl radical. They are extremely reactive chemicals produced during normal metabolism. Normally, they are dealt with by complex antioxidant enzyme systems, but they can cause oxidative damage to cells. ⇒ Ageing (cellular theories).

Antioxidants are substances that delay the process of oxidation. Some minerals (e.g. zinc) and vitamins A, C and E contained in a balanced diet function as antioxidants and help to minimize free radical oxidative damage to cells.

FUNGI

Fungi are simple plants, the Mycophyta, which include mushrooms, yeasts, moulds and rusts.

FUNGAL DISEASES

Fungal infections in humans may be superficial or systemic.

ASPERGILLOSIS

Aspergillosis is an opportunist infection, most frequently of the lungs, caused by any species of *Aspergillus*. *A. fumigatus* is a fungus that is found mainly in animal manure and rotting vegetation. The spores can be inhaled into the lungs and cause chronic infection or disseminated aspergillosis, where invasive lung infections by *Aspergillus* occurs. Allergic bronchopulmonary aspergillosis (ABPA) can develop in people who have an allergic response to *Aspergillus*. Patients who develop ABPA develop asthma and are treated with prednisolone to treat the wheeze, and anti-fungals (e.g. itraconazole and amphotericin) to treat the infection.

BLASTOMYCOSIS

Blastomycosis is caused by *Blastomyces*, a genus of pathogenic fungi. A granulo-matous condition caused by *B. dermatitidis* affects the lungs, lymph nodes, the skin, viscera, bones and joints. Treatment is with itraconazole, ketoconazole or ampho-tericin.

CANDIDIASIS AND/OR CANDIDOSIS (MONILIASIS, THRUSH)

Candidiasis are infections caused by a species of *Candida*, usually *C. albicans*. Infection may involve the mouth, gastrointestinal tract, skin, nails, respiratory tract or genitourinary tract (vulvovaginitis, balanitis), especially in individuals who are debilitated (e.g. cancer, diabetes mellitus or immunosuppressed) and after long-term or extensive treatment with antibiotics, which upsets the microbial flora, and other drugs (e.g. corticosteroids). Oral infection can be caused by poor oral hygiene, including carious teeth and ill-fitting dentures. Antifungal drugs used include nystatin, amphotericin, fluconazole or itraconazole. Systemic infections should be treated with i.v. amphotericin or amphotericin plus flucytosine, or flu-conazole. ⇒ Infections of female reproductive tract, Sexually transmitted and/or acquired infections.

COCCIDIOIDOMYCOSIS

Coccidioidomycosis is an infection caused by the fungus *Coccidioides immitis*. It may be asymptomatic, but otherwise affects the lungs, lymph nodes and the skin. It occurs in Central and South America, and the southern US. Amphotericin, itra-conazole, ketoconazole or fluconazole may be helpful, but relapse is common.

CRYPTOCOCCOSIS

Cryptococcosis is the disease that results from infection with the yeast *Cryptococcus neoformans*, which is present in soil and pigeon excreta. It most commonly causes meningitis, but may also affect the lungs, skin and bones. Immunocompromised individuals, such as those with human immunodeficiency virus (HIV) infection, are at increased risk. Treatment is i.v. amphotericin and oral fluconazole.

HISTOPLASMOSIS

Histoplasmosis is an infection caused by the fungus *Histoplasma capsulatum* or *H. duboisii*. It is found throughout East, Central and West Africa. The visceral form is often fatal. Life-threatening histoplasmosis can occur in people with HIV infec-tion. Treatment is with oral itraconazole or ketoconazole or i.v. amphotericin.

TINEA

⇒ Skin (skin disorders).

GAG REFLEX

The gag or pharyngeal reflex is contraction of the pharyngeal muscles and eleva-tion of the palate when the soft palate or posterior pharynx is stimulated. It is used to check the functioning of two cranial nerves, the vagus (X) and glossopharyn-geal (IX).

> **Practice application – taking steps to avoid initiating the gag reflex**
> The gag reflex, which is an unpleasant sensation, is sometimes experienced when the dentist works on back teeth. In people with extra-sensitive mouths this reflex can be troublesome when cleaning the teeth. Care should be taken when cleaning patients' mouths because eliciting the reflex, apart from being unpleasant, may induce vomiting.

G

GALACTOSAEMIA

Galactosaemia is an excess of galactose in the blood and other tissues. Normally lactase (an enzyme) in the small intestine converts lactose into glu-cose and galactose. In the liver another enzyme system converts galactose into glucose. Galactosaemia is the result of a congenital enzyme deficiency in this system (two types) and is one cause of learning disability. ⇒ Learning dis-ability.

GAMETOGENESIS

Gametogenesis is the production of gametes (oocytes and spermatozoa). Its pur-pose is to produce haploid gametes from diploid germ cells. Haploid describes the chromosome complement after the reduction division of meiosis. This set rep-resents the basic complement of 23 (n) unpaired chromosomes in humans (22 auto-somes and 1 sex chromosome). Diploid describes a full set of paired chromosomes. In humans the diploid number is 46 chromosomes (44 autosomes and 2 sex chro-mosomes) arranged in 23 pairs. ⇒ Chromosomes, Genes and genetics, Meiosis, Mitosis.

OOGENESIS

Oogenesis is the formation and maturation of oocytes in the ovary. All the oocytes are present at birth, albeit in an immature state. Oogenesis is a complex process that involves mitosis, a first meiotic division that is interrupted by a long resting stage, and a second meiotic division that is only completed if the secondary oocyte is fertilized by a spermatozoon (*Fig. 88*).

SPERMATOGENESIS AND SPERMIOGENESIS

Spermatogenesis and spermiogenesis, respectively, describe the formation and maturation of spermatozoa in the testes (*Fig. 89*). Maturation involves the change in shape of the spermatocytes (sperm cell) into the characteristic form.

GANGRENE

Gangrene is death of part of the tissues of the body. It is usually the result of inad-equate blood supply, but occasionally it is caused by direct injury (traumatic gan-grene) or infection (e.g. gas gangrene – see below). Deficient blood supply may result from:

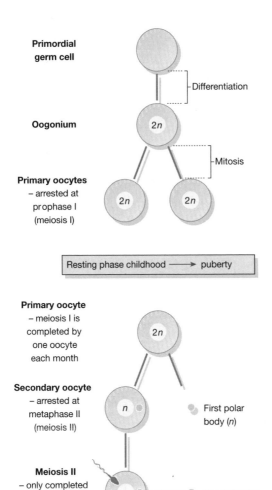

Primordial germ cell

Differentiation

Oogonium

$2n$

Mitosis

Primary oocytes
– arrested at prophase I (meiosis I)

$2n$ $2n$

Resting phase childhood ⟶ puberty

Primary oocyte
– meiosis I is completed by one oocyte each month

$2n$

Secondary oocyte
– arrested at metaphase II (meiosis II)

n First polar body (n)

Meiosis II
– only completed if spermatozoon penetration occurs

n Second polar body (n)

n

Ovum

$2n$ = Diploid number of chromosomes
n = Haploid number of chromosomes

NB Polar bodies eventually degenerate with the ovum

Fig 88 Oogenesis

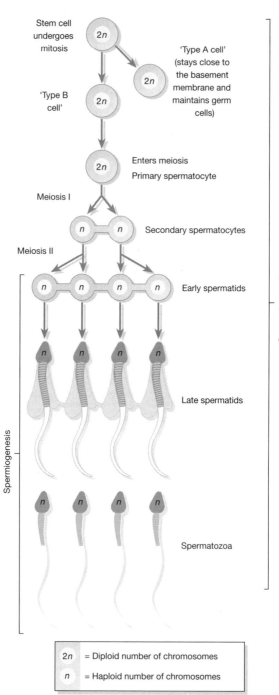

Fig 89 Sperm production

- Pressure on the blood vessels (e.g. tourniquets, tight bandages and swelling of a limb);
- From obstruction within healthy vessels (e.g. arterial embolism, frostbite when the capillaries become blocked);
- From spasm of the vessel wall (e.g. ergot poisoning);
- From thrombosis caused by disease of the vessel wall (e.g. arteriosclerosis in arteries, phlebitis in veins).

Dry gangrene occurs when the drainage of blood from the affected part is adequate; the tissues become shrunken and black. *Moist gangrene* occurs when venous drainage is inadequate so that the tissues are swollen with fluid.

GAS GANGRENE

Gas gangrene is a serious wound infection caused by anaerobic organisms of the genus *Clostridium*, especially *C. perfringens (welchii)*, a soil microbe often present in the intestine of humans and animals.

GASTROINTESTINAL TRACT (ALIMENTARY TRACT)

The gastrointestinal (GI) tract is a muscular tube approximately 9 m in length that consists of the mouth, pharynx, oesophagus, stomach, small intestine (duodenum, jejunum and ileum), large intestine (colon and large bowel), the rectum and anal canal (*Fig. 90*, which also shows the liver and pancreas). The GI tract is controlled by the autonomic nervous system. It is responsible for the breakdown, digestion and absorption of food and the removal of solid waste in the form of faeces from the body. It does this by allowing foods to pass through each sec-

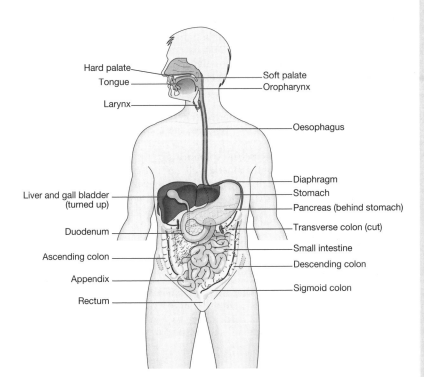

Fig 90 The organs of the digestive system

tion and subjecting them to the action of various digestive fluids and enzymes. The fluids and enzymes are secreted by a variety of glands and organs, such as the salivary glands, the stomach, small intestine, the pancreas and the liver (*Table 19*). It is this secretion of fluids that helps to maintain the function of the tract. ⇒ Defecation, Nutrition (nutritional support), Peritoneum.

GASTROINTESTINAL DISORDERS

A brief overview of some gastrointestinal disorders is provided here. Some conditions (e.g. colorectal cancer, etc.) are covered in more detail. ⇒ Anorectal problems, Endoscopy, Food problems (coeliac disease, food poisoning), Hernia, Oral (oral problems), Stoma.

ACHALASIA

Achalasia is the loss of oesophageal peristalsis and failure of lower oesophageal sphincter relaxation.

APPENDICITIS

Appendicitis is inflammation of the vermiform appendix.

CANCER

Cancer may occur in the oesophagus, when it often presents with dysphagia and weight loss. Patients with gastric (stomach) cancer often have symptoms that suggest an ulcer (but do not improve), anorexia and weight loss.

Colorectal cancer

Colorectal cancer is the second most common cause of cancer deaths in the UK. It can affect any part of the large bowel, although it is more common in the sigmoid colon and the rectum. Symptoms may only become apparent when the cancer is at an advanced stage. Symptoms and signs depend on the site affected, but include:
- Altered bowel habit, rectal bleeding and tenesmus (a feeling that the bowel is not emptied), a mass felt when rectal examination is performed;
- Abdominal pain and weight loss, signs of anaemia;
- Fistula, abdominal mass, bowel obstruction, perforation and haemorrhage.

Following investigations the cancer is staged using the Dukes' or TNM classification, as follows:
- Grade A – confined to mucosa and submucosa;
- Grade B – involves part of the muscle wall, but not the lymphatic system;
- Grade C – involves the wall and regional lymph nodes;
- Grade D – tumour that has metastasized to distant sites.

Depending upon the grade, radiotherapy, chemotherapy and/or surgery (curative or palliative) is carried out. The type and extent of the surgery undertaken depends upon the site of the cancer and patients may require a temporary or permanent stoma. ⇒ Cancer, Stoma.

DIVERTICULAR DISEASE

Diverticulosis is a condition in which there are many diverticula (sing., diverticulum – pouch or sac protruding from the wall of a tube or hollow organ), especially in the intestines. Colonic diverticula increase in frequency with age. It may be asymptomatic, bleed, become infected or perforate. Diverticulitis is inflammation of a diverticulum.

Table 19 Summary of the sites of digestion and absorption of nutrients

	Mouth	Stomach	Small intestine		Large intestine
			Digestion	Absorption	
Carbohydrates	*Salivary amylase:* cooked starches to disaccharides	Acid denatures and stops action of salivary amylase	*Pancreatic amylase:* cooked starches to disaccharides *Sucrase, maltase, lactase* (in enterocytes): disaccharides to monosaccharides (mainly glucose)	Into blood capillaries of villi	–
Proteins	–	*Acid:* pepsinogen to pepsin Pepsin: proteins to polypeptides	*Enterokinase* (in intestinal mucosa): chymotrypsinogen and trypsinogen (from pancreas) to chymotrypsin and trypsin *Chymotrypsin and trypsin:* polypeptides to di- and tripeptides; *Peptidases* (in enterocytes):di- and tripeptides to amino acids	Into blood capillaries of villi	–
Fats	–	–	*Bile* (from liver): bile salts emulsify fats *Pancreatic lipase:* fats to fatty acids and glycerol *Lipases* (in enterocytes): fats to fatty acids and glycerol	Into the lacteals of the villi	–
Water	–	Small amount absorbed here	–	Most absorbed here	Remainder absorbed here
Vitamins	–	Intrinsic factor secreted for vitamin B_{12} absorption	–	Water-soluble vitamins absorbed into capillaries; fat-soluble ones into lacteals of villi	Bacteria synthesize vitamin K in colon; absorbed here

G

Dyspepsia

Dyspepsia is indigestion, and can be a symptom of a GI disorder.

Enteritis

Enteritis is inflammation of the intestines.

Gastritis

Gastritis is inflammation of the lining mucosa of the stomach. It may be acute or chronic (see below, peptic ulcer).

Gastroenteritis

Gastroenteritis is food poisoning with inflammation of mucosa of the stomach and the small intestine, usually caused by micro-organisms, but it may be caused by chemicals, poisonous fungi, etc. There is vomiting and diarrhoea because of either the multiplication of micro-organisms (invasive intestinal gastroenteritis, such as *Campylobacter jejuni, Salmonella typhimurium, S. enteritidis, Listeria monocytogenes, Bacillus cereus*) and viruses (such as Norwalk virus, rotovirus ingested in food), or from food contaminated with bacterial toxins (intoxication), such as from *Escherichia coli 0157, Staphylococcus aureus, Clostridium botulinum* and *C. perfringens*.

Gastroenteritis is generally transmitted by the faecal–oral route, either directly or indirectly, however droplet spread is a feature of some viruses. ⇒ Communicable disease (notifiable diseases), Escherichia, *Salmonella* (enteric fevers).

Gastrointestinal bleeding

Haematemesis is the vomiting of blood, which may be bright red after recent bleeding. Otherwise it is of 'coffee ground' appearance because of the action of gastric juice. The bleeding is usually from the GI tract and causes include peptic ulcer, oesophageal varices, cancers, drug erosions and coagulation defects, but blood swallowed from elsewhere may be vomited.

Melaena is the passage of black, tar-like stools, and is evidence of GI bleeding.

Gastro-oesophageal reflux disease

Gastro-oesophageal reflux disease (GORD) consists of an incompetent and/or malfunctioning lower oesophageal sphincter, which allows the stomach contents to move into the oesophagus. In children this results in vomiting, oesophagitis, scarring and stricture. There is also the danger of aspiration pneumonia. The exact cause is unknown, but predisposing factors include gastric distension, increased abdominal pressure caused by coughing, central nervous system disease, delayed gastric emptying, hiatus hernia and gastrostomy placement.

In adults GORD typically causes heartburn. Complications also include Barrett's oesophagus in which mucosal changes predispose to oesophageal cancer.

Ileitis

Ileitis is inflammation of the ileum.

Ileus

Ileus is an intestinal obstruction. The term is usually restricted to paralytic as opposed to mechanical obstruction and characterized by abdominal distension, vomiting and the absence of pain. It can occur with peritonitis, after GI surgery, etc.

INFLAMMATORY BOWEL DISEASE

Inflammatory bowel disease (IBD) is an idiopathic intestinal inflammation. It results mainly from ulcerative colitis and Crohn's disease. ⇒ Stoma.

Crohn's disease

Crohn's disease is a chronic recurrent granulomatous disease that usually affects the terminal ileum, but lesions occur elsewhere in the small bowel and in the colon, rectum and anus. It affects young adults mainly and is characterized by a necrotizing, ulcerating inflammatory process. There can be healthy bowel ('skip' area) intervening between two diseased segments. It causes pain, diarrhoea, steatorrhoea, malabsorption, anaemia, weight loss and pyrexia. Complications include abscess formation, obstruction, fistula formation and bowel perforation.

Management includes high protein and/or energy diet, enteral or parenteral feeding, correction of anaemia and vitamin deficiency, antidiarrhoeal drugs, corticosteroids, an aminosalicylate (e.g. sulfasalazine or mesalazine), the immunosuppressant azathioprine and metronidazole, an antimicrobial drug. Recently, treatment with a monoclonal antibody was introduced for severe forms of Crohn's disease. Surgery is indicated where medical treatment fails or to treat complications, such as obstruction.

Ulcerative colitis

Ulcerative colitis is an inflammatory and ulcerative condition of the rectum and colon. Characteristically, it affects young and early middle-aged adults and causes diarrhoea with blood and mucus, pain, tenesmus, anaemia, weight loss and serious complications that include toxic dilatation (megacolon), perforation, dehydration, electrolyte disturbances, malignant changes and liver damage.

Management may include general supportive measures, such as parenteral nutrition, and drugs, such as the corticosteroids (rectal and systemic), sulfasalazine and an immunosuppressant ciclosporin or azathioprine. Surgery is indicated where medical treatment fails or as an emergency treatment for toxic dilatation, haemorrhage or bowel perforation.

INTESTINAL FAILURE

The intestine can fail to absorb adequate fluid and nutrients to sustain metabolic requirements because of disease or resection. ⇒ Nutrition (nutritional support).

INTESTINAL OBSTRUCTION

Intestinal obstruction is not a disease in itself. The causes may be:
- Mechanical (e.g. strangulated hernia, bowel disease, adhesions, tumours outside the bowel);
- Neurological, partial or complete loss of peristalsis (e.g. paralytic ileus);
- Vascular, when the blood supply to a segment of bowel is cut off (e.g. embolism, atheroma with thrombosis and strangulated hernia).

IRRITABLE BOWEL SYNDROME

Irritable bowel syndrome (IBS) covers functional intestinal symptoms not explained by organic bowel disease. Symptoms include abdominal pain, bloating and change in bowel habit (alternating constipation and diarrhoea). It is important to exclude pathology such as colorectal cancer.

PEPTIC ULCERATION

Ulceration of the GI mucosa is caused by disruption of the normal balance of the corrosive effect of gastric juice and the protective effect of gastric mucus.

The most common sites are the duodenum and the stomach. Peptic ulcers may be acute such as those associated with severe stress (e.g. serious illness, shock, burn, etc.) or chronic illness.

Duodenal ulcer

A duodenal ulcer is a peptic ulcer that occurs in the duodenal mucosa. The majority are associated with the presence of the bacterium *Helicobacter pylori* in the stomach. Other factors include nonsteroidal anti-inflammatory drugs (NSAIDs), smoking and genetic factors. Epigastric pain may occur some time after meals or during the night. The pain may be relieved by food, antacids and vomiting. The ulcer can bleed, which leads to haematemesis and/or melaena, or it can perforate. Severe scarring after chronic ulceration may produce pyloric stenosis and gastric outlet obstruction.

Management includes:

- General measures such as smoking cessation, avoiding foods that cause pain, avoiding aspirin and NSAIDs;
- Antibiotic drugs to eradicate *H. Pylori*;
- Drugs to reduce gastric acid, such as H_2-receptor antagonists (e.g. ranitidine), proton pump inhibitors (e.g. omeprazole) and antacids based on calcium, magnesium or aluminium salts;
- Rarely, surgical treatment (e.g. after perforation).

POLYPOSIS

In polyposis there are numerous intestinal polyps. Familial adenomatous polyposis is a dominantly inherited condition in which multiple polyps occur throughout the large bowel. It invariably leads to colon cancer. Polyps also occur in the stomach and duodenum.

PYLORIC STENOSIS

Narrowing of the pylorus may be congenital or acquired. Congenital hypertrophic pyloric stenosis results from a thickened pyloric sphincter muscle. Pyloric stenosis may be caused by scar tissue formed during the healing of a peptic ulcer.

VARICES

Varices are dilated, tortuous veins. Those that occur in the oesophagus and stomach result from hepatic portal hypertension. These varices can bleed and may cause massive haematemesis.

TYPES OF GASTROINTESTINAL SURGERY

ABDOMINOPERINEAL RESECTION

Abdominoperineal (AP) resection involves extensive surgery in which the sigmoid colon is brought out as a colostomy, and the rectum and anus are removed. A permanent colostomy is usually performed, although some specialist centres offer total anorectal reconstruction as an alternative to a colostomy.

ANTERIOR RESECTION

Anterior resection is an operation performed for high rectal or low sigmoid cancers. This involves radical removal of the tumour and anastomosis (joining together) of the left side of the colon to the distal bowel end. The surgeon may create a colonic pouch, which allows patients to have a 'normal' bowel function, or a temporary stoma, which allows the anastomosis time to heal.

APPENDICECTOMY (APPENDECTOMY)

An appendicectomy is the surgical removal of the appendix.

CARDIOMYOTOMY

Cardiomyotomy involves cutting or dissection of the muscular tissue at the gastro-oesophageal junction for achalasia.

COLOSTOMY

⇒ Stoma.

FUNDOPLICATION

Fundoplication is folding of the gastric fundus to prevent reflux of gastric contents into the oesophagus.

GASTRECTOMY

Gastrectomy is removal of a part or the whole of the stomach. It is usually used for cancers, but may be used for gastric ulcers that do not respond to drug therapy. *Billroth I gastrectomy* is a partial gastrectomy in which the remaining portion of the stomach is anastomosed to the duodenum. *Polya's partial gastrectomy* (known in the US as *Billroth II gastrectomy*) involves removal of part of the stomach and duodenum and anastomosis of the remaining part of the stomach to the jejunum. *Total gastrectomy* is a radical operation that may be performed for cancer in the upper part of the stomach.

GASTROENTEROSTOMY

Gastroenterostomy is a surgical anastomosis between the stomach and small intestine.

GASTROJEJUNOSTOMY

Gastrojejunostomy is a surgical anastomosis between the stomach and the jejunum.

GASTRO-OESOPHAGOSTOMY

Gastro-oesophagostomy is an operation in which the oesophagus is joined to the stomach to bypass the natural junction.

GASTROSTOMY

Gastrostomy is a surgically established fistula between the stomach and the exterior abdominal wall, used for feeding. ⇒ Nutrition (nutritional support).

GASTROTOMY

Gastrotomy is an incision into the stomach during an abdominal operation for such purposes as removing a foreign body, securing a bleeding blood vessel and approaching the oesophagus from below to pull down a tube through a constricting growth.

ILEOCOLOSTOMY

An ileocolostomy is a surgically made fistula between the ileum and the colon, usually the transverse colon. It is most often used to bypass an obstruction or inflammation in the caecum or ascending colon.

Ileosigmoidostomy

Ileosigmoidostomy is an anastomosis between the ileum and sigmoid colon.

Ileostomy

⇒ Stoma.

Oesophagectomy

Oesophagectomy is an excision of part or the whole of the oesophagus.

Oesophagogastrectomy

Oesophagogastrectomy is the removal of part of the oesophagus and stomach.

Oesophagostomy

Oesophagostomy is a surgically established fistula between the oesophagus and the skin in the root of the neck. It may be used temporarily for feeding after excision of the pharynx for malignant disease.

Oesophagotomy

Oesophagotomy is an incision into the oesophagus.

Proctocolectomy

Proctocolectomy is a surgical excision of the rectum and colon.

Pyloromyotomy (syn. Ramstedt's operation)

Pyloromyotomy is an incision of the pyloric sphincter for congenital pyloric stenosis.

Pyloroplasty

A pyloroplasty is a plastic operation on the pylorus designed to widen the passage.

Practice application – gastric aspiration

Gastric aspiration is used to keep the stomach empty of contents. A tube (usually nasogastric) is passed into the stomach and suction applied using either a syringe or a pump. It is usually performed in the following circumstances:
- Intestinal (bowel) obstruction;
- Paralytic ileus;
- Preoperatively for gastric or some abdominal surgery;
- Postoperatively (e.g. partial gastrectomy).

Continuous aspiration can be carried out by some form of pump, the recommended suction pressure being 20–25 mmHg. A lower pressure is ineffective and a higher pressure can damage the gastric mucosa.

Sometimes, usually postoperatively, a drainage bag and tubing may be attached to the end of the nasogastric tube. If the drainage bag is placed lower than the person's stomach, the stomach contents siphon into the bag.

Intermittent aspiration can be performed by pump or catheter-tipped syringe. Between aspirations, a clean disposable spigot should be used to occlude the end of the tube. It is important to observe and measure all aspirate. The amount is charted as appropriate, usually on a fluid chart, and changes in volume or colour are documented and reported. For example, decreasing amounts may indicate the resumption of normal gastric emptying, or increasing blood in the aspirate may indicate internal bleeding.

Further reading

Jamieson E, McCall J and Whyte L (2002). *Clinical Nursing Practice*, pp. 161–164. Fourth Edition. Edinburgh: Churchill Livingstone.

GENDER

Gender is more than just the biological sex. The term encompasses the socially constructed views of feminine and masculine behaviour within individual cultural groups. ⇒ Sexuality.

GENES AND GENETICS

Genes are hereditary factor located at a specific place (locus) of a specific chromosome, consisting of DNA. Genes are responsible for determining specific characteristics or traits and the precise replication of proteins.

Genes may be recessive or dominant. A dominant gene has the capacity to overpower other recessive genes. Dominant genes are expressed in both the homozygous state (inherited from one parent) and the heterozygous state (inherited from both parents). Examples of dominant characteristics and diseases include freckles, normal skin and hair pigmentation, and Huntington's disease.

Recessive genes are only expressed when the specific allele that determines it is present at both paired chromosomal loci (i.e. in the homozygous state). When the specific allele is present in a single dose, the characteristic is not manifest, as its presence is concealed by the dominant allele at the partner locus. The exception is for X-linked genes in males, in which the single recessive allele on the X-chromosome expresses itself so that the character is manifest.

GENETIC CODE

Genetic code is the information carried on the DNA molecules of the chromosome. It is in this coded form that the information contained in the genes is transmitted to the cells to determine their activity through the precise replication of proteins.

GENETIC IMPRINTING

Genetic imprinting is a form of inheritance caused by structural alterations to chromosomes during gametogenesis that may affect the way a particular allele is expressed. The effects depend on whether the chromosome is paternal or maternal. It results in two distinct conditions that arise from the same mutation (e.g. chromosome 15 change results in Prader–Willi syndrome if inherited via paternal chromosomes and Angleman syndrome when the chromosome is maternal).

GENETIC DISEASES

There are many genetic diseases. ⇒ Cystic fibrosis, Haemoglobin (haemoglobinopathies), Learning disability (Angleman syndrome, fragile X syndrome, Prader–Willi syndrome), Phenylketonuria. They include those inherited as:

- Autosomal dominant traits, single major gene defects (e.g. Huntington's disease, achondroplasia), or two or more major gene defects [e.g. breast cancer (familial, early onset), polycystic kidney disease];
- Autosomal recessive traits, e.g. cystic fibrosis, phenylketonuria, sickle cell disease, beta-thalassaemia, etc.;
- X-linked, e.g. haemophilia A and B, Duchenne's muscular dystrophy, fragile X syndrome;
- Imprinted gene (e.g. Prader–Willi syndrome and Angleman syndrome);
- Mitochondrial DNA abnormalities (e.g. hereditary optic atrophy).

GERMAN MEASLES

⇒ Communicable diseases (rubella).

GERONTOLOGY

Gerontology is the scientific study of ageing. ⇒ Ageing.

GILLICK COMPETENCE

In Gillick versus West Norfolk and Wisbech Area Health Authority (1985) 3 all ER 402, the House of Lords ruled that children under 16 years of age can give legally effective consent to medical treatment providing they can demonstrate that they have the *"sufficient maturity and intelligence to understand the proposed treatment"*. Parental power is transferred to competent children, not shared with them. The Children Act (1989) supports this by stating that adults *"should have regard in particular to the ascertainable wishes and feelings of the child concerned"*. The Gillick ruling has enabled children to have the right to be consulted about decisions that affect them, such as medical treatment, residence, contact with parents, their education, religion and welfare ..., *"if the child is of sufficient understanding to make an informed decision"*.

Further reading

Moules C and Ramsay J (1998). *The Textbook of Children's Nursing Module 8*: *Legal and Ethical Issues*. London: Stanley Thornes.

GLASGOW COMA SCALE

The Glasgow Coma Scale (GCS) was first developed by Teasdale and Jennet (1974). It consists of a 15-point scale to assess conscious level by evaluating three behavioural responses.:
- Eye opening (E);
- Verbal response (V);
- Motor response (M).

Each of these categories is assessed individually and the observed responses are recorded on a neurological observation chart. Only part of the chart constitutes the GCS. The rest of the chart is used to record other observations, such as respiration, pupil response, etc. ⇒ Head injury (Practice application – holistic assessment in acute brain injury), Nervous system, Pupillary response.

Different levels of response in each of the above categories are afforded a numerical value, which may then be documented. On occasions these figures are summed and a 'coma score' is calculated; however, it is better to document the score achieved from each of the subdivisions separately (e.g. E-4, V-5, M-6). The coma score is sometimes used to define specific levels of consciousness and a patient with a GCS of 8 or below and no eye opening may be defined as being in a coma.

The GCS is an adult scale, but has also been adapted for children in recognition that verbal and motor responses must be related to the child's age (Campbell and Glasper 1995; *Table 20*).

ASSESSING EYE OPENING

Within this category, the subdivisions are eyes open spontaneously, response to speech, to pain or no responses (*Table 21*). When assessing consciousness it may be necessary to apply a painful stimulus to elicit a response. Painful stimuli should be applied with care and only after training, observation and supervised practice.

Table 20 Paediatric Glasgow Coma Scale (modified from NICE 2003)

Response	Score
Eye opening (4)	
Spontaneous eye opening	4
Eye opening in response to speech	3
Eye opening in response to pain	2
No response	1
Verbal response (5): check with parents and/or carers about best usual verbal response	
Alert, communicates to usual ability level (i.e. sentences, words, coos or babbles)	5
Less than usual ability and/or spontaneous irritable cry	4
Inappropriate crying	3
Occasional moaning and/or whimpering	2
No response	1
Grimace response (5): the orofacial response is used as an alternative to the verbal response for babies who are pre-verbal and when the patient is intubated	
Spontaneous normal facial/oromotor activity	5
Less than usual spontaneous ability or only responds to touch	4
Vigorous grimace to painful stimuli	3
Mild grimace to painful stimuli	2
No response to painful stimuli	1
Motor response (6)	
Spontaneous movements or obeys verbal command	6
Localizes to painful stimuli or withdraws in response to touch	5
Withdrawal from pain	4
Abnormal flexion in response to pain (decorticate)	3
Abnormal extension in response to pain (decerebrate)	2
No motor response to painful stimuli	1

The methods used include supraorbital pressure and pressure at the jaw margin (Woodward 1997a).

ASSESSING VERBAL RESPONSE

Within this category, the subdivisions are orientated, confused, inappropriate words, incomprehensible sounds and none (*Table 22*).

Table 21 Assessing eye opening

Response	Score	Behaviour
Spontaneously	4	Document this response for patients who have their eyes open as you approach them, without any further stimulation
To speech	3	This response is recorded for patients who open their eyes if you ask them to, or as you speak to them. Initially, use your normal tone of voice, but do not be afraid to raise your voice or be persistent to elicit a response. It is also acceptable to shake patients gently by the shoulder. This is the same level of neurological stimulation and overcomes a possible misinterpretation of response if the person is deaf
To pain	2	For patients who do not open their eyes when you touch or gently shake them, you need to apply a painful stimulus
None	1	Record this response for patients who do not open their eyes at all, even if you apply pain

Note: Some patients will be unable to open their eyes because of periorbital swelling, rather then because of a reduced level of consciousness. This is recorded on the chart with a letter C.

ASSESSING MOTOR RESPONSE

The subdivisions within this category are obeys commands, localizes to pain, withdrawal from pain, flexion to pain, extension to pain and no response (*Table 23*).

GLUCOSE

Dextrose, a monosaccharide, is the form of glucose in which carbohydrates are absorbed through the intestinal tract and circulated in the blood. The amount in the blood is controlled by hormones that include insulin and glucagon. It is stored as glycogen in the liver and skeletal muscle. Some terms used to describe the processes of glucose metabolism are defined in *Box 14*.

Box 14 Glucose metabolism

Glycogen – the main carbohydrate (polysaccharide) storage compound in animals. It is formed as many glucose molecules are linked together in a process called glycogenesis, which occurs in the liver and skeletal muscle. The conversion of liver glycogen back into glucose is called glycogenolysis.
Glycogenesis – glycogen formation from blood glucose.
Glycogenolysis – the breakdown of glycogen to glucose.
Glycolysis – a metabolic pathway whereby glucose is broken down to form pyruvic acid and some energy (adenosine triphosphate).
Glucogenesis – production of glucose.
Gluconeogenesis – the formation of glucose from noncarbohydrate sources (e.g. amino acids, lactate, etc.).

Table 22 Assessing verbal response

Response	Score	Behaviour
Orientated	5	To record that patients are orientated, they must be orientated to time, place and person. They must be able to tell you who they are, where they are and at the very least correctly identify the month and year
Confused	4	The person who is able to converse, but is unable to answer the above, even when questioned further, is recorded as confused
Inappropriate words	3	In this case, patients answer using only one or a few words that make little sense. If the only response is swearing, this is also considered inappropriate, but needs to be taken in context. Patients who are woken repeatedly in the middle of the night may respond initially by swearing, but if they are really orientated they will understand what you are doing and usually respond appropriately once they are fully roused
Incomprehensible sounds	2	If you are unable to elicit any comprehensible words from a patient, but some vocalization is heard (e.g. moans and/or groans) this is the response recorded on the chart. You may elicit this response either when you speak to patients or, if their level of consciousness is slightly worse, when you apply a painful stimulus. Either way, if any sounds are produced, this is the response recorded
None	1	If no words or sounds are uttered from a patient in response to either speech or pain, this response should be documented

G

Practice application – oral glucose tolerance test
After a period of fasting, a measured quantity (75 g) of glucose is taken orally; thereafter, blood samples are tested for glucose levels at intervals. A blood glucose equal to or greater than 11.1 mmol/L 2 hours after the oral glucose meets the diagnostic criteria for diabetes mellitus (*Fig. 91*). ⇒ Diabetes mellitus.

Impaired glucose levels between 7.9 and 11.0 mmol/L after a 2 hour glucose load indicate a pre-diabetic state and confer a significantly increased risk of cardiovascular disease.

G

Table 23 Assessing motor response

Response	Score	Behaviour
Obeys commands	6	To assess whether patients are obeying commands, ask them to stick their tongue out. Always use a command that requires movement of muscle above the neck. It is obvious to the observer if they have obeyed and it enables you to assess patients who may have a spinal injury that prevents them from moving limbs. Be aware that asking patients to squeeze fingers to command may elicit a primitive grasp reflex from the touch of your fingers within the patient's palm, which may be confused with an appropriate response
Localizes to pain	5	If patients do not obey commands then you need to apply a painful stimulus. If they are localizing to pain, they purposefully move an arm in an attempt to remove the cause of the pain. If you have applied pain above the neck, this is obvious. If other sites have been used, it is more difficult to differentiate localizing from flexion. Patients may also be seen to be localizing in an attempt to remove uncomfortable nasogastric tubes, etc. If you have observed patients localizing to the painful stimulus when applied to assess eye opening, there is no need to inflict pain again to assess motor response
Withdrawal from pain	4	Patients pull their limb away from the painful stimulus
Flexion to pain	3	If patients do not localize, you may observe a purposeless general flexion of the arms in response to the painful stimulus. If this has not been observed, then increased pressure is required
Extension to pain	2	If patients have not flexed their elbow away from the painful stimulus, you may observe the arm being extended by straightening the elbow and sometimes internally rotating the shoulders and hands
None	1	If the arms do not move at all in response to speech or pain this response is documented

Note: Applying painful stimuli to the lower limbs may not be reliable in assessing consciousness. Any response elicited may be the result of a spinal reflex, rather than a cortical function.

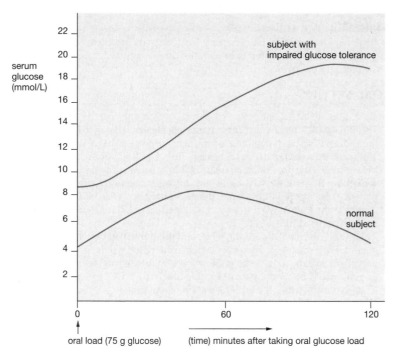

Fig 91 Glucose tolerance test

GLYCOSIDES

Glycosides are complex substance that contain a sugar found in some plants. Many contain pharmacologically active substances, such as digitalis from foxgloves.

CARDIAC GLYCOSIDES

Digoxin is an example of a glycoside. It increases myocardial contractility and is described as being a positive inotrope. Digoxin slows heart rate by increasing vagal activity and by partially blocking impulse conduction. It inhibits the sodium–potassium pump, causing calcium to accumulate in the myocardial fibres, which increases contractility and improves cardiac output. It is used in heart failure with atrial fibrillation and other atrial arrhythmias.

However, it has a narrow therapeutic index (an indicator of the difference between a therapeutic dose and one that causes toxicity). Regular serum digoxin levels should be assessed and if a patient presents with symptoms of digoxin toxicity, the drug should be discontinued.

> **Practice application – digoxin therapy**
> Although digoxin is a very useful therapeutic agent it does have serious side-effects, such as nausea and vomiting, heart block and other serious arrhythmias, such as ventricular tachycardia, and it can also accumulate in the body because it has a long half-life. As it may cause bradycardia, the apex beat and the radial pulse should be determined prior to administration. Should the apical rate fall below 60 beats/min the dose is withheld and medical advice is sought.

GOALS

To set goals for care it is first necessary to identify the problems or needs. Once the goals are set the next step is to plan the care necessary to meet the goals. ⇒ Integrated care pathway.

GOAL-SETTING

Goals should be SMART, that is:
- Specific – which means that they must state clearly what is to be achieved. For example, instead of stating 'encourage fluids', a SMART goal would say 'For (*patient's name*) to drink 1.5 litres of fluid by 20.00 hours'.
- Measurable – the goal must be quantifiable in some way and if it concerns something that is not measurable (e.g. anxiety), it should focus on how the patient expresses it. For example, the goal might say '(*Patient's name*) will state that she knows what to expect and feels less anxious before the premedication is administered'.
- Achievable and realistic – it must be something that can be achieved by the patient. For example, if a woman suffers from chronic pain, it would be unrealistic to expect her to be pain-free at all times. An achievable and realistic goal would be for the patient to state that her pain is at an acceptable level 30 minutes after the administration of analgesics.
- Time-orientated – there must be an indication of when the goal should be achieved so that it is possible to evaluate whether this has happened.

GRAFT

A graft is transplanted living tissue, or to implant or transplant such tissue (e.g. skin, bone, bone marrow, cornea and organs, such as kidney, heart, lungs, pancreas and liver). Grafts may be:
- *Autologous*, when tissue is moved from one site to another in the same individual;
- *Isografts* between genetically identical individuals;
- *Allogenic (homografts)* where tissue is obtained from a suitable donor;
- *Xenografts (heterograft)* between different species.

Transplantation customarily refers to the surgical operation of grafting a suitable organ, which has been removed from a person who has been declared brain-dead, or from a living matched donor. If the recipient's malfunctioning organ is removed and the transplant is placed in its bed, it is referred to as an *orthotopic transplant* (e.g. liver and heart). If the transplanted organ is not placed in its normal anatomical site, the term *heterotopic transplant* is used. ⇒ Haemopoietic stem cell transplantation (graft versus host disease), Renal failure (renal replacement therapies).

GRIEF

Grief and its expression are very individual phenomena and each person who is suffering must be helped in the ways most suited to his or her needs. The determinants of grief identified by Parkes (1975) in the Harvard Study are:
- Mode of death;
- Nature of attachment;
- Who the person was;
- Historical antecedents;
- Personality variable;
- Social variables.

THE GRIEVING PROCESS

Engel (1964) identified the stages of grief as follows:
• Numbness and disbelief, often with a sense of unreality and slow motion;
• Anger and guilt;
• Depression and sadness;
• Grief pangs;
• Readaptation (resolution).
Engel (1964) takes the view that losing a loved one is as psychologically traumatic as being seriously injured oneself. He argues that normal grief reactions are a threat to one's mental health. In the same way that physical healing is necessary to help the body restore its equilibrium, thus a time is required to allow grieving to occur.

Stages in the grieving process apply equally to anticipatory (before the event) grief and the feelings experienced when a loved one actually dies. The reactions of relatives to a poor prognosis and the death of their loved one can be many and varied, ranging from frozen to histrionics. Judging the relative who does not appear unduly moved as coping well is often erroneous.

Worden (1991) identified the tasks of mourning as being able to:
• Accept the reality of loss;
• Experience the pain of loss;
• Adjust to the environment where the deceased is missing;
• Move on with life.
Where a death has been anticipated and the family have observed the gradual decline in health of the significant person who is dying, the loss is an observable phenomenon. In the case of sudden death, particularly where there is no body, as in a major maritime disaster, accepting the loss can be extremely difficult. Parents bereaved through sudden infant death syndrome often return to the hospital to see the baby several times to reassure themselves that it is their baby who has died.

As nurses and as fellow human beings, watching individuals who are suffering and not being able to stop the hurt is very difficult. However, severe psychological problems can result if someone is not allowed to grieve. Unresolved grief can lead to psychological disturbance and mental ill health. The pain is needed to allow healing. Although we recognize the needs of bereaved people to explore the loss, often many times over, it is very difficult to facilitate this and people cannot then share the distress they feel.

The third task in mourning involves adjusting to an environment in which the deceased is missing. Worden (1991) recognizes that the survivor does not always realize all of the roles performed by the deceased until some 3 months have elapsed from the time of the death. The survivor has to learn skills that were previously the responsibility of the deceased. Through doing this, the bereaved person may well restore the damage to their feelings of self-worth.

Finally, the bereaved person needs to carry on with living. The deceased will always be remembered and significant, but the time has now come to love and live again. ⇒ Bereavement.

Further reading

Kubler Ross E (1975). *Death: The Final Stage of Growth*. London: Prentice Hall.

GROUP C MENINGOCOCCAL DISEASE

Group C meningococcal disease is a serious infection caused by *Neisseria meningitidis* of the serological group C. It causes meningococcal meningitis and life-threatening septicaemia in children and young adults. Effective immunization in the form of injectable vaccine is included in the routine immunization programme. It is offered to high-risk groups – infants, preschool children, school children and young people entering further and higher education. ⇒ Defence mechanisms (active artificially acquired immunity – immunization), Nervous system (meningitis), Septicaemia.

GUSTATION (TASTE)

Gustation is the chemical sense of taste. ⇒ Oral (oral assessment, oral hygiene), Taste.

GYNAECOLOGICAL EXAMINATION

Gynaecological examination is a fundamental investigation in determining causes for gynaecological disorders. It is one of the most intimate and potentially embarrassing investigations a woman will ever undergo.

BIMANUAL VAGINAL EXAMINATION

A bimanual vaginal examination is used to ascertain the origins and degree of pelvic pathology and pain. Two forefingers are gently placed in the woman's vagina, and the examiner's other hand is placed on the abdomen. Both hands are then used together to feel for abnormalities of the internal genitalia, such as ovarian cysts or fibroids.

SPECULUM EXAMINATION OF THE VAGINA AND CERVIX

The woman is placed flat on her back with her knees bent and ankles together. Then she is asked to separate her knees so that a Cusco (bivalve) speculum can be inserted gently into the vagina (*Fig. 92A*). The blades of the speculum are separated to stretch the vaginal walls and visualize the cervix. The examination is used to assess the cervix for disease or bleeding and to obtain a sample of cervical cells for cytological examination, etc. A Sims' speculum (*Fig. 92B*) is used to assess vaginal or uterine displacements and to remove foreign objects from the vagina. The speculum is inserted into the vagina with the woman lying on her left side. All investigations of the vagina and cervix involve the use of a speculum.

HIGH VAGINAL SWABS

High vaginal swabs (HVS) are taken to investigate the presence of any pathogenic bacteria that may affect the woman's health. For most bacteria, a dry cotton bud is inserted high into the vagina, using a speculum, and a gentle sweep of the tissues is made. The swab is then removed and placed in transport medium and sent for microbiological examination. To investigate for the presence of chlamydia, another swab is inserted into the cervical os and gently turned to capture some endocervical cells. This swab must be placed in a special solution before sending it to the microbiology laboratory.

CERVICAL CYTOLOGY

Cervical cytology involves removing a sample of cells from the cervix, using a Cusco speculum to visualize the cervix. In the newer technique, liquid-based cytology, the cells are removed with a brush that is then transported to the cytology laboratory in a vial of liquid preservative. The traditional smear or 'Pap' test uses a spatula (usually wooden), rotated against the cervix to scrape off a thin layer of cells. These cells are smeared onto a glass slide and alcohol fixative added to prevent the cells drying.

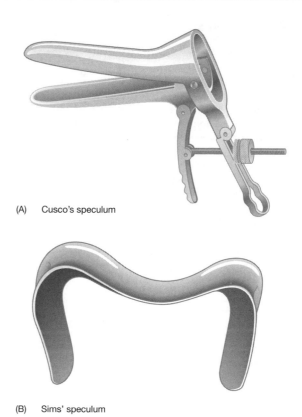

(A)   Cusco's speculum

(B)   Sims' speculum

Fig 92 Vaginal specula: (A) Cusco's, (B) Sims'

This procedure can be uncomfortable and embarrassing for the woman so the nurse must explain it thoroughly and try to put the woman at ease. At the end of the procedure, the woman must be informed of the expected time before the results are available to minimize anxiety experienced while waiting.

COLPOSCOPY

An abnormal cervical screening result may require the woman to be referred for a colposcopic examination, depending on the grade of the abnormality. The woman is referred to a specialist colposcopy clinic where her cervix can be examined closely using a low-powered microscope, known as a colposcope, which magnifies the cells of the cervix. During the consultation, a specially coated metal speculum is used that is compatible with electrical diathermy treatment, if required. The cervix is viewed through the colposcope for abnormalities. Abnormal cells are detected by applying acetic acid and iodine to the cervix and observing for any colour change. ⇒ Cervix (cancer of the cervix).

Further reading

Brooker C and Nicol M (2003). *Nursing Adults. The Practice of Caring*, pp. 711–715. Edinburgh: Mosby.

Haematological tests

⇒ Blood (*Box 3*), Bone marrow sampling, Coagulation, Haemostasis.

Haemoglobin

Haemoglobin is the red respiratory pigment in red blood cells. A molecule comprises four globin chains (two alpha chains and two beta chains) and four haem groups, each with an atom of ferrous iron. Haemoglobin readily binds with oxygen when it is in an oxygen-rich environment, such as the lungs. Conversely, haemoglobin releases oxygen in an oxygen-poor environment, such as the body tissues. By this mechanism, oxygen is transported from the lungs to the tissues for cellular respiration. As body tissues take up oxygen, they release carbon dioxide. This is transported to the lungs for excretion either as bicarbonate ions in the plasma or combined with the haemoglobin. The haemoglobin molecule also helps to prevent changes in pH by acting as a buffer.

HAEMOGLOBINOPATHIES

The haemoglobinopathies are inherited disorders that affect haemoglobin production. They are associated with considerable long-term health problems, including chronic haemolytic anaemia.

Thalassaemia

Thalassaemia can occur in people of all ethnic backgrounds, but is most commonly found in those with Mediterranean ancestry. It occurs when the gene responsible for globin production is faulty. People who inherit the faulty gene from both parents are said to have thalassaemia major, whereas those who inherit a faulty gene from only one parent have thalassaemia trait.

In thalassaemia, the synthesis of alpha- or beta-globin chains, essential for haemoglobin production, is reduced because of a genetic abnormality. This leads to fragility of red cells, with impaired oxygen-carrying abilities, which are more rapidly destroyed by the spleen.

The management of thalassaemia includes:
- Regular blood transfusions;
- Splenectomy;
- Haemopoietic stem cell transplantation is the only curative option (only recommended for children who have a suitable sibling donor);
- The risk of organ damage from iron overload after regular transfusion can be minimized by the long-term administration of iron-chelating drugs, such as desferrioxamine, which bind to iron and enable it to be excreted in urine.

Sickle cell disease

Sickle cell disease is an inherited haemoglobin disorder caused by an abnormality in the beta-globin gene. If a person inherits a gene for normal adult haemoglobin (HbA) from one parent and a gene for sickle haemoglobin (HbS) from the other, he or she is said to have sickle cell trait. People with sickle cell trait are carriers of sickle cell disease, but have no clinical problems and have normal blood counts. The inheritance of an HbS gene from both parents, on the other hand, results in sickle cell disease (HbSS).

Sickle cell disease is most commonly found in people of African, African Caribbean or African–American descent, but can also be found in those with Indian, Middle Eastern, Far Eastern and southern European ancestry. The high prevalence of the abnormal gene in people of African ancestry appears to result from the protection that sickle cell trait offers against falciparum malaria in childhood.

When HbS becomes deoxygenated, crystals are formed within the red cells. The cells become distorted and take on a characteristic sickle shape ('sickling'). When red cells are oxygenated they can return to their normal shape. However, with time, affected cells become increasingly rigid and inflexible and are destroyed prematurely by the cells of the mononuclear–macrophage system in the spleen and liver. The life span of an HbSS cell is around 5–30 days (120 days in normal red cells).

The management of sickle cell disease includes:

- Haemopoietic stem cell transplantation is the only curative option;
- Dealing with sickle cell crises (pain control, rehydration and oxygen therapy) – sickling crisis that affects the lungs may require exchange transfusion whereby some of the patient's blood is removed and donated blood is transfused by apheresis;
- The cytotoxic drug hydrocarbamide is given to some people, as it may reduce the frequency and severity of crises.

Practice application – managing sickle cell disease and maintaining as normal a lifestyle as possible

The following includes some general recommendations of the UK Sickle Cell Society (http://www.sicklecell.co.uk):

- Maintain general health and nutrition;
- Avoid situations that may trigger a crisis, including sports such as scuba diving and skydiving;
- Treat infections early;
- Consider taking prophylactic penicillin and having pneumococcal vaccination;
- Consider taking folic acid supplements;
- Undergo regular blood tests;
- Carry a haemoglobinopathy card or letter that gives details of the condition.

HAEMOLYSIS

Haemolysis is the breakdown of red blood cells, with liberation of the contained haemoglobin. The causes include red cell defects, infections, drugs, chemicals, incompatible blood transfusion, antibodies, overactive spleen, etc. ⇒ Blood (blood transfusion), Erythrocyte (anaemia).

HAEMOLYTIC DISEASE OF THE NEWBORN (SYN. ERYTHROBLASTOSIS FETALIS)

Haemolytic disease of the newborn is a pathological condition in the newborn child caused by Rhesus incompatibility between the child's blood (Rhesus positive) and that of the mother (Rhesus negative). Fetal red blood cell destruction occurs with anaemia, often jaundice and an excess of erythroblasts or primitive red blood cells in the circulating blood. *Hydrops fetalis* is severe oedema that occurs in the fetus, and it is associated with severe haemolytic disease of the newborn. Severe jaundice or *icterus gravis neonatorum* is one of the clinical forms of haemolytic disease of the newborn. *Kernicterus* is staining of brain cells, especially the basal nuclei (ganglia), with bilirubin. It is a complication of jaundice that affects pre-term babies and haemolytic disease of the newborn. It can lead to a severe encephalopathy with resultant learning disabilities. ⇒ Jaundice.

Treatment of affected infants may include phototherapy, blood transfusion and exchange transfusion in severe cases. ⇒ Blood (Rhesus blood group).

ANTI-D

Anti-D is the antibody formed when rhesus negative individuals are exposed to rhesus positive blood, such as during pregnancy. Immunization of Rhesus negative women at risk, using anti-D immunoglobulin, can prevent haemolytic disease of the newborn. Anti-D (Rh_0) immunoglobulin is a sterile solution of globulins derived from human plasma that contains antibody to the erythrocyte factor Rh(D); it is used to prevent formation of the anti-D antibody by rhesus negative women in circumstances that include during pregnancy, after delivery or following a spontaneous miscarriage or termination of pregnancy.

HAEMOPHILIAS

⇒ Coagulation, Haemostasis (disorders).

HAEMOPOIESIS

In the fetus, blood cell formation, or haemopoiesis, commences in the yolk sac, liver and spleen. Towards the end of pregnancy, the bone marrow becomes the primary site for haemopoiesis and blood cell formation occurs in all bones. During childhood much of this active red marrow is replaced by fat; it is then termed yellow marrow. By adulthood, the red haemopoietic marrow is confined to the pelvis, vertebrae, sternum and the ends of the long bones.

Pluripotent stem cells are found within the red marrow. Stem cells are able to self-replicate, but they can also differentiate into mature blood cells. A single stem cell can differentiate through several stages to become any type of blood cell (*Fig. 93*).

Normal haemopoiesis requires sufficient supplies of energy, protein, vitamins and minerals. It is regulated by a series of growth factors that act upon the stem cells and cause them to differentiate into specific cell types. Growth factors can also speed up the maturation process. Many growth factors have been isolated and some are used therapeutically to enhance specific blood cell production. Erythropoietin (EPO) stimulates red cell production. ⇒ Erythrocytes (erythropoiesis, erythropoietin and the control of erythropoiesis).

Granulocyte colony-stimulating factor (G-CSF) and granulocyte–macrophage colony stimulating factor (GM-CSF) stimulate the production of white blood cells and can be used therapeutically following haemopoietic stem cell transplantation. They can also limit the period of neutropenia (reduced neutrophil count) after cytotoxic chemotherapy.

HAEMOPOIETIC STEM CELL TRANSPLANTATION

Haemopoietic stem cell transplantation (HSCT) or bone marrow transplant (BMT) enables normal blood cell production to be re-established in patients whose bone marrow function is inadequate or has failed as a result of disease or its treatment.

HSCT is used to treat a range of haematological conditions, including leukaemia, lymphoma, myeloma, aplastic anaemia, thalassaemia and sickle cell disease.

There are two main types of HSCT – autologous and allogeneic. In autologous transplants, the patient's own stem cells are collected and later re-infused after myeloablative doses of chemotherapy and/or radiotherapy. This procedure is sometimes called stem cell rescue. When the bone marrow is the primary site of disease, or in cases where there is pre-existing bone marrow failure, allogeneic transplantation may be indicated. In allogeneic transplants, stem cells are obtained from a human leucocyte antigen (HLA) compatible donor. The healthy stem cells are infused into the patient and serve to repopulate the bone marrow.

The toxic effects of allogeneic HSCT mean that these treatments are only suitable for people who are relatively young and fit. The use of better-tolerated

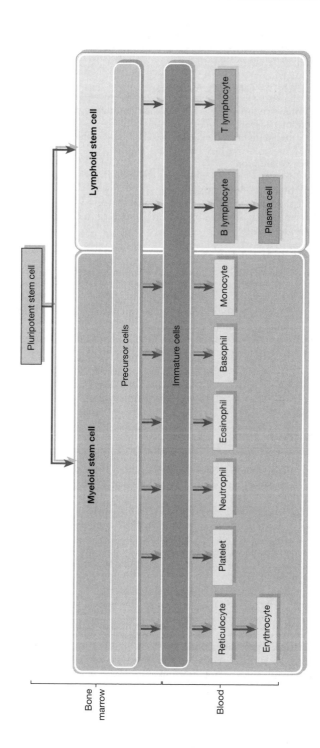

Fig 93 Haemopoiesis

nonmyeloablative transplants that suppress the recipient's immune system sufficiently to allow engraftment of the donated marrow means that a wider range of patients can benefit. However, the longer-term effectiveness of these transplants has still to be evaluated.

SIDE-EFFECTS AND COMPLICATIONS

Side-effects are related primarily to the cytotoxic and immunosuppressive effects of conditioning regimens. They include:
- Profound neutropenia (neutrophil count $<1.0 \times 10^9/L$) in which even minor everyday infections can prove life-threatening, so protective isolation is needed after transplantation;
- Red blood cell and platelet production is also inhibited – requires blood transfusion and blood product support;
- Other side effects of cytotoxic chemotherapy, such as nausea and vomiting, mucositis, diarrhoea, fatigue and alopecia, are common and can be severe.
⇒ Immunocompromised patient.

GRAFT VERSUS HOST DISEASE

Graft versus host disease (GVHD) is an immune reaction whereby T-cells in the transplanted marrow, or graft, attack the recipient's cells. GVHD most commonly affects the cells of the skin, gut or liver. GVHD may simply manifest as a minor skin rash, but in extreme cases it can cause severe cell destruction that leads to widespread ulceration of the skin or gut, profuse diarrhoea, bleeding, infection and liver failure. Severe GVHD often proves fatal. ⇒ Erythrocyte (anaemia), Haemoglobin (haemoglobinopathies), Leukaemia, Lymphoma.

Further reading

Brooker C and Nicol M (2003). *Nursing Adults. The Practice of Caring*, pp. 474–475. Edinburgh: Mosby.

HAEMORRHAGE

Haemorrhage is loss of blood from a vessel, but usually refers to serious rapid blood loss. This may lead to hypovolaemic shock with tachycardia, hypotension, rapid breathing, pallor, sweating, oliguria, restlessness and changes in conscious level. ⇒ Shock.

Haemorrhage can be classified in several ways, which include:
- According to the vessel involved, arterial, venous or capillary;
- Timing – *primary haemorrhage* occurs at the time of injury or operation, *reactionary haemorrhage* occurs within 24 hours of injury or operation and *secondary haemorrhage* occurs within some days of injury or operation and is usually associated with sepsis;
- Whether it is internal (concealed) or external (revealed).

Haemorrhage may also be named for the site of bleeding (e.g. subarachnoid haemorrhage, gastrointestinal haemorrhage, etc.).

> **Practice application – pressure points**
> A pressure point is a place at which an artery passes over a bone, against which it can be compressed, to stop bleeding (*Fig. 94*).

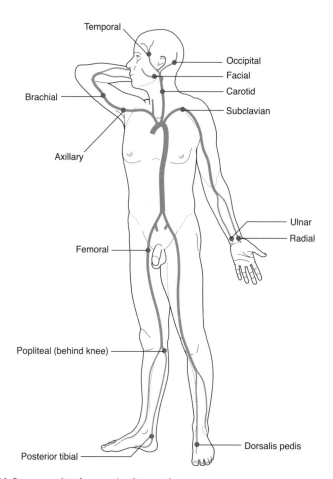

Fig 94 Pressure points for arresting haemorrhage

HAEMORRHAGIC DISEASE OF THE NEWBORN

Haemorrhagic disease of the newborn is characterized by gastrointestinal, pulmonary or intracranial haemorrhage that occurs from the second to the fifth day of life. It is caused by a physiological variation in blood clotting that results from a transient deficiency of vitamin K, which is necessary for the formation of some clotting factors. It responds to the administration of vitamin K.

HAEMORRHAGIC FEVERS

Haemorrhagic fevers occur mainly in tropical areas, are often transmitted by mosquitoes or ticks and may have a petechial skin rash. They include chikungunya, dengue, ebola, Lassa fever, Marburg disease, Rift valley fever and yellow fever.

HAEMOSTASIS

Haemostasis is the process by which blood clots at the site of an injury, and thus prevents excessive blood loss. It is a complex and carefully orchestrated process often explained in terms of four overlapping phases, *vasoconstriction, platelet plug formation, coagulation* and *fibrinolysis* (*Fig. 95*). ⇒ Anticoagulant, Blood, Coagulation.

When a blood vessel is first injured, vasoconstriction occurs to reduce blood flow to the affected area. Platelets immediately begin to adhere to the damaged endothelium, and to swell and aggregate around the site of injury. This creates a primary haemostatic plug and temporarily halts blood loss. The intrinsic coagulation pathway is initiated when granules within the platelets break down and release chemical substances into the bloodstream, while substances released by the damaged endothelium initiate the extrinsic coagulation pathway. These pathways interconnect within the coagulation cascade.

A feedback mechanism exists to limit clot formation to the area of damage after coagulation has been established. Once formed, fibrin absorbs thrombin to halt the coagulation process. As tissue damage is repaired, the fibrinolytic system is activated to dissolve the clot. This occurs through the action of the proteolytic enzyme plasmin.

DISORDERS OF HAEMOSTASIS

Disorders of haemostasis may result from reduced or abnormal platelet production or abnormalities in the coagulation process. Several disorders arise from these factors.

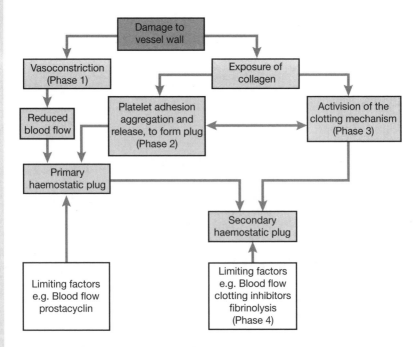

Fig 95 An outline of the main events in haemostasis

THROMBOCYTOPENIA

Thrombocytopenia is an abnormally low platelet count (normal range of 150–400 $\times 10^9/L$). Spontaneous bleeding tends to occur when the platelet count falls below $10 \times 10^9/L$. Physical examination may reveal petechiae. Other symptoms can include spontaneous bruising, nosebleeds and bleeding gums. Women may complain of menorrhagia.

Platelet counts can be reduced temporarily as a result of infection, alcohol consumption and the use of common medications such as penicillin, heparin and quinine. In the longer term, thrombocytopenia is most often caused by inadequate platelet production, such as in aplastic anaemia, or increased platelet destruction, which is often immunological in nature. There may, however, be no obvious underlying cause, as in chronic idiopathic thrombocytopenic purpura (ITP) in which antibodies target platelets and mark them for destruction.

DISSEMINATED INTRAVASCULAR COAGULATION

Disseminated intravascular coagulation (DIC) results from the simultaneous over-activation of both the coagulation and fibrinolytic pathways, which leads to widespread clotting and thrombus formation throughout the body. As clotting factors become exhausted, generalized bleeding can also occur. ⇒ Shock, Systemic inflammatory response syndrome.

HAEMOPHILIA

Haemophilia is an inherited disorder that results in a lifelong deficiency of one of two essential coagulation factors, factor VIII (Haemophilia A) or factor IX (Haemophilia B or Christmas disease). The severity of haemophilia is in direct proportion to the level of factor deficiency. The genes for both factor VIII and factor IX are found on the X chromosome. This means that inheritance is sex-linked and the vast majority of people with haemophilia are males, while females are carriers (*Fig. 96*).

In haemophilia, the activated partial prothrombin time (APTT) is prolonged. This means that people bleed for longer after trauma or surgery, including relatively minor procedures such as dental extraction. In severe cases, spontaneous

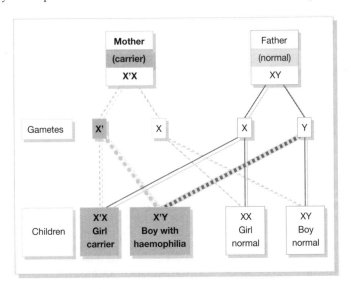

Fig 96 The inheritance of haemophilia

bleeding may also occur, the effects of which can be serious. Repeated bleeds into muscles or joints can cause severe pain, swelling and deformity, as well as long-term arthritic changes and mobility problems.

The management includes:

- Human factor VIII and IX – bleeding is usually treated by intravenous injection of the deficient factor. People with severe haemophilia, those undergoing surgery and children may also use coagulation factors prophylactically. In the past, use of nonheat-treated human products was linked to the spread of serious blood-borne viral infections, such as human immunodeficiency virus (HIV) and hepatitis C. Genetically engineered recombinant clotting factors are now available and, because these are not derived from human sources, the chances of viral contamination are negligible
- Milder forms of haemophilia A may respond to treatment with desmopressin (DDAVP), which can be given by intravenous injection or nasal spray.
- Antifibrinolytic agents, such as tranexamic acid, may be used to promote clot stability (e.g. after dental surgery).
- People with haemophilia are advised to carry a medic-alert card.

Further reading and resources

Brooker C and Nicol M (2003). *Nursing Adults. The Practice of Caring*, pp. 476–478. Edinburgh: Mosby.
Haemophilia Society, http://www.haemophilia.org.uk

Hair

There are three types of hair:

- Lanugo – the soft, downy hair sometimes present on newborn infants, especially when they are pre-term;
- Vellus – short downy hair found on most hair-bearing parts of the body, except the scalp, axillae and external genitalia;
- Terminal hair – coarse pigmented hair of the scalp and eyebrows. During puberty, terminal hair replaces the vellus hair of the axillae and external genitalia in both sexes and forms body and facial hair in males.

Hair growth is cyclical – a period of growth, then a resting phase before the old hair is shed and new hair develops. Individual hair follicles remain active for varying times and those on the scalp may function for years. ⇒ Skin.

ABNORMAL HAIR GROWTH

Hair may fall out, or grow excessively, or grow in an abnormal site, all of which can lead to distress.

ALOPECIA

Literally, alopecia means a fall of hair. Several different types are described, such as male pattern baldness, telogen effluvium caused by stress, serious illness, childbirth or drug induced (e.g. cytotoxic drugs), alopecia areata (*Fig. 97*) and traumatic (twisting or pulling of hair, etc.).

Practice application – supporting people with alopecia

Hair (including eyebrows, lashes and beard) is very much part of the human identity and self-esteem, so hair loss causes great psychological distress and thus reassurance and support is required. In the short term the person may benefit from having a wig fitted. Any treatment programme should be explained fully, as well as the importance of completing the course of therapy.

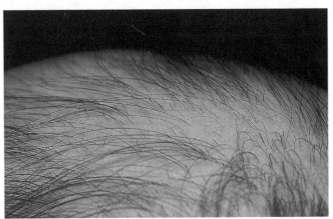

Fig 97 Alopecia areata. Marked hair loss with diagnostic exclamation mark hairs

H

HIRSUTISM

Hirsutism is excessive terminal hair growth in an androgenic (male) pattern (e.g. face, chest, inner thighs, external genitalia, etc.) because of increased androgen activity in a female.

Management depends on the cause, for example systemic anti-androgen drugs or local cosmetic interventions, such as hair removal (shaving, depilatory creams, waxing, electrolysis) or bleaching.

HYPERTRICHOSIS

Hypertrichosis is excessive terminal hair growth in a nonandrogenic pattern, and can occur in either sex. Depending on the underlying cause (possible malignancy), investigations and treatment chosen need to be fully explained with realistic outcomes, so as not to give false hope.

Electroylsis treatment is prolonged and people often resort to bleaching the hair or using cosmetic products.

HALLUCINATIONS

Hallucinations are false perceptions in the sense that there is usually no adequate external stimulus to account for the experience ⇒ Perception (illusion). However, some may be triggered as, for example, the young man who heard the police talking about him while listening to music. Hallucinations can occur in any sense (i.e. hearing, smell, touch, etc.). Hallucinations do not necessarily imply mental illness. For example, fleeting hallucinations are fairly common after bereavement (those affected see or hear the lost person, etc.). Pathological hallucinations are typically grouped according to the sensory modality affected – auditory, visual, tactile, gustatory (taste) and olfactory (smell). They may be highly invasive, frequent and interfere with virtually all normal function, or they may occur largely in the background with little apparent impact on ordinary function.

Auditory hallucinations may involve noises, such as the sound of an engine running, electrical hums or rumbling. There may be voices speaking directly to sufferers (second person) or talking about them, either commenting on their behaviour, etc., or having a conversation with another 'voice' (third party). The nature of the 'voice' may be congruent with mood, so, for example, tending to be deprecatory with depressive delusions.

Visual hallucinations may be fleeting and fragmentary (e.g. flashes of light), formed objects or even vivid and complex scenes. Visual hallucinations are particularly associated with organic brain disease, such as temporal lobe epilepsy and delirium, but also occur in schizophrenia and other functional psychoses.

Olfactory hallucinations include simple hallucinations of perfume or burning, and others with delusional elaboration, such as patients who can smell the poison gas pumped into the room by their persecutors.

Tactile hallucinations include feelings of touch as well as more noxious insertions of wires or needles into the body.

Gustratory hallucinations include tastes of poison in food.

CHARLES BONNET SYNDROME

Some people who are blind experience visual hallucinations, a rare condition known as Charles Bonnet syndrome. Those affected report 'seeing' events and worry that they have a mental health problem. Nurses should provide support, explanation and reassurance that this is not the case.

HAND–ARM VIBRATION SYNDROME (SYN. SECONDARY RAYNAUD'S PHENOMENON)

Hand–arm vibration syndrome (HAVS) is a progressive chronic condition that arises after prolonged use of handheld vibrating equipment. Early signs are 'white finger', which is caused by constriction of and damage to the digital arteries. Other symptoms include tingling and loss of sensation caused by involvement of the digital nerves leading to loss of manual dexterity.

HEAD INJURY (BRAIN INJURY)

Head injury (brain injury) refers to any injury to the scalp, skull or brain that is of sufficient magnitude to interfere with normal function and require hospital treatment. ⇒ Glasgow coma scale, Persistent vegetative state.

PRIMARY BRAIN INJURIES

CEREBRAL CONTUSIONS (COUP AND CONTRE-COUP)

Cerebral contusions are bruises on the brain caused at the time of the injury as the brain tissue rocks backwards and forwards within the skull – coup injuries as the brain hits the front of the skull and contre-coup as it hits the back.

HAEMORRHAGE

Haemorrhage also occurs at the time of the injury and bleeding can occur in several different layers within the brain and meninges, which leads to clot formation (haematoma). It may be extradural (outside the dura), subdural (under the dura), subarachnoid (bleeding into the subarachnoid space) or intracerebral where bleeding occurs into the brain tissue.

SKULL FRACTURES

Skull fractures may occur at any point from a blow. There may be an associated wound that increases the risk of infection. The fracture may be depressed and push downwards into the brain tissue. Fractures of the base of skull are potentially very serious with the risk of meningitis, as a route of entry for infection exists. Basal skull fracture should be suspected if cerebrospinal fluid is leaking from the nose (rhinorrhoea) or the ear (otorrhoea).

SHEARING

Shearing occurs as a result of mechanical forces after deceleration, which results in disruption to and tearing of axonal fibres.

CONCUSSION

Concussion is a temporary disruption in cerebral function that results from the injury. Consciousness may fluctuate and there may be other temporary losses in neurological function.

SECONDARY BRAIN INJURIES

Secondary sequelae include further bleeding, seizures, hydrocephalus, infection, hypoxia, infarction and cerebral oedema (swelling of the brain), many of which result in a raised intracranial pressure (ICP, see below).

RAISED INTRACRANIAL PRESSURE

Apart from cerebral oedema after trauma and brain injury, the many other causes of raised ICP include brain tumours, cerebral haemorrhage and abscess, and non-neurological events.

BRAIN SHIFTS (HERNIATION SYNDROMES) AND 'CONING'

As a lesion expands within the skull, the surrounding brain tissue becomes compressed. Pressure gradients are established and cause brain tissue to shift from an area of high pressure to one of low pressure. In other words, brain tissue swells and is compressed against the point of least resistance (*Fig. 98*).

The clinical features of raised ICP include:

- Deterioration in level of consciousness, one of the earliest signs of raised ICP;
- Focal neurological deficits may also develop quite early on as specific areas of brain tissue become compressed (e.g. limb deficits);
- Later, changes in pupillary response to light become evident; a pupil that is becoming oval, enlarging or losing the ability to react to light may be an indication of rising ICP. This often occurs before a pupil becomes fixed and dilated (often referred to as a 'blown' pupil), although this process can be rapid and the intermediate stages missed. Changes may also be seen in systemic observations, such as increasing blood pressure with a widening gap between systolic and diastolic pressures (see Practice application). These, however, are late signs of raised ICP and indicate that brain herniation is occurring. ⇒ Pupillary response.

Practice application – holistic assessment in acute brain injury

Holistic assessment is vital, as patients can experience problems with any body system as a result of the injury, which may lead to complications that increase the risk of secondary brain damage. Assessment includes:

- Neurological assessment, of which Glasgow Coma Scale, pupil response and limb movement are the most important nursing assessments performed and must be documented accurately, with changes reported immediately. Patients who have suffered an apparently mild head injury can also deteriorate within 24 hours after the injury and so may be admitted for observation. Patients may also experience headache, so pain assessment should be undertaken. Worsening headache, increasing drowsiness or vomiting should be reported immediately, as this may indicate development or worsening of cerebral damage and haemorrhage.

H

- Respiratory assessment is also important, as alterations in respiratory pattern can result in cerebral hypoxia. Respiratory rate and depth should be observed and pulse oximetry may be performed to monitor oxygen saturation. Patients are also at risk of aspiration, so should be positioned in such a way as to protect their airway. Patency of the airway should be assessed on a regular basis
- Cardiovascular problems, such as cardiac arrhythmias and hypo- or hypertension, may develop for a variety of reasons after head injury. Assessment of vital signs (blood pressure, pulse and temperature) is therefore important.

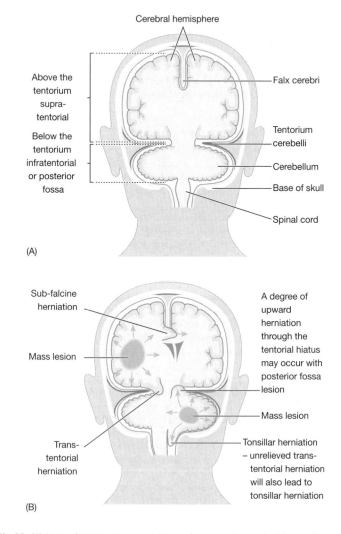

Fig 98 (A) Normal structures – note the gap between the cerebral hemispheres and tentorium cerebelli, and between the base of the cerebellum and the floor of the skull, (B) brain shifts

Further reading

Brooker C and Nicol M (2003). *Nursing Adults. The Practice of Caring*, pp. 297–303 Edinburgh: Mosby.

Headache

Headache is the most common neurological symptom reported and is something that most people suffer. Headaches may be experienced as a one-off event or may be recurrent, acute or chronic.

Headaches may fall into one of the following categories, each having its own specific causes and mechanism of onset:
* Tension headaches (most common);
* Migraine;
* Cluster headaches;
* Temporal (giant cell) arteritis;
* Headache associated with raised intracranial pressure (e.g. head injury);
* Non-neurological headache (e.g. sinus problems).

H

Practice applications – headaches: nursing interventions

One of the main nursing interventions is assessment of the pain to assist in evaluation of the headache type and the effectiveness of treatment. It may be useful to assist the person in keeping a headache diary, noting the time of onset, any precipitating factors that may be associated with the onset and any accompanying symptoms, such as vomiting. The nurse also needs to assess the pain itself, noting the quality, quantity and site. ⇒ Pain.

Once a diagnosis has been made, the main nursing interventions include administration of prescribed medication and other therapies and patient education. The aimed is to prevent and minimize the frequency of attacks, such as avoiding precipitating factors. However, during an attack, people often appreciate a dark, quiet environment in which to rest until the analgesic begins to relieve the pain.

People with tension headaches often benefit from relaxation and stress management techniques. Advice about posture can be useful. Some people find relief from gentle massage to the shoulders and neck, often given by a partner or family member.

Migraine sufferers have been found to have lower levels of the mineral magnesium. As well as dietary advice about foods to avoid (having identified the precipitating factors by using the headache diary), nutritional advice about good sources of magnesium can also be given (e.g. green leafy vegetables, legumes, nuts, seeds and whole grains). Nurses can also advise people to cut down on exposure to bright or fluorescent lighting. A regular routine for going to bed, waking and eating have been found to reduce the frequency of headaches.

Some people have also reported benefit from complementary therapies such as acupuncture.

Health

Health is generally understood to identify a state of being to which we all aspire. The most common usage is health being the absence of disease or illness, the opposite of being sick. Health is thus a negative term, defined more by what it is not than what it is. There is also a positive definition interpreted by the World Health Organization in its constitution in 1948 as 'a state of complete physical, mental and social well-being'. Modern society views the body holistically and within its social, environmental and economic context. Health is thus seen broadly as encompassing a person's social and psychological resources as well as his or her physical capacities. An understanding of what constitutes good health may vary from one individual to another and from place to place, as well as at different times. Health is therefore a very subjective concept.

HEALTH DEVELOPMENT AGENCY

The Health Development Agency is a statutory body that works to improve health and reduce inequalities. It is concerned with identifying evidence for ways to improve health and placing that evidence into practice, and works with health professionals and government to produce guidance.

HEALTH ECONOMICS

Various definitions exist, but Jefferson *et al.* (2000) describe health economics as 'a logical and explicit framework to aid healthcare workers, decision-makers, governments, or society at large, to make choices on how best to use resources'.

Health economics and its application can be complex, so an outline of important terms and concepts is given here:

- Average unit cost – an average cost for a specific activity (e.g. a scan or a home visit). It is calculated by dividing the total cost of the service by the number of outputs.
- Avoided costs – an assessment of the costs avoided by the introduction of a particular intervention (i.e. the disease and/or ill health avoided).
- Direct and indirect costs – direct costs, such as for treatment, are those met by the health service or communities and individuals. Indirect costs may be tangible (e.g. loss of wages) or intangible, such as pain.
- Fixed costs – those incurred regardless of the level of activity (e.g. related to buildings, etc.).
- Marginal cost – the cost of providing the extra resources required to carry out activity above a baseline figure.
- Opportunity cost – the cost of a service viewed in terms of the opportunities lost to use the resource for alternatives. For example, any decision to fund an expensive treatment for a few people must consider the benefits of funding a slightly cheaper treatment for more people.
- Variable costs – depend on the level of activity (e.g. the cost of extra drugs if more people are treated).
- Economic evaluation – the methods used to study the cost and results of specific healthcare interventions. For example, counselling compared with antidepressants in primary care.
- Cost–benefit analysis (CBA) – a complex method of analysing the costs (as opportunity costs) of the provision and the benefits of a particular health intervention in terms of money. The cost of each benefit (cost–benefit ratio) is calculated, with some difficulty because of the subjectivity of judging quality-of-life measures, which allows comparisons to be made between different interventions.
- Cost–effectiveness analysis – an assessment of efficiency. The comparison of measurable health gains (outcomes) with the net cost of the healthcare intervention (input).
- Cost-minimization analysis – an analysis that aims to achieve the agreed output at minimum cost (cost efficiency). For example, comparing two treatments may show them to be equally effective, but treatment 'A' costs twice as much as treatment 'B'.

- Cost–utility analysis – a method whereby costs are measured in monetary terms and benefits are measured in quality-adjusted life years (QALYS). This allows the cost of a QALY to be calculated.
- Quality-adjusted life years (QALYs) – used as a method to evaluate health-care outcomes by looking at quality of life, such as the degree of dependency, as well as life expectancy (the extra years of life). QALYS are used to inform decisions regarding the use of resources for particular interventions.
- Value for money (VFM) – is a way to obtain the best quality of service within resource limits. The term embraces 'the three Es': economy, efficiency and effectiveness. *Economy* means that as little resource as possible is spent, while still maintaining the appropriate quality of service. *Efficiency* is the term that describes the relationship between resource input and workload output. Efficiency can be improved by either increasing outputs while using the same amount of resource, or by maintaining the output while reducing the amount of resources used. *Effectiveness* describes using the resources to achieve the intended outcome.

HEALTH EDUCATION

Health education aims to empower people to make and sustain healthy actions and equip them with the skills to exercise choice. It may include a wide range of activities at different levels. For the individual, it may involve advice on how to follow a treatment schedule. For the wider population, it may involve a campaign to raise awareness about the importance of physical activity. A main focus of health education is to modify those aspects of behaviour known to impact on health. The process includes imparting knowledge, clarifying attitudes and developing skills. Simply conveying information about risks is not effective. People's health behaviour may be a response to, and maintained by, the environment in which they live. Understanding their health beliefs and their perceptions about their own susceptibility and the seriousness of the disease is an important task of health education. ⇒ Disease (disease prevention).

HEALTH PROMOTION

Health promotion is an umbrella term used to describe any measure aimed at health improvement in individuals, communities or the population as a whole. The health improvement may increase the length of life or the number of years people spend free of illness and it may narrow the health gap between the worst and better-off in society. Health promotion embraces many approaches, which include:

- Education and information to empower people to make informed decisions about healthy ways of living;
- Personal counselling to support people to make changes in their health behaviour;
- Legislative and fiscal measures to develop the capacity of communities to become involved in health decisions that affect them.

The World Health Organization (WHO 1986) identified the broad components of a health-promotion strategy as building public policy, creating supportive environments for health, strengthening community action, developing personal skills and reorienting health services from treatment to prevention. ⇒ Disease (disease prevention).

HEALTHCARE SYSTEM

The healthcare system is the national or local organizations that provide medical and/or healthcare. The structure of the system has to accommodate progress in medical interventions, consumer demand and economic efficiency. Criteria for a successful system have been formulated:
- Adequacy and equity of access to care;
- Income protection (for patients);
- Macro-economic efficiency (national expenditure measured as a proportion of gross domestic product);
- Micro-economic efficiency (balance of services provided between improving health outcomes and satisfying consumer demand);
- Consumer choice and appropriate autonomy for care providers.

There are four basic types of healthcare systems – socialized (UK NHS), social insurance (Canada, France), mandatory insurance (Germany) and voluntary insurance (US).

HEARING

HEARING ASSESSMENT (AUDITORY ACUITY)

Hearing can be assessed in several ways.

VOICE

Although voice tests are not diagnostic in themselves, they allow nurses to identify patients who are at risk of a hearing loss who can then be referred quickly and appropriately to the local audiology department for advanced screening.

TUNING FORK TESTS

There are two well-established tuning fork tests in regular use – Rinne's and Weber's – and they test both air and bone conduction of sound. A 512 Hz tuning fork is used for both tests.

AUDIOMETRY

An audiometry test is ideally performed in a soundproof room, usually with headphones for air conduction and with an instrument like an Alice band abutting the mastoid process for bone conduction. Different frequencies are tested with varying intensities of sound measured in decibels (dB). Each ear is tested in turn for both air conduction and bone conduction.

TYMPANOMETRY

Tympanometry involves introducing a sound into the external auditory canal (EAC), at the same time varying the pressure in the EAC. The amount of sound reflected from the tympanic membrane is measured, which allows its compliance to be calculated. Tympanometry can provide a quick, easy method of discovering whether there is a problem within the middle ear.

BRAINSTEM-EVOKED RESPONSES

Brainstem-evoked responses (BSERs) measure different electrical potentials from electrodes placed on the head and mastoid prominences in response to varying intensities of sound. A characteristic waveform is produced if the vestibulocochlear nerve is stimulated. This test is used to examine thresholds of hearing and also to investigate for acoustic neuromas. ⇒ Neonatal (neonatal checks).

Otoacoustic emission testing

Otoacoustic emission (OAE) testing is a hearing screening-test performed on new-born babies, using a small probe linked to a computer. ⇒ Neonatal (neonatal checks).

Hearing impairment

Classically, two types of hearing loss are described, *sensorineural* and *conductive* hearing loss. However, there can be significant overlap between the two and a mixed hearing loss is not uncommon. A conductive loss is incurred if there is any obstruction to the conduction of sound through the external and middle ear (e.g. excess wax, otosclerosis), while a sensorineural hearing loss is incurred if there is disruption of the transmission of sound from the inner ear onwards to the brain. ⇒ Ear.

Presbycusis

Presbycusis is hearing loss caused by age-related degenerative changes of the inner ear. It results from degeneration of the inner and outer hair cells of the inner ear and of the cerebral components of hearing.

Noise-induced hearing loss

Hearing loss as a result of excess noise is an increasingly important problem. In recent years, people have become more aware of the complications of loudness levels in both occupational and recreational situations:

- Occupational exposure occurs in people who work with heavy machinery, etc., where noise exposure is continuous;
- Recreational exposure occurs during leisure activities, such as shooting and discos.

It is postulated that the hair cells in the inner ear suffer metabolic exhaustion because of an overload of work and, with further exposure, they are thought to become permanently nonfunctional.

Practice application – improving communicating with people who have hearing problems (adapted from Robins and Mangan 1999)

Nurses should establish how hearing-impaired people wish to communicate (e.g. by lip-reading, using sign language via an interpreter or family member, using pen and paper or computer).

Suggestions for improving communication are outlined here:

- Ensure that any hearing aids are available and working;
- Try to find a quiet location if possible;
- Reduce the effects of background noise, such as the television, and remember that hearing aids amplify all noises;
- Make sure that the person can see your face – sit or stand facing the light and maintain eye contact (taking account of what level is culturally appropriate);
- Sit or stand at the same level as the person, at a distance of 1–2 m;
- Speak clearly and slightly slower than usual;
- Shouting causes distortion and makes it even more difficult for the person to hear what you are saying;
- Make sure that you do not cover your face when talking (e.g. with your hand);
- Gestures and other nonverbal communication can be helpful, but excessive use of exaggerated facial expressions is best avoided;
- Use the level of language that is appropriate for the person, not the person's level of hearing.

Further reading and resources

Brooker C and Nicol M (2003). *Nursing Adults. The Practice of Caring*, Ch 16. Edinburgh: Mosby.
Royal National Institute for the Deaf (RNID) – http://www.rnid.org.uk

HEART

The heart is a muscular pump that circulates blood around the systemic and pulmonary circulations. The adult heart weighs around 300 g. It is roughly cone-shaped with its base uppermost and the apex inclined to the left. It is situated between the lungs in the mediastinal area of the thoracic cavity and extends from the second to the fifth intercostal spaces. The base is level with the second costal cartilage and the apex can normally be located just medial to the mid-clavicular line in the fifth intercostal space. ⇒ Circulation, Pulse.

STRUCTURE OF THE HEART

H

The wall of the heart comprises three layers (*Fig. 99*):
- The outer pericardium encloses the heart. There is a fibrous outer layer and a double serous layer.
- The myocardium is made up of specialized striated cardiac muscle. The muscle cells work together to create the forceful contraction needed to pump blood into the circulation.
- The innermost endocardium lines the four chambers and covers the valves. In health the endocardium is smooth and helps to prevent blood cells sticking and clotting together.

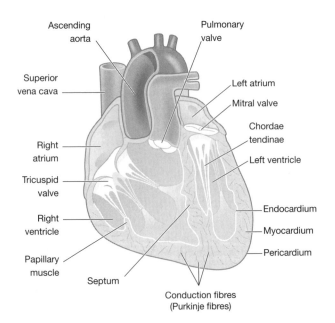

Fig 99 The heart – showing the wall, chambers and valves

The heart has four chambers – two upper receiving chambers, called atria, and two lower pumping chambers, called ventricles. These are divided into the right and left sides by the septum. The atria are separated from the ventricles by atrioventricular (AV) valves – the mitral valve on the left and the tricuspid valve on the right. At the opening of the ventricles lie the semilunar valves – the pulmonary valve between the right ventricle and the pulmonary artery and the aortic valve (not shown on *Fig. 99*) at the point where the aorta leaves the left ventricle. The valves are important in ensuring that blood flows in one direction only.

CORONARY CIRCULATION

The coronary vasculature traverses the heart and is composed of coronary arteries (that branch from the aorta), coronary veins and the capillary network. These supply the myocardium with oxygen and nutrients, and remove the waste products of metabolism. Three major coronary arteries supply the myocardium with oxygen – the right coronary artery, the left anterior descending and the circumflex arteries (*Fig. 100*). The arteries form a dense network of arterioles and capillaries that traverse the external surface of the heart and penetrate the myocardium. Once the muscle has been supplied with oxygen, the blood returns to the right atrium of the heart, via the coronary sinus.

The coronary arteries primarily fill with blood during diastole when the heart muscle is relaxed – an important point to remember when considering the effects of cardiac disorders that cause a shortening of diastole.

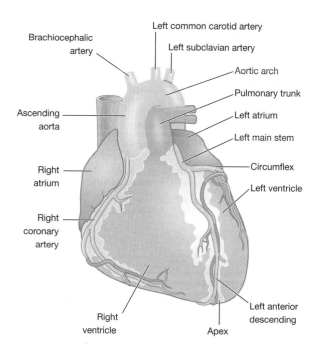

Fig 100 The coronary circulation

ELECTRICAL CONDUCTION SYSTEM

The electrical conduction system comprises four main structures:
- Sinus or sinoatrial (SA) node, on the posterior surface of the right atrium;
- Atrioventricular (AV) node, at the junction of the right atria and right ventricle;
- AV bundle (bundle of His) and branch bundles, which lie in the septum between the two ventricles;
- Purkinje fibres, which spread out through the ventricular muscle mass.

The sinus node is the pacemaker of the heart and beats at its own intrinsic rate of 60–100 beats/min (bpm). From the sinus node, the impulse passes to the AV node and results in atrial systole (contraction). The impulse then passes to the Bundle of His, the right and left bundle branches and the Purkinje fibres. This causes the ventricular muscle fibres to contract and expel the blood.

HEART DISEASE

An overview of cardiac disorders is provided here. Coronary heart disease (CHD) is covered in a separate entry because of its importance as a leading cause of morbidity and premature death in developed countries. ⇒ Congenital defects (congenital heart disease), Coronary heart disease, Deep vein thrombosis, Hypertension, Peripheral vascular disease.

DISORDERS OF ELECTRICAL CONDUCTION – SELECTED CARDIAC ARRHYTHMIAS

⇒ Electrocardiogram.

Sinus bradycardia

In sinus bradycardia there is normal heart rhythm, but the heart rate is below 60 bpm (see pacemaker below).

Sinus tachycardia

In sinus tachycardia there is normal rhythm, but the heart rate is above 100 bpm at rest.

Atrial fibrillation

In atrial fibrillation (AF) the heartbeat does not originate in the sinus node, but in cells throughout the atria. This leads to a disorganized pattern of impulses reaching the AV node, which are then conducted sporadically to the ventricles. Ventricular contraction is irregular and frequently fast (*Fig. 101A*). AF may lead to a decreased cardiac output (see synchronized DC cardioversion below).

Supraventricular tachycardia

Supraventricular tachycardia (SVT) is the term used for any tachycardia that originates from a focus above the ventricles, but for which the exact origin is uncertain. The heart rate is greater than 100 bpm and may be as fast as 280 bpm. The P wave is unclear or not present. The QRS complex may be normal if the ventricular cells can conduct the rhythm or, as is more commonly seen, narrow (*Fig. 101B*). Many of the causes of SVT are benign, such as excessive caffeine intake, alcohol, smoking and stress. It can, however, warn of CHD (see synchronized DC cardioversion below).

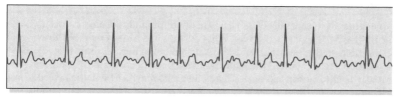

(A)

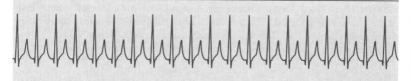

(B)

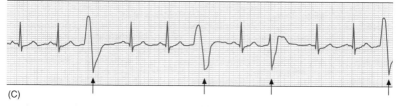

(C)

Fig 101 Cardiac arrhythmias: (A) atrial fibrillation has a wavy baseline of fibrillating waves, (B) supraventricular tachycardia has a narrow QRS complex, (C) ventricular ectopic beats have broad bizarre QRS complexes with no preceding P wave (arrows) between normal sinus beats

Wolff–Parkinson–White syndrome

Wolff–Parkinson–White (WPW) syndrome is an arrhythmia that results from an abnormal conduction pathway between the atria and ventricles. It usually produces supraventricular tachycardia.

Premature ventricular contraction (ventricular extrasystoles or ectopic beats)

Premature ventricular contraction (PVC) arises from an abnormal focus in the ventricles that depolarizes early and the impulse is conducted abnormally through the ventricles. On the electrocardiogram (ECG) this is seen as a QRS complex with a broad and bizarre shape that is not preceded by a P wave (*Fig. 101C*). It is only when they become more frequent than about 10 bpm, if they originate from multiple sites (multifocal) or they occur in salvoes (runs of three or more), that PVCs are considered dangerous. PVCs are probably one of the most common arrhythmias, but in the absence of CHD they are usually benign and may result from exposure to stress or excessive caffeine, alcohol or nicotine intake. However, they may also indicate heart disease. PVCs frequently pass unnoticed and only occasionally does the person complain of palpitations. Healthy people tend to notice the palpitations more often when at rest.

Ventricular tachycardia

Ventricular tachycardia (VT) is a serious arrhythmia and is usually associated with heart disease. There is a risk of sudden death. VT is caused by rapid firing from ectopic foci in the ventricles and results in a rapid ventricular rate (see *Fig. 39A*). The speed of the rhythm means the reduction in cardiac output is severe and may rapidly lead to unconsciousness. The pulse rate may not be palpable (pulseless VT) or it may be fast and thready. The blood pressure is likely to fall rapidly.

Treatment must be started as soon as possible. If the patient has no discernible pulse, defibrillation should be used and advanced life support (ALS) commenced. Patients with VT, and who are haemodynamically stable, are treated with i.v. lidocaine. Those with recurrent VT or ventricular fibrillation can have an implantable defibrillator inserted. ⇒ Defibrillation (implantable defibrillator).

Radiofrequency ablation of the abnormal pathways may be used for symptomatic VT.

Ventricular fibrillation

H

In ventricular fibrillation (VF) the ventricles no longer contract. Instead, there is a characteristic fast quiver of the ventricles, which fails to produce any cardiac output. There are rapid, fibrillatory waves seen on the ECG (see *Fig. 39B*). Patients do not have a blood pressure or pulse rate. Without immediate resuscitation, VF becomes a fatal arrhythmia. Treatment is commenced as soon as possible with defibrillation and ALS. ⇒ Advanced life support, Cardiac arrest.

CARDITIS

Carditis is inflammation of the heart, and a word seldom used without the appropriate prefix (endo-, myo-, peri-).

CARDIOMYOPATHY

Cardiomyopathy is a disease of the myocardium associated with cardiac dysfunction. It is classified as dilated cardiomyopathy, hypertrophic cardiomyopathy, arrhythmogenic right ventricular cardiomyopathy or restrictive cardiomyopathy. Management includes treatment of the cause (if possible), treatment of heart failure and sometimes heart transplantation.

INFECTIVE ENDOCARDITIS

Infective endocarditis (IE, previously referred to as acute, subacute or chronic bacterial endocarditis) results from a microbial infection of a heart valve or endocardial lining of the heart. The infection is usually bacterial, and the organisms responsible include *Staphylococcus aureus*, *S. epidermidis*, *Streptococcus faecalis* and *Str. viridans*. More rarely the infection may be caused by fungi, *Rickettsia* or *Chlamydia*.

The population at risk includes people with diseased heart valves, those with replacement valves, i.v. drug misusers, patients with an i.v. or central line *in situ*, etc.

Vegetation (fibrin, micro-organisms and platelets) grows on the heart valve or on the endocardium itself. When micro-organisms stick to this vegetation, the process of IE commences. Part of the vegetation may break off and form emboli, which may travel to the brain or other systemic sites.

Management includes intravenous antibiotics (after blood cultures) for at least 6 weeks and oral antibiotics for 4–6 weeks to ensure the infection has cleared. The prophylactic use of antibiotics for those at risk of IE (see above) should be encouraged whenever they undergo a procedure in which the mucous membranes may be breached. Such procedures include dental interventions, body piercing and tattoos.

VALVULAR HEART DISEASE

Valvular heart disease (VHD) is often divided into categories that depend upon whether the valve is stenosed or regurgitant (incompetent). These categories are further divided to describe the affected valve. More commonly, these include mitral stenosis, mitral regurgitation, aortic stenosis and aortic regurgitation.

Rheumatic fever

Acute rheumatic fever is a systemic inflammatory disease that damages the endothelial lining of the heart as well as the skin and connective tissue. It occurs mainly in children and young adults.

The aetiology of acute rheumatic fever is infection with certain strains of group A beta-haemolytic *Streptococcus* that cause upper respiratory tract infections.

It causes carditis, which may involve individual layers, but it is the involvement of the endocardium that leads to rheumatic heart disease. There is also joint inflammation with arthritis, and skin involvement. Sometimes late involvement of the central nervous system leads to chorea.

Management includes:
- Antibiotics;
- Drugs to reduce pain and inflammation (e.g. aspirin, not for children under 16 years);
- Corticosteroids may be prescribed for carditis, or severe joint inflammation;
- Specific treatment for pericarditis and myocarditis;
- Supportive treatment for arrhythmias and heart failure.

SELECTED CARDIOVASCULAR SURGERY AND PROCEDURES

⇒ Coronary heart disease (coronary artery bypass graft, percutaneous myocardial revascularization, percutaneous transluminal coronary angioplasty).

ABLATION

Ablation is a technique used to interrupt abnormal conduction pathways with radiofrequency energy delivered through a transvenous catheter. Used for SVT, WPW syndrome and to treat other atrial and junctional tachycardias.

ANGIOPLASTY

Angioplasty is the surgical reconstruction of blood vessels.

EMBOLECTOMY

Embolectomy is the surgical removal of an embolus from a vessel.

LEFT VENTRICULAR ASSIST DEVICE

Left ventricular assist device (LVAD) is a mechanical pump used to increase the output of blood from the left ventricle of the heart. It may be used in the short term to support critically ill patients, those waiting for a heart transplant or to give the heart time to recover.

PACEMAKER

A pacemaker is an electrical device to maintain myocardial contraction by stimulating the heart muscle (e.g. in symptomatic sinus bradycardia). A pacemaker may be permanent or temporary, and can be programmed in a variety of modes. Nowadays, pacemakers can be programmed to alter their rate in response to physical activity.

CARDIOPULMONARY BYPASS

Cardiopulmonary bypass (CPB) uses a machine that temporarily acts as the heart and lung. Blood is pumped around the body and gaseous exchange takes place through an oxygenator.

HEART TRANSPLANTATION

Heart transplantation may be used for patients with severe heart failure, such as that caused by cardiomyopathy.

SYNCHRONIZED DC CARDIOVERSION

Cardioversion is the use of direct current (DC) electricity to convert an arrhythmia, such as AF or SVT, to normal sinus rhythm. A controlled electric shock momentarily stops the heart, allowing the natural pacemaker of the heart (the sinus node) to initiate the heartbeat and thereby allow the sinus rhythm to be restored.

Cardioversion requires a general anaesthetic. Patients are attached to an electrocardiograph and the lead identified where the characteristics of the arrhythmia are clearest. This is normally lead II. Two paddles are placed on the chest wall, one on each side of the heart (one towards the apex, and the other towards the base). The paddles are charged to between 100 and 150 joules. ⇒ Defibrillation.

VALVE SURGERY

Surgery includes valve replacement using either a mechanical (metal) valve or a biological (tissue) valve. Valvoplasty is a plastic operation on a valve, usually reserved for the heart, and must be distinguished from valve replacement or valvotomy. Valvotomy (valvulotomy) is the incision of a stenotic valve, by custom referring to the heart, to restore normal function.

HEIMLICH MANOEUVRE

The Heimlich manoeuvre, also known as abdominal thrusts, is a first-aid measure to dislodge a foreign body (e.g. food) that obstructs the glottis. If the person is still standing, the first aider should stand behind the victim, place his or her arms round the victims abdomen with the clenched fist supported by the other hand just below the diaphragm, and give a sharp compression inwards. This should force air under pressure through the airway to dislodge the obstruction (*Fig. 102A*). It may also be performed with the victim lying down, the first aider straddling the victim and placing his or her hands, clasped one on top of the other below the diaphragm and giving a short, sharp push upwards (*Fig. 102B*). If the manoeuvre is unsuccessful, the victim requires immediate hospitalization for emergency treatment to secure an airway and endoscopic removal of the foreign body.

HELMINTHIASIS

Helminthiasis is a condition that results from infestation with parasitic helminths (worms).The most common parasitic helminth in Britain is the nematode *Enterobius (Oxyuris) vermicularis* or threadworm. Other worms that may be acquired in Britain include *Toxocara canis* (causing toxocariasis, which leads to fever, hepatomegaly and possible blindness), *Echinococcus granulosus* (causing hydatid disease with cysts in the liver, lungs, bone and brain) and *Fasciola hepatica*, the endemic fluke of sheep.

CLASSES OF HUMAN PARASITIC HELMINTHS

Human parasitic helminths include cestodes, nematodes and trematodes.

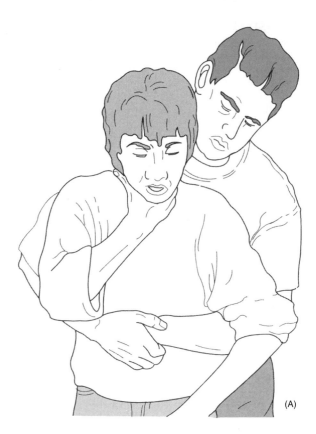

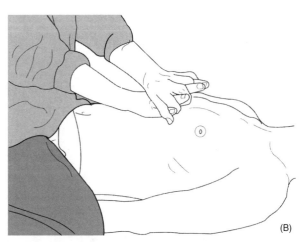

Fig 102 Heimlich manoeuvre: (A) standing position, (B) with victim lying down

Cestodes (tapeworms)

Cestodes can be intestinal, such as *Taenia saginata* (beef tapeworm), *Taenia solium* (pork tapeworm), *Diphyllobothrium latum* (freshwater fish tapeworm), or tissue-dwelling cysts or worms (larval stage), such as *Taenia solium* (cysticercosis) and *Echinococcus granulosus* (tapeworm of dogs and wild canines).

Nematodes (roundworms)

Nematodes are divided into three groups:

- Intestinal human nematodes, such as *Enterobius (Oxyuris) vermicularis* (threadworm), *Ascaris lumbricoides* (roundworm), *Trichuris trichiura* (whipworm), *Ancylostoma duodenale* (hookworm) and *Strongyloides stercoralis*.
- Tissue-dwelling human nematodes include the filarial worms *Wuchereria bancrofti, Brugia malayi, Loa loa* and *Onchocerca volvulus*, which all cause filariasis, and *Dracunculus medinensis* (guinea worm).
- Zoonotic nematodes such as *Toxocara canis* (from dogs) and *Trichinella spiralis* (from pigs and rats).

Trematodes (flukes)

The three species of the genus *Schistosoma* (*S. haematobium, S. mansoni* and *S. japonicum*) are found in the blood and cause schistosomiasis (bilharziasis), which is an important cause of morbidity in tropical regions. Flukes also affect the lungs (*Paragonimus* species), the hepatobiliary system (*Clonorchis sinensis, Opisthorchis felineus* and *Fasciola hepatica*) and intestine (*Fasciolopsis buski*).

ANTHELMINTICS

Anthelmintics are a large group of drugs that act against parasitic worms. An overview is provided in *Box 15*.

Box 15 Anthelmintics
Ancylostoma duodenale (hookworm) – mebendazole.
Ascaris lumbricoides (roundworm) – levamisole, mebendazole, piperazine.
Echinococcus granulosus (hydatid disease) – albendazole (combined with surgery).
Enterobius vermicularis (threadworm) – mebendazole, piperazine.
Onchocerca volvulus – ivermectin.
Schistosoma species– praziquantel.
Strongyloides stercoralis – tiabendazole, ivermectin.
Taenia solium (tapeworm) – niclosamide.
Toxocara canis – albendazole.
Wuchereria bancrofti, Brugia malayi, Loa loa – diethylcarbamazine.

Further reading

Haslett C *et al.* (1999). *Davidson's Principles and Practice of Medicine*, Eighteenth Edition, pp. 164–182. Edinburgh: Churchill Livingstone.

Heredity

Heredity is the transmission from parents to children of genetic characteristics by means of the genetic material, the process by which this occurs and the study of such processes. ⇒ Chromosomes, Genes and genetics, Meiosis.

HERNIA

The abnormal protrusion of an organ, or part of an organ, through an aperture in the surrounding structures – commonly the protrusion of an abdominal organ through a gap in the abdominal wall.

Bowel, for example, may protrude through a weak point in the musculature of the anterior abdominal wall or an existing opening. This occurs when there are intermittent increases in intra-abdominal pressure, most commonly in men who lift heavy loads at work. The possible outcomes include:

- Spontaneous reduction when intra-abdominal pressure returns to normal;
- Manual reduction by applying slight pressure;
- Strangulation, which leads to venous congestion, ischaemia, gangrene and intestinal obstruction.

The sites for hernias are diaphragmatic (hiatus), inguinal, femoral, umbilical and incisional (*Fig. 103*).

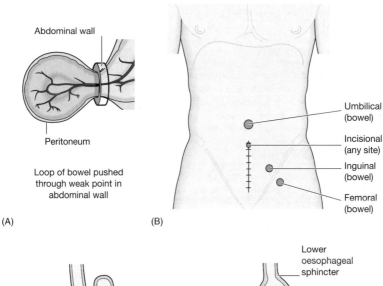

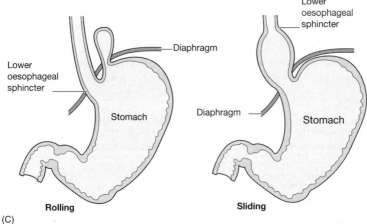

Fig 103 Hernias: (A) strangulated hernia formation, (B) common sites of herniation, (C) diaphragmatic (hiatus) hernia

SURGICAL TREATMENT FOR HERNIAS

HERNIOPLASTY

Hernioplasty is an attempt to prevent recurrence by refashioning the structures to give greater strength.

HERNIORRHAPHY

In herniorrhaphy the weak area is reinforced by some of the person's own tissues or by some other material.

HERNIOTOMY

Herniotomy is an operation to cure hernia. It involves the return of its contents to their normal position and the removal of the hernial sac.

HERPESVIRUSES AND HERPES

The herpesviruses are a group of DNA viruses that include cytomegalovirus (CMV), Epstein–Barr virus (EBV), varicella-zoster virus (VZV) and herpes simplex virus (HSV).

CYTOMEGALOVIRUS

CMV infection can be latent and asymptomatic. It is passed to the fetus and may cause miscarriage, stillbirth or serious neonatal disease, including encephalitis and microcephaly with learning disability, or death. In adults it causes an illness similar to infectious mononucleosis and pneumonia. The virus is a serious threat to immunocompromised individuals.

EPSTEIN–BARR VIRUS

The EBV causes infectious mononucleosis (glandular fever). It is also linked with the formation of some malignant tumours, including Burkitt's lymphoma and nasopharyngeal cancer.

VARICELLA-ZOSTER VIRUS

The VZV causes varicella (chicken pox) and herpes zoster. ⇒ Communicable diseases (varicella), Nervous system (herpes zoster).

HERPES SIMPLEX VIRUS

There are two types of HSV, HSV-1 and HSV-2. HSV-1 is associated with orolabial herpes and HSV-2 with genital herpes, but either type can cause genital herpes.

HERPES

Herpes is a vesicular eruption caused by infection with the HSV. HSV-1 produces blisters around the mouth (herpes labialis – cold sores). The severity of infection depends on the state of the person's immune system – the effects may be much more severe in debilitated individuals, especially the immunocompromised and those at the extremes of age. The virus can also cause conjunctivitis and oesophagitis. *Eczema herpeticum* is a serious condition that occurs when existing eczema becomes infected with HSV-1. It can be life-threatening and patients may need to be hospitalized, nursed in isolation and treated with antiviral drugs.

Genital herpes is a sexually transmissible infection, caused by either HSV-1 or HSV-2, and associated with painful, tender superficial ulcers of the genitalia or anal region. Without treatment first-episode lesions heal within about 1 month (antiviral therapy shortens the duration of the lesions). Recurrences are common, particularly with HSV-2, but the duration of lesions is shorter than during the initial episode. An individual can transmit the virus to a sexual partner even when there are no apparent genital or orolabial lesions.

Neonatal herpes is acquired during vaginal delivery from a mother actively shedding HSV. It is a devastating illness with a 75% mortality rate and a high incidence of severe neurological sequelae among survivors. ⇒ Sexually transmitted (acquired) infections.

HOLISTIC HEALTH AND CARE

To understand the web of influences upon someone's health and well-being involves taking a 'holistic' approach (from the Greek *holos*, meaning 'whole'). The holistic health approach incorporates a belief in people's responsibility for their own lives, a willingness to co-operate with others and an emphasis on developing meaningful relationships and a positive outlook on life.

Nurses who apply the holistic approach to healthcare place emphasis on the whole person, taking into account each person's physical, emotional, intellectual, spiritual and sociocultural background. Therefore, health has five components:

- Social health, the ability to interact well with people and the environment – satisfying interpersonal relationships;
- Mental health, the ability to learn – a person's intellectual capabilities;
- Emotional health, the ability to control emotions so that someone feels comfortable expressing them when appropriate and expresses them appropriately – the ability not to express emotion when it is inappropriate to do so;
- Spiritual health, a belief in some unifying force – for some this is nature, for some it is the sciences and for others a god-like force;
- Physical health, the ability to perform daily tasks without fatigue – biological integrity of the individual (Greenberg 1992).

All aspects of health need to be balanced and integrated for a high degree of 'wellness' to be present.

HOMEOSTASIS

The composition of the internal environment is maintained within narrow limits, and this fairly constant state is called *homeostasis*. It describes a dynamic, ever-changing situation kept within a narrow range. When this balance is threatened or lost, there is a serious risk to the well-being of the individual. Many factors in the internal environment must be maintained within narrow limits (e.g. temperature, electrolyte concentrations, pH, blood glucose, blood pressure, etc.).

Homeostasis is maintained by control systems that detect and respond to changes in the internal environment. A control system has three basic components – detector, control centre and effector. The *control centre* determines the limits within which the variable factor should be maintained. It receives an input from the *detector (sensor)*, and integrates the incoming information. When the incoming signal indicates that an adjustment is needed the *control centre* responds and its output to the *effector* is changed.

NEGATIVE FEEDBACK MECHANISMS

In systems controlled by negative feedback the effector response decreases or negates the effect of the original stimulus, restoring homeostasis (thus the term negative feedback). Body temperature is a physiological variable controlled by negative feedback (*Fig. 104*). When body temperature falls below the pre-set level,

H

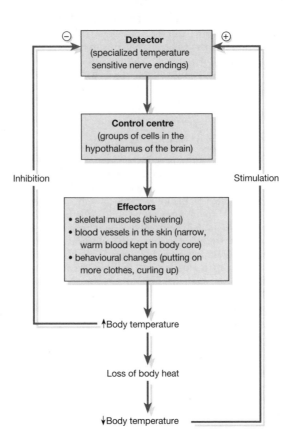

Fig 104 Example of a physiological negative feedback mechanism: control of body temperature

this is detected by specialized temperature-sensitive nerve endings. They transmit this input to cells in the hypothalamus of the brain, which form the control centre. The output from the control centre activates mechanisms that raise body temperature (effectors). These include:

- Shivering;
- Vasoconstriction of vessels in the skin;
- Behavioural changes (e.g. putting on more clothes).

When body temperature rises to within the normal range, the temperature-sensitive nerve endings no longer stimulate the cells of the control centre and therefore the output of this centre to the effectors ceases.

Most of the homeostatic controls in the body use negative feedback mechanisms to prevent sudden and serious changes in the internal environment.

POSITIVE FEEDBACK MECHANISMS

Only a few of these *amplifier* or *cascade systems* occur in the body. In positive feedback mechanisms, the stimulus progressively increases the response, so that as long as the stimulus is continued the response is progressively amplified. Examples include blood clotting and uterine contractions during labour.

During labour, uterine contractions are stimulated by the hormone oxytocin. These force the baby's head onto the cervix, which stimulates stretch receptors. In response to this, more of the hormone oxytocin is released, further strengthening the contractions and maintaining labour. After the baby is born the stimulus (stretching of the cervix) is no longer present and the release of oxytocin stops.

Further reading

Watson R and Fawcett T (2003). *Pathophysiology, Homeostasis and Nursing*. London: Routledge.

Hormones

⇒ Endocrine, Homeostasis.

Hospital-at-home

Hospital-at-home is a scheme whereby complex and often 'high-tech' care is delivered to patients in their own homes (e.g. children with chronic conditions or adults with chronic respiratory conditions). These schemes, which are often nurse-led, aim to avoid unnecessary admissions to an acute hospital.

Human immunodeficiency virus

The human immunodeficiency virus (HIV) currently designates the acquired immune deficiency syndrome (AIDS) virus. There are two types – HIV-1 (many strains), mainly responsible for HIV disease in Western Europe, North America and Central Africa, and HIV-2, which causes similar disease, but mainly in West Africa. HIV is a retrovirus, which means that it contains RNA that, by reverse transcriptase enzymes, makes a viral DNA copy of the RNA. This is able to integrate into the host cell DNA, where it changes the chromosomes and further replication of viral RNA occurs.

HIV depletes T cells (specifically, T_{helper} cells) of the immune system that normally stimulate the immune response. Without the means to mount an immune response the host is open to a wide variety of opportunistic infections that do not normally produce disease. It is these infections that are so detrimental to patients. However, not all HIV patients develop AIDS, which implies there is some resistance to HIV-associated immune system suppression.

HIV is transmitted through sexual contact, in blood or blood products and other body fluids and by vertical transmission perinatally. ⇒ Acquired immune deficiency syndrome, Sharps.

CLINICAL PRESENTATION

Infection with HIV can cause nonspecific illnesses, such as fever, malaise, lymphadenopathy and rashes. Within 6 weeks antibodies can be observed, although some evidence indicates that these antibodies can take longer to develop. Antibodies can be detected (once expressed) by blood tests, such as enzyme-linked immunosorbent assay (ELISA), but this is not highly specific for HIV infection, and a positive test is usually repeated and followed by the more specific Western blot test to confirm the diagnosis.

Patients may remain asymptomatic in the early stages of the disease process, but may have generalized lymph node swelling. Opportunistic infections can follow and commonly affect mucous membranes (e.g. candidiasis, affecting the mouth, oesophagus and lungs). Other opportunistic infections include pneumonia caused by *Pneumocystis carinii*, tuberculosis, cytomegalovirus infection and

Cryptococcus neoformans (which causes meningitis and lung disease). As the disease develops, weight loss, fevers and night sweats are commonly found.

Patients with HIV are also prone to develop malignancies such as Kaposi's sarcoma (characterized by new blood vessel growth that produces red, brown or purple lesions, often on the skin, but with metastatic potential), non-Hodgkin's lymphoma, etc.

MANAGEMENT

The management of HIV is drug based. Treatment is with antiviral drugs, but additional aims of treatment include prevention of (or treatment of) opportunistic infections, such as fluconazole for candidiasis, augmentation of the immune system and support to patients. Antiviral drugs are usually given in different combinations depending on the stage of the disease. The different types of antiviral drugs include:
- Nucleoside reverse transcriptase inhibitor (antiretroviral), such as zidovudine (azidothymidine AZT), didanosine (DDI) and zalcitabine (DDC);
- Protease inhibitors (e.g. amprenavir, ritonavir, saquinavir, etc.);
- Non-nucleoside reverse transcriptase inhibitors (e.g. efavirenz and nevirapine).

Further reading

Adler MW (2001). *ABC of AIDS*, Fifth Edition. London: BMJ Publishing Group.

HUMAN PAPILLOMA VIRUS

There are many types of human papilloma virus (HPV), including several associated with anogenital warts (particularly types 6 and 11), and a few types (particularly 16 and 18) associated with genital tract malignancy, such as cervical carcinoma. ⇒ Cervix (cancer of the cervix).

HUMAN NEEDS

The concept of human needs has been widely used in nursing, and is based on Maslow's (1974) analysis of human needs (*Fig. 105*). The basic physiological needs for food, breathing and eliminating are at the bottom of the hierarchy and have to be at least minimally fulfilled before motivation can be established to deal with safety and security needs; then love and belonging, and self-esteem needs are attended to; and at the top level, achievement of self-actualization brings satisfaction with living and a sense of fulfilment.

HUMANISM

Humanism is a philosophical movement that focuses on the nature and essence of the human individual. It explores and promotes the central importance of the human individual and underpins the reasonings behind human rights movements, patients' rights campaigns and patient-centred approaches to healthcare. It is one of the main philosophical movements to underlie current theories of nursing practice.

HYPERSENSITIVITY REACTIONS

⇒ Allergy.

HYPERTENSION

Systemic hypertension is a common condition in which the systolic blood pressure persistently exceeds 140 mmHg and the diastolic blood pressure 85 mmHg.

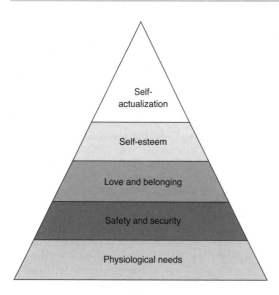

Fig 105 Maslow's hierarchy of human needs

H

The underlying cause of secondary hypertension is unknown in the vast majority of patients (over 95%), and is called *essential hypertension*. Hypertension has a multifactorial aetiology – the factors associated with hypertension include obesity, diabetes, high salt (sodium) intake, alcohol misuse and smoking. Genetic factors are also important. Certain racial groups have a higher prevalence of hypertension, such as African–Americans and the Japanese.

Blood pressure rises with age and hypertension is rarely seen in the age group under 25 years, unless they have a primary illness, such as renal failure.

The known causes of secondary hypertension are outlined in *Box 16*. ⇒ Blood pressure, Pregnancy.

Box 16 Known causes of secondary hypertension
- Pre-eclampsia;
- Coarctation of the aorta;
- Renal artery stenosis;
- Renal diseases;
- Certain drugs (e.g. corticosteroids);
- Endocrine disorders, such as Cushing's disease, acromegaly and phaeochromocytoma.

Frequently, hypertension is diagnosed from a routine medical examination, in a person who is asymptomatic. However, if symptoms do occur they include headaches, dizziness or burst blood vessels in the eyes. Hypertension over a prolonged period of time may lead to what is referred to as end-organ damage, that is damage to the kidneys (renal failure), eyes (cataracts and conjunctival haemorrhage), central nervous system (papilloedema, transient ischaemic attacks and strokes), heart (heart failure and atheroma) and blood vessels (aneurysm; see Practice application).

Diuretics, such as bendroflumethiazide or furosemide, and angiotensin-converting enzyme (ACE) inhibitors, such as captopril, are prescribed frequently. Other antihypertensive drugs include beta-adrenoceptor antagonists (beta-blockers), such as atenolol, that block the sympathetic nervous system response and cause vasodilation. Calcium channel blockers (amlodipine or nifedipine) may be prescribed.

Other drugs that may be used include alpha$_1$-adrenoceptor antagonists (prazosin), vasodilator drugs (such as hydralazine) or drugs that act centrally (such as clonidine).

Practice application – reducing the risk of end-organ damage

Once hypertension is diagnosed, the main aim of treatment must be to reduce the risk of end-organ damage by reducing blood pressure. People should be encouraged to eat a low salt and low fat diet, and reduce alcohol intake if appropriate. They may need advice about losing weight and starting a regular exercise programme. Smoking cessation should be encouraged. Relaxation techniques and the use of biofeedback have been found to combat hypertension associated with the life-style stresses. Primary prevention, especially among those with a family history is important.

Individuals should be taught to record their blood pressure at home, usually while sitting, as blood pressure values vary with posture. They should also become familiar with any symptoms or signs that may indicate a worsening of their condition. These include deteriorating eyesight, burst blood vessels in the eyes or a cerebrovascular incident. People encouraged with self-monitoring may adapt to their chronic illness in a more positive way.

Further reading

Ramsey L, Williams B, Johnston G, *et al.* (1999). British hypertension society guidelines for hypertension management: summary. *Br Med J.* **319**: 630–635.

HYPOTENSION

Hypotension is low blood pressure insufficient for adequate tissue perfusion and oxygenation; it may be primary or secondary (e.g. reduced cardiac output, hypovolaemic shock, Addison's disease) or postural (orthostatic). $\Rightarrow$ Adrenal glands (adrenal insufficiency), Shock.

Practice application – postural hypotension

Postural hypotension is a sudden fall in blood pressure on standing up quickly from a sitting or lying position. It occurs most commonly in older people. It may be caused by a delay in the physiological mechanisms that normally compensate for changes in posture. Postural hypotension can also occur when patients are being treated with antihypertensive drugs, especially when the most appropriate dose is being established. Nurses should advise patients to avoid sudden changes in posture. When patients have been lying or sitting for some time, healthcare staff must anticipate the potential for a sudden fall in blood pressure when they stand up, and ensure that they stand gradually and safely.

ILLNESS BEHAVIOUR

In very simplistic terms, illness behaviour can be divided into that which occurs in response to organic malfunctions or that which occurs when there are no organic manifestations. The perception of illness where there is no obvious organic cause has been termed abnormal illness behaviour.

Pilowsky (1978) developed a useful questionnaire that distinguished between various patterns or styles of illness behaviour. The *Illness Behaviour Questionnaire* (IBQ) was based on a sample of 100 chronic pain patients. The subjects were an average age of 49.1 years, the pain was experienced for an average of 7.4 years, and all subjects had not responded to medical treatment. On the basis of their scores, the following clusters were observed:
- General hypochondriasis – patients have a general anxiety about their health and a distinct fear of contracting disease;
- Disease conviction – there is a conviction that disease is present, rather than a fear of contracting it, so patients reject medical advice and are abnormally preoccupied with their bodily functions;
- Psychological perception of illness – patients are willing to attribute the cause of their disorder to psychological factors or their own behaviour;
- Affective inhibition – a reluctance to express negative emotions, such as anger, to other individuals;
- Affective disturbance – patients are anxious and depressed (dysphoric);
- Denial of problems – patients tend to deny any financial or family problems and think that their illness is the only difficulty in their lives;
- Irritability – there is a tendency to be quick to anger, which often places a strain on interpersonal relationships.

Pilowsky (1978) cluster-analysed scale profiles of the 100 patients and was able to classify six types of patients – three were adaptive forms of illness behaviour and three were maladaptive forms of illness behaviour (*Box 17*).

Box 17 Illness behaviour
Adaptive:
- Capacity to use denial adaptively;
- Use of denial, but less effective in employing strategy;
- Irritability and interpersonal friction with denial of problems other than physical health.

Maladaptive:
- Somatic preoccupation and rejection of reassurance;
- High disease conviction and many life problems;
- Anxious hypochondriacal concern with health.

The questionnaire provides a useful classification of abnormal illness behaviour, but does not make any predictions about how illness is likely to be perceived by different individuals. ⇒ Behaviour, Somatization.

IMAGING TECHNIQUES

Diagnostic techniques used to investigate the condition and functioning of organs and structures. ⇒ Urinary system (urinary disorders, *Box 41*).

COMPUTED TOMOGRAPHY

Computed tomography (CT) is a computer-constructed imaging technique of a thin slice through the body, derived from X-ray absorption data collected during a circular scanning motion.

MAGNETIC RESONANCE IMAGING

Magnetic resonance imaging (MRI) is a noninvasive technique that does not use ionizing radiation (i.e., X-rays). It uses radiofrequency radiation in the presence of a powerful magnetic field to produce high-quality images of the body in any plane. Sometimes called nuclear magnetic resonance (NMR).

POSITRON EMISSION TOMOGRAPHY

Positron emission tomography (PET) uses isotopes of extremely short half-life that emit positrons. PET scanning is used to evaluate physiological function of organs (e.g. the brain).

RADIOGRAPHIC EXAMINATION

A radiographic examination of an image (radiograph is the correct term for an 'X-ray' image) formed by exposure to X-rays. It is used, for example, to diagnose fractures or pneumonia, etc.

RADIONUCLIDE SCANS

A radionuclide scan is an imaging technique that produces a pictorial representation of the amount and distribution of radioactive isotope (radioisotope or radionuclide) present in a particular organ.

Radioisotopes are forms of an element that undergo spontaneous nuclear disintegration to emit radiation. When taken orally or by injection, they can be traced by a Geiger counter.

SINGLE PHOTON EMISSION COMPUTED TOMOGRAPHY

Single photon emission computed tomography (SPECT) produces three-dimensional images of organ structure and function, such as the brain.

ULTRASONOGRAPHY

Ultrasonography is the formation of a visible image by the use of ultrasound. A controlled beam of sound is directed into the relevant part of the body. The reflected ultrasound is used to build up an electronic image of the body structures. It is offered routinely during pregnancy to monitor progress and detect fetal and placental abnormalities. Real-time ultrasonography involves rapid pulsing to enable continuous viewing of movement to be obtained, rather than stationary images.

IMMUNE RESPONSE AND IMMUNITY

⇒ Defence mechanisms.

IMMUNOCOMPROMISED (IMMUNOSUPPRESSED) PATIENT

Immunocompromised patients have defective immune responses, which can be inherited or acquired. ⇒ Immunodeficiency.

Depending on the immune defect, different patterns of infection result. Patients with cellular defects are likely to develop infections with opportunistic organisms such as *Candida, Pneumocystis carinii* and *Cryptococcus neoformans*. Patients with antibody defects are more liable to infections with encapsulated bacteria, such as pneumococcus.

Treatment with drugs or irradiation often immunocompromises patients, and immunocompromisation also occurs in some patients with cancer and other diseases that affect the lymphoid system.

Defective immune responses are also caused by having myeloablative doses of chemotherapy and/or radiotherapy for (most commonly) haematological cancers prior to having a haemopoietic stem cell transplant (HSCT). ⇒ Haemopoietic stem cell transplantation.

Practice application – minimizing infection risk in patients with neutropenia

It is impossible to eliminate all risk of infection for neutropenic patients (neutrophil count $<1.0 \times 10^9/L$), but various strategies may reduce this risk. In the past, neutropenic patients were often nursed in strict protective isolation. However, such measures are not always necessary and may have a detrimental psychological impact. Nowadays, people tend to be nursed in less stringent isolation, or even may remain at home, depending on the intensity of the treatment and the duration of the neutropenia.

Most centres now adopt a common-sense approach to infection control, whereby normality is preserved as far as possible while risk is minimized. The general principles are that:

- Neutropenic patients should be nursed away from infected patients – clean single room, or some centres have a sterile laminar air flow environment in which positive pressure filters sterile air through the room;
- Strict hand washing should be observed by all personnel who enter the patient's room and before any care episode;
- Staff or visitors with an obvious infection, or those who have been in contact with an infectious illness, should avoid contact with the patient;
- Special care should be taken during any invasive procedures.

The general environment should be kept meticulously clean and patients should also be encouraged to maintain high standards of personal hygiene and mouth care. Good general hygiene with regard to food preparation should also be maintained. Thus, food should be stored correctly and should be consumed well within its expiry date. Foods should be cooked thoroughly, as the process of cooking destroys most micro-organisms. Raw vegetables, salads and nuts are best avoided. Fruit is only recommended if it has been peeled. Soft cheeses, raw eggs and unpasteurized dairy products should not be eaten when patients are neutropenic. That said, a degree of common sense should be used when advising patients about diet. The risk of infection from food is relatively small in comparison to the patients' need for good nutrition. It is also psychologically important for patients to eat foods that they desire and feel able to tolerate.

IMMUNODEFICIENCY

Immunodeficiency is the state of having defective immune responses, which leads to increased susceptibility to infection.

IMMUNODEFICIENCY DISEASES

Immunodeficiency diseases are inherited or acquired disorders of the immune system. Inherited disorders include severe combined immunodeficiency that affects both B and T cells (lymphocytes) and X-linked agammaglobulinaemia (XLA), a primary immunodeficiency disorder that affects boys. In XLA a gene mutation results in absent B cells (lymphocytes) and hence absent immunoglobulin production.

Acquired or secondary immunodeficiency disorders may be caused by drugs (such as cytotoxic chemotherapy), radiation and micro-organisms, including the human immunodeficiency virus (HIV). ⇒ Defence mechanisms, Human immunodeficiency virus.

IMPOTENCE

⇒ Sexuality (*Box 36*, Sexual dysfunction).

INCIDENT AND ACCIDENT REPORTING

Any nonroutine incident or accident that involves a patient and/or client, relative, visitor or member of staff must be recorded by the nurse who witnesses the incident or finds the patient and/or client afterwards. Incidents include falls, needlestick accidents, drug errors, a visitor fainting or a member of staff being assaulted.

Careful documentation of all incidents and accidents is important for clinical governance (continuous quality improvement, learning from mistakes and managing risk, etc.), to fulfil legal requirements to report incidents and accidents under the relevant legislation and in case of a complaint or legal action.

In the UK the information can be used by the Health and Safety Executive (HSE) to monitor occupational incidents nationally. For nurses, accurate reporting protects individual rights and benefits in the event of loss of income or personal injury. Occupational injuries should be reported to the occupational health department and injured workers may require an assessment of fitness before returning to work. ⇒ Drug (Practice application – drug errors), Moving and handling, Risk assessment and management, Sharps.

Practice application – good practice in incident and accident reporting
- An incident or accident form should be completed as soon as possible after the event;
- Be concise, accurate and objective;
- Record what you saw and describe the care you gave, who else was involved and the person's condition;
- Do not try to guess or explain what happened (e.g. record that side rails were not in place, but not that this was the reason the patient fell out of bed);
- Record the actions taken by other nurses and doctors at the time;
- Do not blame individuals in the report;
- Always record the full facts.

INCONTINENCE

Control of bladder and bowels is fundamental to the developmental stage shift from infant to child. To lose control over the most intimate of bodily functions is humiliating and distressing at any age. Maintaining continence and managing incontinence are vitally important in nursing, so readers are advised to consult the Further reading suggestions. ⇒ Catheters and urinary catheterization, Continence (Practice application – maintaining continence), Defecation, Micturition.

THE IMPACT OF URINARY INCONTINENCE

The impact of incontinence on the emotional, social, physical and economic well-being of individuals and their carers should not be underestimated. The experience of incontinence has a profound impact on an adult's psychological well-being. Fear of this loss of control being witnessed by others leads people to curtail their social and public activities. People who are incontinent describe a range of emotions, including increased levels of depression, irritability, anxiety and feelings of hopelessness.

TYPES OF URINARY INCONTINENCE

A number of different types of urinary incontinence are classified by the International Continence Society (Abrams *et al.* 2002).

OVERACTIVE BLADDER (ALSO KNOWN AS DETRUSOR INSTABILITY AND URGE INCONTINENCE)

The overactive bladder is a symptomatic diagnosis that comprises the symptoms of frequency of micturition (more than eight times in 24 hours) and urgency with or without urge incontinence, occurring either singly or in combination.

The overactive bladder is a chronic condition defined by urodynamic investigations as detrusor overactivity, and characterized by involuntary bladder contractions during the filling phase of the micturition cycle (Abrams *et al.* 2002). It is the most common cause of urinary incontinence in older people.

STRESS INCONTINENCE

Stress incontinence is defined as urine loss coincident with an increase in intra-abdominal pressure, in the absence of a detrusor contraction or an overdistended bladder. Clinically, it presents as the involuntary loss of urine on coughing, sneezing, laughing or performing physical activities. It occurs in about 85% of women who present with incontinence (Cardozo 1991). It is usually associated with bladder outlet incompetence caused by weakness of the supporting pelvic floor muscles and insufficiency of the urethral sphincter. In women this is usually, but not always, the result of childbirth; in men it can occur after prostate surgery.

MIXED INCONTINENCE

It is not uncommon for people to complain of both urge and stress symptoms, termed mixed urinary incontinence, and particularly common in postmenopausal women. The most important aspect of this type of incontinence is to identify the most 'bothersome' symptom, which should then be targetted.

OVERFLOW INCONTINENCE

This term is used to describe the involuntary loss of urine associated with overdistension of the bladder. It can be caused by a number of different conditions, including bladder outlet or urethral obstruction, which is most commonly seen in men with prostatic hyperplasia. This type of incontinence is less common in women, but may occur as a complication after surgery to correct incontinence or because of severe pelvic organ prolapse.

An underactive or acontractile detrusor muscle can also lead to overdistension and overflow. The causes include neurological disorders, such as strokes or multiple sclerosis, diabetes and medication side-effects. In some individuals it is idiopathic.

VOIDING INEFFICIENCY

Voiding inefficiency means that the bladder fails to empty completely, which leads to the involuntary loss of urine associated with overdistension. Voiding inefficiency is a common problem in individuals with neurological problems, such as multiple sclerosis or Parkinson's disease, or in those who have had strokes. Individuals who have diabetes can also have voiding inefficiency because of autonomic neuropathy. Benign prostatic hyperplasia in men may lead to obstruction that can cause voiding inefficiency, and women may have an obstruction caused by a pelvic organ prolapse.

NOCTURIA AND NOCTURNAL ENURESIS

Individuals who have to wake up one or more times at night to void have nocturia. Nocturnal enuresis is when individuals wet the bed at night. Nocturia can be a normal phenomenon in older people because they have small bladder capacities and a reduced excretion of antidiuretic hormone overnight. In addition, heart failure can lead to an increased diuresis at night, as the fluids in the tissues returns to the circulation when they are elevated and this is voided overnight. Nocturnal enuresis occurs commonly in children; however, sometimes this continues into adulthood. In addition, those individuals who have overactive bladders can have nocturnal bedwetting if they sleep through the impulse to void.

Practice application – assessment of urinary incontinence

A complex interaction of factors contributes to the development of urinary incontinence, especially in the frail older person. Identification and management of problems, such as an inability to undress in time at the lavatory, need as much attention as the diagnosis of the underlying pathology. Thus, a systematic assessment of all potential factors is required, preferably using a single-assessment, evidence-based protocol or care pathway customized to the particular area. A thorough assessment is crucial, and should preferably be multidisciplinary (Baylis *et al.* 2001). The following key aspects of assessment should be covered:

- Presenting symptoms and history of incontinence – a detailed exploration of the symptoms is important, as is clarifying the most bothersome symptoms, which helps lead to a preliminary nursing diagnosis of what type of incontinence problems the patient might have.
- Impact on the person's quality of life (e.g. reducing social contact outside the home, impact on sexuality, evidence of depression).
- Past medical history (e.g. whether the onset was during or after childbirth, or whether it was after surgery, such as a prostatectomy or hysterectomy. Other medical history is also relevant, such as heart disease that requires treatment with diuretics and could lead to continence symptoms. If an individual has asthma and a related cough, this may worsen stress incontinence symptoms.
- Associated disease, such as dementia, diabetes, neurological disease (e.g. multiple sclerosis, etc.), can lead to incontinence symptoms. Spinal cord disease or injury can also be a predisposing factor. Arthritis can lead to mobility problems that may influence whether an individual can reach the lavatory in time.
- Environmental factors, such as whether the lavatory is too low or too high. Furthermore, for individuals with mobility problems lavatories located some distance from where they are sitting, or upstairs, can lead to difficulty reaching them on time and thus to maintaining continence. Many people with continence symptoms find it difficult to leave the house because of the lack of public toilet facilities.
- Current medications and drug use, such as diuretics, alcohol consumption and smoking, etc.
- Dietary intake and fluids (e.g. how much and what type of fluids are drunk). Caffeine, alcohol and fizzy and diet drinks are known to aggravate continence symptoms. In addition, many people with continence symptoms tend to restrict their fluid intake, which can lead to urine becoming concentrated and cause bladder irritation. Conversely, if they drink large quantities of fluids this can also aggravate bladder symptoms.

FAECAL INCONTINENCE

The impact of faecal incontinence mirrors and amplifies those described for urinary incontinence. Underestimates of prevalence are common because of the reluctance to admit to this symptom. People tend to find it a distasteful topic to discuss; it is a taboo subject that is often hidden by patients.

CAUSES OF FAECAL INCONTINENCE

Faecal incontinence is more common in women than in men and more common in older adults. It is not, however, a normal part of ageing. Faecal incontinence can have several causes, as described below.

DAMAGE TO THE ANAL SPHINCTER MUSCLES

Faecal incontinence is most often caused by injury to one or both anal internal and/or external sphincters that lie at the bottom of the anal canal. In women, this damage most often happens during childbirth. The risk of injury is greatest during an instrumental delivery or if a midline episiotomy is performed. Surgery for haemorrhoids can also damage the sphincters.

DAMAGE TO THE NERVES OF THE ANAL SPHINCTER MUSCLES OR THE RECTUM

If the sensory nerves are damaged, there is no sense that stool is in the rectum and faecal leakage occurs. Nerve damage may be caused by childbirth, a long-term straining to pass stool, stroke and chronic conditions that affect the nerves, such as diabetes and multiple sclerosis.

LOSS OF STORAGE CAPACITY IN THE RECTUM

Rectal surgery, radiation treatment and inflammatory bowel disease can cause scarring of the rectal walls, which makes them stiff and less elastic. The ability of the rectum to hold stool is then compromised, and faecal incontinence may result.

DIARRHOEA

Diarrhoea, or loose stool, is more difficult to control than solid stool. Even people who do not have faecal incontinence can be incontinent of faeces when they have diarrhoea.

PELVIC FLOOR DYSFUNCTION

Pelvic floor dysfunction includes a decreased perception of rectal and anal sensation, rectal prolapse and generalized weakness of the pelvic floor. This may be more pronounced in later life. When the cause of pelvic floor dysfunction is childbirth, incontinence does not usually present until the fifth decade.

CONSTIPATION

The most common cause of faecal incontinence in older adults is believed to be constipation (Petticrew *et al.* 1998). ⇒ Defecation (constipation).

Further reading

Brooker C and Nicol M (2003). *Nursing Adults. The Practice of Caring*, Ch 12. Edinburgh: Mosby.

INDUSTRIAL DISEASES

⇒ Occupational health (occupational diseases).

INEQUALITIES IN HEALTH

Inequalities in health are the differences in the distribution of health associated with social class or poverty (as opposed to physiological processes, such as age, sex and constitution). A considerable body of evidence shows a clear relationship between poor health and deprivation (measured by income, level of education and type of employment or unemployment). Measures of inequality include differences in standardized mortality ratios, life expectancy and infant and maternal mortality rates. Low-income individuals are more likely to die prematurely, suffer acute and chronic illnesses and experience long-term disability. ⇒ Epidemiology, Ethics (equity), Health, Mortality.

DEPRIVATION INDICES

Deprivation indices are a set of census variables and weightings used to assess levels of deprivation within a specific community or population. They include levels of unemployment, lone-parent households, pensioners who live alone and households without a car, etc.

JARMAN INDEX

In the UK, the Jarman index is the system for weighting general practice populations according to social conditions. It is a composite index of social factors that general practitioners (GPs) considered important in increasing workload and pressure on services. These factors were identified through a survey of one in ten GPs in the UK in 1981. An underprivileged area (UPA) score was then constructed based on the level of each variable in each area, weighted by the weighting assigned from the national GP survey. Eight variables were used:
- Elderly living alone;
- Children under five years of age;
- Unskilled;
- Unemployed (as a percentage of the economically active);
- Lone parent families;
- Overcrowded accommodation (more than one person per room);
- Mobility (moved house within 1 year);
- Ethnic origin (new Commonwealth and Pakistan).

TOWNSEND INDEX

In the UK, the Townsend index is a composite index of deprivation in the population. It is the sum of the standardized values of the percentages of households without cars, households not owner occupied, overcrowded households and the unemployed in an electoral ward. The components (socioeconomic variables) are drawn from census information.

INFECTION

Infection is defined as the successful invasion, establishment and growth of microorganisms on or in the host tissues, which leads to an associated tissue reaction.

If there is no tissue reaction in the host or it is subclinical (i.e., there are no overt symptoms of infection), it is termed '*colonization*', which means that the microorganism is carried but, as there is an absence of any host response, it may not be identified as being present. Colonization in a number of patients may indicate that an organism is spreading in a ward or unit, as seen in many outbreaks of methicillin-resistant *Staphylococcus aureus* (MRSA). Colonized patients spread the organism to both healthcare workers and other patients, but this may go unnoticed unless somebody exposed to it becomes infected clinically.

Sepsis refers to the presence of inflammation, pus and other signs of infection. Infective illnesses are sometimes described using terms that refer to the site of infection (e.g. pneumonia for the lungs and tonsillitis for the tonsils) or, alternatively, as a specific disease (such as tuberculosis).

Contamination refers to the presence of organisms on inanimate objects or living material that may have harmful infectious or unwanted matter.

RESERVOIRS OF INFECTION

Micro-organisms have a reservoir in which they live. For some, particularly viruses that cannot replicate outside living cells, the human body is the reservoir and they survive by passing from person to person. The human body is also the reservoir for bacteria and fungi that colonize the bowel, skin and respiratory tract.

Animals provide a reservoir for some micro-organisms that do not cause disease in the animal, but establish infection when passed to humans.

Other micro-organisms (e.g. *Clostridium* and *Legionella*) normally inhabit the environment in soil, dust or water.

MODE OF TRANSMISSION AND PORTALS OF ENTRY

For cross-infection to occur, a means or mode of transmission and a portal of entry are required. In healthcare settings, the mode of transmission is often the hands of healthcare workers; the portal of entry varies. For example, if micro-organisms from infectious diarrhoea are on a healthcare worker's hands and those hands go around or inside the healthcare worker's mouth, the organisms could then be swallowed and ingested into the gut, and the healthcare worker becomes symptomatic within a period of hours. In the same way, a wound infection may be spread to another wound (portal of entry) on a healthcare worker's hands (mode of transmission).

Direct contact spread refers to the transfer of infection to a patient via direct contact with an infected person. *Indirect contact* refers to the acquisition of organisms, such as blood-borne pathogens, from needles and instruments, or micro-organisms from bedding, dirt and dust or food, and it must also include the unwashed hands of hospital staff.

Vertical transmission of infection [e.g. human immunodeficiency virus (HIV)] can occur from mother to fetus, via the placenta, during the delivery or via breast milk.

Regardless of the way in which organisms are spread, for pathogenic organisms to take hold and cause an infection they require a susceptible host. This may be another patient, an informal carer or a healthcare worker.

TYPES OF INFECTION

⇒ Superinfection.

CROSS-INFECTION (EXOGENOUS) INFECTION

Cross-infection occurs when the micro-organism that causes an infection is acquired from another person (patient, healthcare worker, carer) or the environment (i.e. from an exogenous source). Examples are a wound infection caused by a member of staff who is a *Staphylococcus* carrier, or who may have boils or septic lesions or, more commonly, who may have failed to wash his or her hands properly.

ENDOGENOUS OR SELF-INFECTION

Self-infection occurs when a micro-organism that has colonized a site on the host enters another site and establishes an infection, such as bowel micro-organisms that cause infection in a wound or urinary tract.

HOSPITAL-ACQUIRED INFECTION (HAI)

A nosocomial or hospital-acquired infection (HAI) occurs in a patient who has been in hospital for at least 72 hours and who had no signs and symptoms of such infection on admission. The most common HAI is urinary tract infection.

OPPORTUNISTIC INFECTION

An opportunistic infection is a serious infection with a micro-organism that normally has little or no pathogenic (ability to produce disease) activity, but causes disease where host resistance is reduced by serious disease, invasive treatments or drugs [e.g. *Pneumocystis carinii* pneumonia in patients with HIV and/or acquired immunodeficiency syndrome (AIDS)].

PREVENTION AND CONTROL OF INFECTION

Patients are afforded protection against infection in three principal ways:
- By application of the principles of asepsis (use of a nontouch technique and sterile gloves) and by having high standards of environmental hygiene, the purpose of which is to remove the sources, or potential sources, of infection (i.e. to remove the disease-producing organisms). This includes the treatment of infected patients as well as the cleaning, disinfection and sterilization of equipment, contaminated materials and surfaces (Ayliffe *et al.* 1992).
- By blocking the routes of transfer of bacteria from their potential sources and reservoirs to uninfected patients. Methods include isolation of infected or susceptible patients, application of the principles of asepsis and effective hand hygiene, and the use of protective clothing. ⇒ Asepsis (aseptic technique).
- By enhancing the patient's resistance to infection, especially during surgical operations. For example, by the careful handling of tissues and removal of slough (necrotized tissue) and foreign bodies, and (when indicated) by prophylactic antimicrobial therapy (e.g. prior to bowel surgery). All of these factors, however, are influenced most widely by the patient's overall physical health, including nutritional status and susceptibility to infection.

UNIVERSAL AND/OR STANDARD PRECAUTIONS

Universal and/or standard precautions are the routine precautions taken by healthcare workers during contact, or the possibility of contact, with blood and any body fluids. The measures include:
- Regular hand washing or decontamination;
- Wearing protective clothing, such as gloves, plastic aprons, masks, eye protection, etc.;
- Covering wounds with waterproof dressings, safe use of sharps (avoiding their use where possible), proper procedures for dealing with spillages of blood and body fluids;
- Proper disposal of contaminated waste and the cleaning, disinfection and sterilization of equipment. ⇒ Sharps.

HAND WASHING

Hand washing (also referred to as hand hygiene) is the single most important procedure related to infection control and yet we know it is still not carried out properly (Ayliffe *et al.* 1992). Hand hygiene may be achieved by washing with liquid soap or antiseptic detergent soap and water, or by the use of alcohol-based hand rubs. For hands that are visibly soiled, washing with liquid detergent soap is required before the application of an alcohol-based hand rub. *Fig. 106* illustrates the areas most frequently missed during hand washing.

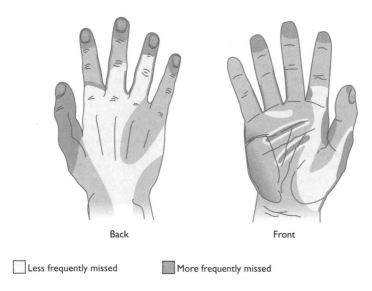

Back   Front

☐ Less frequently missed   ■ More frequently missed

Fig 106 Area of hand surface missed during hand washing

Practice application – hand disinfection
Surgical hand disinfection should take 3 minutes and social (hygienic) hand disinfection 30–60 seconds. Thorough drying of the hands, with disposable hand towels, is important as moist environments encourage the growth of micro-organisms.

For both hygienic hand disinfection and surgical hand disinfection, the same antiseptic soaps are used. The two most commonly used are chlorhexidine and iodine-based products. The difference is in the procedure and the length of time it takes. Alternatives to chlorhexidine and iodine-based products are hexachlorophene and triclosan. These are used less frequently, but remain good alternatives if any member of staff shows an allergic reaction to either chlorhexidine or iodine. Repeated use of antiseptic soaps reduces resident bacteria to low levels.

As previously discussed, hands are one of the main routes of spread of infection. Effective hand washing and disinfection therefore comprise probably the single most important infection-control measure. Various studies have identified that healthcare workers do not wash their hands as often as they should (Ayliffe *et al*. 1992). To improve compliance, it is essential that all products (liquid soap, antiseptic disinfectant, alcohol hand rubs or gels and hand towels) are acceptable to the users, otherwise they are simply not used. Running water from elbow-operated mixer taps should be used so that the appropriate temperature can be maintained, as should a hand towel that is soft and does not damage the hands when drying them.

ROLE OF THE INFECTION-CONTROL NURSE

The role of the infection-control nurse (ICN) is to provide an advisory service on all aspects of the prevention and control of infection, utilizing methods that are evidence-based, practical and cost-effective. Audit, research and education are key aspects of this role. ICNs and their teams have a major role in managing outbreaks of infection.

INFECTIONS OF THE FEMALE REPRODUCTIVE TRACT

Infections that affect the female reproductive tract can cause serious ill health. It is important that they be diagnosed and treated appropriately to prevent further complications developing, such as pelvic infection and infertility. Some infections are outlined below.

VAGINITIS

During the reproductive years, the vagina normally produces acid secretions that help to prevent infection. Infections tend to be more common when the pH is modified, such as at puberty or after the menopause, during pregnancy or with antibiotic therapy, etc.

TRICHOMONIASIS

Trichomoniasis is an infection caused by the protozoon *Trichomonas vaginalis*. ⇒ Sexually transmitted and acquired infection.

CANDIDIASIS (THRUSH)

Candidiasis is a fungal infection usually caused by the yeast *Candida albicans*. ⇒ Sexually transmitted and acquired infection.

BACTERIAL VAGINOSIS

Bacterial vaginosis is an infection caused by overgrowth of the vaginal commensal micro-organisms, such as *Gardnerella vaginalis*. Women complain of a grey–white vaginal discharge that has a 'fishy' odour. The nature of the discharge can be very distressing and women are embarrassed and acutely aware of the associated odour. This type of infection might be associated with an increased risk of late miscarriage or preterm delivery. Treatment is with oral metronidazole or clindamycin cream vaginally.

CERVICITIS AND ENDOMETRITIS

Sexually transmitted and acquired infections can cause cervicitis (e.g. gonorrhoea can infect the cervix then ascend to infect the uterus and uterine tubes). Chlamydia can cause the same problems, but is often asymptomatic, so women are often not diagnosed. ⇒ Sexually transmitted and acquired infection.

Acute endometritis can develop from ascending infection from the external genitalia or the presence of retained products of conception, which result in a smelly vaginal discharge and some abdominal pain. Pus can collect in the uterine cavity (pyometria) and often requires draining surgically. In all cases, antibiotics are required.

SALPINGITIS AND PELVIC INFLAMMATORY DISEASE

Salpingitis (inflammation and/or infection that affects the uterine tubes) develops from ascending infection(as described above) and can cause acute abdominal pain. Early diagnosis is essential, otherwise women can develop acute inflammation of the uterine tubes or pelvis, a condition known as pelvic inflammatory disease (PID).

In the acute phase, this can result in severe abdominal pain and fever, which may require women to be admitted as an emergency and treated with intravenous antibiotics. Long-term damage to pelvic organs can result, which can cause infertility, among other things. ⇒ Infertility.

TOXIC SHOCK SYNDROME

Toxic shock syndrome (TSS) can occur when an infection develops in the genital tract and the bacterial toxins produced cause septicaemia and toxic shock. It has been associated with tampons left in the vagina for extreme lengths of time. The absorption of toxins into the bloodstream can result in hypotension, shock and multiple organ dysfunction, and so must be treated promptly. ⇒ Shock, Systemic inflammatory response syndrome.

TSS is a rare illness caused by bacterial infection, which (although seen in immunocompromised patients) is associated with menstruating women who use high-absorbency tampons. The most common bacterium to cause this infection is *S. aureus*. Although the use of tampons is not necessarily a cause itself, it is thought to facilitate the condition. This is particularly true for high-absorbency tampons that may be left in the vagina for prolonged periods. TSS is not exclusively linked to tampon use. *S. aureus* may enter the blood by other routes to cause TSS in men and nonmenstruating women.

Symptoms can occur suddenly and include pyrexia (38.8°C or higher), a rash that resembles sunburn, dizziness and light-headedness, muscle aches and watery diarrhoea.

Immediate emergency treatment comprises fluid replacement and i.v. antibiotic therapy, plus appropriate supportive therapy for organ dysfunction.

Practice application – avoiding toxic shock syndrome; advice to women
TSS can be prevented by good hygiene while menstruating:
- Hands must be washed before inserting a tampon into the vagina, particularly if the type used does not have a disposable applicator;
- Tampons should be changed regularly and not just when there is leakage, which is why the use of tampons with minimum absorbency should be advocated (many manufacturers of tampons now include an information leaflet with their product);
- If a woman has ever suffered from TSS, she should not use tampons, but instead she should use external protection, such as pads. The new generation of sanitary pads are extremely absorbent, less bulky and more acceptable to women, and their use should be encouraged.

INFERTILITY

Infertility is also known as subfertility and can be defined as the inability of a couple to conceive spontaneously. The length of time a couple have been trying for a pregnancy is important, and it is usually considered to be a problem if they have not conceived after 1 year of unprotected intercourse. It is further defined as:
- Primary infertility – the couple have not had a pregnancy previously;
- Secondary infertility – the couple, either together or with other partners, have previously conceived, although that pregnancy may not have continued to produce a live baby.

It is estimated that up to one in four couples may experience problems achieving a pregnancy at some time, and up to one in six couples seek specialist advice. In some instances, no actual cause can be found. These figures demonstrate the large scale of this problem, and in recent years major advances in healthcare technology have provided many more treatment options for both sexes. Many of these advances have major moral and ethical implications that must be considered with the couple when treatment options are being discussed.

In normal conception, a sperm is required to pass through the cervix, uterine cavity and uterine tubes to meet and fertilize a 'ripe' oocyte that has been released from the ovary. The fertilized ovum needs to pass through the uterine tube and implant in the hormone-prepared endometrium lining the uterus. Although this sounds relatively straightforward, all the factors in this pathway must be present to achieve a successful pregnancy. If one or more of these factors is absent or not functioning correctly, the couple is unable to conceive.

INVESTIGATIONS

Investigations into the possible causes of infertility are based around discovering which part of the pathway may be preventing conception. These can be divided into two areas:
- Hormonal – whether the gametes are being produced;
- Mechanical checks that there are no obstructions to the gametes meeting.

Practice application – infertility; initial assessment

Initially, the couple are seen together, as this is a problem that affects the couple, not just the woman or man, and both must be fully included and investigated. An accurate history is taken from both partners; it includes their medical history, previous surgery, sexual activity (both current and past), previous sexually acquired infections (SAIs), family history, alcohol consumption, smoking habits, use of recreational drugs and lifestyle and/or exercise. In addition, details are recorded of the woman's menstrual, obstetric and contraceptive history, and of any previous pregnancies caused by the man. Each partner undergoes a full physical examination that includes inspection of the external genitalia and a pelvic examination of the woman. The information sought from the couple can be extremely embarrassing for them and so questions must be handled in a sensitive manner. However, individuals may not have disclosed details of previous pregnancies, terminations, SAIs and past sexual activities to each other, so sometimes this sort of information is divulged only when the couple are apart (e.g. during a specific test).

After the initial assessment, more specific investigations are planned. These are designed to look at:
- Ovulation, such as a blood test (progesterone peak on day 21 of the menstrual cycle), ultrasound scan, etc.;
- Tubal patency (e.g. laparoscopy to check the pelvis and reproductive structure) and tubal dye test;
- Spermatozoa production – semen analysis is undertaken, to check the volume of semen, the number of spermatozoa present, their motility and the percentage of abnormal spermatozoa.

MANAGEMENT OF INFERTILITY

All UK infertility units, both NHS and private, must be licensed by the Human Fertilization and Embryology Authority (HFEA) and must comply with their standards to be able to practise.

Management of the disorder depends on the cause, if one is discovered. There are many treatment options, all of which are termed assisted conception. These are outlined in *Table 24*.

Table 24   Common assisted-conception treatments

Disorder	Treatment	Description of treatment
Ovulatory disorder	Clomifene	Nonsteroidal anti-oestrogen oral tablet. Acts on hypothalamus and increases pituitary gonadotrophin production. Effective in inducing ovulation in approximately 80% of women, up to 50% of whom conceive
	Follicle-stimulation hormone (FSH)	Daily injections to induce ovulation. Follicles mature, human chorionic gonadotrophin (hCG) injection to release eggs, followed by intercourse
Tubal blockage	Tubal surgery salpingostomy	Can be done laparoscopically or by laparotomy to remove blockages, particularly at fimbrial end. Salpingostomy involves stitching back the fimbrial ends to form an opening at the end of the tube
Pelvic adhesions	Division of adhesions	Can often be done laparoscopically, but may need to undergo open surgery via laparotomy. Adhesions are divided to free up the tubes and ovaries so both can be aligned
Unexplained infertility	Artificial insemination by partner	The woman is given treatment to induce ovulation, and produce up to three oocytes. Semen is introduced through the cervix
Low or absent sperm count	Donor insemination (DI)	Semen from screened donor introduced through the cervix
Unexplained infertility	Gamete intrafallopian transfer (GIFT) – one tube must be functional	The woman has ovulation induction using gonadotrophins to produce several follicles. Oocytes are collected before ovulation either transvaginally or laparoscopically under general anaesthetic. A maximum of three oocytes plus a medium that contains motile sperm are transferred to the functional uterine tube. Thus fertilization occurs in the normal site
	Zygote intrafallopian transfer (ZIFT) – one tube must be functional	As for GIFT, but this time fertilization occurs in the laboratory (in vitro). The fertilized oocyte is transferred to the functional tube about 18–24 hours after insemination. A further variation is tubal embryo transfer (TET) in which the transfer takes place 48 hours after insemination
Unexplained infertility, tubal blockage	In vitro fertilization (IVF)	Known as 'test-tube baby'. Ovulation is induced using gonadotrophins to produce several follicles. Oocytes are collected before ovulation either transvaginally or laparo-scopically under general anaesthetic. The best sperm is selected from a fresh sample and added to the oocytes in the laboratory. The resultant embryos (up to the maximum allowed) are introduced into the uterus at the

Table 24 (*Cont*). **Common assisted-conception treatment**		
Disorder	*Treatment*	*Description of treatment*
		4–8 cell stage for implantation. Donor eggs can also be used if there are problems with ovulation. Additional embryos can be frozen for use at a later date
Sperm disorder	Intracytoplasmic sperm injection (ICSI)	Sperm is obtained via ejaculate or directly from the testis. In the laboratory a single sperm is injected into the centre of an oocyte obtained as an IVF procedure

Specialist nurses have developed skills in both counselling and undertaking procedures in infertility clinics that enable couples to receive continuity of care throughout their treatment.

INFESTATIONS

An infestation is the presence of animal parasites in or on the human body. ⇒ Helminthiasis.

PEDICULOSIS

Pediculosis is infestation with lice:
- Head louse (*Pediculus humanus capitis*);
- Body and/or clothing louse (*P. humanus humanus*);
- Pubic (crab) louse (*Phthirus pubis*).

The body louse is a major carrier of diseases, such as epidemic typhus, etc. Infestation with body lice is rare in developed countries, except in rough sleepers and others unable to change and launder their clothing. In contrast, the head louse maintains a high profile among schoolchildren everywhere and affects all socioeconomic groups, and adults may also be affected.

Pubic lice are transmitted almost entirely by sexual contact.

HEAD LICE

Head lice transmission is primarily by head-to-head contact. Pruritus is the main symptom but may only be apparent with large numbers of lice. Persistent scratching may result in secondary bacterial infection and lymphadenopathy. Eggs (nits) can be seen cemented to the hair shaft; initially, the main sites are behind the ears and the nape of the neck. Live adult insects are often not seen on clinical examination, as they are hard to detect if they have just had a blood meal. There may be bite reactions and excoriations.

Practice development – detection of head lice and treatment

The best way to find lice is by using a fine-tooth (detector) comb on damp, conditioned clean hair. The hair is combed into sections. The fine-tooth comb is carefully drawn through each section of hair over a sheet of white paper. Any lice present can be seen on the comb or the white paper. This physical removal of the lice does not remove the eggs, but may damage them.

Treatment is only needed if live lice are found. Both chemical and physical methods can be used.

Chemical treatment is with lotions (e.g. malathion). Individuals with eczema and/or asthma should use aqueous solutions instead of those in alcohol. The community pharmacist should be consulted as to the current chemical of choice. The instructions for use should be followed exactly and the nurse should be able to explain these to parents and/or carers and ensure that enough treatment is given to treat all cases. All family members should be checked and all those with live lice treated at the same time.

Repeated physical removal – 'bug busting' – is a safe method of treating, as it breaks the life cycle by constantly removing immature lice (nymphs) as they hatch. It is not effective against eggs and needs to be repeated every 3–4 days for a period of 2 weeks.

BODY AND PUBIC LICE

The treatment of pubic lice is best done with aqueous solutions of the same chemicals used for head lice, as alcoholic solutions may irritate the genitalia. The instructions included with the treatment should be complied with and repeated after 7–10 days.

Eyelash infestation is treated by the application of petroleum jelly (e.g. Vaseline). Clothes are laundered in a high-temperature wash and ironing the seams of clothing to kill both lice and eggs. Bathing the host removes any live lice from the body.

SCABIES

Scabies is caused by infestation with a minute arthropod mite, *Sarcoptes scabiei* var. *hominis* (itch mite). The mite is passed from person to person during close physical contact, and in severe infestations from contaminated clothing and bedding. The effects of infestation might take up to 4 weeks to be obvious, so it is possible to be infected in the absence of any symptoms.

Scabies usually affects the finger webs, natural skin folds and pressure areas. In time, all areas of the body may be affected, except the head, neck and soles of the feet. 'At risk' groups include immunocompromised individuals, those in institutions (e.g. prisons and nursing homes) and individuals whose personal hygiene and lifestyle put them at risk.

Infestation with scabies is characterized by the following:
• Characteristic burrows;
• Intense itching;
• Eczematous changes and secondary infection from chronic itch–scratch cycle;
• Papules – caused by scratching.

MANAGEMENT

The treatment of scabies consists of using chemical pesticides, such as aqueous preparations of permethrin or malathion, which need only one application if applied effectively. Topical corticosteroid may be applied to ease the irritation caused by treatment. All clothing and bedding used during the treatment time should be laundered. The ordinary wash cycle of a machine suffices. It may be necessary to repeat these procedures 5–7 days later.

INFLAMMATION AND INFLAMMATORY RESPONSE

⇒ Defence mechanisms.

INFLUENZA

Influenza is an acute viral infection of the nasopharynx and respiratory system that occurs in epidemics or pandemics. Complications include pneumonia, which may lead to death, especially in the very young, older adults and individuals with immunosuppression, chronic respiratory disease, diabetes mellitus, renal disease and cardiovascular disease.

In most cases, influenza is an unpleasant but self-limiting illness. For otherwise-fit individuals treatment is symptomatic and those affected should stay at home, rest and drink plenty of fluids.

Vaccination is available and is the best way to prevent the illness (see Practice application – flu vaccination). Antiviral drugs (e.g. oseltamivir and zanamivir) are only recommended for adults in the high-risk groups (mentioned above) who can start the drug within 48 hours of the start of symptoms. Oseltamivir can be used for at-risk children within 48 hours of the start of symptoms. Amantadine can be prescribed prophylactically for nonimmunized individuals in high-risk groups and for key staff, such as healthcare personnel when influenza A is within the community.

Practice application – flu vaccination

Vaccination against influenza ('flu' vaccine) is recommended for certain groups and needs to be administered annually between late September and early November.

- Flu vaccine should be offered to all people over 65 years of age;
- Vaccination is also recommended for people of any age who have underlying conditions (see above) that put them at higher risk of serious illness from flu, and for those in long-stay residential accommodation;
- The aim is to increase the uptake each year until a 70% uptake in people over 65 years of age is achieved;
- Strategic health authorities are being asked to work with their local general practitioners and Primary Care Trusts to contact all people over 65 years of age, and to achieve the target uptake.

INFORMATICS

Informatics is a term that covers information management and technology (IM&T).

Practice application – information management

Information management encompasses the management of any sort of information. Information is a resource needed to ensure the effective running of any organization. Data (singular datum) are pieces of material that, when compiled appropriately, form information. This information may be managed in a number of different ways. Increasingly, information is managed via information technology (IT), but other means may be more appropriate for the target group and/or recipient. For example, telephone calls, meetings and notice boards are all ways in which information might be managed. Use of an inappropriate management technique results in the information not being received by those for whom it is intended. Information sent via technology is of no use to those groups who do not have the means or skills to access technology.

Information management is achieving a higher profile in healthcare, as the public is more information-aware in every way. There is commitment to 'transparent systems' and patients and clients expect to be kept well informed. Information is important in ensuring a quality service.

INJECTION

An injection is the introduction of fluid material into the body under pressure, usually by syringe. It may be intra-arterial (into an artery), intra-articular (into a joint), intradermal (into the skin), intramuscular (into a muscle), intrathecal (usually into the subarachnoid space of the meninges), intravenous (into a vein), subcutaneous (beneath the skin) or into a hollow structure or cavity. The term is also applied to the medication being injected.

The sites commonly used for intramuscular and subcutaneous injection are illustrated in *Fig. 107.* ⇒ Diabetes mellitus (insulin therapy), Intrathecal, Sharps (needle-stick injuries – prevention).

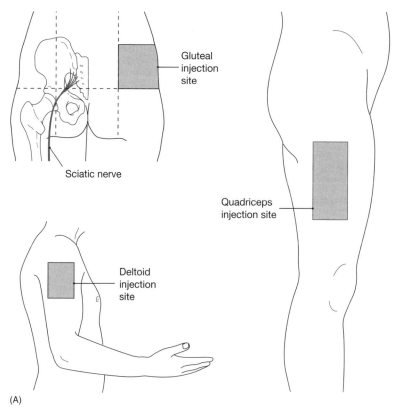

(A)

Fig 107 Sites for injection: (A) sites for intramuscular injection

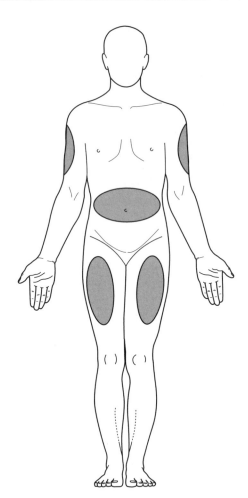

(B)

Fig 107 Sites for injection: (B) sites commonly used for subcutaneous injection

---

Practice application – Z-track injection technique

A Z-track intramuscular injection technique may be required with certain medications that can stain the skin (e.g. iron) or a particularly irritant (Workman 1999):

- Using the nondominant hand, apply a shearing movement to the skin so that the skin and subcutaneous tissue slide over the underlying muscle. With the dominant hand, insert the needle two-thirds in, at an angle of 90°, to ensure that the needle is inserted into the muscle (*Fig. 108A*).
- After injecting the drug in the usual way, withdraw the needle smoothly and quickly. Release the tension on the skin and subcutaneous tissue to permit the tissues to return to their pre-injection position. This creates an internal seal over the muscle entry point and so prevents leakage of the medication into the superficial tissues (*Fig. 108B*).

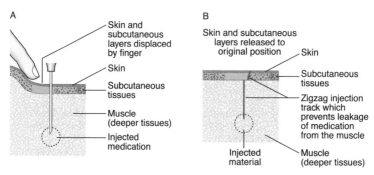

Fig 108 Z-track injection technique: (A) during injection, (B) after injection

---

Practice application – needle phobia

Many children and young people who require medical intervention are most concerned about needles. Some of these children develop an extreme fear or phobia, with manifestations of neurogenic shock when exposed to needles, a reaction that can spread so that the child also fears objects or situations associated with needles. All children need to be prepared for interventions that require the use of a needle.

Preparation involves physical and psychological interventions:

• For most needle procedures topical anaesthetic cream can be used to numb the site, most effectively used in conjunction with psychological preparation, as the frightened child's fear will not be allayed merely by numbness of the site;

• Give information, in an appropriate age-related way, to the child and family about the procedure, being honest about the physical and sensory effects of the procedure;

• Provide a supportive environment by allowing parental presence in child-friendly surroundings with staff who are empathetic;

• Help the child to cope by using distraction, play therapy, relaxation, etc., during the procedure;

• Provide positive reinforcement to the child after the procedure with the use of bravery certificates or stickers, as well as verbal encouragement of their coping skills.

INOTROPES

Inotropes are substances, such as drugs, that have an effect on myocardial contractility. Those that increase contractility are *positive inotropes*, which include digoxin and beta$_1$-adrenoceptor agonists (sympathomimetics), such as dopexamine, adrenaline (epinephrine), etc. ⇒ Glycosides.

Note that dopamine has positive inotropic effects when given in higher doses; it is also commonly used at lower doses when its effects are limited to the enhancement of renal perfusion.

Practice application – positive inotrope therapy

Positive inotropes, including dobutamine, adrenaline (epinephrine), dopexamine and dopamine, are used therapeutically to improve myocardial contractility in:

- Heart failure;
- Cardiogenic shock – post-myocardial infarction or cardiac surgery;
- Sepsis.

The nursing management includes:

- As positive inotropes are given to improve blood pressure, continuous blood pressure monitoring is required, usually via an indwelling arterial cannula;
- Before starting inotrope therapy, ensure that patients have an adequate circulating volume, as giving inotropes to hypovolaemic patients is dangerous and can cause cardiac arrhythmias;
- Inotropes have a short half-life and consequently need to be given as a continuous infusion. Accuracy is also important and an infusion-regulating device should always be used. These drugs (with the exception of dobutamine) require central venous access because of their profound vasoconstrictive effect in peripheral blood vessels. ⇒ Arterial cannula or line.

The *negative inotropes* reduce myocardial contractility. They include beta$_1$-adrenoceptor antagonists (e.g. atenolol) and calcium antagonists (channel blockers, e.g. nifedipine and verapamil).

INTEGRATED CARE PATHWAY

An integrated care pathway (ICP) is an outline or plan of anticipated clinical practice for a group of patients (client group) with a particular diagnosis or set of symptoms (e.g. 'cardiac chest pain and/or suspected myocardial infarction'). The ICP provides a multidisciplinary template of the plan of care to lead each patient towards a desired objective. ⇒ Multidisciplinary team and working.

In simple terms, the ICP document is a matrix that places interventions (tasks) on one axis and time (hours, days and weeks) and/or milestones (specific stages of recovery) on the other.

The fundamental principle of ICPs is to make explicit the most appropriate care for a patient group, based on the available evidence and consensus of best practice. The intention of ICPs is to ensure evidence-based care is delivered to the patient by the right individual, at the right time and in the right environment, and thus help to reduce unnecessary variations in treatment and outcome. ⇒ Evidence-based practice.

A number of elements make up the ICP model of care, which can be described as:

- Patient groups;
- Scope;
- Multidisciplinary collaboration;
- Sequential and appropriate care;
- Patient-focused care;
- Single record of care;
- Analysis of variations.

INTERMEDIATE CARE

Intermediate care is a broadly defined concept that incorporates the care of patients who do not need acute care in hospitals, but are not yet sufficiently independent to be self-caring within their own homes. The form intermediate care takes can vary, but it is frequently offered in community hospitals and may be primarily nurse-led, with an emphasis on rehabilitation.

COMMUNITY HOSPITALS

Community hospitals are NHS hospitals that provide intermediate care for a local community. Nurses, general practitioners and therapists manage care. Patients may receive all their necessary care in a community hospital for a period or may use it as a 'step-down' facility between an acute hospital episode and independent living at home or in a long-term care.

INTERNATIONAL CLASSIFICATION OF DISEASE

⇒ Disease (disease classification).

INTRAOSSEOUS

Intraosseous literally means inside a bone.

INTRAOSSEOUS ROUTE FOR FLUID ADMINISTRATION

The intraosseous route developed as a way to give fluids when the rapid establishment of systemic access is vital and venous access is impossible. It provides an alternative route for the administration of drugs and fluids until venous access can be established. This route can safely administer any intravenous drug or fluid required during paediatric resuscitation. Onset of action and drug levels are similar to those achieved when using the intravenous route.

Paediatric advanced life support (PALS) courses recommend that the intraosseous access should be established if reliable venous access cannot be achieved within three attempts or 90 seconds, whichever comes first.

An intraosseous needle is a wide-bore needle inserted into the medullary cavity of a long bone. The preferred site for children under 6 years of age is the flat anteromedial surface of the tibia, 1–3 cm below the tibial tuberosity. In children of this age the marrow cavity is very large, which minimizes potential injury to adjacent tissues. The main contraindication to this route is a fracture of the pelvis, or the extremity proximal to or of the chosen site. ⇒ Advanced life support (paediatric advanced life support).

INTRATHECAL

Intrathecal pertains to the lumen of a sheath or canal, and most often means within the meninges, usually the subarachnoid space. It is a route used to administer certain drugs, such as analgesic drugs after surgery. ⇒ Anaesthesia (spinal and epidural blocks), Injection.

INTRAVENOUS THERAPY AND/OR INFUSION

An intravenous (i.v.) infusion is used to administer sterile fluid into the circulation when the enteral route is not appropriate (e.g. pre- and postoperatively and after major trauma). The fluid may be infused for several reasons:
- To maintain fluid and electrolyte balance;
- To restore fluid and electrolyte balance;
- For nutritional purposes, when it is referred to as parenteral nutrition;
- To administer drugs.

Fluids infused are described as either crystalloid or colloid. *Colloid* solutions contain solute particles that remain in the bloodstream, as they are too large to cross capillary membranes. They include gelatin solutions, hydroxyethyl starch, albumin and blood. *Crystalloids* are clear fluids that readily cross cell membranes and pass between the circulation and the tissue fluid. They are used to manage fluid and electrolyte balance.

The tonicity of i.v. fluids is important as it affects their destination within the fluid compartments. Isotonic fluids (e.g. normal saline) have the same concentration of solutes as plasma. They maintain extracellular fluid (ECF) volume and prevent movement of water from the ECF to the intracellular fluid (ICF). Hypotonic solutions (e.g. 5% dextrose) have a lower osmolality than plasma and infusion results in movement of water into the body cells (ICF). In contrast, hypertonic solutions have a greater concentration of solutes than plasma and infusion causes movement of water from the body cells (ICF) to the ECF.

Normal daily requirements of fluids and electrolytes are met by providing 1 L of 0.9% saline and 2 L of 5% dextrose plus 60 mmol of potassium chloride. More is required to compensate for losses as a result of pyrexia, diarrhoea and intestinal obstruction. ⇒ Electrolyte, Fluid balance and body fluids (disorders of fluid balance).

MAINTAINING SAFETY AND COMFORT DURING INTRA-VENOUS INFUSIONS

A cannula is inserted into a peripheral vein, usually in the forearm or dorsum of the hand, and secured in place according to local policy. The fluid container is connected to an administration set and connected to the cannula. The system must be patent and kept closed to avoid introducing contaminants (*Fig. 109*).

Aseptic technique and universal or standard precautions are required when the system is open. Intravenous fluids should be changed every 24 hours using aseptic technique. The giving set is changed according to local policy. The site is checked regularly for signs of complications (see below). Intravenous fluids and any additives must be prescribed and volumes recorded on the fluid balance chart.

Accurate calculation and control of the flow rate are the nurse's responsibility. Flow rate is checked at least hourly. Common causes of obstruction or inadequate flow rate include:

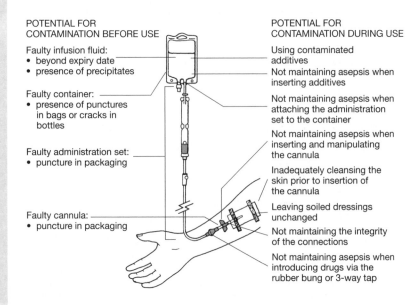

POTENTIAL FOR CONTAMINATION BEFORE USE

Faulty infusion fluid:
• beyond expiry date
• presence of precipitates

Faulty container:
• presence of punctures in bags or cracks in bottles

Faulty administration set:
• puncture in packaging

Faulty cannula:
• puncture in packaging

POTENTIAL FOR CONTAMINATION DURING USE

Using contaminated additives

Not maintaining asepsis when inserting additives

Not maintaining asepsis when attaching the administration set to the container

Not maintaining asepsis when inserting and manipulating the cannula

Inadequately cleansing the skin prior to insertion of the cannula

Leaving soiled dressings unchanged

Not maintaining the integrity of the connections

Not maintaining asepsis when introducing drugs via the rubber bung or 3-way tap

Fig 109 Potential routes for contamination associated with intravenous infusion

- The height of the infusion container is too low;
- Kinking of the giving set tubing;
- Position of the cannula in the vein.

Infusion control devices (pumps) are used to regulate the flow rate for accuracy when small volumes are prescribed or drugs are added and when there is danger of rapid over-infusion. The nurse is responsible for using this equipment safely and requires training for each type of pump used in the clinical setting to ensure familiarity with its correct use.

COMPLICATIONS OF INTRAVENOUS THERAPY

Complications can be minor or major with serious consequences. The effects of complications are local or systemic.

LOCAL COMPLICATIONS

- Infection caused by contamination of any part of the system.
- Infiltration of the tissues occurs when fluid infuses into the tissues instead of the circulation.
- Extravasation occurs when irritant solutions enter the tissues and can cause severe damage, including tissue necrosis. Such substances may be hypertonic (e.g. 8.4% sodium bicarbonate) or contain vasoconstricting drugs (e.g. dopamine) and are normally given through a central line to minimize this potential problem. ⇒ Inotropes.
- Phlebitis (see Practice application).

SYSTEMIC COMPLICATIONS

- Circulatory overload occurs when fluid, especially normal saline, is infused too quickly, which increases the blood volume and venous pressure, and may result in cardiac failure and acute pulmonary oedema. Infusion-control devices are therefore used in susceptible patients. Regular checks of the flow rate are made to detect this potential problem, which often happens when the cannula is 'positional' (i.e. when the position of the arm affects the flow rate).
- Fluid volume deficit caused by overly slow infusion of fluid.
- Septicaemia – when pathogenic bacteria invade the bloodstream. This is especially dangerous when large numbers of virulent bacteria are present in an immunocompromised host.
- Pulmonary embolism is a rare but life-threatening complication. The risk is minimized by using a filter to administer blood or particulate solutions and using only gentle pressure to flush a cannula. ⇒ Pulmonary embolism.
- Air embolism is another rare and potentially life-threatening complication (most likely during the insertion of a central line).
- Allergic reactions may occur during blood transfusion or with some intravenous drugs.

Practice application – minimizing phlebitis associated with intravenous infusions

Phlebitis is inflammation of the inner layer of the vein. The aetiology may be:
- Mechanical – caused by the cannula in the vein;
- Chemical – caused by the substances infused;
- Bacterial – caused by local infection.

Signs:
- Inflammation, often with pain and redness at the site;
- Redness may track from the cannula along the course of the affected vein towards the heart;

- In thrombophlebitis there is also an intravascular blood clot usually associated with a palpable cord.

Causes:
- Cannula is too large, an unsuitable vein used or poor insertion technique;
- Cannula moving within the vein;
- Infusion of irritant solutions (e.g. hypertonic, etc.);
- Contamination of the system (see *Fig. 109*).

Prevention or early detection:
- Secure cannula firmly in place to avoid movement in the vein;
- Infuse irritant solutions slowly, and dilute irritant solutions whenever possible;
- Inspect the site frequently for signs of inflammation;
- Remove cannula if phlebitis is present and re-site if necessary;
- Maintain aseptic technique to minimize the risk of contaminating the system.

Further reading

Dougherty L and Lamb J (1999). *Intravenous Therapy in Practice*. Edinburgh: Churchill Livingstone.

NTUBATION

Intubation is the placing of a tube into a hollow organ (e.g. into the trachea). Tracheal intubation is used to ensure an airway, during anaesthesia and for short-term respiratory support using mechanical ventilation. ⇒ Airway, Anaesthesia, Endotracheal, Respiratory system.

NTUSSUSCEPTION

Intussusception is a condition in which one part of the bowel telescopes (invaginates) into the adjoining distal bowel, which causes severe colic, intestinal obstruction, vomiting and the passage of blood and mucus rectally ('redcurrant jelly' stools; *Fig. 110*). The invaginated portion is called the intussusceptum.

Intussusception occurs most commonly in infants around the time of weaning, and presents as an acute emergency. The intussusception may be reduced by performing a nonsurgical hydrostatic reduction, usually by barium enema, but may sometimes require surgical treatment.

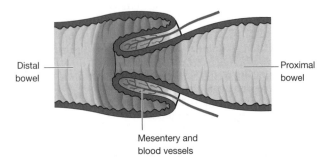

Distal bowel

Proximal bowel

Mesentery and blood vessels

Fig 110 Intussusception

INVESTIGATIONS

The purpose of medical investigation is to acquire information about the extent to which an organ is performing in relation to the norm. The results of investigations are like pieces of a puzzle – they fill in some gaps, but they can only provide a partial view of the whole picture. Thus, the results of investigations contribute, along with other information (e.g. physical examination) to confirm or reject a diagnosis. Investigations are classified as invasive (e.g. endoscopy) or noninvasive (i.e. taking the blood pressure using a sphygmomanometer).

It is important that nurses understand the common investigations, and any requirement for specific physical preparation and aftercare. This allows them to provide explanation and reassurance to patients and to ensure that patients are prepared adequately, and the investigation is safe and successful. Nurses must ensure that patients have sufficient information to allow them to give informed consent. All investigations have the potential to increase patient anxiety, and research has shown that well-informed patients are less anxious. Nurses should provide information about what will happen, any machines involved, what will be expected from the patient, who will be present and, very importantly, when the results will be available. In some situations arrangements for patients to visit the department to see equipment, such as scanning machines, can reduce anxieties.

The healthcare professional who will perform the investigation must ensure that patients fully understand the potential risks attached and obtain written consent, where appropriate, for certain invasive procedures. Increasingly, nurses are performing invasive investigations, such as gastroscopy, and they become responsible for obtaining written consent from patients.

JAUNDICE – TYPES, HYPERBILIRUBINAEMIA

Jaundice is not a disease in itself. It is a sign of abnormal bilirubin metabolism and excretion that results in an accumulation of bilirubin in the blood (hyperbilirubinaemia). Serum bilirubin may rise to 34 µmol/L before the yellow colouration of jaundice is evident in the skin, mucous membranes and sclera (normal 3–13 µmol/L). The discolouration is usually first seen in the sclera and is often accompanied by pruritus (itching). For people with a darker skin colour, the palms of the hands and the soles of the feet are yellow.

Jaundice develops when there is an abnormality at some stage in the metabolic sequence caused by one or more factors. Jaundice is classified as (*Table 25*):
- Pre-hepatic or haemolytic – there is excess haemolysis of red blood cells with the production of more bilirubin than the liver can deal with;
- Hepatic or hepatocellular – there is abnormal liver function that may cause incomplete uptake of unconjugated bilirubin by hepatocytes, ineffective conjugation of bilirubin or interference with bilirubin secretion into the bile;
- Post-hepatic or obstructive (cholestatic) – bile flow is obstructed after it leaves the liver.

⇒ Haemolytic disease of the newborn, Pruritus.

Practice application – pruritus in jaundice

Pruritus, caused by an accumulation of bile salts in the skin, is often the most distressing symptom of jaundice for the patient. The itching can be severe, and the scratching behaviour can be very distressing. Patients may have disturbed nights and the lack of sleep can be detrimental to well-being. It can also affect other family members, who feel helpless. The physical trauma to the skin causes the release of chemicals (e.g. histamine) that stimulate further itchiness. The patient's skin should be kept clean and dry, and the use of perfumed toiletries avoided. Encourage the patient to keep the nails short and not to scratch. Observe the skin for areas of redness, bruising or breakdown – moisturizers can be used if the patient has dry skin.

JET LAG

⇒ Biorhythm.

JOINT

A joint is the articulation of two or more bones. Joints can be classified according to a combination of structural and functional characteristics:
- Fibrous (synarthroses) – immovable joints (e.g. sacrum);
- Cartilaginous (amphiarthrosis) – slightly movable joints of two types, synchondrosis (formed from the epiphyseal plates of the long bones during growth) and symphysis (e.g. pelvis);
- Synovial (diarthrosis) – freely movable joints (e.g. hip).

Note that no joint is truly freely movable, but rather has a specific broad range of movement or motion (ROM). The fibrous joint capsule, associated ligaments and the design of the particular bones that comprise the joint restrict the particular movement of any joint.

Ligaments are strong, tough collagenous fibres that serve to reinforce the joint capsule through binding the articular ends of bone together. They may be inside (intra-articular) and/or outside (extra-articular) the joint capsule.

In synovial joints there is an interfacing layer of articular hyaline cartilage, and a synovial capsule surrounds the joints. A synovial membrane lines the capsule

Table 25 Types and causes of jaundice

Types of jaundice	Possible causes	Urinalysis Colour	Urinalysis Bilirubin	Urinalysis Urobilirubin	Faeces	Degree of jaundice
Pre-hepatic or haemolytic	Blood transfusion reactions Haemolytic anaemia Physiological jaundice of the newborn	Normal	Slight	++++	Normal to dark in colour	Mild jaundice – lemon colour to skin
Hepatic or hepatocellular	Carcinoma of the liver, excessive drug use, alcoholic cirrhosis or hepatitis, poisons	Dark	Slight	Normal	May be paler and fatter	Variable
Post-hepatic or obstructive	Cancer of the head of pancreas, gallstones, strictures or inflammation of the biliary system	Very dark	+++	Nil	Pale, fatty and offensive	Severe – green tinge to skin

J

and covers all the nonarticular surfaces inside the joint; therefore, in health the bones in such a joint do not have direct contact (*Fig. 111*). This membrane secretes a clear, oily, lubricating fluid into the synovial cavity. Thus, during movement of the joint, cartilage and synovial fluid protect bone tissue. The effect of this is to dampen vibration, reduce shock and friction, and create smooth movement.

Fibrous sacs filled with synovial fluid, known as bursa, also help to reduce friction and facilitate movement. They are located near joints in muscle, between tendons and bone, and between bone and skin. The different types of synovial joint, with examples and the possible movements, are summarized in *Table 26*.

The stability of joints is determined by the nature of the articular surface, sockets and grooves, the number of stabilizing ligaments (i.e. the more ligaments, the stronger the joint) and the amount of muscle tone. The presence of looser, stretchable joint ligaments is often termed 'double-jointed'.

The various types of movement that joints can perform are gliding, angular, circular and special. ⇒ Mobility.

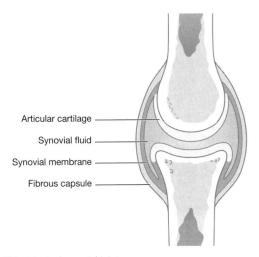

Articular cartilage
Synovial fluid
Synovial membrane
Fibrous capsule

Fig 111 A typical synovial joint

JOINT INJURIES

Injuries to joints may be caused by sporting activities, falls, accidents at home and work, road accidents, etc., and may be associated with other injuries such as ligament tears. The three types of joint injury are subluxation, dislocation and fracture dislocation.

SUBLUXATION

Subluxation is a partial dislocation for which active treatment is often not required.

DISLOCATION

Joint dislocation is displacement of the articular surfaces of a joint, so that apposition is lost. The joint must be reduced and immobilized until the soft tissues heal, and in some cases the joint may require open repair.

FRACTURE DISLOCATION

A fracture dislocation often requires fixation of the bony fragment. ⇒ Fracture.

Table 26 Types of synovial joints

Type of synovial joint	Movement	Example
Gliding	Short, gliding movements; back-and-forth or side-to side movements	Wrist, ankle, vertebra
Hinge	Angular movement allowed in one direction only	Elbow, interphalangeal, knee
Pivot	Limited to rotation around an axis of one bone on another bone	Ring of the atlas around the peg of the axis (cervical vertebrae) Proximal radioulnar joint allows for rotation of the forearm (supination and pronation)
Condyloid	No rotation allowed, back-and-forth or side-to side movement	Metacarpophalangeal joint
Ball and socket	Allows the greatest range of motion	Hip, shoulder
Saddle	Permits a wide variety of movements	Carpometacarpal joint of the thumb

JOINT DISEASES

⇒ Musculoskeletal disorders (sprains and strains), Rheumatic disorders (rheumatoid arthritis).

ANKYLOSING SPONDYLITIS

Ankylosing spondylitis is a progressive inflammatory disease of unknown aetiology. There is gradual stiffening of the axial skeleton, sacroiliac joints and pubic symphysis with loss of joint space and fusion. It primarily involves the spine, but may involve other joints. It primarily affects men under 30 years of age.

The thoracic spine becomes stiff and 'rounded' and the cervical spine grows rigid. The spinal changes lead to reduced chest expansion and vital capacity, which affect breathing. There is debilitating pain and decreased mobility. Ankylosing spondylitis also affects the heart and eyes, and many sufferers have inflammatory bowel disease as well.

Management includes nonsteroidal anti-inflammatory drugs (NSAIDs), intravenous antibiotics for chest infections, analgesics, sleeping on a firm mattress, wearing a spinal orthosis to maintain the best possible alignment of the affected areas and an exercise programme designed to increase muscle. Surgery (spinal or hip arthroplasty) may be indicated in some people.

OSTEOARTHRITIS (OSTEOARTHROSIS)

Osteoarthritis is sometimes termed degenerative arthritis, although the disease process is much more than simply 'wear and tear'; it may be primary or it may follow injury or disease that involves the articular surfaces of synovial joints. The articular cartilage becomes worn, osteophytes form at the periphery of the joint surface and loose bodies may result. The joints most commonly affected are the knees, hips, spine and hands. There is pain, joint disruption and loss of mobility.

Management includes activity modification, physiotherapy to improve muscle strength, hydrotherapy, analgesics, NSAIDs, weight loss as appropriate, mobility aids, intra-articular injections of a corticosteroid and surgery. Surgical treatment often involves joint replacement arthroplasty, most commonly for the hip, knee, elbow or shoulder (see Practice application).

Practice application – advice after total hip replacement arthroplasty

Things to do

- Do the exercises you have been taught twice a day, if possible;
- Continue to lie flat on your back for a short period daily (30 minutes twice a day) for a couple of weeks after leaving hospital;
- Use your walking stick(s), especially outside the house – it is best to use one stick for 6 weeks;
- Be critical of your own posture in sitting, standing and walking;
- Sleep on the side of your new hip, if you want to, and put a pillow between your legs for comfort;
- Use the equipment you have been given to put on socks, stockings and shoes;
- Ask advice if in doubt about any activity.

Things to avoid

While the surrounding muscles and other tissues take time to heal and strengthen, your new hip is at risk of dislocating. To minimize this risk you must take the following precautions for at least 6 weeks after your operation:

- Don't cross your legs;
- Don't sit on a low chair or lavatory;
- Don't sleep on your unaffected side for 2 months;
- Don't squat or bend to pick up things from the floor;
- Don't try to bend the affected leg up to your chest;
- Don't attempt to climb in to or out of the bath for 6 weeks after the operation;
- Don't drive until 6 weeks after the operation.

SEPTIC ARTHRITIS (PYOGENIC OR SUPPURATIVE)

Septic arthritis is joint inflammation caused by micro-organisms, usually pus-forming bacteria. The micro-organism enters the joint from the bloodstream, or through a penetrating joint injury or during joint injection or surgery. Management includes immediate drainage either by arthroscopic lavage or at open arthrotomy and intravenous antibiotics.

GOUT

Gout is a form of metabolic disorder in which blood levels of uric acid are raised (hyperuricaemia). Acute arthritis can result from inflammation in response to urate crystals in the joint. The big toe is characteristically involved and becomes acutely painful and swollen. If gout is untreated the deposition of urate crystals can cause chronic arthritis, nodules (e.g. in the ear) and kidney damage.

Gout can result from abnormal purine metabolism or increased intake, increased uric acid production and reduced renal excretion of uric acid. Gout may also occur in situations in which there is increased purine turnover, such as in some types of leukaemia, chemotherapy and severe psoriasis.

Management involves NSAIDs, colchicine and corticosteroids during an acute episode. Long-term control and prophylaxis are with allopurinol and the urico-suric agents probenecid and sulfinpyrazone. Patients are advised to rest the affected part and to limit their intake of purine-containing foods, such as offal, and restrict alcohol intake.

LABELLING AND STIGMA

Labelling is grouping according to general or specific characteristics – categorization. Within a sociological perspective, labelling has been considered one of the methods by which individuals who are 'different' or who fail to conform to societal norms and expectation can be segregated from that society. A special status – criminal, schizophrenic, prostitute – is awarded by an authoritative body and this label generates stigma and often weighty moral condemnation.

As a result of illness or surgery, labels such as 'diabetic', 'mental patient' or 'amputee' may be applied. Therefore, the labelled individual is marked as different from the rest of society and may evoke negative social reactions (stigma). The negative social response to conditions that attract stigma are related to feelings such as fear or disgust associated with certain labels and the attribution of stereotypical traits to individuals. Therefore, people who use wheelchairs are often viewed as both mentally and physically disabled, while someone with a mental health problems is considered to be potentially violent.

Stigmatized ideas are determined culturally, that is they are based on the society's norms and values, which are learnt early in life and reinforced through everyday conversations and the media. Individuals with stigmatizing illnesses may be viewed as socially inferior and may also be subject to discrimination and socially disadvantaged. The imposition of such social disfavour may result in poor self-concept and identity. ⇒ Ageism, Body image, Discrimination, Fair and antidiscriminatory practice, Racism.

LABOUR

⇒ Pregnancy.

LACTOSE INTOLERANCE

⇒ Food problems.

LARYNX

The larynx or voice box is located at the top of the trachea and is responsible for producing sound. It is a specialized section of the trachea and is formed by the hyoid bone and the thyroid, cricoid and arytenoid cartilages (*Fig. 112*).

During swallowing the airway is protected, as the epiglottis covers the larynx. The larynx contains the true vocal cords or folds. Their length varies, which is why men, with longer cords, have deeper voices than women. At the front of the larynx, the vocal cords are joined together at approximately the level of the Adam's apple (thyroid prominence) and are anchored firmly to the thyroid cartilage. Posteriorly, the vocal cords are attached to moveable cartilages, which allow their position to be altered depending on the function of the larynx. An opening (the glottis) between the true vocal cords allows air movement through the larynx.

DISORDERS OF THE LARYNX

LARYNGITIS

Laryngitis is inflammation of the larynx. Acute laryngitis often occurs after an acute upper respiratory infection and generally resolves fairly promptly. Chronic laryngitis is more common in the winter and often follows a cold or influenza. Other precipitating factors include smoking, drinking alcohol and over-use of the voice.

There may be hoarseness, dysphonia (difficulty speaking) or aphonia (complete voice loss), and a sore throat may also occur. The larynx looks red and dry and often there is stringy mucus between the vocal cords.

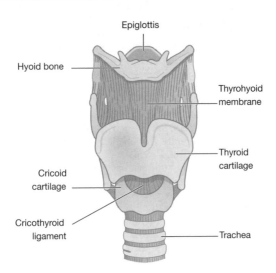

Fig 112 Anterior view of the larynx

LARYNGOTRACHEOBRONCHITIS

Laryngotracheobronchitis is inflammation (usually viral) of the larynx, trachea and bronchi. It may be very serious when it occurs in small children (croup). The viral infection leads to laryngeal narrowing. The child has 'croupy', stridulous (noisy or harsh-sounding) breathing. Narrowing of the airway that gives rise to the typical attack with crowing inspiration may result from oedema or spasm, or both.

LARYNGOSPASM

Laryngospasm is the convulsive involuntary muscular contraction of the larynx, usually accompanied by spasmodic closure of the glottis.

LARYNGEAL OBSTRUCTION

The causes of laryngeal obstruction include tumours, acute infection or inhaled foreign bodies. The most striking sign of laryngeal obstruction is stridor (a hard, high-pitched respiratory sound). Patients may be restless and anxious. Dyspnoea and cyanosis may be present.

The airway is secured with endotracheal intubation or tracheostomy as required. ⇒ Airway, Tracheostomy.

CANCER OF THE LARYNX

Cancers of the larynx are generally squamous cell carcinomas, which often affect males of age 55–65 years and with a history of heavy smoking. The presentation depends on the tumour site. Hoarseness is common. Dyspnoea, dysphagia and referred otalgia (earache) may also occur. Cervical lymph nodes may be enlarged.

Management depends on the extent of the disease. Radiotherapy may be indicated, but where this fails or the cancer recurs, radical surgery may be the only option. Surgery involves laryngectomy (removal of the larynx) in most cases, with part or all of the thyroid gland. The tracheal 'stump' is then sutured to the skin of the neck and the patient breathes via this stoma.

Practice application – communication after laryngectomy
Assistance and encouragement with communication is vital, as speech is lost. Rudimentary measures, such as providing pen and paper, may be of most help in the initial stages and a nurse call bell should be available at all times. Voice rehabilitation is necessary and considerable input from the speech and language therapist is essential. Measures available to enable speech after a total laryngectomy include oesophageal speech, use of an artificial larynx or tracheo-oesophageal speech using a voice prosthesis.

Family and partners should be involved in all aspects of care from the diagnosis on. Such collaboration reduces isolation for the patient, reduces the fear involved in caring for a patient with a tracheostome and encourages acceptance of altered body image and functioning for all concerned.
⇒ Tracheostomy.

LATEX SENSITIVITY

Latex sensitivity is an allergic reaction to natural latex or one of the components used in the production of latex equipment, such as in medical gloves, airways, intravenous tubing, elastic bandages, catheters, etc. Latex allergy is becoming more common in healthcare workers because of the increased use of gloves after the rise in the incidence of blood-borne viruses. Latex allergies are also more common in patients and any sensitivity to latex should be established and documented.

Avoiding contact with latex is the most important intervention. The establishment of a latex-free environment is being accomplished in many healthcare facilities in which staff and patients are at high risk (such as those having repeated exposure to latex). Where possible, latex-free products should be substituted, such as vinyl gloves for latex gloves. In healthcare settings and in the community it is important to use products with the lowest potential risk of sensitizing patients and staff.

Individuals with latex sensitivity should be advised about nonmedical items in the home and the wider community that may contain latex, such as kitchen gloves, condoms, elastic on clothing, etc. Consideration should be given to the wearing of some form of allergy identification, such as a Medic-Alert bracelet.

LAW

CIVIL LAW

Civil law is the law that relates to noncriminal matters. A civil action involves the proceedings (litigation) brought in the civil courts. A claim form (previously called a writ) is the commencement of a civil action. The person who brings legal action to obtain compensation or other redress for an alleged civil wrong is called the claimant (previously known as the plaintiff).

A civil wrong is an act or omission that can be pursued in the civil courts by the person who has suffered the wrong. The term tort describes a civil wrong, excluding breach of contract. It includes negligence, nuisance, breach of statutory duty and defamation.

The standard of proof required in civil cases is the balance of probabilities.

COMMON LAW

Common law is the law that derives from decisions made by judges, case law and judge-made law.

CRIMINAL LAW

Criminal law is the law that deals with offences heard in the criminal courts, such as theft. A criminal wrong is an act or omission that can be pursued in the criminal courts. To secure a conviction in criminal proceedings, the prosecution must establish beyond reasonable doubt the guilt of the accused.

EMPLOYMENT LAW

Employment law is the law, common law and statute that relates to the relationship of employer and employee. Continuous service is the length of service required before an employee is entitled to certain statutory and contractual rights.

HEALTH AND SAFETY LAW

Health and safety law is the law, common law and statute that covers health and safety duties. The Health and Safety at Work Act 1974 sets out the responsibilities of the employer in relation to the workforce, work environment, equipment and substances, and those of individual employees to themselves and others.

STATUTE LAW

Statute law is made by Acts of Parliament, such as The Misuse of Drugs Act (1971).

LEARNING DISABILITY

Learning disability is a general term used to describe the inability to develop intellectually. Individuals may often have problems integrating into society. Learning disability encompasses many conditions that range from specific learning disorders, such as dyslexia, through to problems of global intellectual impairment. Some types of learning disability are associated with varying degrees of physical or sensory impairment. ⇒ Autism, Dyslexia, Galactosaemia, Haemolytic disease of the newborn.

AETIOLOGY OF LEARNING DISABILITY

Conditions that can cause learning disability may occur prenatally, intranatally and postnatally. They include:
- Prenatal – chromosome abnormalities (e.g. Down's syndrome), damage to genes (e.g. untreated phenlyketonuria), maternal infections (e.g. rubella, etc.), maternal substance misuse, etc.;
- Intranatal – developmental abnormality associated with preterm and low birthweight infants, and birth injuries (e.g. hypoxia) that lead to brain damage;
- Postnatal – infections (e.g. encephalitis), trauma (e.g. physical abuse, etc.), deprivation and neglect, toxins (e.g. lead), adverse drug reactions, solvent misuse, etc.

SOME DISORDERS THAT GIVE RISE TO LEARNING DISABILITY

ANGLEMAN SYNDROME

Angleman syndrome is an inherited condition that arises from mutations in the maternal chromosome 15. Features include 'puppet-like' gait, learning disability, brachycephaly (short, broad skull), inappropriate emotional outbursts, tongue protrusion and hooked nose. ⇒ Prader–Willi syndrome.

Down's syndrome

Down's syndrome is caused by chromosomal abnormality, either a third chromosome or trisomy involving chromosome 21, or in about 5% of cases a fused chromosome. The last is inherited from a carrier parent, whereas the risk of trisomy rises with maternal age (as high as 1 in 50 when the mother is 44 years of age or older). Both types of chromosomal abnormality produce multisystem disorders. These include generalized disturbances of growth, which lead to:

- Characteristic facial features, such as an upward slant of the eyes and a fold around the angle of the eyelids;
- Poor muscle tone;
- Overall average weight of the brain decreased by 10–20%;
- Intellectual disability shows as a delay in the achievement of developmental milestones, although there is considerable variability in overall intellectual attainment.

Other problems associated with the syndrome are congenital heart disease, conductive deafness, thyroid disease and acute lymphatic leukaemia.

Fragile X syndrome

The fragile X syndrome form of learning disability is mainly, but not exclusively, found in men. The cause is a defect in the X chromosome (a sex chromosome). In many cases the condition is passed from a carrier mother to an affected son. The physical features that show in around 80% of adult men who have the condition are enlarged testes and ears, a long and narrow face, and (in a smaller percentage) very smooth skin, flat feet and mitral valve prolapse. The physical features tend to come to prominence after puberty and learning disability is usually the most notable feature in childhood. It can range from borderline to severe. As it is an inheritable disorder, genetic counselling for affected families is important.

Prader–Willi syndrome

Prader–Willi syndrome is an inherited condition that arises from mutations in the paternal chromosome 15. There is learning disability, hypotonia, short stature, hyperphagia and obesity (see Angleman syndrome above).

Retts's syndrome

Rett's syndrome is a neurodegenerative disorder that occurs in girls. It is a chromosomal condition (X-linked dominant inheritance), with progressive neurological and developmental regression from early childhood. Death occurs by the second or third decade.

THE ROLE OF THE LEARNING DISABILITY NURSE

The role of the learning disability nurse in enabling the person with a learning disability to reach his or her own 'balance and highest potential' is vitally important. In a sense, the role of the learning disability nurse is no different from that of any other speciality of nursing. However, the nurse in learning disability works within a multidisciplinary team (MDT) in a variety of settings. For example, nurses within the speciality can be found in hospitals, community learning disability teams, community homes, special schools, etc.

Specifically, the role of the learning disability nurse is to promote:
- The health of the person with a learning disability, such as access to screening tests (e.g. mammography);
- Communication and interpersonal skills, including alternative methods of communicating;

- Independence through teaching life-skills;
- Advocacy and self-advocacy;
- Philosophy of social role valorization (normalization);
- Rights, risks and responsibilities associated with being a citizen;
- Dignity and respect;
- Leisure, recreation and stimulation;
- Meaningful work opportunities;
- Lifelong learning;
- Working in partnership with families;
- Harmonious working relationships within the MDT for the enhanced care of a person with learning disability.

Practice application – chaining

Chaining is a technique that may be used when helping people with learning disabilities to master complex sequences of behaviour. The idea is to reward each stage of the process so that it sets up a positive link in a whole chain of actions. There are two forms of chaining, forward and backward.

Forward chaining means analysing a behaviour, such as eating a meal, by starting with sitting at an appropriate place, then picking up one utensil, then another, etc. On successful accomplishment of each stage the individual receives a reward, praise in the early stages, enjoyment of the food later on. In contrast, backward chaining starts at the end of a complex chain of behaviour and uses rewards to create links with the stage before. So when teaching dressing, one might begin by encouraging the individual to perform only the final step, putting on the second shoe and then rewarding with praise and an admiring glance in a mirror to see the process completed. Next time the encouragement is to put on the first shoe and then the second with the same reward at the end of the chain. The advantage of this approach is that the overall goal is usually a strong reward and is seen as achievable from beginning to end.

Further reading

Department of Health (2001). *Valuing People. A New Strategy for Learning Disability for the 21st Century*. London: The Stationery Office. Online, available at http://www.dh.gov.uk/learningdisabilities/strategy.htm

LEG ULCERS

Ulceration of the lower leg is a common chronic condition that frequently recurs and causes considerable distress. All leg ulcers result from an insufficiency of the blood supply to the lower limb. The majority occur because of poor venous return, which causes oedema and eventual skin breakdown (venous ulcers, *Fig. 113A*). The remainder (arterial ulcers) result from inadequate arterial supply to the foot, which causes ischaemia and a breakdown of the soft tissues (*Fig. 113B*). A comparison of the venous and arterial leg ulcers is provided in *Table 27*.

ANKLE BRACHIAL PRESSURE INDEX

The use of a vascular assessment method, such as the Doppler ultrasound, can increase the accuracy of patient assessment. The Doppler test produces a reading that is the index of the brachial systolic blood pressure divided by the ankle systolic blood pressure. This reading is called the ankle brachial pressure index (ABPI). An ABPI reading of 1.0 is normal and indicates that 100% of the blood flow is reaching the extremities, whereas a value of 0.8 indicates a reduced peripheral

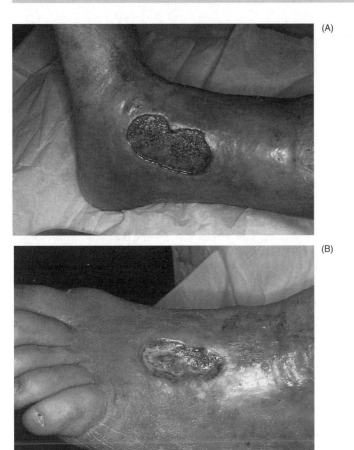

(A)

(B)

Fig 113 Leg ulcers: (A) venous, (B) arterial

tissue perfusion as only approximately 80% of blood flow is reaching the affected foot. Although approximately 70% of leg ulcers are of venous origin, it is recognized that many of these patients, especially older adults, have coexisting arterial disease and an ABPI reading of below 0.9. Some ulcers have a combined aetiology, which results from venous insufficiency and arterial impairment, and have the combined features of both types of ulcer.

The use of a Doppler assessment in isolation is of no value. The aetiology of the ulcer should be established on the basis of the patient history and physical assessment. Doppler assessment aids the management of venous ulcers by indicating whether or not standard compression therapy can be applied. Ulcers that appear to be venous in origin may be associated with some degree of arterial impairment. It is therefore important to determine the status of the arterial circulation of the limb prior to the application of compression bandages. The force applied by compression bandages on people with ischaemic legs may cause additional skin damage, as the arteries become occluded. It is currently best practice that patients with Doppler readings of 0.8 and below do not have compression bandaging applied (Royal College of Nursing 1998).

Table 27 Comparison of clinical presentation of venous and arterial leg ulceration

	Venous ulceration (Fig. 113A)	Arterial ulceration (Fig. 113B)
Previous medical history	Deep vein thrombosis (DVT), varicose veins or family history of leg ulcers	Cerebrovascular accident (CVA) angina, peripheral, vascular disease, hypertension, diabetes
Site and/or position	Often near the ankle or between the ankle and knee	Usually on the foot and between the toes, or close to the ankle
Appearance	Typically, large shallow wounds producing copious exudate	Often smaller, deeper wounds producing less exudate
Surrounding skin condition	Characteristic pigmentation – lipodermatosclerosis (brown staining), atrophe blanche (white patches) Contact dermatitis and eczema are common	Hairless, shiny skin Skin colour ranges from white to dusty pink and purple Dusty pink feet turn pale when raised above the heart In darker-skinned individuals, ischaemic skin ranges from a paler colour to a dark mottled appearance Thickening of nail beds is sometimes seen
Pain and/or discomfort	Aching or heaviness in legs often related to localized oedema Localized pain, tenderness of ulcer	Intermittent claudication (pain on exertion) Rest pain, severe constant pain, often worse at night

L

Experienced nurses may perform Doppler assessment provided they are competent in this procedure. All patients with leg ulcers should have their ABPI calculated prior to commencement of treatment. As arterial impairment can occur over time it is important to reassess it every 3 months (Vowden *et al.* 1996). ⇒ Doppler technique.

PRINCIPLES OF LEG ULCER MANAGEMENT

VENOUS ULCERS

The primary aim of venous leg ulcer management should focus on the reversal of venous and capillary hypertension. General management principles for patients with venous leg ulcers include:
- Accurate assessment of the underlying ulcer aetiology;
- Reduction of the high pressure exerted on the superficial venous system;
- Improving venous return to the heart;
- Maintenance of patient compliance with treatment;
- Prevention of complications.

It is widely accepted that sustained graduated compression from the toes to the knee is the treatment of choice for uncomplicated venous leg ulcers (ABPI must be ≥0.8, Vowden *et al.* 1996). Compression therapy can be provided using a variety of different methods, but needs to be sustained for at least a week.

Once a venous ulcer is healed, it is important that the patient wear a below-knee support stocking to prevent ulcer recurrence (see Practice application). Compression hosiery maintains a compression force of 30–40 mmHg at the ankle and therefore continues to maintain venous return. However, some patients find high-compression stockings uncomfortable and prefer to wear stockings that provide lower levels of support. Hosiery must be fitted correctly and patients need to be measured accurately before being supplied. All stocking manufacturers provide instructions and sizing charts to aid measurement. ⇒ Wounds and wound care.

Practice application – minimizing the recurrence of venous leg ulcers
Hosiery
- Wear compression hosiery during the day;
- Apply and remove hosiery carefully to avoid skin damage and / or irritation;
- Renew compression hosiery every 6 months.

Exercise
- Walk as much as possible;
- Avoid prolonged standing;
- Move toes and ankles several times an hour, even when resting;
- Avoid sitting with legs crossed.

Skin care
- Wash legs in warm water;
- Use emollient creams in the water and apply to the skin after washing;
- Take special care of feet and toenails – podiatry (chiropody) referral may be necessary.

Elevation
Position ankles higher than the buttocks by:
- Resting on a bed with feet on a pillow;
- Sitting on the sofa with feet resting on one of the arms;
- Using a stool and pillows.

ARTERIAL ULCERS

Management of arterial ulcers is usually conservative and is concerned with the relief of symptoms. If arterial insufficiency results from local arterial occlusion, surgical intervention may be appropriate. Arterial ulcers are common in patients with diabetes (combination of peripheral vascular disease and diabetic neuropathy).

The treatment objectives for patients with arterial ulcers focus on symptom relief, local wound management, patient education and psychological support. The management principles of caring for patients with arterial ulcers are:
- Daily examination of the legs and feet, looking for any skin breaks or signs of ischaemia;
- Regular foot and nail assessment by a podiatrist;
- Maximization of arterial blood flow to the feet by avoiding constrictive clothing or shoes and resting the legs in a dependent position;
- Avoidance of mechanical trauma and prevention of any further deterioration in the condition of the limb;
- Effective pain control;
- Maintenance of skin hygiene and rehydration of dry skin.

LEGIONNAIRES' DISEASE

Legionnaires' disease is a severe, acute pneumonia caused by the bacterium *Legionella pneumophila*, a small Gram-negative bacillus. The micro-organism was discovered in 1976 after an outbreak of disease at a convention of the American

Legion. There is headache, myalgia, high fever, confusion, dry cough, pleurisy, pneumonia and often nonpulmonary involvement, such as gastrointestinal symptoms and hepatitis. Treatment is with antibiotics (e.g. erythromycin) and supportive measures, such as respiratory support. The mortality rate has been as high as 20% in some outbreaks. It is a cause of both community and hospital-acquired pneumonia, and is associated with an infected water supply in public buildings, such as hospitals and hotels. There is no person-to-person spread.

LEPROSY

Leprosy (Hansen's disease) is a chronic communicable disease, endemic in warmer climates and characterized by granulomatous formation in the peripheral nerves or on the skin, mucous membranes and bones with tissue destruction. It is caused by *Mycobacterium leprae* (Hansen's bacillus) and there are two forms – tuberculoid and lepromatous. Bacille Calmette–Guérin (BCG) vaccination conferred variable protection in different trials. Management includes specific care (such as that required for impaired sensation), plastic surgery and long-term treatment with various antimicrobial drugs, including dapsone and rifampicin.

LEPTOSPIROSIS

Leptospirosis is infection of humans by bacteria (spirochaetes) of the genus leptospira found in rats and other rodents, cattle, dogs, pigs and foxes. *Leptospira* are very thin, finely coiled bacteria that are common in water as saprophytes, and pathogenic species are numerous in many animals. *L. interrogans* serotype *icterohaemorrhagiae* causes Weil's disease in humans and *L. interrogans* serotype *canicola* infects dogs and pigs, and is transmissible to humans.

Transmission is via the infected urine of rats and other animals and those at risk of infection include abattoir and agricultural workers and water sports enthusiasts. Presentation varies according to which leptospira is responsible, but may include high fever, headache, conjunctival congestion, rash, anorexia, jaundice, severe muscular pains, rigors and vomiting. Severe infections may cause hepatitis, myocarditis, renal tubular necrosis and (less frequently) meningitis with an associated mortality rate of up to 20%.

LEUCOCYTES

Leucocytes (also called white blood cells) function as a defence against infection and in surveillance for abnormal cells such as cancer. The total white blood cell count is $4.0–11.0 \times 10^9/L$. $\Rightarrow$ Blood (*Box 3*). Leucocytes are nucleated and may be classified as myeloid cells or lymphocytes. $\Rightarrow$ Defence mechanisms (phagocytosis).

MYELOID CELLS

Myeloid cells e are subdivided into neutrophils, eosinophils, basophils and monocytes. Collectively, the neutrophils, eosinophils and basophils are known either as polymorphonuclear (polymorphs) cells because they have multilobed nuclei, or as granulocytes, which reflects the presence of granules in their cytoplasm.

NEUTROPHILS

Neutrophils (*Fig. 114*) are the most numerous of the white cells (40–70%) and provide the first line defences in many infections, but are relatively short-lived. Neutrophils help to control infection by phagocytosis. They are attracted to a site of infection by chemicals released by infected or damaged cells. Huge numbers of neutrophils can congregate at a site of infection, forming pus.

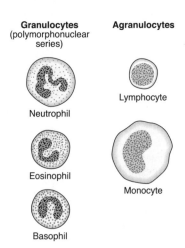

Granulocytes
(polymorphonuclear series)

Agranulocytes

Neutrophil

Eosinophil

Basophil

Lymphocyte

Monocyte

Fig 114 Types of leucocytes

EOSINOPHILS

The eosinophils (*Fig. 114*) account for less than 5% of the total white cell count. Eosinophils are less actively phagocytic than are neutrophils; their specialized role is to deal with parasites, such as worms, and with immune responses that involve allergies and immmunoglobulin E (IgE).

Eosinophils are often found at sites of allergic inflammation, such as the asthmatic airway, where they promote tissue inflammation by releasing chemicals stored in their granules. They may also dampen down the inflammatory process by releasing other chemicals.

BASOPHILS

Basophils (*Fig. 114*) make up less than 1% of the total white cell count. Basophils, which are closely associated with allergic reactions, contain granules packed with histamine, heparin and other chemicals that promote inflammation. Usually, the stimulus that causes basophils to release the contents of their granules is an allergen (antigen-causing allergy) of some type.

A cell type very similar to basophils, except that it is found in the tissues, not in the blood, is the mast cell. Masts cells release their granule contents within seconds of binding to an allergen, which accounts for the rapid onset of allergic symptoms after exposure (e.g. pollen in hay fever). ⇒ Allergy.

MONOCYTES

Monocytes (*Fig. 114*) form 2–10% of the white blood cells. As they mature, they move out of the blood and into the tissues, where they become macrophages. Macrophages can destroy pathogens by phagocytosis and can enhance the immune response. They also remove and break down ageing or damaged cells (see monocyte–macrophage system below).

Monocyte–macrophage system

The monocyte–macrophage system, which is sometimes called the *reticuloendothelial system*, consists of the body's complement of monocytes and macrophages. Some macrophages are mobile, whereas others are fixed. These include:

- Histiocytes in connective tissues;
- Microglia in the brain;
- Kupffer's cells in the liver;
- Alveolar macrophages in the lungs;
- Those in the spleen, lymph nodes and thymus gland, etc.

Macrophages are actively phagocytic and, if they encounter large amounts of foreign or waste material, they tend to multiply at the site and 'wall off' the area, isolating the material (e.g. in the lungs when foreign material has been inhaled).

LYMPHOCYTES

Lymphocytes (*Fig. 114*) form around 30–40% of the total white cell count in the peripheral bloodstream. Large numbers are also found within the lymph nodes. Lymphocytes can be subdivided into T cells and B cells:

- T cells mature in the thymus gland, where they are 'programmed' to react with specific foreign antigens, such as a cancer cell or virus-infected cell, rather than body cells. They play an important role in cell-mediated immunity.
- B cells mature in the bone marrow. Some B cells differentiate into plasma cells that produce immunoglobulins and play an important role in humoral immunity.

⇒ Defence mechanisms.

LEUCOPOIESIS

Leucopoiesis describes the formation of leucocytes from pluripotent stem cells. ⇒ Haemopoiesis.

DISORDERS OF LEUCOCYTES

LEUCOCYTOSIS

Leucocytosis is an increase in the number of leucocytes in the blood. One or more of the different types of white cell is involved. It is often a response to infection, but other causes include leukaemia, tissue damage (e.g. inflammation, myocardial infarction, burns), heavy smoking, etc.

LEUCOPENIA

Leucopenia is a decreased number of white blood cells in the blood. Granulocytopenia is a general term used to indicate an abnormal reduction in the number of circulating granulocytes (polymorphonuclear leucocytes), commonly called neutropenia because most granulocytes are neutrophils. Neutropenia predisposes to severe infections, septicaemia and death. The pathogens are commonly commensals, such as those in the bowel, which are normally present in the body, but do not usually cause infection. Extreme shortage or absence of granulocytes is called agranulocytosis. Inadequate production of granulocytes may be caused by:

- Drugs (e.g. cytotoxic chemotherapy);
- Irradiation damage to the bone marrow;
- Severe microbial infections.

⇒ Haemopoietic stem cell transplantation, Immunocompromised patient, Leukaemia.

LEUKAEMIA

The leukaemias are neoplastic diseases of the haematopoietic tissue with, most commonly, abnormal proliferation of white cells (leucocytes). Uncontrolled proliferation of the leukaemic cells causes secondary suppression of other blood components, and anaemia and thrombocytopenia result. The lack of mature white cells increases the risk of infection, thrombocytopenia increases the risk of bleeding and anaemia is also characteristic. Causes include ionizing radiation, previous chemotherapy, retroviruses, chemicals and genetic anomalies (e.g. Down's syndrome). The classification is according to cell type (lymphocytic or myelocytic) and the course (acute or chronic). The chronic leukaemias may enter a 'blast crisis' or acute phase.

ACUTE LEUKAEMIA

Acute leukaemia can be divided into two broad categories – acute myeloid leukaemia (AML) and acute lymphoblastic leukaemia (ALL). Patients usually present with a short history of weight loss, bruising, bleeding, pallor, fatigue and repeated infection. A full blood count often reveals anaemia and thrombocytopenia. White cell counts can be elevated or very low. Leukaemic blast cells are visible on the blood film. A definitive diagnosis is usually made from bone marrow biopsy.

ACUTE MYELOID LEUKAEMIA

AML is rare in childhood and the incidence increases with age. Secondary AML is sometimes seen in people previously treated with cytotoxic chemotherapy or radiotherapy. Treatment for AML involves:

- Intensive chemotherapy – a combination of cytotoxic agents is given in a number of courses or cycles;
- Haemopoietic stem cell transplantation may be used in certain circumstances.

The intensive chemotherapy causes profound bone marrow suppression, leaving patients severely pancytopenic (decrease in all blood cells) until normal bone marrow function recovers. Frequent blood and platelet transfusion is often required after chemotherapy. However, infection can be the most serious complication of treatment. ⇒ Immunocompromised patient.

ACUTE LYMPHOBLASTIC LEUKAEMIA

ALL is the most common form of haematological malignancy in children. ALL does, however, occur in adults, with the incidence increasing with age.

Many of the signs and symptoms of ALL are similar to those of AML and result largely from bone marrow failure. Patients also have specific manifestations that include enlarged lymph nodes (lymphadenopathy), enlarged liver and spleen (hepatosplenomegaly) and infiltration into the central nervous system (CNS).

ALL is treated with a very complex drug regimen that includes both cytotoxic and immunosuppressant drugs. Some of the cytotoxic drugs are given intravenously, some by intramuscular injection and some intrathecally via the spinal canal to treat CNS disease. Patients tend not to be rendered so profoundly neutropenic as those who have treatment for AML. However, they do remain at risk of serious infection. As with AML, haemopoietic stem cell transplantation may be an option in certain circumstances

NURSING SUPPORT AFTER A DIAGNOSIS OF ACUTE LEUKAEMIA

A diagnosis of acute leukaemia is clearly devastating for both patients and their families. The situation can be compounded because, once the diagnosis is confirmed, treatment should commence as soon as possible, usually within 24 hours. Skilled nursing is required to support the patients and their relatives in coming to terms with the diagnosis. At the same time, nurses must provide them with a great deal of complex information about the disease and its treatment. Patients should be made aware of the short-term (e.g. pancytopenia, nausea and vomiting, and hair loss) and long-term (e.g. infertility) effects of treatment prior to its commencement.

Practice application – nausea and vomiting with cytotoxic drugs

Nausea and vomiting are distressing symptoms that can produce a range of additional effects, such as anxiety, fatigue, anorexia and fluid and electrolyte imbalance. Anxiety can exacerbate symptoms and may precipitate anticipatory nausea, which is very difficult to control. Frequent retching can cause discomfort and potentiate bleeding in patients with thrombocytopenia or mucositis. Nurses should therefore ensure that all patients who undergo cytotoxic chemotherapy receive effective anti-emetic cover. A variety of anti-emetics may be prescribed, depending on the chemotherapy regimen and its potential to cause emesis. In regimens where there is a relatively low risk of emesis, symptoms may be well controlled by the use of anti-emetics such as metoclopramide. Regimens with a higher risk of emesis may require the use of 5-HT$_3$-receptor antagonists (5-hydroxytryptamine), such as ondansetron or tropesitron, in combination with the corticosteroid dexamethasone. Patients who are nauseated should be encouraged to maintain a good oral fluid intake. Food may be better tolerated if the principle of 'little and often' is adhered to. Distraction and relaxation therapies may also help.

CHRONIC LEUKAEMIA

CHRONIC MYELOID LEUKAEMIA

Chronic myeloid leukaemia (CML) is a stem-cell disorder that results in the unregulated production of myeloid white cells. The aetiology is unknown, but it is generally associated with a specific, acquired chromosome abnormality, the Philadelphia (Ph) chromosome. CML can affect any age group, but mainly affects people between the ages of 40 and 60 years. CML has an insidious onset and is frequently diagnosed by a routine blood test. The usual clinical features include anorexia, weight loss, anaemia and hepatosplenomegaly. A full blood count reveals a high white cell count.

The initial treatment involves:

- Lowering the white cell count using apheresis and oral cytotoxic drugs, such as hydroxycarbamide or busulfan;
- Subcutaneous interferon-alpha can help to correct any chromosomal abnormality;
- The drug imatinib, which targets Ph chromosome positive cells to prevent abnormal cell proliferation, is used during some stages;
- Allogeneic haemopoietic stem cell transplantation is the main curative option for those with CML.

CHRONIC LYMPHOCYTIC LEUKAEMIA

Chronic lymphocytic leukaemia (CLL) is a proliferative disorder of the lymphocytes. These cells accumulate in the blood, bone marrow, lymph nodes and spleen. CLL is the most common form of leukaemia and usually occurs in later life; 95% of cases are seen in people over the age of 50 years.

In the early stages, the symptoms of CLL are mild and include fatigue, weight loss and some enlargement of lymph nodes, liver and spleen. However, the disease is marked by a slow, but progressive bone marrow failure.

Treatment is generally delayed until symptoms become troublesome, often for a period of years. If symptoms do progress, oral cytotoxic agents (e.g. chlorambucil) can help to control the disease and reduce symptoms. Eventually, the disease is likely to progress and require more aggressive treatments. These include:

- Fludarabine (cytotoxic drug);
- Combination chemotherapy regimens such as CHOP (cyclophosphamide, hydroxydoxorubicin, vincristine and prednisolone);

- Haemopoietic stem cell transplantation may be offered to some relatively young patients.

L IPIDS

Lipids are a large, diverse group of fat-like organic molecules that include neutral fats [e.g. triacylglycerols (triglycerides)], phospholipids, lipoproteins, fat-soluble vitamins, steroids, prostaglandins, leukotrienes and thromboxanes. They consist of carbon, oxygen and hydrogen, and some contain phosphorus and nitrogen. They are insoluble in water, but they can be dissolved in organic solvents such as alcohol. Lipids are important in the body, both structurally and functionally. Fat deposits provide an energy store, insulate and offer some protection. Other lipids are important constituents of cell membranes (phospholipids), are precursors for steroid hormones, act as regulatory molecules (e.g. leukotrienes, prostaglandins, thromboxanes – *Box 18*) and transport fats around the body (lipoproteins), and the fat-soluble vitamins are concerned with blood clotting, vision and antioxidant functions. ⇒ Cholesterol, Fat, Vitamins.

> **Box 18 The role of regulatory lipids**
> *Leukotrienes* – regulatory lipids derived from arachidonic acid (fatty acid). They function as signalling molecules in the inflammatory response and in some allergic responses.
> *Prostacyclin* – a substance derived from prostaglandins. It inhibits platelet aggregation and is a potent vasodilator. It is important in preventing intravascular clotting of blood.
> *Prostaglandins* – a large group of regulatory lipids. They are found in most body tissues, where they regulate physiological functions, such as smooth muscle contraction, inflammation, gastric secretion and blood clotting. They are used therapeutically to terminate pregnancy, induce labour, prevent platelet aggregation during haemodialysis and in the treatment of asthma and gastric hyperacidity.
> *Thromboxanes* – regulatory lipids derived from arachidonic acid. They are released from platelets and cause vasospasm and platelet aggregation during platelet plug formation. ⇒ Haemostasis.

L IPOPROTEIN

⇒ Cholesterol.

L ISTERIOSIS

Listeriosis is an infection caused by *Listeria*, a genus of bacteria present in animal faeces and soil. For example, *L. monocytogenes* causes meningitis, septicaemia, and intrauterine or perinatal infections. The infection is transmitted via contaminated soil, contact with infected animals and by eating unpasteurized foods, such as soft cheeses that may be infected. It may lead to a flu-like illness, but serious consequences may occur in infants, older people, debilitated or immunocompromised individuals and pregnant women. Infection during pregnancy may lead to miscarriage, stillbirth, premature labour, septicaemia and neonatal meningitis.

L ITERATURE SEARCHING AND REVIEW

A literature review is a thorough, systematic, comprehensive and critical examination of the articles relevant to a particular topic. The literature reviewed can be from both published articles and unpublished dissertations, theses and reports.

Indeed, a PhD thesis is often a very valuable resource in that the literature review may be more up to date than anything that is published (often there is a time-lag between the article being written and its acceptance for publication).

The first step in reviewing the literature is to decide on the purpose of the review and the subject to be reviewed. Individuals who conduct a review for their own interest or for an assignment may not be concerned with clarifying the purpose and therefore need only decide on the topic. However, researchers use the literature in different ways and for slightly different purposes, depending on the approach taken. Broadly speaking, a review of the literature enables the researcher to determine:

- What previous work has been done on the topic;
- The level of knowledge and theory development that relates to the subject;
- The research methodologies employed and the strategies that might be employed during the proposed study.

A successful search and review of the literature demands enthusiasm, curiosity and interest. Whatever subject you choose, it must be of interest to you.

BIBLIOGRAPHIC DATABASES

Bibliographic databases are available at libraries, typically on CD-ROM. However, many of these are available on the Internet, some for free. For example, Medline is available via the National Library of Medicine (among others) for no charge. Bibliographic databases provide details of articles, etc., but abstracts and full articles are sometimes available. The various bibliographic databases relevant to nursing practice include:

- Allied and Complementary Medicine (AMED) – literature relevant to a multidisciplinary team;
- Cumulative Index to Nursing and Allied Health Literature (CINAHL) – literature relevant to nursing and allied health;
- Medline – medical science literature;
- PsycLIT Journal Articles Database (PsycLit) – summaries of literature in psychology and related disciplines;
- Sociological Abstracts and Social Planning Policy and Development Abstracts (SOPODA) – literature relevant to sociology and social policy.

Practice application – using bibliographic databases

In the UK the Royal College of Nursing (RCN) bibliographies may be more useful to nursing students than the computerized databases, since they concentrate on reviewing journals that are likely to be easily available and are more informative than the North American publications. Some libraries have their own database and review all the journals that are stocked. This is particularly useful because it may mean that you can actually obtain the articles easily.

To maximize your literature search it is a very good idea to ask the librarian for help with the use of CD-ROMs and on-line searches. CD-ROMs often give abstracts with the reference, making it easier to determine the nature and usefulness of the paper. Whatever method of reference collection is used, it is crucial to note the full reference and gather as much information as possible about the literature before sending off for it.

THE REVIEW

There is no set way to write a review. The style and presentation are likely to be influenced by the purpose of the review and the research methodology. However, most authors include an introduction, some discussion of the concepts and/or theories addressed in the literature, a critical evaluation of the current level of knowledge and identify gaps in the literature. If you are writing the review as part of a research project, then you need to give an overview and justification for your study and design, as well as indicate where your study fits along the spectrum of knowledge of the topic.

People are usually able to write a descriptive review of the literature, but the aim is to demonstrate critical thinking throughout the review. Readers need to have some indication of the value of a particular study before spending time and money to obtain it. ⇒ Evidence-based practice (critical appraisal of evidence, Practice application – sources of evidence for nursing practice), Referencing and citation systems.

LIVER

The liver is a remarkable organ, as it plays a vital role in the body's metabolism through the synthesis, processing and/or storage of many of the substances essential to normal body functioning. It is the largest gland and solid organ in the body and is situated in the right upper quadrant of the abdomen (see *Fig. 30*). Functionally, it is divided into two parts (left and right) and then subdivides into eight sectors, each with its own blood supply (some authors still describe the liver as having four lobes – right, left, caudate and quadrate).

The liver is a highly vascular organ, receiving approximately 28% of the body's total blood flow. It receives its blood supply from two sources:
- Hepatic artery, which delivers oxygenated arterial blood from the aorta;
- Hepatic portal vein, which carries partly deoxygenated blood from the stomach, intestines, spleen and pancreas.

Blood leaves the liver via the hepatic vein. This dual blood flow ensures that the liver is able to play its key role in the metabolism and synthesis of vital substances. The pressure in the hepatic portal vein is normally low (5–10 mmHg), but if there is an obstruction in the liver, portal pressure rises, which leads to portal hypertension.

Each sector is subdivided into lobules, which are microscopic hexagonal units made up of columns of liver cells called hepatocytes. These are separated by numerous blood vessels and fibrous strands. Each lobule contains a central venule, surrounded by branches of the hepatic artery, hepatic portal vein and bile duct (together known as the 'portal triad', *Fig. 115*).

Surrounding the hepatocytes (within the cell membrane) is a network of minute tubules called bile canaliculi, which secrete bile. The lobular bile ducts unite to form the hepatic duct, which joins the cystic duct to form the common bile duct. The blood vessels between the cells are lined with phagocytic cells, called Kupffer's cells, that play a vital role in phagocytosis and antibody production.

The functions of the liver include:
- Bile production – yellow–green or brown fluid concerned with the emulsification of fats and absorption of lipids and fat-soluble vitamins, but which also deodourizes faeces. Bile pigments (bilirubin, biliverdin) are formed during the breakdown of eythrocytes and food. Some bile is excreted in the faeces. The remainder is absorbed by the terminal ileum in a recycling process, passes to the liver and is re-excreted into the bile (enterohepatic circulation). ⇒ Biliary tract.
- Metabolism of carbohydrates, proteins and fats. The liver is central to blood glucose homeostasis.
- Storage of energy – mostly as glycogen. ⇒ Glucose.
- Synthesis of blood components, such as plasma proteins (mostly albumin), clotting factors and erythrocytes (in the fetus and at times of extra demand).
- Destruction of worn-out erythrocytes.
- Detoxification of drugs, chemicals and hormones.
- Heat production.

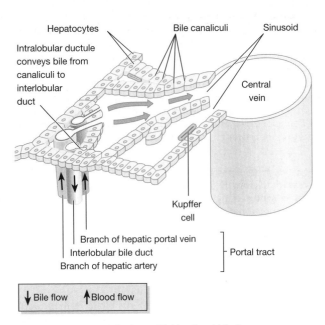

Hepatocytes

Bile canaliculi

Sinusoid

Intralobular ductule
conveys bile from
canaliculi to
interlobular
duct

Central
vein

Kupffer
cell

Branch of hepatic portal vein
Interlobular bile duct
Branch of hepatic artery

Portal tract

↓ Bile flow   ↑ Blood flow

Fig 115 Cellular structure of the liver with blood and bile flow

Liver function is assessed using a variety of blood tests (*Table 28*).

DISORDERS OF THE LIVER

An overview of viral hepatitis, tumours and cirrhosis is provided below. Further coverage of these and other conditions can be found in the suggestion for Further reading. ⇒ Alcohol (alcohol misuse), Jaundice.

HEPATITIS

Hepatitis is inflammation of the liver, commonly associated with viral infection, but can result from toxic agents (e.g. alcohol, drugs and chemicals) or metabolic disorders (e.g. Wilson's disease).

Viral hepatitis is a serious public health problem. A number of types of hepatitis are associated with the different hepatitis viruses.

Hepatitis-A

Hepatitis-A (HAV) is caused by an RNA enterovirus. It is the least serious type and is relatively common. It may cause epidemics, especially in institutions (e.g. schools). The virus is transmitted by the faeco-oral route, caused by poor hygiene or contaminated food.

Hepatitis-B

Hepatitis-B (HBV) is caused by a DNA virus. It is usually transmitted sexually (vaginal or anal intercourse) through the administration of infected blood and/or blood products, or via contaminated equipment, such as needles or dialysis, or from infected women to their young children. Individuals at high risk include intravenous drug users, homosexual or bisexual men, prostitutes and healthcare

Table 28 Common blood tests for disorders of the liver

Blood test	Normal range	Interpretation
Bilirubin	2–17 µmol/L	Conjugated bilirubin increases with biliary obstruction Nonconjugated bilirubin increases with excessive erythrocyte haemolysis
Cholesterol	3.5–6.5 mmol/L	Elevated when secretion blocked by bile duct obstruction Reduced in severe liver damage
Albumin	36–53 g/L	Decreased in chronic liver disease because of impaired protein synthesis
Ammonia	<1 mg/L	Elevated when severe hepatocellular damage reduces the synthesis of urea from ammonia
Aspartate aminotransferase (AST)	7–40 U/L	Released from damaged liver cells, heart, kidney and muscle cells; prolonged elevation in liver disease may be the first indicator of chronic active hepatitis
Alanine aminotransferase (ALT)	10–40 U/L	As above
Alkaline phosphatase (ALP)	25–115 U/L	Increased in biliary obstruction and liver disease (cirrhosis, metastases)
γ-Glutamyl transferase (GGT)	Male 11–50 U/L Female 7–33 U/L	Elevation of GGT and ALP is a significant indication of liver disorders and bile duct disease; alcohol ingestion causes a rise in GGT
Hepatitis viral studies	Negative	Used to identify known antigens and anti-bodies associated with the hepatitis viruses
Platelets	$150–400 \times 10^9$/L	May fall when spleen is enlarged by hepatic portal hypertension
Prothombrin time (PT)	12–15 seconds	Prolonged in acute liver damage and cirrhosis
International normalized ratio (INR of clotting time)	1	Prolonged with (i) decreased synthesis of prothrombin caused by liver disease or (ii) decreased vitamin K absorption caused by bile duct obstruction
α-Fetoprotein (AFP)	<10 µg/L	Usually only synthesized by the fetus – raised AFP levels in adults usually indicate hepatocellular cancer

professionals through needle-stick injuries (see Practice application). Hepatitis-B virus may persist, causing chronic hepatitis, or a carrier state can develop. An effective vaccine exists.

Practice application – hepatitis B: protecting staff and patients

- Handwashing – the most effective way to reduce cross-infection, this should be carried out before and after all care;
- Treat all body fluids as potentially infected;
- Wear protective clothing (disposable gloves and aprons) whenever contact with blood, faeces, urine or other body fluids is likely – masks are not advocated unless there is a risk of being splashed in the face, in which case glasses and/or goggles afford additional protection in this situation;
- Specimens – bottled samples of blood, urine, sputum or faeces must be enclosed in a sealed plastic bag with the request form kept separately, and be labelled clearly as a biohazard, to alert and protect laboratory staff;
- Contaminated linen – should be double-bagged and clearly labelled, as should blood-stained clinical waste;
- Disposal of any clinical waste should always be as close to the point of use as possible;
- Spillages of blood, urine and faeces should be cleaned wearing plastic gloves and an apron – disinfect the area with paper towels soaked in 1% hypochlorite solution and, if possible, leave for 30 minutes (Rogers et al. 1998);
- Reporting – any untoward incidents that involve patients with hepatitis should be reported, no matter how minor;
- Immunization should be offered to all healthcare workers – offers protection for up to 90% of recipients (Department of Health 1998b). It is not a substitute for good infection-control practices. ⇒ Infection, Sharps.

Hepatitis-C

Hepatitis-C (HCV) is caused by an RNA virus and is most common in intravenous drug users and in those who have had a transfusion of blood or blood products. The virus can remain in the blood for many years and infected people can develop chronic hepatitis, cirrhosis, liver failure and possibly liver cancer. Some people become carriers of the virus.

Hepatitis-D

Hepatitis-D (HDV) can only replicate in the presence of hepatitis-B and is therefore found infecting simultaneously with hepatitis-B, or as a superinfection in chronic carriers of hepatitis-B. Delta virus may increase the severity of a hepatitis-B infection, which increases the risk of chronic liver disease.

Hepatitis-E

Hepatitis-E (HEV) is transmitted via the faeco-oral route and has been reported in travellers returning from areas that include the USA, Mexico, Asia and Africa.

Other viruses

Other viruses known to cause hepatitis include Epstein–Barr virus (EBV), cytomegalovirus (CMV) and Hepatitis-G (HGV).

Treatment of viral hepatitis

The treatment of viral hepatitis tends to centre around symptom control and supportive therapy. The patient's medications are reviewed and reduced wherever possible. Drugs deactivated by the liver (e.g. oral contraceptives and morphine) should be avoided. Patients should also avoid alcohol. Interferon-alpha is used to reduce progression to liver failure in patients with chronic HBV and HCV. End-stage liver disease caused by HCV is a common indication for liver transplantation.

TUMOURS

Liver tumours may be benign or malignant. Benign tumours are usually single and small; patients are usually asymptomatic and the tumour is often discovered accidentally. Surgical removal is not usually necessary, unless patients experience pain.

Malignant tumours may be primary or (more commonly) secondary. The liver is the most frequent site of blood-borne metastases from cancers elsewhere in the body. Most primary tumours are associated with an already diseased liver – the highest frequency is among African and Far Eastern races (from the underlying cirrhosis). The condition is increasing in Europe and North America, related to the prevalence of HBV and HCV infections. Alcohol misuse also increases the risk of primary cancer of the liver.

The management of primary tumours may involve surgery, but large liver resections carry high morbidity and mortality rates. However, small localized tumours may be removed by less radical surgery. Chemotherapy (e.g. 5-fluorouracil) may be part of treatment. For the majority of patients, however, treatment is restricted to symptom control and the prognosis is bleak.

CIRRHOSIS

Cirrhosis is a serious liver disease characterized by the destruction of hepatocytes and the formation of dense fibrous scar tissue. Although symptoms may not occur for many years, structural changes gradually lead to total liver dysfunction. The early signs of cirrhotic changes often go unnoticed, because the liver has a large reserve capacity. Impaired liver function may gradually appear over a long period of time, sometimes even years. Symptoms may include the following:

- Initial stages – lethargy and fatigue, vague digestive disturbances (anorexia, flatulence, nausea), weight loss;
- Later stages – jaundice, dependent oedema, anaemia, ascites and increased girth, spider naevii (dilated branching cutaneous arteries), bleeding, epistaxis, melaena, haematemesis and endocrine abnormalities [e.g. gynaecomastia (breast development) and erectile dysfunction in males, amenorrhoea and infertility in females] may develop;
- Advanced stages – splenomegaly (enlarged spleen), hepatic coma, haemorrhage from oesophageal varices (enlarged tortuous veins in the lower oesophagus).

The care patients receive depends largely on the cause and severity of the disease and the presence of any complications. The first priority is to treat the underlying cause (e.g. exposure to toxins, use of alcohol, biliary obstruction, etc.). Complications of cirrhosis are usually inevitable and, for many patients, the only chance of a full recovery is to have a liver transplant. The management of the effects of cirrhosis is detailed in *Table 29*.

Further reading

Brooker C and Nicol M (2003). *Nursing Adults. The Practice of Caring*, pp. 622–638 Edinburgh: Mosby.

Table 29 Cirrhosis – effects, causes and medical management

Effect	Cause	Medical management
Hepatic portal hypertension	Increased vascular resistance leading to the development of an efficient collateral system with back-flow into the vessels of the spleen, oesophagus and intestines	Beta-blockers (e.g. propranolol) – reduced hepatic portal blood flow and thus the risk of re-bleeding
Ascites	Increased resistance to blood flow and decreased lymphatic protein filtration – force protein into the peritoneal space Dehydration – causes adrenal glands to secrete aldosterone, causing water and sodium retention	Restrict sodium and water Diuretics: loop (furosemide) aldosterone antagonist (spironolactone) Paracentesis Replace albumin Peritoneovenous shunt
Oesophageal varices	Portal hypertension causes distension and rupture of vessels in the oesophagus – the excessive blood loss is life-threatening. Compounded by disruption to the liver's normal role in the blood-clotting process	Vasoconstrictive agents Balloon tamponade Sclerotherapy Vitamin K
Encephalopathy	Failure by the liver to metabolize and detoxify nitrogenous substances, especially ammonia	Lactulose Neomycin

L IVING WILL

⇒ Advance directive.

L OCUS OF CONTROL

Locus of control is a concept in health psychology. It is a behaviourist theory to describe individual differences in perceived control over events in people's lives. Some people feel that events in their lives are beyond their control, a belief in an external locus of control. This consequently determines their response to stress and health-seeking (illness) behaviour with an over-reliance on medical intervention for improving health. Others may feel that they do exercise a degree of control over events, a belief in an internal locus of control. This is more likely to lead to self-help – altered behaviour to reduce the risk of ill health, adoption of healthier lifestyles and adherence to medical advice.

L OW BIRTHWEIGHT

⇒ Preterm and/or premature infants.

LYMPHATIC SYSTEM

All body tissues are bathed in tissue (interstitial) fluid, which consists of the diffusible constituents of blood and waste materials from cells. Some tissue fluid returns to the capillaries at their venous end and the remainder diffuses through the more permeable walls of the lymph capillaries and becomes lymph.

Lymph passes through vessels of increasing size and a varying number of *lymph nodes* before returning to the blood. The lymphatic system (*Fig. 116A*) consists of:

- Lymph – clear fluid identical in composition to tissue (interstitial) fluid;
- Lymph vessels – the capillaries and larger lymph vessels that eventually join together to form two large ducts, the *thoracic duct* and the *right lymphatic duct*, that empty lymph into the subclavian veins (*Fig. 116B*);

L

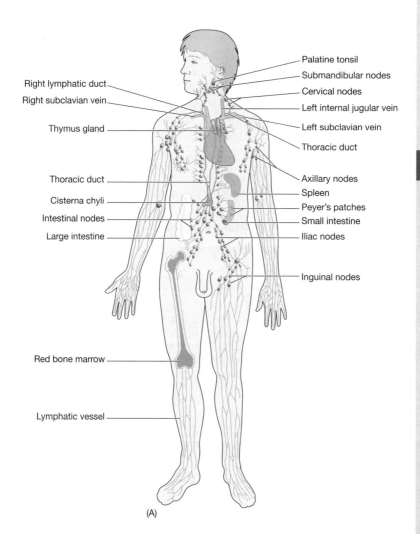

Right lymphatic duct
Right subclavian vein
Thymus gland
Thoracic duct
Cisterna chyli
Intestinal nodes
Large intestine
Red bone marrow
Lymphatic vessel

Palatine tonsil
Submandibular nodes
Cervical nodes
Left internal jugular vein
Left subclavian vein
Thoracic duct
Axillary nodes
Spleen
Peyer's patches
Small intestine
Iliac nodes
Inguinal nodes

(A)

Fig 116 (A) The lymphatic system

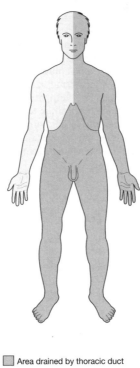

Area drained by thoracic duct
Area drained by lymphatic duct

(B)

Fig 116 (B) lymph drainage

- Lymph nodes – arranged, often in groups, along the length of the lymph vessel, the nodes filter lymph as it passes through, such that particulate matter (e.g. micro-organisms), worn out cells and cancer cells are destroyed by macrophages and antibodies;
- Lymph organs (e.g. spleen and thymus) ⇒ Spleen, Thymus gland;
- Diffuse lymphoid tissue or mucosa-associated lymphoid tissue (MALT), such as tonsils, Peyer's patches (lymphoid tissue in the small intestine) ⇒ Tonsils;
- Bone marrow (lymphocytes are produced in the bone marrow).

Functions of the lymphatic system include:

- Tissue drainage. Every day, around 21 L of plasma fluid, which carries dissolved substances and some plasma protein, escape from the arterial end of the capillaries and into the tissues. Most of this fluid is returned directly to the bloodstream via the capillary at its venous end, but 3–4 L of it are drained away by the lymphatic vessels. Without this, the tissues would rapidly become waterlogged, and the cardiovascular system would begin to fail as the blood volume falls.
- Absorption in the small intestine. Fat and fat-soluble materials (e.g. the fat-soluble vitamins) are absorbed into the central lacteals (lymphatic vessels) of the villi.
- Immunity. The lymphatic organs are concerned with the production and maturation of lymphocytes, the white blood cells that are primarily responsible for the provision of immunity. ⇒ Defence mechanisms.

LYMPHATIC DISORDERS

LYMPHADENITIS

Lymphadenitis is inflammation of a lymph node. It may be secondary to a number of conditions, such as infectious mononucleosis (see below), measles, typhoid fever, wound and skin infections, etc.

INFECTIOUS MONONUCLEOSIS

Infectious mononucleosis (glandular fever) is a contagious self-limiting disease caused by the Epstein–Barr virus (EBV). It mainly affects teenagers and young adults and is characterized by tiredness, headache, fever, sore throat, enlarged lymph nodes, splenomegaly and the appearance of atypical lymphocytes that resemble monocytes. Specific antibodies to EBV are present in the blood, as well as an abnormal antibody that forms the basis of the Paul–Bunnell test, which confirms the diagnosis. Clinical or subclinical infection confers life-long immunity.

LYMPHANGITIS

Lymphangitis is inflammation of a lymph vessel, such as when the microbes in the lymph that drains from an infected area spread along the walls of the lymph vessels (e.g. in acute *Streptococcus pyogenes* infection of the hand, a red line may be seen to extend from the hand to the axilla).

LYMPHOEDEMA

Lymphoedema is excess fluid in the tissues from an abnormality or obstruction of lymph vessels that blocks or interrupts lymph drainage. There is swelling of (usually) a limb, increased risk of cellulitis and possible loss of limb function. In women with breast cancer the removal of the axillary lymph nodes is a contributory factor in the development of lymphoedema (see Practice application). The axilla is not irradiated after axillary clearance, as this increases the risk of lymphoedema. Untreated, the inflamed tissue becomes fibrosed and the skin becomes hard, with loss of elasticity.

Lymphoedema, together with skin changes (elephantiasis), can result from lymph vessel blockage caused by filarial worms (tissue-dwelling nematodes). ⇒ Helminthiasis.

Practice application – management of lymphoedema in breast cancer

Lymphoedema is a distressing and disabling condition, with no predictability regarding its onset. A woman may experience pain or discomfort that may cause her to use the limb less, which compromises her ability to perform normal activities of living or maintain independence. There may be a cost and time impact as she is forced to visit the hospital for treatment. Physical problems often lead to psychological problems, as a result of altered body image.

Lymphoedema responds much better when detected early and when women follow their treatment regimen. Any management must include continuous assessment, which involves regular limb measurement and assessment of hosiery for a correct fit, patient education, treatment and evaluation.

There are four main areas of treatment, which should be used simultaneously:
- Skin care – aims to prevent infection and inflammation. Patients should be advised about how to minimize risks, such as avoiding minor skin injuries (e.g. having blood taken from the arm), treating cuts immediately and consulting a doctor if the arm becomes infected, and keeping hands and nails clean.

- Exercise – normal use of the limb should be encouraged to improve lymph drainage. Passive or specific exercise can be used to increase joint mobility, but excessive use may cause vasodilatation and increased lymph flow.
- Massage – the technique used is not vigorous, as this would increase blood flow to the area, but a gentle technique known as manual lymphatic drainage (MLD). Fluid will re-accumulate if containment hosiery is not used.
- Containment hosiery or bandaging – this increases the interstitial pressure and aids absorption by the pumping action of the muscles. It is not intended to force fluid out of the limb by compression and is therefore used in conjunction with massage and exercise. Hosiery (elastic arm sleeve) is used long-term for mild uncomplicated lymphoedema. Bandaging is used for more complicated lymphoedema and gross swelling. The aim of treatment is to restore the limb to a more reasonable shape, size and condition so that hosiery can be used (Badger 1987). Indications for bandaging are *lymphorrhoea* (leakage of lymph through the skin), oedematous fingers and broken skin.

LYMPHOMAS

The lymphomas are a group of malignant tumours that develop in lymphoid tissue. Lymphomas are classified, according to histological appearances, into either *Hodgkin's lymphoma* or *non-Hodgkin's lymphoma* (NHL). Lymphoma is characterized by lymph node enlargement, night sweats and/or swinging pyrexia, pain from splenic enlargement and/or infarction, hepatomegaly, weight loss, pruritus, alcohol-related bone pain (Hodgkin's), malaise or recurrent infection. The aetiology is largely unknown, although genetic and environmental factors may be implicated. Certain viruses, particularly EBV and human T-cell leukaemia virus (HTLV-1), may also be a factor. People who are immunocompromised appear to be susceptible to NHL.

Burkitt's lymphoma is a highly malignant lymphoma, frequently of the jaw, but in other sites as well. Until recently, it was a very rare disease associated with EBV infection and predominately found in children of African origin. There is an increasing incidence of Burkitt's lymphoma among adults in Europe and North America, which is often associated with HIV infection.

Therapy for lymphomas includes:

- Hodgkin's lymphoma – radiotherapy for early-stage, then cytotoxic chemotherapy.
- NHL – depends on the type. Generally, a conservative 'wait-and-see' approach for indolent (low-grade) NHL. If treatment is given, the options include localized radiotherapy or chemotherapy, but these are not very effective. However, newer agents include fludarabine, interferon-alpha and monoclonal antibodies. Conversely, people with highly aggressive (high-grade) NHL respond well to chemotherapy.
- Burkitt's lymphoma is highly aggressive and requires complex and intensive chemotherapy regimens, which comprise chemotherapy with intrathecal central nervous system (CNS) treatment and haemopoietic growth factor support.
- Relapsed lymphoma – second-line chemotherapy. Nowadays, people may also opt for further high-dose chemotherapy followed by autologous peripheral blood stem cell rescue or allogeneic stem cell transplantation. A promising new treatment licensed for selected forms of lymphoma is anti-CD20 monoclonal antibody therapy.

MACRONUTRIENTS

Macronutrients are those nutrients (protein, carbohydrate and fats) required by the body in relatively large amounts that can be metabolized to produce energy. Each fulfils a vital role and the relative amounts of each taken in the diet are important. They consist of carbon, oxygen and hydrogen in different proportions – proteins contain nitrogen, and some amino acids contain phosphorus and sulphur. ⇒ Carbohydrates, Fat, Micronutrients, Nutrition, Protein.

MALARIA

Malaria is a serious disease caused by protozoa of the genus *Plasmodium* and carried by infected mosquitoes of the genus *Anopheles*. It occurs in tropical and subtropical regions and is encountered in people who have returned from malarial areas. The parasite causes haemolysis during a complex life cycle. *P. falciparum* causes the most severe disease, with complications that include anaemia, shock and organ damage. *P. malariae* causes quartan [symptoms, such as fever, recur every 72 hours (fourth day)] malaria. *P. ovale* and *P. vivax* cause tertian (symptoms recur every 48 hours) malaria.

The signs and symptoms depend on the type of malaria, but include bouts of fever, rigors, headache, vomiting, cough, anaemia, jaundice and hepatosplenomegaly (enlarged liver and spleen). Relapses are common in malaria.

Various antimalarial drugs are available for both prophylaxis (e.g. chloroquine, proguanil hydrochloride, doxycycline hyclate, etc.) and treatment (e.g. quinine, mefloquine, etc.). Drug resistance has occurred and many of the drugs have serious side-effects (e.g. mefloquine can cause side-effects that include depression and panic attacks, cardiac arrhythmias, etc.). The choice of drug depends on the region and the risk of exposure, drug effectiveness, side-effects, level of resistance and particular features of the person (e.g. pregnancy, etc.).

In addition to adhering to prophylactic drug regimens, individuals are advised to take precautions against being bitten by mosquitoes (see Practice application). Efforts to eliminate the mosquito and its habitat are also important in prevention.

Practice application – general measures for antimalarial prophylaxis
Depending on the particular circumstances the measures include:
- Sleeping under mosquito nets treated with the insecticide permethrin;
- Use of insect repellents (e.g. sprays, vaporizers);
- Lotions and/or sprays that contain diethyltoluamide for skin application;
- Wearing clothes that cover as much skin as possible (i.e. trousers and tops with long sleeves);
- Household screens to prevent mosquitoes gaining entry.

MALNUTRITION

Malnutrition is the state of being poorly nourished because the diet contains incorrect amounts of a micro- or macronutrient. It can result from malabsorption (e.g. cystic fibrosis) or an inability to utilize the nutrients. Malnutrition can result in disease, such as scurvy (malnutrition through inadequate dietary intake of vitamin C), or obesity (malnutrition through excessive energy intake). ⇒ Nutrition (nutritional assessment).

OBESITY

Obesity is the most common nutritional disorder world-wide, and its incidence is increasing and differs with socioeconomic status and racial group. Obesity involves the deposition of excessive fat around the body, particularly in the subcutaneous tissue. It develops when the intake of food is in excess of the body's energy requirements.

Obesity is the cause of preventable ill health, including type 2 diabetes mellitus, coronary heart disease, hypertension, stroke, gallstones, osteoarthritis, sleep apnoea, some cancers and psychological disorders. Obesity is usually diagnosed from body mass index (BMI). Other methods of assessment include measurement of waist and hip circumference, bioelectrical impedance and skin-fold thickness measurement.

The WHO (1998b) classifies obesity and overweight according to BMI:
- Underweight – BMI <18.5
- Normal range – BMI 18.5–24.9
- Overweight – BMI >25.0
- Pre-obese – BMI 25.0–29.9
- Obese Class 1 – BMI 30.0–34.9
- Obese Class 2 – BMI 35.0–39.9
- Obese Class 3 – BMI >40.0

The causes of obesity include a high fat diet, high sugar diet, physical inactivity, endocrine disorders, genetic make up, psychosocial factors, etc.

TREATMENT

The treatment of obesity centres on lifestyle changes, such as dietary change and exercise, which usually needs to be accompanied by behaviour therapy to be successful. Surgery and drug treatments are considered as a last resort.

PROTEIN-ENERGY MALNUTRITION

Protein-energy malnutrition (PEM) is a form of malnutrition caused by an insufficient intake of protein and energy, such as in famine situations or anorexia. PEM occurs, all too frequently, in hospitalized individuals who develop a negative nitrogen balance because protein is being used primarily to produce energy. A negative balance is associated with starvation or any severe physiological stress that increases protein catabolism (e.g. burns, sepsis, major surgery and multiple injuries; see Practice application).

Practice application – malnutrition in hospital

The consequences of malnutrition include:
- Delayed wound healing;
- Increased risk of pressure ulcers;
- Loss of muscle strength;
- Low mood and apathy;
- Increased incidence of postoperative complications;
- Impaired immune responses;
- Increased risk of death.

Many of these consequences, such as risk of pressure ulcers, also apply to individuals in other care settings.

The nursing role in preventing or minimizing the problem includes:
- Recognition of the malnourished person by use of standardized screening tools;
- Identifying those people at risk of malnutrition;
- Making appropriate referrals to the dietician;
- Ensuring that dietary intake is sufficient to meet nutritional needs.

KWASHIORKOR

Kwashiorkor is a form of PEM that occurs when children are weaned on to a low protein diet with adequate amounts of energy from carbohydrate sources. It is characterized by a miserable child who fails to thrive. Weight loss may not be marked, but the child fails to grow. There is generalized oedema, ascites, anaemia, changes in hair and skin pigmentation, diarrhoea and hepatomegaly.

MARASMUS

Marasmus is a severe form of PEM caused by insufficient protein and energy (calories) in the diet. It affects young children who become very thin with muscle wasting. Growth is retarded, the skin is wrinkled and hair is lost. It is rarely seen in developed European and North American societies, but is still common in developing countries when famine occurs.

MALPRACTICE

Malpractice in the healthcare context means improper or injurious treatment from a health professional, such as medical or nursing treatment. It is professional practice that falls short of accepted standards and causes harm. It may involve unethical professional behaviour, negligence, abuse or criminal activities. ⇒ Abuse, Negligence.

MEASLES

⇒ Communicable diseases (morbilli).

MEDICAL JURISPRUDENCE

⇒ Forensic.

MEDICINES

⇒ Controlled drugs, Drug, Pharmacokinetics and pharmacodynamics.

MEDICINES AND HEALTHCARE PRODUCTS REGULATORY AGENCY

The Medicines and Healthcare Products Regulatory Agency (MHRA) is an executive agency of the UK Department of Health formed from a merger between the Medicines Control Agency (MCA) and the Medical Devices Agency (MDA). Its main function is to promote and protect public health and the safety of patients by ensuring that all medicines, healthcare products and medical devices and equipment meet suitable standards of safety, quality, performance and efficacy, and are used in a safe manner.

MEIOSIS

Meiosis is the two-stage reduction cell division that occurs during gametogenesis when the chromosomes of a gamete are halved [reduced from *diploid* ($2n$) to *haploid* (n)] in preparation for the union of egg and sperm at fertilization. Each human cell, including the primitive gametes, contains 46 chromosomes (23 pairs). Each pair of chromosomes consists of two structurally similar chromosomes (*homologues*), one of maternal origin and the other paternal (see *Fig. 43*).

The first event of meiosis (*Fig. 117*) is the replication of deoxyribonucleic acid (DNA) in each homologue to form *double-stranded DNA*. The two chromosomes of each pair come together and some reshuffling of genetic material occurs

M

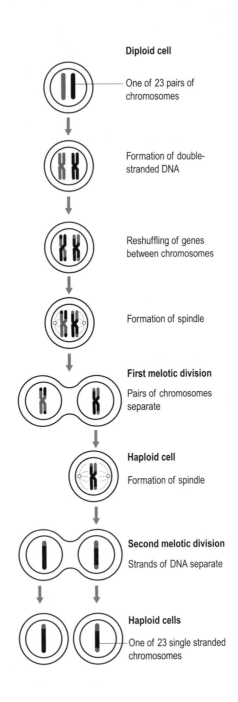

Fig 117 The process of meiosis

between them. When the *first meiotic division* begins, the 23 pairs of chromosomes line up around the middle of a spindle of microtubules formed between the two poles of the cell. The members of each pair of chromosomes separate, 23 being drawn to one pole and 23 towards the other. The cell divides to form two daughter cells that each contain 23 chromosomes only, half the usual number.

The daughter cells divide for a second time (*second meiotic division*). The chromosomes again line up at the middle of the spindle of microtubules, but this time the two strands of DNA in each chromosome separate and each is drawn to opposite poles of the cell along the spindle and the cell divides to form two daughter cells. As two cells were produced at the first meiotic division, the second meiotic division results in four mature gametes that each contain only 23 chromosomes. The second meiotic division is similar to mitosis, but differs in that only 23 chromosomes are involved from start to finish, instead of 46. The four resulting daughter cells are the mature gametes. ⇒ Cell (cell cycle), Chromosomes, Gametogenesis (oogenesis, spermatogenesis and spermiogenesis), Mitosis.

MEMORY

At a very basic level, memory can be described as the ability to retain and recall prior learning (information and events). It is a very complex process that includes different types of memory (*Box 19*). Memory processing depends on two forms of rehearsal of facts:

*   *Maintenance rehearsal*, in which information re-enters short-term memory (STM) by repetition (such as repeating a telephone number) – each time the information enters STM appears to increase its chance of being stored in long-term memory (LTM);
*   *Elaborative rehearsal* processes information in STM so that it can be coded for storage in LTM, for which it may use sensory characteristics, such as sound, or focus on the meaning of the information.

Hypermnesia describes an extraordinarily good memory. It is an exaggerated memory with the individual being able to recall minute detail.

Box 19 Types of memory
*   Episodic memory is the part of LTM that stores personal experiences. It is organized with respect to when and where the experience happened (e.g. an episode from your first day in a new job).
*   Long-term memory (LTM) is the part of memory that deals with the retention of information for longer periods. It is potentially permanent and has a much greater capacity than STM.
*   Procedural memory is the part of memory that stores information needed to do things (e.g. take a blood pressure or make a cup of tea).
*   Semantic memory is the part of memory that stores general information about the world (e.g. where polar bears are found).
*   Short-term memory (STM) is the part of memory that deals with the retention of information for a few seconds only. It can only be retained if it is rehearsed or moved to LTM (also known as working memory). The process of *chunking* describes the organization and coding of chunks of information that allows us to increase the effective capacity of STM, which can only store around seven items of information. The loss of pieces of information from STM, as new information is added, is called *displacement*.

MEMORY PROBLEMS

AGE-ASSOCIATED MEMORY IMPAIRMENT

See Practice application.

ECMNESIA

Ecmnesia is an impaired memory for recent events with a normal memory for remote ones. It is common in old age and in early cerebral deterioration.

MEMORY LAPSES

Many adults have episodes of memory loss and some time later retrieve the appropriate information. The lapses often occur when individuals are under stress and typically increase with age. ⇒ Amnesia, Confusion and delirium, Dementia.

Practice application – age-associated memory impairment

A classic stereotype of old age is the loss of memory, and it is true that, as we age, we suffer a decline in memory. Clearly, there is some interplay between STM and LTM, as recent events may become stored, eventually, in the LTM while others are forgotten. It is STM that declines with age, but, while this can be a significant inconvenience for older people, it does not usually have an adverse effect on their lives. Older people learn to compensate for any decline in STM and it is often the case that this feature of ageing is barely noticeable, especially in familiar surroundings. However, some people do have age-associated memory impairment, and memory loss is a cardinal feature of dementia. It is unclear, however, whether normal memory that declines with age, age-associated memory impairment and dementia lie on a continuum. If they do, the conclusion must be that longevity ultimately leads to memory failure. If they do not, then age-associated memory impairment and dementia are distinct conditions.

MENSTRUAL CYCLE

The menstrual (uterine) cycle describes the events that occur as the endometrium responds to ovarian hormones (*Fig. 118*). Menstrual cycles usually start at the age of 12–13 years (the menarche) in developed countries and cease around the age of 50 years (menopause, a single event that occurs during the climacteric).

The menstrual cycle corresponds to the ovarian cycle and is normally repeated every 28 days or so (range 21–35 days) during the reproductive years (except during pregnancy). It is all about preparing the endometrium in case an oocyte is fertilized, and is usually described in three distinct phases – proliferative, secretory and menstrual. By convention the first day of menstrual bleeding is counted as day 1 of the cycle, although the menstrual phase is at the end of the cycle, so as to provide an obvious landmark.

The *proliferative phase* corresponds to the follicular phase of the ovarian cycle and commences when menstrual bleeding has stopped. Oestrogen causes the regeneration of the stratum functionalis. This phase ends with the maturation of a Graafian follicle and ovulation around day 14.

The *secretory phase* starts after ovulation, corresponds to the luteal phase of the ovarian cycle and lasts about 14 days. The endometrium is now influenced by progesterone. The glands enlarge and secrete glycogen, which is intended to sustain an embryo during implantation. The endometrium is now 5 mm thick. Without fertilization, the reduction in hormones from the corpus luteum leads to spasm in the spiral arteries, caused by prostaglandins that are normally inhibited

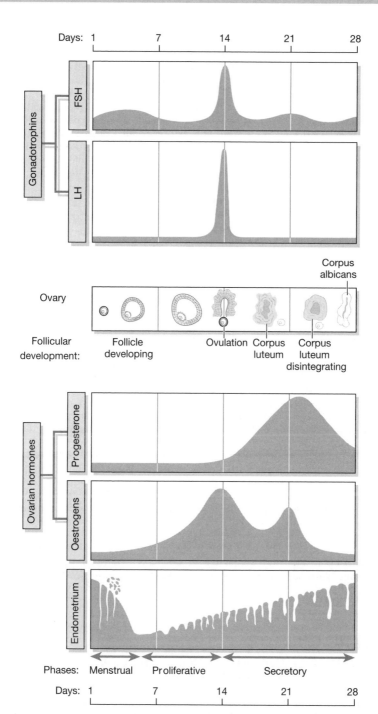

Fig 118 Menstrual (uterine) cycle (with hormonal and ovarian events); FSH, follicle-stimulating hormone; LH, luteinizing hormone

by progesterone and oestrogen. Arterial spasm causes the endometrium to degenerate as it is deprived of nutrients and, later, autodigestion by enzymes. This leads (about 24 hours later) to menstrual bleeding.

The *menstrual phase* is the last phase of the cycle (but remember it is taken as day 1 of the cycle). Menstrual flow (*menses*) contains blood, other fluids and endometrial debris, and usually lasts for 3–6 days. Vaginal loss during menstruation, which is usually around 75 mL (only half is blood), varies considerably and is extremely difficult to assess objectively. To replace this blood loss, women need more dietary iron than men during the reproductive years. Fibrinolysins stop menstrual blood clotting within the uterus, which ensures that the redundant stratum functionalis is completely discharged through the cervix. ⇒ Climacteric, Infections of female reproductive tract (toxic shock syndrome), Reproductive systems, Uterus and vagina (uterine and vaginal disorders).

Some menstrual disorders are outlined in *Box 20*.

Box 20 Disorders of menstruation

Amenorrhoea – absence of the menses. When menstruation has not been established at the time when it should have been, the term *primary amenorrhoea* is used (e.g. chromosomal defects or *cryptomenorrhoea* where bleeding is hidden in the uterine cavity); absence of the menses after they have commenced is referred to as *secondary amenorrhoea* (e.g. pregnancy, anorexia nervosa, ovarian cysts, etc.).

Oligomenorrhoea – irregular infrequent menstruation. The causes include endocrine disorders and polycystic ovary syndrome (PCOS).

Dysmenorrhoea – painful menstruation. This may be *spasmodic* or *primary dysmenorrhoea* and most often affects young women once ovulation has become established, or it may be *congestive* or *secondary dysmenorrhoea*, which usually affects women in their late twenties and may be associated with pelvic pathology, such as fibroids or endometriosis.

Menorrhagia – heavy bleeding during a regular cycle. The causes include dysfunctional uterine bleeding (no organic cause is found), uterine fibroids and polyps, endometriosis and thyroid disorder.

Metrorrhagia – heavy uterine bleeding, usually irregular and frequent. It may be caused by uterine fibroids, polyps or dysfunctional uterine bleeding.

Postmenopausal bleeding (PMB) – not strictly a menstrual disorder, as it is vaginal bleeding that occurs after the menopause. The causes include endometrial cancer, polyps and atrophic vaginitis. The risk of endometrial cancer means that any woman who presents with PMB must be investigated urgently to exclude cancer.

Premenstrual syndrome (PMS) – a group of physical (e.g. fluid retention, breast pain, etc.) and mental (e.g. mood changes and poor concentration) changes that occur any time between 2 and 14 days before menstruation. The cause(s) are unknown, but may be linked to endocrine imbalance and/or fluid retention.

MENTAL HEALTH

Mental health can be defined as a sense of well-being in the emotional, personal, spiritual and social domains of people's lives. ⇒ Anxiety, Attention-deficit hyperactivity disorder, Autism, Child and adolescent mental health, Commission for Healthcare Audit and Inspection, Community (community mental health teams), Dementia, Disorders of mood, Eating disorders, Obsessive–compulsive disorder, Phobias, Schizophrenia, Somatization, Suicide and deliberate self-harm.

MENTAL HEALTH NURSING

Mental health nursing is a branch of nursing concerned with helping people to enhance, maintain or improve their emotional, personal, spiritual and social lives. It is an area of care that was first called 'mental nursing' and then 'psychiatric nursing'. Mental health nurses, increasingly, care for people in the community as the UK government's policy of community care continues. Mental health nursing concentrates, particularly, on the enhancement or maintenance of mental health, and one of the aims of mental health nursing is to prevent the onset of breakdown or illness, where this is possible. The skills of a mental health nurse include a range of interpersonal and therapeutic skills, such as listening, responding, problem-solving, crisis management and enabling the release of emotion. The *Butterworth Report* (Department of Health 1994) highlighted the need for a flexible response to future mental health needs. Its recommendations include:

* Greater understanding of racial and cultural needs;
* More research;
* Representation and participation of service users;
* Links with the criminal justice system;
* Focus on severe mental illness;
* Availability of mental health nursing skills to the primary care team;
* Clinical supervision;
* Development of a framework for good practice.

Mental health nursing skills are important to achieve the mental illness target of reducing deaths from suicide and undetermined injury by at least one-fifth by 2010, set out in the government report *Saving Lives: Our Healthier Nation* (Department of Health 1999b).

Approaches to mental health in the UK today often combine a range of approaches to clients (drug, electroconvulsive or psychological therapies). Although medical treatment still dominates, the roles of social circumstances in the genesis and maintenance of mental distress and illness have been recognized. This has had a considerable influence on clinical practice, particularly by those who pursue psychosocial models of care. These attempts at a more integrated approach to care often involve a team of professionals, including psychologists, occupational therapists, counsellors and nurses, as well as psychiatrists. ⇒ Antidepressants, Antipsychotics, Anxiolytics, Cognition (cognitive behavioural therapy), Counselling, Electroconvulsive therapy.

ASSESSMENT TOOLS IN MENTAL HEALTH (CLIENT AND CARER)

In addition to holistic assessment skills, mental health nurses use a variety of formal assessment tools in their practise, such as:

* Health of the Nation Outcome Scale (HoNOS) is a 12-item health and social functioning scale. It measures risk behaviours, physical problems, deterioration and/or improvement in symptoms and social functioning. It can be completed by the mental healthcare team and/or the individual practitioner.
* Camberwell Assessment of Need (CAN) was developed to provide a comprehensive assessment of the client's health and social needs, and the extent to which these are being met by the client's carers and services.
* Hopelessness Scale (Beck Hopelessness Scale) was developed to provide information about suicidal intent. It takes a few minutes to complete and may be given to the client on a regular basis to monitor the risk of suicide.
* Beck Anxiety Inventory (BAI) is a questionnaire that measures the degree of anxiety felt by clients. It includes an evaluation of both cognitive and physical manifestations of anxiety.
* Caregiver Strain Index (CSI) is used to assess caregiver strain, using a simple questionnaire. Predetermined questions (13) are answered yes or no by interviewee. It has the benefit of being quick and simple, although crude.

- Carers Assessment of Managing Index (CAMI) is used by mental health nurses and others to assess coping styles and management of stress by questionnaire. Carers are given examples of coping strategies, and asked if they use these and if they are effective. It is important as it assumes carers have coping strategies that can be enhanced.
- Relatives Assessment Interview (RAI) is based on the Camberwell Family Interview, but modified for clinical use. It is used by mental health nurses and others to obtain essential information that helps to direct family intervention work. It covers seven main areas, summarized as client's family background and contact time, chronological history of the illness, symptoms of current problems, irritability, relatives' relationship with client and the effects of the illness on relatives. ⇒ Expressed emotion.

MENTAL DEFENCE MECHANISMS

Mental defence mechanisms are unconscious mental processes or coping patterns that lessen the anxiety associated with a situation or internal conflict. A nurse who understands mental defence mechanisms has an increased self-awareness of her or his own use of such mechanisms, and is also sensitive to the use of them by patients and colleagues.

Some mental defence mechanisms are outlined in *Box 21*.

Box 21 Mental defence mechanisms

Compensation – used to cover up a weakness, by exaggerating a more socially acceptable behaviour trait.

Displacement – the redirection of a drive from one focus to an alternative target (looking for an easier option), such as a motorist unconsciously directing anger at a parking attendant because they are angry with themselves for being late for an interview.

Identification – in which individuals take on the characteristics of an admired role model figure.

Intellectualization – people attempt to detach themselves from painful emotions or difficult situations by dealing with the issues in an abstract, intellectual manner.

Isolation – occurs when a drive becomes detached from the emotions commonly associated with a particular situation.

Projection – occurs in normal people unconsciously, and in an exaggerated form in some mental health problems, whereby the person fails to recognize certain motives and feelings in him- or herself, but attributes them to other people.

Rationalization – a person justifies his or her actions, so it looks more positive, rational or socially acceptable.

Regression – reversion to an earlier stage of development (perceived as being more safe), becoming more childish (e.g. to avoid making a difficult decision).

Repression – distressing events, unacceptable thoughts and impulses are impelled into, and remain in, the unconscious mind, such as the denial of drastically changed circumstances (e.g. sudden incapacitating illness or terminal illness).

Sublimation – undesirable drives are unconsciously redirected to, and expressed through, personally approved and socially accepted behaviour, such as aggression redirected to sporting activity.

Suppression – people do not respond to conscious awareness of difficult or painful drives. They ignore a situation and hope that it will just go away.

MENTORSHIP

Mentorship is a system that usually provides support to students during their training. A mentor (a qualified and experienced nurse in this context) works with the student on clinical placements, ensuring he or she receives the appropriate experience. The mentor offers advice and support while the overall aim is to promote learning and development. Mentors also act as a role model. ⇒ Preceptorship.

METABOLISM

Metabolism constitutes all the chemical reactions that occur in the body, using absorbed nutrients to:
• Provide energy by the chemical oxidation of nutrients;
• Make new or replacement body substances.
Two types of processes are involved – catabolism and anabolism.

CATABOLISM

Catabolism is the process whereby large molecules are broken down into smaller ones to release chemical energy, which is stored as adenosine triphosphate (ATP), and heat.

ANABOLISM

Anabolism is the building up, or synthesis, of large molecules from smaller ones and requires a source of energy, usually ATP.

METABOLIC PATHWAYS

Anabolism and catabolism usually involve a series of chemical reactions, known as *metabolic pathways*. Both processes occur continually in all cells, which maintains an energy balance. Much of the metabolic effort of cells is concerned with energy production to fuel cellular activities. ⇒ Adenosine.

Certain common pathways are central to this function. Fuel molecules enter three central energy-producing pathways and, in a series of steps (during which a series of intermediate molecules are formed and energy is released), these fuel molecules are broken down chemically. The preferred fuel molecule is glucose, but alternatives should glucose be unavailable include amino acids, fatty acids and glycerol. Each of these may enter the central energy-producing pathways and be converted into energy (ATP), carbon dioxide and water. The three central metabolic pathways are:
• Glycolysis – break down of glucose to form pyruvic acid and some energy;
• Citric acid (Krebs) cycle – the final common pathway for the oxidation of fuel molecules;
• Oxidative phosphorylation – a mitochondrial process, whereby adenosine diphosphate (ADP) is converted into ATP by the addition of a phosphate group.
Fig. 119 summarizes the fates of the three main energy sources in the central metabolic pathways.

BASAL METABOLIC RATE

The basal metabolic rate (BMR) is the energy consumed at complete rest for essential physiological functions. It is influenced by nutritional status, age, gender, weight, disease, certain drugs and ambient temperature.

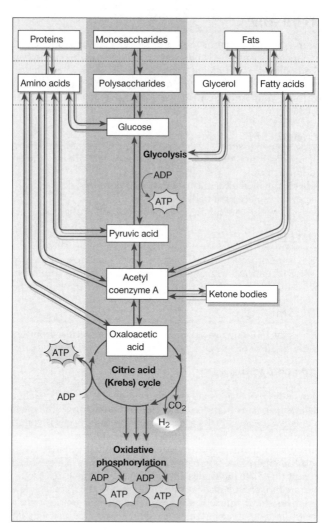

Fig 119 Summary of the fates of the three main energy sources in the central metabolic pathways

ABSORPTIVE STATE

The absorptive state is the normal metabolic state immediately after a meal, which continues for about 4 hours. Absorbed nutrients are used as an energy source or to build up other substances through anabolic processes such as glycogenesis (formation and storage of glycogen).

POSTABSORPTIVE STATE

The postabsorptive state is the normal metabolic state that exists between meals, such as late afternoon and at night. Fuel molecules for immediate energy use are in short supply and the body uses catabolic processes, such as glycogenolysis (conversion of glycogen into glucose), to break down complex substances to provide energy.

ABNORMAL METABOLIC STATES

Hypermetabolic states may occur in a variety of disorders, whereby energy demands are increased but not met, such as sepsis, severe trauma, cancer, etc. There is a greatly increased metabolic rate. The body mobilizes stores of energy by glucogenolysis and later lipolysis (breakdown of fat stores). The utilization of fat for energy is limited and catabolism of muscle protein occurs to provide amino acids for gluconeogenesis (production of glucose from noncarbohydrate sources). This ensures a constant supply of glucose for tissues such as the brain.

Without an adequate energy intake to conserve proteins the hypermetabolic and/or hypercatabolic state leads to protein-energy malnutrition and eventually severe cachexia (extreme wasting).

MICRONUTRIENTS

The micronutrients are vitamins and minerals (including trace elements), of which daily amounts are required for cellular function and health. The amount required of each varies from micrograms to grams and reflects the activity of the substance, its toxicity and evidence of disease caused by deficiency. Reference nutrient intakes (RNIs) for vitamins and minerals have been calculated and take into account age, gender and bioavailability (Department of Health 1991a). Vitamins and trace elements are usually only required in minute quantities. ⇒ Dietetics (dietary reference values), Minerals, Vitamins.

MICRO-ORGANISMS (SYN. MICROBE)

A micro-organism is an organism (plant or animal) that is usually microscopic. It is often synonymous with bacterium, but also includes chlamydia, fungus (some of which are not microscopic), protozoon, rickettsia and virus.

NORMAL FLORA

The normal flora comprises the micro-organisms that usually colonize the surfaces of the body (e.g. *Staphylococcus epidermidis*) on the skin, which protects against invasion by pathogens through competition for nutrients (*Table 30*). The micro-organisms of the normal flora are *commensals*; that is, they do not harm their hosts and could even be described as *symbiotic* because they benefit their host by preventing other, harmful micro-organisms from occupying the surfaces. Commensal micro-organisms are harmless in their normal site, but may cause disease if they are transferred to a different part of the body (e.g. *Escherichia coli* from the bowel causes urinary and wound infection) or when the host's normal defences are impaired (e.g. *S. aureus* in the nose may cause infection if transferred to damaged skin).

Table 30 The normal flora of the body

Site of body	Common commensal micro-organisms
Skin	*Staphylococcus epidermidis*, *Streptococcus* spp., *Corynebacterium* spp., *Candida*
Throat	*Strep. viridans*, *Neisseria* spp., diphtheroids
Mouth	*Strep. viridans*, *N. catarrhalis*, *Actinomyces* spp., spirochaetes
Respiratory tract	*Strep. viridans*, *N.* spp., diphtheroids, micrococci
Vagina	Lactobacilli, diphtheroids, streptococci, yeasts
Intestines	*Bacteroides* spp., anaerobic streptococci, *Clostridium perfringens*, *Escherichia coli*, *Klebsiella* spp., *Proteus*, *Strep. faecalis*

Micro-organisms that cause disease are called *pathogens*. They account for only a small proportion of the total microbial population, but are difficult to define accurately because the ability of some to cause disease depends on the susceptibility of the host. ⇒ Infection (opportunistic infection).

Practice application – effects of hospitalization on normal skin flora
When patients are hospitalized the normal skin flora is often replaced by strains of hospital bacteria that are more resistant to antibiotics (e.g. methicillin-resistant *Staphylococcus aureus, Klebsiella* and *Acinetobacter*) and that can cause serious infection if they enter the body during invasive procedures.

MICTURITION (SYN. URINATION)

Micturition is the act of passing (voiding) urine. The urinary bladder acts as a reservoir for urine. When 300–400 mL of urine have accumulated, afferent autonomic nerve fibres in the bladder wall sensitive to stretch are stimulated. In the infant this initiates a *spinal reflex action* and micturition occurs. Micturition occurs when autonomic efferent fibres convey impulses to the bladder and cause contraction of the detrusor muscle and relaxation of the internal urethral sphincter.

When the nervous system is fully developed the micturition reflex is stimulated, but sensory impulses pass upwards to the brain and there is an awareness of the desire to pass urine. By conscious effort, reflex contraction of the bladder wall and relaxation of the internal sphincter can be inhibited for a limited period of time (*Fig. 120*).

In adults, micturition occurs when the detrusor muscle contracts, and there is a reflex relaxation of the internal sphincter and voluntary relaxation of the external sphincter. It can be assisted by increasing the pressure within the pelvic cavity, achieved by lowering the diaphragm and contracting the abdominal muscles (Valsalva's manoeuvre). Over-distension of the bladder is extremely painful, and when this stage is reached there is a tendency for involuntary relaxation of the external sphincter to occur and a small amount of urine to escape, provided there is no mechanical obstruction. Some problems associated with micturition are outlined in *Box 22.* ⇒ Catheters and urinary catheterization, Urinary system.

Box 22 Disorders of micturition
Dysuria – painful micturition.
Enuresis – incontinence of urine, especially bedwetting. *Nocturnal enuresis* is incontinence at night.
Frequency – the need to pass urine more often than is acceptable to the person, usually more often than had been experienced in the past. The person passes small amounts of urine. It is often associated with urinary tract infection.
Haematuria – blood in the urine.
Hesitancy – a delay in starting to pass urine, even when responding to a strong desire to void. It is a symptom of outflow obstruction, such as with prostatic enlargement.
Intermittency – stopping and starting several times during micturition.
Nocturia – having to get up at night to pass urine. A feature of increasing age as the kidneys lose their ability to produce concentrated urine, but it may be caused by pathology.
Poor stream of urine – often a sign of prostatic enlargement.
Retention – an inability to pass urine that accumulates within the bladder. It has a variety of causes (e.g. physical obstruction, nerve damage, etc.). Retention may occur with overflow.

Strangury – constant painful urge to pass small amounts of urine, as a result of muscle spasm associated with inflammation or irritation.

Urgency – strong desire to pass urine, which, if not responded to immediately, may lead to urge incontinence. ⇒ Continence, Incontinence.

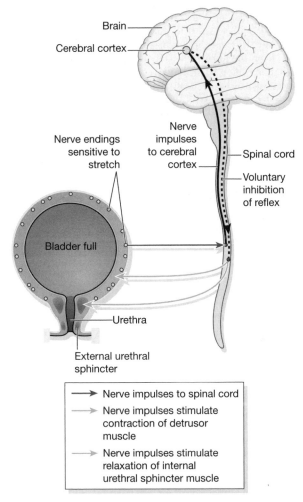

Fig 120 Control of micturition when conscious effort overrides the reflex action

MINERALS

Minerals are the inorganic elements that play a vital role in body structure and functions, and comprise calcium, chloride, iron, magnesium, phosphorus, potassium, sodium and zinc, and the trace elements cobalt, chromium, copper, fluorine, iodine, manganese, molybdenum and selenium. Details of some important minerals and trace elements are provided in Further reading.

ABSORPTION OF MINERALS

The minerals in food often represent the environmental conditions and mineral content of the soil. The more varied the diet from a region, the less likely there is to be mineral deficiency.

However, the absorption of minerals from food is far from straightforward. The bioavailability of minerals may be low, such as iron from nonhaem sources (e.g. cereals, fruit, vegetables, etc.) is absorbed less well than that in meat and offal. Many minerals need other factors to enhance their absorption. Most dietary iron is in the ferric state. However, iron is absorbed more readily in the ferrous form, and reduction from the ferric to the ferrous form is facilitated by gastric juice and also by vitamin C. Another example is calcium absorption, which is facilitated by lactose and protein. The absorption of some minerals is inhibited by the presence of other substances in food. Calcium absorption is inhibited by oxalates, phytic acid, phytates (found, for example, in cereals and rhubarb), and phosphate.

Further reading

Barker H (2002). *Nutrition/Dietetics for Healthcare*, Tenth Edition. Edinburgh: Churchill Livingstone.

MINIMALLY INVASIVE SURGERY

Minimally invasive surgery is known colloquially as 'keyhole surgery', and involves surgical techniques that require minimal access only; the procedure is performed through very small incisions using endoscopic instruments. A variety of procedures are undertaken, such as cholecystectomy. ⇒ Day-care surgery, Endoscopy.

MIOSIS (MYOSIS)

Miosis is the constriction of the pupil of the eye. Drugs that constrict the pupil, such as pilocarpine, are termed miotics (myotics, see *Table 18*).

MISCARRIAGE

⇒ Early pregnancy problems.

MITOSIS

Mitosis is the process of nuclear division, usually followed by division of cytoplasm (cytokinesis), whereby body (somatic) cells replicate themselves. The precise replication of the genetic material of the cell results in two genetically identical 'daughter' cells that retain the diploid ($2n$) chromosome number (46 in humans).

It is not known exactly what triggers cells to divide. In part, this may depend on the attainment of a critical mass and/or nuclear to cell surface ratio, but some cells are able to divide without prior growth in size.

Mitosis is preceded by a period of preparation known as the interphase. The preparations include:
• Replication of the DNA complement of the chromosomes;
• Replication of the centrioles;
• Synthesis of proteins from which the fibres of the mitotic spindle are formed;
• Metabolic production of adequate energy to undergo cell division. ⇒ Cell (cell cycle).

Mitosis is a continuous process, but is usually described as a series of stages (*Fig. 121*):
• Prophase – the chromatin condenses and shortens to form visible chromosomes (there is a double set of chromosomes that result from DNA replication during interphase). The double chromosomes are joined by the

M

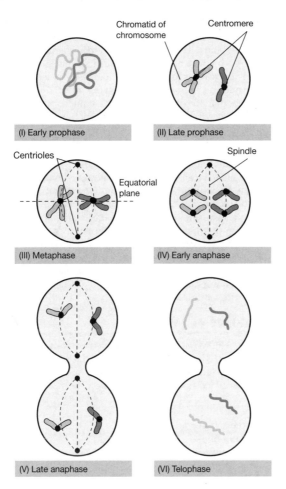

Fig 121 The stages of mitosis – only one chromosome pair is shown

centromere. Each half of this double chromosome is known as a chromatid. The nucleoli start to break down and the nuclear membrane disintegrates. Each pair of centrioles moves to opposite poles of the cell, where they commence the formation of the mitotic spindle, which eventually reaches from one pair of centrioles to the other.

- Metaphase – during metaphase, the double chromosomes move towards the middle of the cell so that their centromeres are arranged along the equator of the mitotic spindle.
- Anaphase – during anaphase the double chromosomes split at the centromere with each chromatid becoming a complete chromosome with its own centromere. The fibres of the mitotic spindle contract, which causes one chromosome from each new pair to be pulled to the opposite pole of the cell.
- Telophase – in telophase the set of chromosomes at each pole uncoils to form the thread-like chromatin. Other changes include the formation of a cleavage furrow that encircles the cell, and reversal of the events that occur during prophase (the nuclear membrane reforms, the mitotic spindle disappears and the nucleoli reform).

Cytokinesis (cytoplasmic division) is a separate process that occurs after mitosis. The cleavage furrow that forms round the cell during late anaphase continues to progress inwards during the telophase. This continues until the original cell is pinched into two 'daughter' cells, each with a nucleus that contains identical genetic material.

Nuclear division is not always followed by cytokinesis, which means some cells have more than one nucleus, such as may be seen in skeletal muscle. The two new cells, which are smaller than the original cell, now commence the cell cycle at interphase and a period of growth before their own division. ⇒ Meiosis.

MOBILITY

In a physical context, mobility refers to a person's ability to walk, rise from and return to a bed, chair, lavatory and so on, as well as movements of the upper limbs needed to undertake the activities of daily living. However, the person's level of mobility, or impaired mobility, can have far-reaching psychological and social effects.

The comprehensive assessment of mobility requires the integrated input of a multidisciplinary team that includes physiotherapists, occupational therapists, nurses and doctors. The assessment process should include range of movement (see below), balance, body alignment, gait and exercise tolerance. Various assessment tools may be used, such as the Barthel ADL scale that measures the degree of dependency. Interventions are designed to promote as near-normal mobility as possible. ⇒ Exercise, Rehabilitation.

RANGE OF MOVEMENT (MOTION)

Range of movements (ROM) are the movements normally possible at a joint. Movement at synovial joints is limited by the shape of the articulating bones and the structure of extracapsular (and sometimes intracapsular) ligaments. Other limiting factors are the strength and tension of adjacent muscles. The movements are (*Fig. 122*):

- Circumduction;
- Rotation;
- Protraction and retraction;
- Abduction and adduction;
- Inversion and eversion;
- Supination and pronation;
- Extension and flexion.

Some disorders of movement are outlined in *Box 23*.

Box 23 Disorders of movement

Ataxia – ill-timed and unco-ordinated movements.

Akathisia – a subjective state of persistent motor restlessness, which can occur as a side-effect of antipsychotic (neuroleptic) drugs.

Akinesia – impairment in initiation of movement or delay in reaction time.

Bradykinesia – abnormally slow or retarded movement associated with difficulty initiating and then stopping a movement, it is typically seen in Parkinson's disease.

Dyskinesia (clumsy child syndrome) – impairment of voluntary movement, or involuntary purposeless movement.

Dysmetria – difficulty in assessing and achieving the correct distance and range of movement that results in undershooting or overshooting a target and the appearance of homing in on it.

Dyspraxia – lack of voluntary control over muscles, particularly the orofacial ones.

Dyssynergia – loss of fluency of movement, poor sequencing and timing of movements, loss of co-ordination of muscles that normally act in unison (particularly the abnormal state of muscle activity caused by cerebellar disease).

M

Dystonia – a movement disorder that involves the abnormal posture of a part of the body, of which examples are spasmodic torticollis and writer's cramp.
Chorea – irregular and jerky dance-like movements that are beyond the patient's control.
Hyperkinesis – excessive movement.
Tic – purposeless involuntary, spasmodic muscular movements and twitchings, partly through habit, but may also be associated with a psychological factor.
Tremor – rhythmic movement disorder that can affect any part of the body, but typically the hands, and that can be seen in Parkinson's disease. *Intention tremor*, a type of tremor that becomes manifest as the hand approaches the target, typically seen in disease of the cerebellum.

MOBILITY AIDS

Mobility aids include walking sticks, tripod sticks, Zimmer frames, crutches and wheelchairs (see Practice application). Nurses must know how to use the aids effectively and safely, and be able to instruct patients and their carers correctly to avoid problems caused by improper usage.

Practice application – safe use of wheelchairs

The nurse has a key role in enabling patients a degree of mobility through the use of wheelchairs, while at the same time ensuring that patient safety is maintained. The following are general principles that relate to safe wheelchair use (the focus is on manual wheelchairs, but the principles apply equally to powered chairs):

- Wheelchairs should only be used if in a good condition;
- Putting heavy loads on the back of a manual wheelchair may alter the balance and increase the likelihood of tipping;
- Beware of caster flutter (rapid side-to-side motion of the caster), which usually happens at high speed (e.g. when going downhill) and can throw the patient forwards out of the chair;
- Always lock the brakes before the patient climbs in or out of the chair;
- Avoid injury by lifting the footplates up before helping the patient in or out of the chair;
- Always point the casters in the forwards position before changing the patient's position (i.e. leaning forwards or to the side) by moving the wheelchair forwards and then reversing it in a straight line;
- Ensure that any removable arms or leg rests are secure before use;
- Do not make any adjustments or modifications to a prescribed wheelchair or cushion;
- Keep loose objects away from the wheel spokes;
- Instruct patients not to move their buttocks (even partially) from the seat to reach forwards when their feet are on the footrests, and explain that patients should not attempt to retrieve objects from the floor by reaching down between the knees;
- Check tyres pressure;
- When transferring to and from a wheelchair, patients should be positioned as close as possible to the seat or bed they are transferring to. Point the casters in the same direction as the seat or bed. Remove or flip back the wheelchair armrests on the transfer side and position the legs in the direction of the wheelchair.

M

M

Circumduction:
A combination of movements that makes a body part describe a circle.

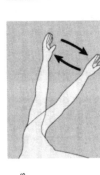

Rotation:
The pivoting of a body part around its axis, as in shaking the head. No rotation of any body is complete (i.e., 360 degrees).

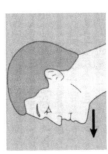

Protraction:
The protrusion of some body part, e.g. the lower jaw.

Retraction:
The opposite of protraction.

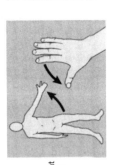

Abduction:
A movement of a bone or limb away from the median plane of the body. Abduction in the hands and feet is the movement of a digit away from the central axis of the limb.
One abducts the fingers by spreading them apart.

Adduction:
The opposite of Abduction, involving approach to the median plane of the body or, in the case of the limbs, to the central axis of a limb.

Fig 122 Types of movement of synovial joints (cont.)

Inversion:
An ankle movement that turns the sole of the foot medially. Applies only to the foot.

Eversion:
The opposite of inversion. It turns the sole of the foot laterally.

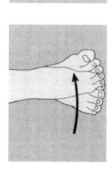
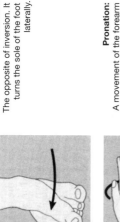

Supination:
The opposite of pronation. When the forearm is in the extended position, this movement brings the palm of the hand upward.

Pronation:
A movement of the forearm that in the extended position brings the palm of the hand to a downward position. Applies only to the forearm.

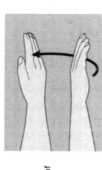
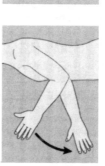

Extension:
The opposite of flexion, it increases the angle between two movably articulated bones, usually to a 180-degree maximum. If the angle of extension exceeds 180-degrees (as is possible when throwing back the head), this action is termed hyperextension.

Flexion:
The bending of a joint; usually a movement that reduces the angle that two movably activated bones make with each other. When one crouches, the knees are flexed.

Fig 122 (cont.) Types of movement of synovial joints

M

POTENTIAL COMPLICATIONS OF IMMOBILITY

Potential complications of immobility are:
- Deep vein thrombosis;
- Chest infection;
- Pressure ulcer formation;
- Increase in body fat;
- Negative nitrogen balance;
- Constipation, faecal impaction with overflow diarrhoea;
- Appetite changes;
- Loss of muscle mass;
- Joint stiffness;
- Contractures;
- Bone reabsorption giving rise to osteoporosis;
- Increased blood levels of calcium (hypercalcaemia);
- Renal calculi;
- Boredom;
- Mood disorders.

⇒ Musculoskeletal disorders (osteoporosis), Deep vein thrombosis, Defecation, Disorders of mood, Pressure ulcers.

MONITORING

Monitoring is sequential recording. The term is also used to describe the regular observation of a patient's condition. Various parameters, such as skin colour, temperature, pulse, respiration, blood pressure, cardiac rhythm or intracranial pressure, are monitored visually, manually or by automatic visual display. ⇒ Observations and observing.

MONOCLONAL ANTIBODIES

Monoclonal antibodies are antibodies derived from a single cell. These highly specific antibodies are used for research, diagnosis and therapy.

Monoclonal antibodies are a fairly recent addition to the range of treatment options for haematological malignancies and other conditions that include some types of inflammatory bowel disease. Monoclonal antibodies harness the body's natural immune system to destroy malignant cells. Different types of cell have specific antigens on their surface. The theory behind monoclonal antibody therapy is that, if the antigens on the surface of tumour cells can be identified, genetically engineered antibodies can be generated to target and destroy the tumour cells. Monoclonal antibodies are an exciting development in cancer care and are being used increasingly alongside standard treatments.

Practice application – monoclonal antibody administration

Monoclonal antibodies are targeted specifically; therefore, they do not cause the same array of side-effects as conventional chemotherapy. Monoclonal antibodies are given by intravenous infusion. The most common complications of treatment are infusion-related reactions. Patients who receive monoclonal antibodies should be observed closely for signs of adverse reaction, such as shivering, fever or dyspnoea. A patient's vital signs should be monitored throughout the infusion. Reactions can usually be treated with paracetamol, antihistamines (e.g. chlorphenamine) or bronchodilators (e.g. salbutamol). As the first dose of a monoclonal antibody can sometimes cause tumour lysis syndrome, patients should have a fluid input of 3 L in 24 hours and their urine output should be monitored. ⇒ Tumour (tumour lysis syndrome).

MONOCYTE–MACROPHAGE SYSTEM

⇒ Defence mechanisms (phagocytosis, inflammatory response), Leucocytes (mononuclear–macrophage system).

MOOD

A general overview of predominant feelings, which includes past and current affective experiences. Variations in mood are normal, but frequent swings from depression to over-excitement may be considered abnormal. ⇒ Disorders of mood.

SEASONAL AFFECTIVE DISORDER

While most individuals feel a little less energetic and enthusiastic as winter months approach, this is usually a subtle change accompanied by a similar slight lowering of mood. However, some individuals find that a significant depressed mood coincides with the onset of winter, only to lift with the arrival of spring. This is seasonal affective disorder (SAD), a condition linked to the amount of melatonin secreted by the pineal body and/or gland (on the surface of the midbrain). Melatonin secretion is light dependent, and hence the treatment of choice for SAD is exposure to bright white light during the autumn and winter, in addition to natural light.

MORTALITY

Mortality is being subject to death (mortal).

DEATH RATE

The annual death rate is expressed as the number of deaths times 1000 and divided by the mid-year population. Various specialized mortality rates and ratios are described in *Box 24*.

M

Box 24 Specialized mortality rates

- Childhood mortality is the number of deaths in children aged 1–14 years in a defined area per 100 000 resident children of that age.
- Infant mortality is the number of infant deaths in the first year of life per 1000 related live births.
- Maternal mortality is the number of women who die from causes associated with pregnancy and childbirth per 1000 total births.
- Neonatal mortality is the number of deaths in the first 4 weeks of life per 1000 related live births.
- Perinatal mortality is the number of stillbirths plus deaths in the first week of life per 1000 total births.
- Postneonatal mortality is the number of deaths in infants from 28 days to 1 year of age per 1000 live births.
- Standardized mortality rate is the number of deaths per 1000 population standardized for age.
- Standardized mortality ratio (SMR) allows comparisons to be made between the death rates in populations with different sex and age structures. It involves the application of national age-specific mortality rates to local populations so that a ratio of expected deaths to actual deaths can be calculated. The figure obtained is multiplied by 100 to give the local SMR. The comparative national figure is, by convention, 100 and, for example, a local figure of 108 means there is an increased risk of 8% and, conversely, a local figure of 92 indicates a risk 8% lower than the national rate.
- Stillbirth rate is the number of stillbirths per 1000 total births to women in that area.

Moving and Handling (Manual Handling)

Many hospitals, other institutions and community trusts are working towards safer-handling or no-lifting policies. This requires proper training and regular updating of all staff in the use of mechanical lifting equipment, such as hoists, as well as sliding transfer aids and other equipment and techniques.

The principles of safe handling are:
- Assess the situation and risks – task, load and client, physical environment, equipment and individual handler;
- Planning – prepare client, equipment and environment;
- Record the task;
- Communicate clearly, so that all involved know what to expect;
- Avoid tensing the muscles;
- Adopt a 'stable' stance – this usually means having your feet about a hip-width apart;
- Keep your knees 'soft' or bent;
- Keep the load as close to your body as possible – avoid stretching;
- Avoid twisting or bending sideways;
- Careful evaluation of the task.

MOVING AND HANDLING EQUIPMENT

Equipment may include (*Fig. 123*):
- Hoists;
- Sliding equipment (e.g. boards, sheets);
- Transfer equipment, belts;
- Turning equipment (e.g. turntables).

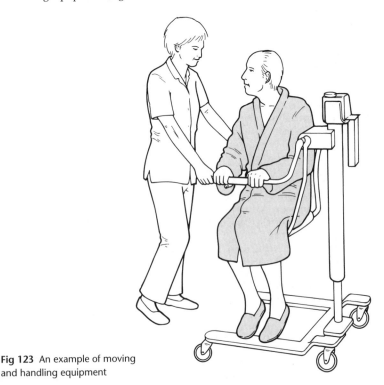

Fig 123 An example of moving and handling equipment

Practice application – assessing risk in moving and handling
It must be acknowledged that assessment tools are simply an aid to nurses. Knowledge and professional judgement are also needed to select the appropriate manoeuvre. Once it is established that the risk is low, medium or high, planning the handling task follows more easily. However, no handling situation is without risk. The risk of injury can only be minimized. Two examples of assessment tools are the Pilling lifting and/or handling risk calculator (Pilling and Frank 1994) and the patient handling assessment form.
The Pilling lifting/handling risk calculator
In assessing mobility, body weight, psychological state, environment, staff, carer and other risk factors, appropriate numerical scores are allocated to the patient and these are added together on a calculator sheet. If the score is over ten, specific actions need to be planned for the patient. The reverse side of the calculator sheet gives carers guidance on actions and aids that may need to be used. Using the score and the guidance offered, carers can begin to formulate a handling plan specific to the client's needs. This form was originally developed for use in the community setting, but can be adapted to any area.
Patient handling assessment form
The patient handling assessment form does not use numerical scoring and is therefore a less objective system than one that does. However, numerical scoring systems can sometimes be inflexible and there may be situations in which it is not justifiable to ignore any risks simply because a set score is not reached.

By not using a numerical score, the nurse needs to account for the whole picture of the patient and has to use professional knowledge of patient handling to make a considered judgement about the level of risk. As such, the more experienced the nurse the more accurate the assessment of risk is likely to be. If when using this form you are in doubt as to the level of risk it is advisable to identify the higher risk and take this into account when planning care.

M

MULTIDISCIPLINARY TEAM AND WORKING

The context of care is changing rapidly (e.g. the needs of an ageing population, increasing care delivery in the community, technological advances, 'new' diseases, etc.). Changes require more effective multidisciplinary teamwork and nurses are required to work flexibly and collaboratively with a range of professionals and agencies. This is as much of a challenge for staff in other disciplines as it is for nurses, but nurses are well placed to foster teamwork, which becomes increasingly important for high-quality healthcare.

The use of integrated care pathways requires multidisciplinary team (MDT) working, bringing together all the professionals involved in delivering care to a chosen patient group. ⇒ Integrated care pathway.

Each professional's role within the care cycle is clearly defined, which helps to improve communication between professional groups and reduces duplication. As patient outcomes are also specified in advance, each member of the team (and the patient and their carer) has a clear view of what is expected of him or her.

The composition of the MDT differs according to the patient group. For example, a person having hip-replacement surgery may have input from the following:
• Primary healthcare team – practice nurse, district nurse, general practitioner, physiotherapist, pharmacist, phlebotomist;
• Social services – social worker, home carer;
• Hospital team – nurses, healthcare assistants, surgeon, anaesthetist, radiologist, operating department practitioner, radiographer, dietician, physiotherapist, occupational therapist, pharmacist, etc.

Multiple Organ Dysfunction Syndrome

Multiple organ dysfunction syndrome (MODS) describes a syndrome in critically ill patients in which more than one organ system (e.g. kidneys, respiratory, coagulation and gastrointestinal) fails to function normally, and which may progress to multiple organ failure. It requires appropriate organ support, such as haemofiltration and mechanical ventilation. ⇒ Haemostasis (disseminated intravascular coagulation), Renal failure, Respiratory system (acute respiratory distress syndrome), Shock, Systemic inflammatory response syndrome.

Munchausen Syndrome

In Munchausen syndrome patients consistently produce false stories so they receive needless medical investigations, operations and treatments.

MUNCHAUSEN SYNDROME BY PROXY

Munchausen syndrome by proxy (MSP) is the term used when a carer (usually the mother, both parents or other carers) produces false stories for the child and falsifies signs and symptoms. Carers feign or create illnesses in children and, as a result, subject them to extensive and unnecessary medical investigation and treatment. MSP usually meets four criteria:
- The child's illness has been fabricated by the parent or carer;
- The child is persistently presented for medical care, which results in multiple investigative procedures;
- The perpetrator denies the cause of the child's illness;
- The acute features of the child's illness are not present in the absence of the perpetrator.

Nurses are in a good position to observe family relationships and the care of the child, and careful record keeping is vital in any suspected case of MSP. Covert videoing has been used to observe parents in hospital, but this method of observation has raised concerns about the invasion of privacy, breach of trust and possible compromise of the role of the health professionals involved.

Allitt Inquiry (Clothier Report 1994)

The Clothier Report is a report of an independent inquiry team into the events that surrounded deaths and injuries to children in the care of one particular nurse in an English hospital. It includes recommendations designed to strengthen procedures that safeguard children in hospital and to prevent any repetition of such events.

Further reading

Clothier Report (19940. *Independent Inquiry Relating to Deaths and Injuries on the Children's Ward at Grantham and Kesteven General Hospital*. London: HMSO.
Crouse K (1992). Munchausen syndrome by proxy: Recognizing the victim. *Paediatric Nursing* **18**(3): 349–352.

Muscle

Muscle is one of four basic body tissues. There are three types of muscle tissue, which consists of specialized contractile cells. ⇒ Tissues.

SKELETAL MUSCLE TISSUE (STRIATED, STRIPED OR VOLUNTARY MUSCLE)

Each cylindrical muscle cell or fibre has several nuclei situated just under the sarcolemma or cell membrane of each muscle fibre (*Fig. 124B*).

The sarcoplasm, the cytoplasm of muscle fibres, contains:
- Bundles of myofibrils (filaments of contractile proteins);
- Many mitochondria, which generate energy;
- Glycogen;
- Myoglobin, an oxygen-binding protein molecule, which stores oxygen within muscle cells.

A myofibril has a repeating series of dark and light bands, which consist of units called sarcomeres (smallest functional unit of a skeletal muscle fibre) and consists of:
- Thin filaments of actin, troponin and tropomyosin;
- Thick filaments of myosin.

The *sliding filament theory* explains the finding that sarcomeres shorten but the filaments remain the same length when skeletal muscle contracts. The thin actin filaments slide past the thick myosin filaments, which increases the overlap of the filaments when contraction takes place. As the sarcomeres shorten, so does the skeletal muscle involved. When the muscle relaxes, the filaments slide apart and the sarcomeres return to their original length (*Fig. 124C*).

An individual skeletal muscle consists of a large number of muscle fibres. In addition to the sarcolemma mentioned above, each fibre is enclosed in a fine fibrous connective tissue called endomysium. Small bundles of fibres are enclosed in perimysium, and the whole muscle in epimysium. The fibrous tissue that encloses the fibres, the bundles and the whole muscle extends beyond the muscle fibres to become the tendon, which attaches the muscle to bone or skin (*Fig. 124A*).

The skeletal muscle mass forms 40–50% of the body weight in an adult. It is divided into nearly 700 individual muscles, such as the deltoid and psoas, which form the musculature of the body.

M

SMOOTH (VISCERAL) MUSCLE TISSUE

Smooth muscle may also be described as nonstriated or involuntary muscle. It is not under conscious control, is found in the walls of hollow organs and it:
- Regulates the diameter of blood vessels and parts of the respiratory tract;
- Propels the contents of the ureters, ducts of glands and alimentary tract;
- Expels the contents of the urinary bladder and uterus.

When examined under a microscope, the cells are seen to be spindle shaped with only one central nucleus. There is no distinct sarcolemma, but a very fine membrane surrounds each fibre. Bundles of fibres form sheets of muscle, such as those found in the walls of the above structures.

CARDIAC MUSCLE TISSUE

Cardiac muscle tissue is found exclusively in the myocardium, and is not under conscious control. Each fibre (cell) has a nucleus and one or more branches. There is very close contact between the ends and branches of adjacent cells (intercalated discs). This arrangement gives cardiac muscle the appearance of a sheet of muscle rather than a very large number of individual fibres. The end-to-end continuity of cardiac muscle cells has significance in relation to the way the heart contracts. A wave of contraction spreads from cell to cell across the intercalated discs, which means that cells do not need to be stimulated individually.

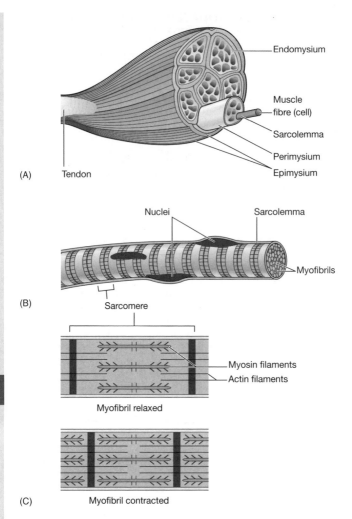

(A) Tendon

(B)

(C) Myofibril contracted

Fig 124 Organization within a skeletal muscle: (A) a skeletal muscle and its connective tissue, (B) a muscle fibre (cell), (C) a myofibril – relaxed and contracted

FUNCTION OF MUSCLE TISSUE

Muscle functions by alternate phases of contraction and relaxation. When the fibres contract they become thicker and shorter. Skeletal muscle fibres are stimulated by motor nerve impulses that originate in the brain or spinal cord and end at the neuromuscular junction. Smooth and cardiac muscle have the intrinsic ability to initiate contraction. In addition, contraction is stimulated by autonomic nerve impulses, some hormones and local metabolites.

When muscle fibres contract they follow the *all-or-none law* (i.e. each fibre contracts to its full capacity or not at all). The strength of contraction (e.g. lifting a weight) depends on the number of fibres that contract at the same time. When effort is sustained, groups of fibres contract in series. Contraction of smooth muscle is slower and more sustained than that of skeletal muscle.

To contract when it is stimulated, a muscle fibre must have an adequate blood supply to provide sufficient oxygen, calcium and nutrients and to remove waste products.

MUSCULOSKELETAL DISORDERS

Musculoskeletal disorders have a variety of origins, which include trauma, inflammatory disorders, muscle disorders, back problems, etc. ⇒ Fracture, Joint (joint diseases, joint injuries), Muscle, Rheumatic disorders, Skeleton, Traction.

SPRAINS AND STRAINS

A *sprain* is an injury to the soft tissues that surround a joint, and results in discolouration, swelling and pain. There is stretching or tearing of a ligament or capsular structure of a joint.

A *strain* is an injury caused by twisting or pulling a muscle or tendon. Severity of a strain ranges from a simple overstretching of the muscle or tendon to a partial or complete tear.

Practice application – the management of sprains and strains

Essentially, treatment for sprains and strains is similar and can be thought of as having two stages.

1 Reduction in pain and swelling – 'RICE' (rest, ice, compression and elevation) regimen for the first 24–48 hours, and nonsteroidal anti-inflammatory drugs (NSAIDs), such as ibuprofen.

2 Rehabilitation (i.e. to improve the condition of the injured part to restore functional ability) for which a physiotherapist usually prescribes an exercise programme designed to prevent stiffness, improve and maintain normal range of movement and restore the joint's normal flexibility and strength.

BONE AND CARTILAGE DISORDERS

Some disorders of bone and cartilage are outlined below.

ACHONDROPLASIA

Achondroplasia is an inherited disorder characterized by restricted growth of the long bones caused by premature ossification of the epiphyseal plates. It results in short stature of varying degrees because the long bones are abnormally 'short', but the trunk and most of the skull develop normally. Inheritance is dominant.

OSTEITIS

Osteitis is the inflammation of bone.

OSTEOCHONDRITIS

Originally described as inflammation of bone cartilage, osteochondritis is usually applied to nonseptic conditions, especially avascular necrosis that involves joint surfaces (e.g. *osteochondritis dissecans*, in which a portion of joint surface may separate to form a loose body in the joint – see Osteochondrosis below).

OSTEOCHONDROSIS

Osteochondrosis is an idiopathic disease characterized by a disorder of the ossification of hyaline cartilage (endochondral). It encompasses a group of syndromes classified on the basis of their anatomical location:

1 Primary articular epiphysis – *Freiberg's disease* and *Köhler's disease*;
2 secondary articular epiphysis – *osteochondritis dissecans* of the talus;
3 nonarticular epiphysis (apophyseal injury) – *Sever's disease*.

The osteochondroses occur during the years of rapid growth. Their aetiology has been linked to hereditary factors, trauma, nutritional factors and ischaemia. The articular osteochondroses, such as Freiberg's and Köhler's diseases and osteochondritis dissecans, are characterized by fragmentation with a centre of ossification.

OSTEOGENESIS IMPERFECTA

Osteogenesis imperfecta is a group of hereditary disorders characterized by fragile bones that result in multiple fractures at birth or during childhood.

OSTEOMALACIA

Osteomalacia is softening of the bone with pain and eventual deformity. There is a failure to mineralize the osteoid. It is caused by lack of vitamin D (dietary or lack of exposure to sunlight; see Rickets below).

OSTEOMYELITIS

Osteomyelitis is inflammation that starts in the marrow of bone, and is usually caused by acute or chronic bacterial infection.

OSTEOPETROSIS (ALBERS–SCHÖNBERG DISEASE, MARBLE BONES)

Osteopetrosis is a congenital abnormality that gives rise to very dense bones that fracture easily. Loss of medullary space and haemopoeitic marrow leads to problems with blood cell production.

OSTEOPOROSIS

Osteoporosis is loss of bone density caused by excessive absorption of calcium and phosphorus from bone, as a result of progressive loss of the protein matrix of the bone. The bones deform and fracture more easily, and fractures of the wrist, vertebrae and neck of femur are especially common. Causes include ageing in both sexes, nutritional deficiencies, immobility, postmenopausal decline in oestrogens, Cushing's disease and corticosteroid therapy.

Practice application – nursing management of osteoporosis
The main aspects of nursing management include:
- Review of the diet, which involves an increased intake of calcium, protein and vitamin D, and is often worthwhile;
- Administration and education relating to medication [e.g. oestrogen hormone replacement therapy (HRT) for woman, or bisphosphonates];
- Advice and encouragement to take weight-bearing exercise and increase general activity;
- Advice about reducing alcohol intake and smoking cessation, as both excess alcohol intake and smoking are associated with osteoporosis;
- Advice aimed at preventing accidents and falls.

Many of these nursing interventions, including advice about accident prevention, are performed by those who work in community settings or outpatient departments.

PAGET'S DISEASE OF BONE (OSTEITIS DEFORMANS)

Paget's disease of bone is associated with increased bone reabsorption and production. Excess of the enzyme alkaline phosphatase causes too rapid bone formation, and consequently bone is thin.

RICKETS

Rickets is a bone disease caused by a lack of vitamin D during infancy and childhood (prior to ossification of the epiphyses), which results from a low dietary intake or insufficient exposure to sunlight. This leads to abnormal calcium and phosphate metabolism with faulty ossification and poor bone growth.

Rickets may be secondary to malabsorption of vitamin D (e.g. in coeliac disease), to defective metabolism (e.g. with certain drugs) and to chronic renal failure. Treatment is with vitamin D and sufficient calcium. Some types of inherited rickets are resistant to treatment (see Osteomalacia above).

TUMOURS OF BONE

Bone tumours may be benign, malignant sarcomas or metastatic carcinomas. In bone there are two potential responses to the tumour. Either increased osteoclast activity with associated bone loss and weakening, or more commonly increased bone formation around the tumour as a consequence of increased osteoblast activity. It is not uncommon for benign tumours to become malignant if left untreated. Osteochondroma is a benign bony and cartilaginous tumour.

MUSCULAR DYSTROPHIES

The muscular dystrophies are a group of genetically transmitted diseases, all characterized by the progressive atrophy of different groups of muscles with loss of strength and increasing disability and deformity.

Duchenne muscular dystrophy (DMD) is an X-linked recessive disorder that affects boys only. The disorder usually begins to show between 3 and 5 years and is characterized by progressive muscle weakness and loss of locomotor skills. Death from respiratory or cardiac failure usually occurs during the teens or early twenties.

Unfortunately, no cure is available and current management focuses on the symptoms. For people with breathing problems an incentive spirometer might improve breathing function, and appropriate antibiotics are prescribed for chest infections.

Treatment for contractures includes physiotherapy, good limb positioning and different kinds of bracing, all used as preventative measures. Baclofen and other skeletal muscle relaxants may be given to reduce the spasticity that contributes to their development. Sometimes surgery is necessary in very severe cases. It may be recommended that people with myopathies try to keep body weight within an acceptable range to avoid overexerting their muscles.

Nurses have a vital role in supporting and educating the patient and their family. Of particular importance is education about drugs, physiotherapy, activity level, diet and teaching carers how to assist with affected activities of daily living. As the disease progresses there is the need to increase health and social care support at home and in other community settings.

Assessment of the home environment and provision of aids to daily functioning is undertaken by the occupational therapist. Genetic counsellors can provide information on the risk of passing on the disease to children. Again, the nurse is in an ideal position to provide referral for this and other specialist services, including local education services.

Patients and family members should be advised on support groups related to their condition.

M

BACK PROBLEMS AND BACK PAIN

Back problems are a major cause of days lost from work, inability to undertake activities of living, inconvenience and pain.

MUSCULOSKELETAL BACK PAIN

The most common type of back pain is musculoskeletal in origin, and results from some mechanical problem with the back muscles, bones, joints or ligaments. It is usually a result of abuse, overuse or underuse of the back. Individuals with occupations that require excessive lifting, bending and heavy work on a routine basis may be more prone to develop this condition. Nurses have been prime candidates for back problems in the past, because of poor handling techniques and lack of specialist equipment. ⇒ Moving and handling.

In addition, the ageing process commonly contributes to the development of back pain. There is pain and, as with any pain, there is decreased mobility in the affected part. Back pain often also occurs as a result of other pathologies (e.g. rheumatoid arthritis, primary and secondary tumour, osteoporosis and infection).

HERNIATED OR PROLAPSED INTERVERTEBRAL DISC

A 'slipped disc', or more correctly a herniated or prolapsed intervertebral disc, most commonly occurs in the lumbar and cervical areas. The pressure that the disc puts on the nerve roots usually causes neurological symptoms in addition to the pain. A person may feel numbness, tingling, burning, aching or a shooting pain down a limb. Some patients may develop motor weakness.

Damage in the lumbar region is often termed *sciatica* because these processes can irritate the sciatic nerve, the largest nerve in the body, which extends down through the buttock and the leg to the foot.

If the herniated disc material compresses the spinal cord itself and not the nerve roots, other symptoms can include weakness along one entire side of the body, numbness and bowel or bladder complications. The particular symptoms depend on which neurological pathways are affected.

MANAGEMENT OF BACK PAIN AND PROBLEMS

Management depends on the cause, and whether the pain is acute or chronic. It includes:

- Restricted bed rest (note that too much bed rest can make the situation worse).
- Appropriate back-strengthening exercise.
- Pain control, such as mild analgesics (e.g. paracetamol and NSAIDs) or stronger prescription drugs for more severe pain. Muscle relaxants (e.g. orphenadrine and diazepam) are often used to treat muscular spasm or related neurological problems and are often combined with NSAIDs for pain relief. Tizanidine is used to treat muscular spasticity as well as chronic back pain, especially musculoskeletal back pain. ⇒ Nonsteroidal anti-inflammatory drugs, Opioids.
- Tricyclic antidepressants (e.g. amitriptyline) are used in low doses for chronic back pain.
- Physiotherapy techniques may include exercises, massage, ultrasound, a cold application (within the first 48 hours) and warmth and spinal manipulation.
- Occupational therapy.

SURGICAL INTERVENTION

Most back pain, especially lower back pain, is self-limiting and disappears with proper care. Clearly, though, some people have more serious conditions and/or still experience pain or other problems despite other forms of therapy. Techniques include:

- Discectomy (termed a microdiscectomy) performed through a small laminectomy (surgical procedure, which includes removal of a portion of the lamina, to provide more room in the vertebral canal) and an operating microscope;
- Spinal fusion (e.g. trauma and spinal instability);
- Implantation of specialized system 'pumps' that deliver a constant rate of medication or stimulation to the spinal area.

MYCOBACTERIUM

A genus of Gram-positive acid-fast bacteria. *Mycobacterium tuberculosis* causes most infections of tuberculosis, but *M. bovis*, which causes tuberculosis in cattle, can be transmitted to humans by milk.

Atypical mycobacteria, which include *M. avium intracellulare* (MAI) and *M. kansasii*, cause both pulmonary and nonpulmonary infection in humans. Individuals who are immunocompromised are particularly susceptible. Disseminated infection with mycobacterium is a problem in patients with human immunodeficiency virus (HIV) and/or acquired immune deficiency syndrome (AIDS). In general, these organisms show *in vitro* resistance to many of the anti-tuberculosis drugs and treatment is often difficult.

Leprosy is caused by *M. leprae*. ⇒ Leprosy, Tuberculosis.

MYDRIASIS

Mydriasis is dilatation of the pupil of the eye. Drugs that dilate the pupil, such as atropine sulphate and phenylephrine hydrochloride, are termed mydriatics (see *Table 18*).

MYELOPROLIFERATIVE DISORDERS

A myeloproliferative disorder is any condition (premalignant or malignant) characterized by a proliferation of one or more of the cellular components of the bone marrow. They include myelofibrosis (formation of fibrous tissue within the bone marrow cavity), primary polycythaemia and thrombocythaemia. ⇒ Erythrocyte (polycythaemia), Platelets (thrombocythaemia).

M

NAIL

The nails are keratinized sheets that protect the distal ends of the digits and are used in some tasks that require fine movements (*Fig. 125*). They are derived from epidermal cells and each nail grows on a vascular nail bed. A nail has a root, a body and a free edge. At the proximal edge, the nail is thickened to form the white lunula covered by the cuticle (eponychium). An abundant capillary network in the dermis means that in health the nail appears pink.

Common nail disorders are outlined in *Box 25*.

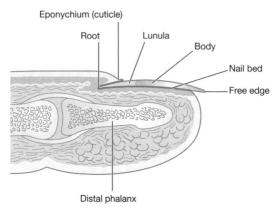

Fig 125 Section through the distal phalynx and nail

Box 25 Nail disorders

Koilonychia – spoon-shaped nails. The normal convex curvature of the nail is lost and it becomes slightly concave. It is associated with iron-deficiency anaemia.

Onychia – acute inflammation of the matrix and nail bed; suppuration may spread beneath the nail, causing it to become detached. It frequently originates from paronychia.

Onychocryptosis (ingrowing nail) – part of the nail pierces the epidermis of the sulcus and penetrates the dermis, most frequently in the hallux of male adolescents. The portion of nail penetrates further into the tissues to produce acute inflammation, which often becomes infected (paronychia), and results in excess granulation tissue.

Onychomycosis (tinea unguium) – a fungal infection of the nail bed and plate. The nail plate becomes thickened, brittle and yellowish brown in colour. Eventually it develops a porous appearance.

Paronychia (whitlow) – inflammation of the tissue around a nail plate, which may be bacterial or fungal. It frequently occurs with onychia.

NAMED NURSE

A concept introduced in the UK in *The Patient's Charter* (Department of Health 1991b), which promises that 'Each patient will be told the name of the qualified nurse or midwife who will be responsible for his or her nursing/midwifery care when admitted to hospital, or midwife, community nurse or health visitor when in need of care in the community.' One qualified nurse, midwife or health visitor is accountable for the care of each patient or client and, wherever possible, the same nurse should care for, or supervise care for, the same patient during the time that person needs nursing, midwifery or health-visiting care. The named nurse concept can be operated within primary nursing, team nursing or the patient-allocation model. ⇒ Primary nursing, Team nursing.

NATIONAL CARE STANDARDS COMMISSION (NCSC)

⇒ Commission for Healthcare Audit and Inspection, Commission for Social Care Inspection.

NATIONAL CONFIDENTIAL ENQUIRIES

The national confidential enquiries were established to examine clinical performance and serious avoidable events. The results of the enquiries now form a key part of the data to be considered by the quality bodies, such as the National Institute of Clinical Effectiveness (NICE). Relevant clinicians have a legal duty to participate in the enquiries. The four enquiries are:
- National confidential enquiry into perioperative deaths (NCEPOD);
- Confidential enquiry into stillbirths and deaths in infancy (CESDI);
- Confidential enquiry into maternal deaths (CEMD);
- Confidential enquiry into suicide and homicide by people with mental illness (CISH).

NATIONAL INSTITUTE FOR CLINICAL EXCELLENCE

The National Institute of Clinical Effectiveness (NICE) is an English special health authority (http://www.nice.org.uk), managed by a director and a small executive. The board consists of key health service professionals and lay representation. It has a range of objectives:
- To produce clinical guidance based on relevant evidence of clinical cost-effectiveness;
- To introduce and disseminate associated clinical audit methodologies and information on good practice and clinical audit;
- To bring together work currently being undertaken by the many professional organisations in receipt of Department of Health funding for this purpose;
- To work with a programme agreed with and funded from current resources by the Department of Health.
⇒ Protocols and policies.

NATIONAL SERVICE FRAMEWORKS

National service frameworks (NSFs) bring together the best evidence of clinical and cost-effectiveness with the views of service users to determine the best ways to provide particular patient and care services. The intention is to reduce the 'postcode lottery' of available care and treatment by setting benchmarks and targets for the care and treatment of specific areas of practice. Existing NSFs include:
- Mental health;
- Coronary heart disease;
- The National cancer plan;
- Older people;
- Diabetes mellitus;
- Renal services (part one Dialysis and Transplantation);
- Children, young people and maternity services.
Work on those for renal services and long-term conditions is on-going.

NECROSIS

Necrosis is the localized death of tissue in response to an interruption to the blood supply (e.g. myocardial infarction), infection, chemical or physical injury (e.g. burns), etc. ⇒ Gangrene.

NECROTIZING ENTEROCOLITIS

Necrotizing enterocolitis (NEC) is a condition that occurs primarily in preterm or low-birthweight neonates. Parts of the gut wall become necrotic, which leads to intestinal obstruction and peritonitis. It is probably caused by a combination of ischaemia and infection.

NECROTIZING FASCIITIS

Necrotizing fasciitis is a rare infection caused by some strains of group A *Streptococcus pyogenes*. There is very severe inflammation of the muscle sheath and massive soft-tissue destruction. Effective treatment may require radical excision or even amputation of the affected tissues. Necrotizing fasciitis has a high mortality rate.

NEEDLE PHOBIA

⇒ Injection (Practice application – needle phobia).

NEGLECT

Neglect of children can be life-threatening, such as not feeding them, not keeping them clean and warm or not protecting them from danger. It can range from children's 'failure to thrive' to failure of parents to take children for medical appointments, which impacts seriously on their health. Approximately 25% of children on child-protection registers in the UK are registered under this category of child abuse. Neglect is often caused by ignorance of childcare, and early education of caregivers about children's fundamental physical and emotional needs can help to prevent this abuse. Nurses can help to identify problems by a thorough nursing assessment, which includes finding out about children's usual routines and activities. Manifestations of neglect include physical and behavioural signs, such as malnutrition, poor personal hygiene, inactivity and passivity. ⇒ Abuse.

NEGLIGENCE

Negligence is used to describe an action that is careless and can be an element in a criminal act or the basis of a civil action. Gross negligence, which results in the death of a person, can be the basis of a charge of manslaughter.

As an action brought in the civil courts for compensation, negligence forms one of a group of civil wrongs known as 'torts'. To succeed in an action for negligence, the claimant must establish that a *duty of care* was owed to him or her by the defendant or the defendant's employees, that there has been a breach of this duty of care and, as a reasonably foreseeable consequence of this breach of duty, the claimant has suffered harm. A duty of care exists in law where it can be reasonably foreseen that unless reasonable care is taken, harm could occur. Thus, a nurse has a duty of care to her patients and a driver has a duty of care to other road users. The law does not require a person voluntarily to assume a duty of care; thus, there is no duty in law to go to the assistance of a person involved in a road accident caused by others. The Nursing and Midwifery Council does, however, consider that all its registered practitioners, though not under a legal duty to offer assistance, have a professional duty under the Code of Professional Conduct (NMC 2002a). If a volunteer does assist, then a duty of care is assumed and all reasonable care is required from the volunteer.

The standard of care required by those under a duty of care is to act in accordance with a practice accepted as proper by a responsible body of professionals skilled in that particular art. This standard was laid down in the case of Bolam v. Friern Hospital Management Committee ([1957] 2 All ER 118) and is known as the *Bolam Test*. Experts are required to give evidence to the court over what would be regarded as the reasonable standard of care in the circumstances of the case and whether what actually took place was in accordance with that standard. It is accepted that there may exist different bodies of competent professional opinion over what is reasonable practice in the circumstances (Maynard v. West Midlands RHA [1984] 1 WLR 634). The House of Lords has emphasized that experts must give evidence of opinion that is reasonable, responsible and respectable and has a logical basis (Bolitho v. City and Hackney HA [1997] 4 All ER 771).

The claimant must show on a *balance of probabilities* that there has been a failure to provide a reasonable standard of care and that this failure was a reasonably foreseeable cause of the harm that has been suffered.

The claimant must also establish that he or she has suffered harm to obtain compensation in an action for negligence. This could include personal injury, pain and suffering, loss of amenity and also loss of or damage to property. Where the loss is loss of life, the action can be brought by the personal representatives of the deceased on behalf of the estate, and by dependants upon the deceased.

NEISSERIA SPECIES

Neisseria are Gram-negative cocci that characteristically occur as pairs of cells called diplococci. A number of harmless species form part of the normal flora of the mucous membranes, including the upper respiratory (*N. catarrhalis*) and genital tracts. The two main pathogens are *N. gonorrhoeae* (gonococcus), which causes gonorrhoea, and *N. meningitidis* (meningococcus), which causes meningococcal meningitis or septicaemia. ⇒ Nervous system (meningitis), Sexually transmitted and acquired infections.

NEONATAL

Neonatal relates to the first 28 days of life. ⇒ Mortality (*Box 24*, neonatal mortality).

NEONATAL RESPIRATORY DISTRESS SYNDROME

Neonatal respiratory distress syndrome (NRDS) is respiratory failure caused by surfactant deficiency in the newborn (surfactant is a mixture of phospholipids that reduces surface tension in the alveoli, allows lung expansion and prevents alveolar collapse between breaths). NRDS most commonly affects premature infants – the more immature the greater the risk of this condition, which may be fatal. The deficiency in surfactant leads to atelectasis and hypoxia, which necessitates assisted ventilation and the intratracheal administration of surfactant in seriously affected infants. ⇒ Preterm and/or premature infants.

NEONATAL CHECKS

All newborn babies are checked for a variety of abnormalities. The examinations and tests are outlined below.

PHYSICAL EXAMINATION

A full physical examination to check for physical problems, such as cleft palate, extra digits, neurological problems, heart defects, etc. All babies are weighed, and their length and head circumference are measured.

Blood tests

Blood tests offered as routine include thyroid hormone levels (to exclude hypothyroidism), Guthrie bloodspot card for phenylketonuria (PKU) and cystic fibrosis. Specific blood tests are offered as appropriate, such as those for the haemoglobinopathies.

Hearing tests

In the UK, neonatal hearing is assessed in the first few days of life, using the otoacoustic emissions test (OAE) and/or the automated auditory brainstem response test (AABR). The OAE test measures sound emissions by placing a small probe in the baby's ear. ⇒ Apgar score, Congenital defects (developmental dysplasia of the hip).

NEONATAL UNIT AND NEONATAL INTENSIVE CARE UNIT

The neonatal unit (NNU) or neonatal intensive care unit (NICU) provides dedicated intensive care for neonates, usually reserved for preterm and small-for-dates babies between 700 and 2000 g in weight and who usually require the use of the high technology available in these units. It is staffed by healthcare professionals with the skills and experience required to meet the highly specialized needs of preterm and seriously ill neonates.

A special care baby unit (SCBU) provides specialist care for premature, sick and small-for-dates babies who need extra care and monitoring, but who do not require very specialized intensive care. ⇒ Preterm and/or premature infants.

Nervous system

The nervous system is classically described structurally as consisting of the central nervous system (CNS), comprising the brain (see below) and spinal cord, and the peripheral nervous system (PNS), which is formed by cranial (12 pairs, *Table 31*) and spinal nerves (31 pairs) throughout the body.

Functionally, it is described as consisting of the somatic nervous system, which is concerned with the external environment, and the autonomic nervous system (ANS), which is concerned with life-support functions and homeostasis. The ANS has two opposing divisions, the sympathetic (body stimulation) and the parasympathetic (normal at rest processes). The nervous system reacts to the information gathered and processed using the motor nerves (or *efferent* fibres). The sensory nerves (or *afferent* fibres) take information towards the CNS.

The nervous system consists of excitable nerve cells or neurons and the supportive glial cells. The neurons vary in structure, but all of them have a nucleated cell body and elongated processes (fibres), called either axons or dendrites depending on their shape and function (*Fig. 126*). Some nerve fibres are covered with myelin (white, fatty material) that insulates the nerve and allows faster transmission of the nerve impulse.

Table 31 Functions of the cranial nerves

	Cranial nerve	Function
I	Olfactory	Afferent – smell
II	Optic	Afferent – vision
III	Oculomotor	Efferent – eye movements (to inferior and superior rectus, internal rectus and inferior oblique muscles, and also to iris and ciliary muscles)
IV	Trochlear	Efferent – eye movements (to superior oblique muscles)

Table 31 Continued

Cranial nerve		Function
V	Trigeminal	Afferent – somatic sense (from anterior half of head, including face, nose, mouth and teeth) Efferent – to muscles of mastication
VI	Abducens	Efferent – eye movements (to external rectus muscles)
VII	Facial	Afferent – taste and somatic sense (from tongue and soft palate) Efferent – to muscles of face (controlling facial expression), plus parasympathetic outflow to salivary glands (submaxillary and sublingual glands)
VIII	Vestibulocochlear	Afferent – hearing and balance
IX	Glossopharyngeal	Afferent – taste and somatic sense (from posterior third of tongue and from pharynx) Efferent – to pharyngeal muscles (controlling swallowing), plus parasympathetic outflow to salivary glands (parotid gland)
X	Vagus	Afferent – taste (from epiglottis) and sensory nerves from heart, lungs, bronchi, trachea, pharynx, digestive tract and external ear Efferent – parasympathetic outflow to heart, lungs, bronchi and digestive tract
XI	Accessory	Efferent – to larynx and pharynx, plus to muscles of neck and shoulder (controlling head and shoulder movement)
XII	Hypoglossal	Efferent – to muscles of tongue and neck

N

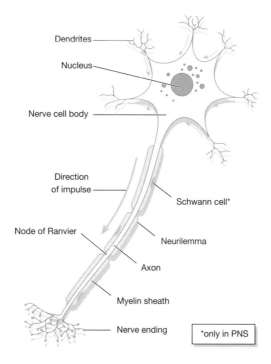

Dendrites

Nucleus

Nerve cell body

Direction of impulse

Schwann cell*

Node of Ranvier

Neurilemma

Axon

Myelin sheath

Nerve ending

*only in PNS

Fig 126 A neuron

The gap between the axon of one neuron and the dendrites of another, or the gap between the axon and a gland or muscle, is called a *synapse*. The synapse permits the nerve impulse across the gap. Most are operated chemically by the release of neurotransmitters, such as acetylcholine.

BRAIN AND SPINAL CORD

The brain is the largest part of the CNS. It is protected within the cranial cavity and comprises the forebrain or cerebrum covered by the cortex, the midbrain and the cerebellum, pons varolii and medulla oblongata, which together form the hindbrain (*Fig. 127*). The midbrain, pons varolii and medulla oblongata are sometimes referred to as the brainstem, which controls vital automatic functions, such as respiratory rate, etc. The lowest part of the brain, the medulla oblongata, becomes the spinal cord as it leaves the cranial cavity through the foramen magnum (opening). The spinal cord is surrounded by the vertebral column.

The brain (and spinal cord) is surrounded by membranes called meninges. There are three meningeal membranes:
- Outer two-layer dura mater that forms a tough inner lining to the skull;
- Middle arachnoid mater, which consists of fine filaments and a subarachnoid space filled by cerebrospinal fluid (CSF);
- Innermost pia mater is a fine membrane that covers the surface of the cerebral cortex.

CSF is formed by specialized capillaries (choroid plexuses) that line the brain ventricles. It enters the subarachnoid space and circulates around the brain and spinal cord and is absorbed into the blood in the cerebral venous sinuses.

CEREBRAL CIRCULATION

The brain needs around 20% of the cardiac output to supply it with oxygen and glucose, without which it would not survive. Blood supply to the brain is mainly via the internal carotid arteries and the vertebral arteries. These arteries unite inside the cranium at the base of the brain to form the circle of Willis. Branches from the circle of Willis distribute blood to the different parts of the brain.

N

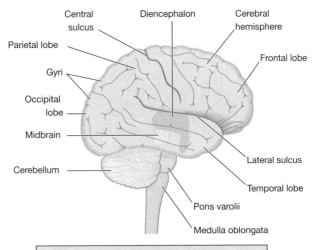

NB The diencephalon and midbrain are shown to indicate their position within the cerebrum

Fig 127 The brain

Venous blood leaves the brain in blood sinuses, which return the blood to the internal jugular vein from where it enters the superior vena cava and so to the heart.

BLOOD–BRAIN BARRIER

The brain and spinal cord are separated from the general circulation by the special arrangement of astrocytes (glial cells) and the capillary endothelium, the blood–brain barrier. This allows only certain substances into the nerve cells and normally maintains the sensitive environment.

NEUROLOGICAL NURSING ASSESSMENT

A comprehensive and accurate nursing assessment is extremely important in the care of patients with neurological problems. It is vital that nurses be alert to the, sometimes subtle, changes in condition that may indicate a worsening of the patient's condition.

In addition to the assessment processes outlined in *Box 26*, nurses should always ascertain the presence of other signs and symptoms that may indicate a neurological problem. These include pain, headache, speech problems, nausea and vomiting, dizziness, weakness, numbness, visual problems (e.g. diplopia), etc. ⇒ Glasgow coma scale, Head injury, Pupillary response.

Box 26 Neurological assessment
- Altered consciousness occurs because of abnormalities within the brain. Consciousness may deteriorate rapidly or more insidiously. A deteriorating level of consciousness is the first sign of raised intracranial pressure (ICP);
- Pupil response;
- Limb response;
- Changes in other observations, such as blood pressure, pulse, temperature and respiratory rate (note that any change in these observations occurs late in response to rising ICP);
- Cognition and confusion;
- Swallowing.

NEUROLOGICAL DISORDERS

Some nervous system disorders are outlined below. Further information about investigations and conditions can be found in separate entries and also in the suggestions for further reading. ⇒ Creutzfeldt–Jakob disease, Dementia (Alzheimer's disease), Group C meningococcal disease, Headache, Paralysis, Persistent vegetative state, Seizure, Spinal problems (spinal injury), Thymus (myasthenia gravis).

BRAIN TUMOURS

Primary tumours may be benign (e.g. meningioma, pituitary and acoustic neuroma) or malignant gliomas. Metastatic spread occurs from cancer of the breast, kidney, bronchus, etc.

The presentation depends on the tumour type and site, and may include raised ICP, seizures or focal changes (such as hemiparesis or diplopia). However, both benign and malignant intracranial tumours cause problems, mainly through compression and raised ICP.

Treatment modalities include surgery, radiotherapy, chemotherapy (e.g. temozolomide), drugs to reduce ICP (e.g. dexamethasone) and anticonvulsant drugs.

CEREBROVASCULAR ACCIDENT

Cerebrovascular accidents (CVAs) are characterized by some disruption to the blood supply to the brain. They include various types of stroke and subarachnoid haemorrhage (SAH). A *transient ischaemic attack* (TIA) is a brief loss of neurological function as a result of a disturbance of blood supply that lasts for minutes to hours.

Strokes may be *haemorrhagic* when there is a bleed within the cranium. The haemorrhage can be into the substance of the brain (an intracerebral haemorrhage) or it can be into the subarachnoid space (SAH).

Ischaemic stroke is caused either by a clot that forms in a cerebral artery (*cerebral thrombosis, thrombotic stroke*) or by a clot or other debris that travels from another part of the body, often the heart, called *embolic stroke*. Thrombotic stroke is more common than embolic stroke.

The *risk factors* for stroke include hypertension, current coronary heart disease, congestive heart failure, peripheral arterial disease and diabetes mellitus. Other risk factors are associated with hypertension and vascular disease, such as obesity and cigarette smoking. Men have a higher rate of stroke in the younger age groups, but women have a higher rate at the older end of the age range. There is a higher proportion of stroke in people of south Asian and African Caribbean origin.

The clinical presentation varies according to the type and severity of the stroke and the area of the brain affected, but includes:

* Altered consciousness;
* Hemiplegia or hemiparesis – the side depends on which cerebral hemisphere is affected, as the left hemisphere controls the right side of the body and vice versa – language problems (deficits) and dysphasia are associated with left hemisphere damage in most people, and therefore dysphasia accompanies right hemiplegia;
* Dysphasia – receptive and/or expressive;
* Dysphagia;
* Loss of sensation as well as motor loss (paralysis);
* Agnosias – various types of perceptual problem can occur in which patients have difficulty in recognizing or identifying objects, people or situations;
* Hemianopia – various patterns of visual field loss depending on the part of the visual pathway affected;
* Loss of the perceptual ability that underlies the sensation – patients are said to have *neglect* or *hemi-inattention*;
* Emotional lability.

Medical and/or surgical management includes:

* Surgery (sometimes) to improve cerebral circulation, such as carotid endarterectomy (atheroma is removed from the artery wall);
* Thrombolytic drugs if the patient has had a thrombus – streptokinase and tissue plasminogen activator (tPa) are given as soon as possible, but only when it is established, by CT scan, that the stroke is not haemorrhagic, as thrombolytic drugs extend the bleed and damage;
* Drugs, such as nimodipine (a calcium-channel blocker), are given as neural protectors because they prevent further brain damage caused by the release of chemicals from ischaemic cells.

Practice application – proper positioning after a stroke
* Neutral alignments should be selected, but the patient's comfort is important.
* Patients should be in a functional position, one that facilitates range of movement and/or motion (ROM) exercises to maintain joint function and prevent contractures.
* The position should be changed frequently to ensure comfort and prevent pressure ulcers.

- Limbs that are weakened or paralysed should be supported with pillows or foam rolls to maintain the best position (*Fig. 128*).
- If splints or other orthotic devices are used, patients should be monitored for pressure and friction damage.
- The patient's head should be aligned to promote upright posture so that the patient looks straight ahead and the neck is aligned with the spine.
- Correct alignment might cause spasticity because, after a stroke, some abnormal reflexes associated with head and neck movements govern abnormal limb postures. These are called the *tonic neck reflexes*. Legs should be placed to avoid contractures and abnormal postures that might limit normal standing and walking on recovery. The upper limbs should be supported to decrease contracture and increase functional use, strength and control, as many normal daily activities, such as eating and washing, depend on the arms and hands.

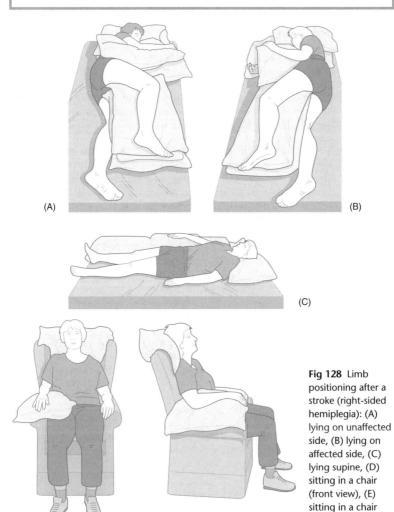

(A)

(B)

(C)

(D)

(E)

Fig 128 Limb positioning after a stroke (right-sided hemiplegia): (A) lying on unaffected side, (B) lying on affected side, (C) lying supine, (D) sitting in a chair (front view), (E) sitting in a chair (side view)

EPILEPSY

The term epilepsy covers a group of conditions that result from disordered electrical activity in the brain and manifesting as epileptic seizures or 'fits'. The seizure is caused by an abnormal electrical discharge that disturbs cerebration and results in a generalized or partial seizure, depending on the area of the brain involved. Epilepsy may be primary (idiopathic) or secondary to head injury, stroke, meningitis, brain cancer, etc.

Anticonvulsant (antiepileptic) drugs include phenytoin, carbamazepine, primidone, ethosuximide, sodium valproate or clonazepam. Different drugs are chosen according to the type of epilepsy and seizure.

Status epilepticus describes epileptic attacks that follow each other almost continuously. It may be life-threatening and requires urgent medical treatment (e.g. diazepam given rectally).

HERPES ZOSTER

Herpes zoster (shingles) is caused by the reactivation of the varicella-zoster virus (VZV) that has remained dormant in a nerve root ganglion since the person had varicella (chickenpox) during childhood. It usually affects middle-aged and older people and those who are immunocompromised.

Shingles is characterized by continuous, severe pain along the distribution of the affected nerve. After a few days, vesicles and reddening are present. Commonly, the sensory nerves that supply the trunk are involved and there is pain and skin eruption on one side of the body. The trigeminal nerve ganglion may be affected and, if the ophthalmic branch is involved, the vesicles are present on the cornea, which may lead to corneal ulceration.

Treatment is based on the early use of oral aciclovir. Topical preparations of idoxuridine may be used on the skin rash or for corneal involvement; however, this is only effective if used at the start of the infection. ⇒ Herpesviruses and herpes.

N

Practice application – shingles; information for patients

Nurses should be alert to the possibility that a client or patient in their care may have shingles, as early treatment is beneficial. This is likely to be in community settings and patients should be encouraged to seek medical advice. Nurses also need to provide information about the link between shingles and chickenpox (i.e. that a patient with shingles can give someone else chickenpox, but that the reverse does not occur).

MENINGITIS

Meningitis is inflammation of the meninges, and may be viral, bacterial or, more rarely, protozoal or fungal in origin. Viral meningitis is the most common type and is usually self-limiting and has no specific treatment. It occurs in both children and adults, and causes severe headache, pyrexia and meningeal irritability (see below). If it is present with encephalitis, it usually requires treatment with an antiviral drug such as aciclovir.

Infections by fungi and protozoa are rare, but immunocompromised patients, such as those with human immunodeficiency virus (HIV) infection, may develop fungal meningitis caused by *Cryptococcus neoformans*.

Bacterial meningitis

Bacterial meningitis may be caused by a number of micro-organisms, including *Neisseria meningitidis* (meningococcal), *Haemophilus influenzae, Escherichia coli, Streptococcus pneumoniae* (pneumococcal) and *Mycobacterium tuberculosis*, although the first two are less common now because of immunization in infancy. Meningitis is usually an acute disease, although *M. tuberculosis* meningitis tends to have a slower onset.

Meningitis may lead to complications, such as septicaemia, and long-term sequelae, including seizures or even death. It is therefore imperative that everyone be alert to the signs of infection and that early, effective treatment is started (see Practice application).

Practice application – recognizing meningitis

The signs and symptoms vary according to the micro-organism involved and the severity of infection. The onset may be very rapid, especially with meningococcal meningitis, in which the person becomes desperately ill within a matter of hours. Typically, patients have headache, pyrexia, meningeal irritation (demonstrated by a positive Kernig's and/or Brudzinski's sign) and neck stiffness. Other presenting features may include:

- Photophobia and phonophobia (intolerance of noise);
- Alterations in conscious level;
- Nausea and vomiting;
- A skin rash (dark red to purple) – petechial spots (small) or purpuric spots (larger) that do not blanch with pressure, disseminated intravascular coagulation and circulatory collapse are associated with meningococcal septicaemia;
- Seizures.

Treatment is with the appropriate antibiotics that cross the blood–brain barrier (e.g. cefotaxime and ceftriaxone). In the community, intramuscular penicillin is given to any suspected cases of meningitis. Management also involves supportive measures, which include intravenous fluid replacement, measures to reduce raised ICP (mannitol, furosemide and dexamethasone) and respiratory support.

Family members and other contacts of meningococcal meningitis are offered prophylaxis with either oral rifampicin or ciprofloxacin.

Motor neuron(e) disease

Motor neuron(e) disease (MND) is a blanket term to cover several similar neurodegenerative conditions that affect the nerves that supply the muscles, and lead to weakness and eventually death.

MND occurs most commonly in people over 40 years of age. The cause is unknown in 90% of cases, but in about 10% there is a familial link. MND is usually fatal within 2–5 years, but some people have survived longer. At present there is no curative treatment available, so patients are treated symptomatically.

Multiple sclerosis (syn. disseminated sclerosis)

Multiple sclerosis (MS) is a variably progressive inflammatory demyelinating disease of the CNS. It is possibly triggered by infection by one or more viruses and most commonly affects young adults. In MS patchy, degenerative changes occur in nerve sheaths in the brain, spinal cord and optic nerves, followed by sclerosis. The presenting symptoms can be diverse, ranging from diplopia to weakness or unsteadiness of a limb, and extreme fatigue, pain, sensory disturbances and disturbances of micturition are common.

Parkinson's disease and parkinsonism

Parkinson's disease is an incurable neurodegenerative condition in which there is a relatively selective loss of dopamine nerve cells in the brain that results in a resting tremor, bradykinesia (slowness of movement) and rigidity in the limbs.

Some people differentiate between idiopathic Parkinson's disease and parkinsonism, the causes of which are multiple and include repeated brain trauma (as in boxing), stroke, atherosclerosis, various toxic agents, viral encephalitis and typical neuroleptic drugs. ⇒ Antipsychotics [tardive (late) dyskinesia], Mobility (*Box* 23 Disorders of movement).

Drug therapy is the mainstay of managing Parkinson's disease and includes dopaminergics (e.g. co-careldopa), dopamine receptor agonists (e.g. bromocriptine), monoamine-oxidase-B inhibitors (e.g. selegiline) and antimuscarinics or anticholinergics (e.g. trihexyphenidyl).

Some surgical approaches to symptom control are offered in a few centres.

In addition to drug therapy, patients may need referrals to the appropriate therapists – physiotherapist, occupational therapist or speech and language therapist.

Further reading

Brooker C and Nicol M (2003). *Nursing Adults. The Practice of Caring*, Ch 14. Edinburgh: Mosby.
Hickey JV (2003). *The Clinical Practice of Neurological and Neurosurgical Nursing*, Fifth Edition. Philadelphia: Lippincott.

Neuroleptics

⇒ Antipsychotics.

Neurosis

Neurosis is an outdated term, as the traditional division between psychosis and neurosis has fallen out of favour. However, the term neurotic disorders is a grouping term for anxiety disorders, phobias and obsessive–compulsive disorder.

Nitrates

Nitrates are used for the prophylaxis and treatment of angina, and in the management of acute left ventricular failure and with other drugs for congestive heart failure. They reduce myocardial oxygen demand by causing peripheral vasodilatation. Their primary action is to relax vascular (and particularly venous) smooth muscle. The pooling of blood in the veins reduces the amount of blood that returns to the heart (preload), and the result is a reduction in cardiac work. They also cause coronary vasodilatation.

Nitrates include *glyceryl trinitrate, isosorbide dinitrate* and *isosorbide mononitrate*. In angina they provide rapid symptom relief and increase exercise tolerance. They may be given as tablets dissolved under the tongue (sublingually) or between the gum and top lip (buccal), as a sublingual aerosol spray or transdermally via a gel or skin patch. Gylceryl trinitrate undergoes extensive first-pass metabolism in the liver and therefore has very little activity when taken orally. Some oral preparations of isosorbide dinitrate and isosorbide mononitrate must be swallowed whole and not chewed. Sustained release and parenteral preparations are available. ⇒ Coronary (ischaemic) heart disease.

Nitrates are metabolized in the body to form the nitrate ion, which generates *nitric oxide* (NO). The latter is thought to be the 'endogenous nitrate' endothelial-derived relaxant factor, which plays an important part in mediating vasodilatation.

Naturally occurring NO is also thought to be involved in areas such as learning, memory, nociception, gastric emptying and penile erection. In pathological conditions, excess production is involved with hypotension in some types of shock, and, because it also acts as a free radical, it is implicated in the brain tissue damage associated with a stroke.

Practice application – advice for patients who take glyceryl trinitrate
- Side-effects include pounding headache, flushing, hypotension and syncope. If side-effects occur after a sublingual tablet is used, the patient is told to either remove the tablet or swallow it once the angina pain has been relieved. Patients should be warned about postural hypotension and advised to get out of bed slowly and avoid abrupt changes in posture, and to avoid dehydration.
- Check the expiry date on the packaging.
- The drug prescription should be renewed every 6 weeks, and tablets should be discarded 8 weeks after the container is first opened.
- Tablets deteriorate with age and a bitter taste may indicate that they have lost their potency.
- Tolerance to the drug may occur, particularly with transdermal preparations.
- Seek medical help if the angina is not relieved by one or two doses, or the pain lasts more for than 15 minutes, because myocardial infarction may be occurring.

NONSTEROIDAL ANTI-INFLAMMATORY DRUGS

Nonsteroidal anti-inflammatory drugs (NSAIDs) are a large group of drugs with varying degrees of anti-inflammatory, antipyretic and analgesic properties. They inhibit two cyclo-oxygenase enzymes (COX-1 and COX-2) needed for the synthesis of prostaglandins (which enhance inflammation and produce pain). NSAIDs can be classed according to the strength of their action. Paracetamol is an example of a weak NSAID, ibuprofen is a moderate NSAID and salicylic acid (aspirin) is a potent agent. They are also classified according to their chemical structures, such as salicylates, oxicams, etc.

NSAIDs have the advantage of reducing pain without causing undue sedation or producing the adverse effects associated with corticosteroids. NSAIDs are used in a variety of conditions, which include:
- Rheumatoid and osteoarthritis;
- Ankylosing spondylitis;
- Acute gout;
- Other inflammatory pain associated with acute or chronic injury;
- Postoperative pain;
- Renal colic associated with ureteric spasm;
- Mefenamic acid is also used in the management of dysmenorrhoea and menorrhagia;
- Indometacin is also used in newborns with certain heart defects to prevent closure of the patent ductus arteriosus.

Most NSAIDs are administered orally, rectally or topically, although some can be given by injection.

Practice application – drug interactions with NSAIDs
NSAIDs can increase the action of several other drugs. This is especially important with anticoagulants, such as warfarin, because bleeding can occur. Sulphonylureas (oral hypoglycaemics) may also be affected, which leads to hypoglycaemia. Other interactions include an increase in plasma concentration of lithium, methotrexate, cardiac glycosides and phenytoin and an increased risk of nephrotoxicity with angiotensin-converting enzyme inhibitors, ciclosporin, tacrolimus and diuretics. NSAIDs can also reduce the antihypertensive effects of some beta-blockers and diuretics. The list is not exhaustive and readers should consult their national formulary.

NOSE AND PARANASAL SINUSES

The nose is part of the respiratory system; it contains the receptors for smell (olfaction) and helps to produce speech. It consists of bone, cartilage and other connective tissue and is divided into two halves by the nasal septum. The lateral wall of the nose comprises three ridges of bone, called turbinates, which increase the surface area of the nasal cavity (*Fig. 129*). The nasal cavity is lined with respiratory mucosa, which enables the nose to moisten, warm and filter inspired air. Filtered particles are trapped in the mucus, which is moved by cilia to be swallowed or expectorated. The other important function of the nose is olfaction, and the area concerned with this is located at the roof of the nasal cavity. ⇒ Smell.

The nose and sinuses receive a good blood supply via branches of the carotid arteries. Little's area, situated at the front of the nasal septum, has a particularly rich blood supply and is the site of many nosebleeds. ⇒ Epistaxis.

The paranasal sinuses – maxillary, frontal, ethmoid and sphenoid – are hollow cavities located in the skull (*Fig. 129*). They are lined with respiratory mucosa. Functions of the sinuses include lightening the skull, reducing the impact of facial trauma and giving the voice resonance. The latter is confirmed by the dull, nasal-sounding voice in a person with a cold.

NASAL AND SINUS DISORDERS

DEVIATED SEPTUM

The nasal septum usually has some degree of bending – indeed, a septum that is perfectly straight and in the midline is rare. Causes of deviation include genetic factors, fractures or birth injury.

NASAL FOREIGN BODIES

Nasal foreign bodies (e.g. beads) are common in children, but they may be encountered in adults. The patient group affected means that removal of the foreign body

N

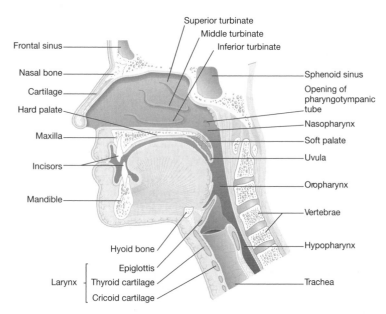

Fig 129 The nose: sagittal section through the head and neck

usually requires a short general anaesthetic (although one attempt under local anaesthetic is normal).

Nasal injuries

Nasal injuries include fractures, septal haematoma and septal perforation. Fractures of the nasal bones and septal haematoma result from facial trauma sustained during sport, assaults, fights or traffic accidents. Septal perforation, usually in the cartilaginous part, can be caused by habitual nose picking, disease, chemicals (e.g. cocaine and industrial exposure to chrome salts) and after nasal packing or surgery.

Nasal polyps

Nasal polyps are pendunculated tumours that arise from the mucosa of the sinuses of the nose. They give rise to nasal obstruction, rhinorrhoea, sneezing and reduced or absent sense of smell. Treatment with topical corticosteroids may be tried. Surgical treatment includes polypectomy or ethmoidectomy.

Rhinitis

Rhinitis may be allergic (hay fever), infective, atrophic (ozena) or vasomotor in origin. Rhinitis is characterized by mucosal inflammation, swelling and increased nasal secretions. Secondary bacterial infection is characterized by mucopurulent (mucus and pus) nasal secretions.

Management of allergic rhinitis is based on allergen avoidance, prophylaxis with sodium cromoglicate and symptomatic treatment with local antihistamine and corticosteroid preparations for use in the nose. Antibiotics may be necessary if bacterial infection is present.

Practice application – information for self-care of allergic rhinitis
Patients with allergic rhinitis are given advice on eliminating or avoiding known irritants (e.g. pollen, animal fur and the house dust mite). Information regarding products available to help with this, such as mattress covers, is offered. Patients should be taught about steam inhalations and the administration of corticosteroids, decongestants and sedatives (e.g. in the form of nasal drops and sprays, *Fig. 130*).

Rhinorrhoea

Rhinorrhoea is nasal discharge. It may be clear, mucopurulent, purulent (greenish-yellow) or bloodstained. It is important to remember that nasal discharge can result from non-nasal causes, such as basal skull fractures. ⇒ Head injury.

Rhinosinusitis

Rhinosinusitis is inflammation of the nose and paranasal sinuses.

Sinusitis

Sinusitis is inflammation of a sinus, and the term is used exclusively for the paranasal sinuses. It may be acute or chronic.

Acute sinusitis is often a sequela to upper respiratory infections, such as the common cold, but can occur secondary to dental problems. Chronic sinusitis may occur from inadequate ventilation of the sinuses caused by nasal obstruction, or it may follow acute sinusitis.

Sinusitis may be managed conservatively with, for example, antibiotics, local decongestants and corticosteroids. If conservative measures fail, there are a number of surgical procedures (e.g. sinus washout, septal surgery, etc.; *Box 27*).

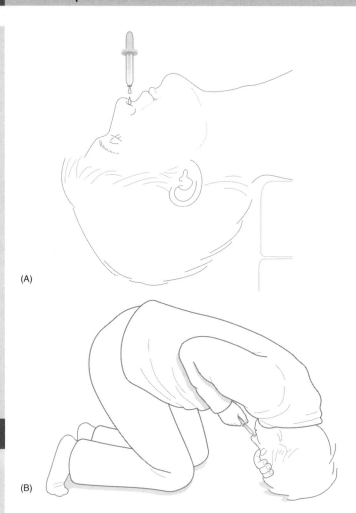

(A)

(B)

Fig 130 Methods of administering nasal drops: (A) with the head tipped back (best achieved by lying on the bed with the head hanging over the edge), (B) with the head tipped forwards (technically more difficult)

Box 27 Nasal and sinus surgery
Antrostomy – surgical opening from the nasal cavity to the maxillary sinus to improve drainage.
Ethmoidectomy – surgical removal of the ethmoid cells from which nasal polyps originate.
Functional endoscopic sinus surgery (FESS) – via a fine nasal endoscope. The sinus openings can be enlarged to improve ventilation and drainage. Diseased tissue within the sinus can be removed.
Polypectomy – removal of a polyp.
Rhinoplasty – plastic surgery of the nasal framework.
Septal or turbinate surgery – improves the airflow to the nose and sinuses and facilitates access for the administration of topical medications.

Septoplasty – conservative operation to straighten the nasal septum. The nasal septum is repositioned in the midline with minimal removal of nasal cartilage. Sinus washout – involves puncturing the maxillary sinus underneath the inferior turbinate. Saline is introduced to displace debris or pus through the ostia. Submucosal resection of the nasal septum – incision of nasal mucosa, removal of deflected nasal septum and replacement of mucosa. Turbinectomy – removal of nasal turbinate bones.

NOTIFIABLE DISEASES

⇒ Communicable diseases.

NUCLEIC ACIDS

The nucleic acids are the largest molecules in the body and are built from components called nucleotides, which consist of three subunits:
- A base;
- A sugar (pentose or 5-carbon);
- One or more phosphate groups linked together.

DEOXYRIBONUCLEIC ACID

Deoxyribonucleic acid (DNA) is the chemical that forms the genes. It is a polymer that consists of nucleotides, which, in turn, are molecules that consist of either a purine or pyrimidine ring [the bases of DNA are adenine (A), thymine (T), guanine (G) and cytosine (C)], a deoxyribose sugar and phosphate. The nucleotide units are bound covalently into long strands that form a double helix with the two strands held together by hydrogen bonds between specific bases – the adenine of one strand always lies opposite the thymine of the other and the same for guanine and cytosine (*Fig. 131*). The double strands of DNA confer its ability to replicate and conserve the genetic code. DNA replicates by unwinding and forming two new strands in which the genetic code is conserved by the base pairing between strands. The genetic code consists of triplets of bases called codons, each of which codes for the incorporation of a specific amino acid into a protein molecule. The genetic code in DNA is transcribed into ribonucleic acid (RNA), which is a template for the translation, by incorporation of specific amino acids, into protein molecules. The processes of replication, transcription and translation are known as the *central dogma* of genetics.

RIBONUCLEIC ACID

Ribonucleic acid (RNA) is a single-stranded chain of nucleotides that contains the sugar ribose instead of deoxyribose found in DNA. It contains no thymine, but uses uracil (U) instead. It is synthesized in the cell nucleus from the DNA template, and carries the message that codes the synthesis of a new protein from the DNA (which cannot leave the nucleus) to the protein-synthesizing apparatus in the cell cytoplasm. Thus, RNA is found in the nucleus, ribosomes and the cytoplasm of cells. There are three types – messenger (mRNA), ribosomal (rRNA) and transfer (tRNA), which perform specific roles during protein synthesis.

PROTEIN SYNTHESIS

The first stage in protein synthesis is *transcription*, which involves the transfer of genetic information (the base sequence) from DNA to mRNA.

N

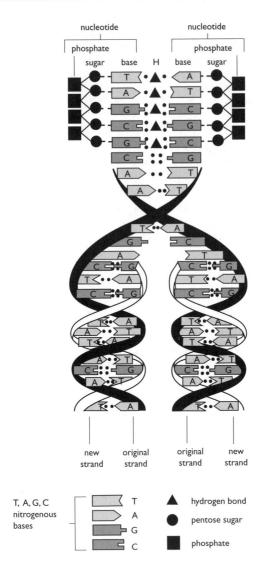

Fig 131 DNA structure and replication

The next stage is *translation*, which involves both tRNA and rRNA. The ribosomes 'read' the message giving the base sequence required to make a new protein, and assemble it by selecting from the free amino acids in the cytoplasm.

NURSE PRESCRIBING

In the UK the Medicinal Products: Prescription by Nurses Act 1992, together with subsequent amendments to the Pharmaceutical Services regulations, allows registered health visitors and district nurses, who have their qualification recorded on the Nursing and Midwifery Council register, to become nurse prescribers after completing appropriate educational programmes. Practitioners whose prescribing status is denoted on the register, and who are approved within their employment setting, may prescribe from the *Nurse Prescribers' Formulary* (NPF). Nurse prescribers must comply with the current legislation and be accountable for their practice. ⇒ Formulary.

Changes from April 2002 have sanctioned the extension of independent nurse prescribing, whereby certain nurses (after specific preparation and training) may prescribe from the Nurse Prescribers' Extended Formulary, which includes some prescription-only medicines (POMs). However, prescribers only prescribe from a limited formulary that relates to their specialist areas. At the time of writing, further changes are planned to allow nurse prescribers to prescribe certain controlled drugs.

Further reading and information sources

Dinesh K Mehta (2002-2003). *Nurse Prescribers' Formulary*. London: British Medical Association and the Royal Pharmaceutical Society of Great Britain in association with Community Practitioners' and Health Visitors' Association and the Royal College of Nursing.
Department of Health (2002). *Extended Independent Nurse Prescribing within the NHS in England: A Guide to Implementation*. London: Department of Health.
http://www.dh.gov.uk/nurseprescribing

NURSING

Nursing has proved difficult to define. Many general dictionaries describe nursing in terms of caring for the sick or injured. Such definitions might go some way towards describing nursing, but they do not really reflect the diversity of roles within the different specialties, the role of nurses who work in schools and colleges and of those whose primary role is health promotion. Neither do they provide any insight into what nurses actually do. Another problem is that caring for sick or injured people is not exclusively the role of registered nurses. Nonregistered nurses, such as healthcare assistants, unpaid carers (e.g. family or friends), parents and volunteers do this every day of the week. Furthermore, many patients care for themselves.

A widely cited definition of nursing is that by Virginia Henderson, an American nurse theorist who, in 1966, defined nursing in terms of the role of the nurse: 'The unique role of the nurse is to assist the individual, sick or well, in the performance of those activities contributing to health and its recovery (or to a peaceful death) that he would otherwise perform unaided if he had the necessary strength, will or knowledge. And to do this in such a way as to help him gain independence as rapidly as possible.' (Henderson 1966)

Although this definition has gained acceptance by many nurses because they can see how the definition 'fits' their role, it does not really explain what nurses actually *do*. It explains *how* they should do it, 'in such a way as to help him gain independence as rapidly as possible,' but it does not define what nurses actually do apart from assist the patient. Perhaps it is impossible to be more explicit; nursing is a complex and dynamic activity.

NURSING ROLES

Nursing roles have undergone massive change in recent years, particularly so in higher level practice roles, which continue to develop at a rapid rate. Some of these newer advanced and specialist roles are outlined below. Boundaries between some roles are blurred and job titles are confusing and sometimes used interchangeably. At the time of writing, the Nursing and Midwifery Council (NMC) is working on a pre-registration framework whereby competencies can be agreed to protect the title of some specialist and advanced practice roles (Nursing and Midwifery Council 2003).

Advanced Nurse Practitioner, Advanced Practice Nurse

Advanced nurse practitioners are those with higher academic qualifications and advanced level knowledge and expertise in a specialist area. There is considerable scope for developing the role to the benefit of clients to provide greater continuity of care, holistic management and improved outcomes.

Clinical Nurse Specialist

A clinical nurse specialist is a nurse who develops skills in relation to a particular group of patients (e.g. those with diabetes or dementia) or in a particular area of nursing (e.g. substance misuse, infection control, pain control, palliative care or intravenous therapy). Clinical nurse specialists work in hospitals and in the community.

Lecturer–Practitioner

A lecturer–practitioner is a health professional, such as a nurse, midwife or health visitor, who has a dual educational and specialist clinical role. The nurse will have undergone higher education and be a role model for colleagues, acting as mentor and educationalist. The lecturer–practitioner has a commitment to a student group at a university, and teaches and undertakes nursing research, in addition to the role of specialist nurse.

Modern 'Matron'

A relatively recent innovation is where some senior nurses take on the role of the modern 'Matron', a post intended to give middle-level nursing managers more authority over hospital matters, and especially control over issues such as cleanliness of the hospital.

Nurse Consultant

The nurse consultant is a relatively new role for experienced clinical practitioners who have the necessary level of expertise in:
- An area of practice;
- Professional leadership and consultancy;
- Education, training and development;
- Practice and service development, research and evaluation.

Those appointed have considerable patient contact and work in diverse areas that include critical care, mental health, continence care, dermatology, spinal injuries, stroke services, accident and emergency, etc.

Nurse Practitioner

A nurse practitioner has undergone specific role preparation to enable him or her to function at an advanced level within a particular working environment. This may be within primary healthcare, in an accident and emergency setting or working with certain client groups, such as homeless people. Nurse practitioners can offer a nurse-led service and invariably have highly developed skills in client assessment.

Nursing and Midwifery Council

The Nursing and Midwifery Council (NMC) came into being in April 2002 and replaced the United Kingdom Central Council for Nursing, Midwifery and Health Visiting (UKCC) as the regulatory body. The role of the NMC is to maintain a register of practitioners (656 000 qualified registered nurses and midwives in 2003), to set standards for nursing and midwifery practice and to safeguard the public.

Part of this role includes hearing cases of alleged professional misconduct and, if found guilty, cautioning, imposing conditions or removing the practitioner from the professional register to prevent him or her practising. New *Fitness to Practise Rules* that include a category of 'lack of competence' as well as misconduct were introduced in 2004. Three new statutory committees (*Investigating Committee, Conduct and Competence Committee* and *Health Committee*) have replaced the existing Preliminary Proceedings Committee, Professional Conduct Committee and Health Committee. In this way the NMC monitors and regulates the profession to ensure that high standards of professional practice are maintained. Nurses are required to re-register every 3 years. ⇒ Postregistration Education and Practice, Professional self-regulation.

NURSING MODELS

A nursing model is based on nursing theory and provides an abstract representation of what nursing is or should be. Together with the nursing process, nursing models guide nurses as they assess, plan, implement and evaluate care (Aggleton and Chambers 2000). There are many models, but in the UK the Activities of living model (Roper *et al.* 1996) is widely used, especially by adult nurses. ⇒ Activities of living model.

For a fuller discussion of the models of nursing, see Further reading.

Further reading

Pearson A, Vaughan B and Fitzgerald M (1996). *Nursing Models for Practice*, Second edition. Oxford: Butterworth–Heinemann.

NURSING PROCESS

To ensure that patients receive appropriate and timely care, irrespective of who is providing that care, it is necessary to have a care plan available to all involved, including the patients themselves. To organize patient care in a systematic way, nurses use a problem-solving approach called the nursing process, which has four stages:
• Assessment;
• Planning;
• Implementation;
• Evaluation.
Some nurses add a further stage to the process, 'nursing diagnosis', which, if used, comes between the assessment and planning stages (see below).

The nursing process is cyclical in nature (*Fig. 132*), which means that evaluation leads to reassessment and the process starts again if the problem is not resolved.

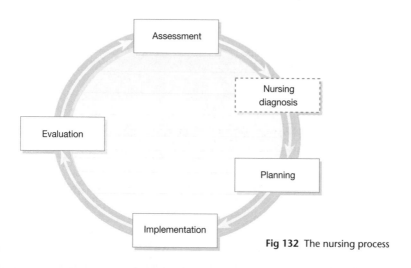

Fig 132 The nursing process

Evaluation is an important stage that enables nurses to determine whether the plan was appropriate and whether the implemented care was effective.

A *nursing diagnosis* is a clinical judgement about individual responses to actual or potential health problems and provides the basis for selecting the appropriate nursing interventions. The North American Nursing Diagnosis Association (NANDA 2001) has developed nursing diagnoses in the USA.

The NANDA nursing diagnoses have not been adopted widely in the UK. However, increasingly nurses include 'nursing diagnosis' or 'nursing opinion' as part of the nursing process. This is because, although the medical diagnosis is clearly important, there may be other issues that require nurse-initiated interventions. Nursing diagnoses explain the effect of the medical diagnosis (e.g. the medical diagnosis may be chest infection, while the nursing diagnosis is 'ineffective breathing pattern'). Each of the NANDA diagnoses is accompanied by a list of recommended nursing interventions. Having established the nursing diagnosis, the nurse then selects the appropriate nursing interventions to plan care.

NUTRITION

Nutrition is the sum total of the processes by which the living organism receives and utilizes the materials (nutrients) necessary for survival, growth and repair of worn-out tissues.

Nutrients are the chemical substances found in food that are digested, absorbed and used to promote body function. The nutrients are carbohydrates, fats, proteins, minerals, vitamins and, of course, water. A particular food often contains more than one nutrient; for example, bread, which we regard as a carbohydrate food, also contains protein, fat, minerals and vitamins. ⇒ Carbohydrates, Dietetics, Eating disorders, Fat, Macronutrients, Malnutrition, Micronutrients, Minerals, Protein, Vitamins.

THE BALANCED DIET

A balanced diet contains all the nutrients required for health in appropriate proportions, and is normally achieved by eating a variety of foods. If any nutrient is eaten to excess, or is deficient, health may be affected adversely. For example, a calorie-rich diet can lead to obesity, and an iron-deficient diet to anaemia. Ensuring a balanced diet requires a certain amount of knowledge and planning. Recommendations for daily food intake sort foods of similar origins and nutritive values into food groups, and advise that a certain number of servings from each group be eaten daily (*Fig. 133*). If this plan is followed, the resulting dietary intake is likely to be well balanced.

The five main food groups are:
• Bread, rice, cereal and pasta;
• Fruit and vegetables;
• Meat, fish, eggs, beans, lentils and nuts;
• Dairy products (e.g. milk and cheese);
• Fats, oils and sweets.

Certain groups of individuals may need a diet different from that outlined in *Fig. 133*. Babies and growing children have higher fat requirements than adults. Pregnant or lactating women also have higher energy requirements to support the growing fetus and milk production. Extra iron is needed by menstruating women to make up that lost in menstrual flow. Nutritional requirement also change during illness, and after major surgery or injury. ⇒ Malnutrition (protein-energy malnutrition).

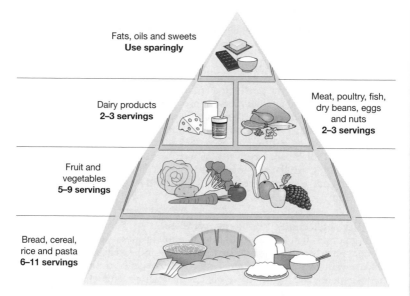

Fig 133 The main food groups and their recommended proportions within a balanced diet

NUTRITIONAL ASSESSMENT

Nutritional assessment is used in a range of situations to determine whether an individual is likely to be suffering from a deficiency of a specific nutrient or general malnutrition (see Further reading). For example:

- To assess the population in famine relief and so ensure the appropriate type of food aid reaches the right people;
- On admission and during a stay in hospital, nursing home, etc.;
- In the community, for instance, when a community nurse takes responsibility for care in the person's home (e.g. the management of leg ulcers).

Nutritional assessment on admission to hospital should be routine, particularly in the care of older people. This is because poor nutrition impairs wound healing, decreases resistance to infection and so increases recovery time and time spent in hospital.

METHODS OF ASSESSING NUTRITIONAL STATUS

The four main methods of nutritional assessment are usually used in conjunction with each other:

- Clinical examination to identify medical conditions that impair nutrient intake and/or absorption (e.g. gastrointestinal surgery, and the specific signs of nutrient deficiency).
- Anthropometric measurement of height, weight, body mass index, skinfold thickness, mid-arm circumference and grip strength – used to identify changes in body weight and muscle mass;
- Diet and nutrient intake history to obtain information about current dietary intake, changes in appetite, unplanned weight loss and any difficulties in the purchase, preparation of food and feeding – swallowing must be assessed, especially after a stroke;

- Serial biochemical measurements, such as creatine height index, 24 hour nitrogen balance, serum proteins (e.g. albumin) and the level of micronutrients in plasma or serum.

NUTRITIONAL SUPPORT

Nutritional support is the prevention and treatment of malnutrition in patients who are unable to eat enough food or absorb sufficient nutrients to meet their nutritional needs. Nurses have an important role in the identification of patients at risk of malnutrition and the provision of nutritional support.

The type of nutritional support used depends on the underlying cause of the malnutrition. Collaboration between the members of the multidisciplinary team is key to ensuring that the nutritional needs of patients are met. The team includes the nutrition nurse specialist, dietician, speech and language therapist, occupational therapist, catering staff, laboratory staff, etc.

Practice application – helping people to eat

It is important that a decision to feed an adult is only taken when all other options have been tried and rejected. To be fed is to return to the total dependence of early childhood, and nurses must help patients to maintain as much independence and dignity as possible. Sometimes it is enough to spend time with the patient at mealtimes to encourage and motivate them to feed themselves.

For some patients, such as those who cannot manage cutlery or have dementia, independence and dignity can be maintained by providing 'finger foods', such as sandwiches, that allow the patient to feed themselves.

Feeding adults

Feeding patients is a basic nursing intervention, but one that requires skill to do well. Prior to feeding a patient it is important that the nurse be competent and that time is set aside for the activity:

- Ask the patients if they would like to go to the lavatory or need a commode, etc.;
- Prepare the immediate environment by removing commodes, bed pans, vomit bowels, sputum pots, etc.;
- Offer handwashing facilities;
- Wash your own hands;
- Protect the patient's clothing with a napkin (paper or cloth) – note that plastic or towelling bibs compromise patient dignity and should not be used;
- Ensure the food is what the patients like and that, where possible, they have been able to choose it;
- Make sure the food is of the correct consistency and temperature, and if it is necessary to liquidize the meal, do each component separately;
- Only have one course on the tray at a time, as patients can feel overwhelmed by the sight of several plates of food – reducing portion size or transferring food to a smaller plate can be less off-putting for patients with small appetites;
- Position patients so that the head, neck and trunk are supported in an upright position;
- Make sure the teeth are clean and that dentures fit and are in place;
- If the mouth is dry, offer sips of water prior to feeding;
- Choose the appropriate feeding utensils (be careful with forks as they can be uncomfortable) – it is not acceptable to use a spoon for the entire meal;

N

- Sit in such a way (e.g. at 90° to the patient) that allows communication and the provision of appropriate physical assistance;
- If communication is difficult, establish a method by which patients can give you information such as 'that is enough';
- Describe the food prior to feeding;
- Do not use pepper and salt or sauces, etc., without first asking the patient, and checking any special dietary requirements, such as restricted salt;
- Offer small amounts, allowing plenty of time for chewing and swallowing;
- Offer drinks;
- Allow time for feeding, but do not offer food that has become cold and unpalatable;
- Record all food and fluids consumed;
- Evaluate and reassess whether nutritional intake can be maintained totally from feeding.

DIETARY SUPPLEMENTATION AND FOOD FORTIFICATION

Dietary supplementation and food fortification are used for individuals who have a functioning gastrointestinal (GI) tract, but who are unable to consume large volumes of food (e.g. older people with a poor appetite). Nutritional support is provided as sip feeds (commercially produced protein-energy nutritional supplements), additional between-meal snacks and by fortifying foods, such as soups, with milk or cream to increase their energy and protein content.

ENTERAL NUTRITION

Enteral feeding is used for those who have a functioning GI tract, but who are unable to swallow (e.g. severe dysphagia after a stroke) or take in sufficient nutrition by the oral route (e.g. a child with renal failure or liver disease). Nutritional requirements are met by using a liquid feed that is nutritionally complete. It is usual to use a nasogastric tube for short-term feeding and a gastrostomy tube (*Fig. 134*) or jejunostomy tube for long-term feeding.

PARENTERAL FEEDING

Parenteral feeding should only be used in patients whose GI tract is nonfunctional. A sterile nutrient solution that does not need to be digested is delivered directly into the circulatory system via a central venous catheter or a catheter passed into a central vein via a peripheral vein. Hypertonic nutrient solutions should be administered into a central vein only, where rapid transport occurs and blood flow is sufficient to dilute the solution. Infusing nutrient solutions into smaller peripheral veins can cause inflammation of the endothelial lining of the vein.

Further reading

Brooker C and Nicol M (2003). *Nursing Adults. The Practice of Caring*, pp. 222–225. Edinburgh: Mosby.

Elia M (2003). *Screening for Malnutrition: A Multidisciplinary Responsibility. Development and Use of the Malnutrition Universal Screening Tool (MUST) for Adults*. Maidenhead: British Association for Parenteral and Enteral Nutrition. Copies of MUST are available Online: http://www.bapen.org.uk.

Lennard-Jones JE (1992). *A Positive Approach to Nutrition as Treatment*. London: King's Fund Centre.

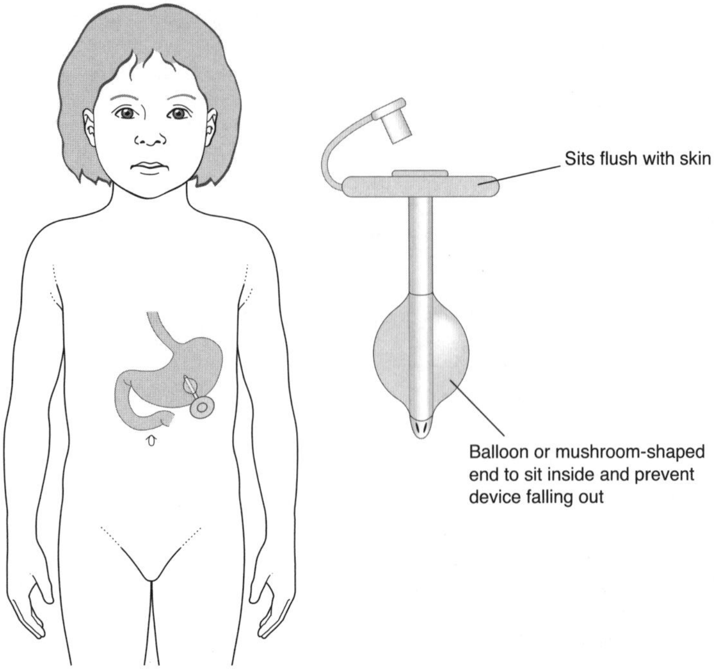

Sits flush with skin

Balloon or mushroom-shaped
end to sit inside and prevent
device falling out

Fig 134 Gastrostomy tube – skin-level 'button' or 'key' device

N

OBSERVATIONS AND OBSERVING

In a nursing context, observations and observing is the regular measurement of the patient's physiological status – blood pressure, temperature, pulse and respiration, and features such as mood or behaviour. ⇒ Monitoring.

Observing is one of the complex skills required by nurses. Most of the nurse's senses must be used to assess the situation and to collect data required to plan individualized care. For example, in assessing skin condition the nurse assesses using vision (redness, pallor, etc.), touch (temperature, oedema), smell (odour associated with infection), hearing [crackling sound associated with air in the subcutaneous tissues (surgical emphysema)]. The sense of taste is not used in modern healthcare, but in much earlier times the only way a physician could diagnose diabetes was to taste the patient's urine for sweetness.

OBSESSIVE–COMPULSIVE DISORDER

Obsessive–compulsive disorder (OCD) is the term reserved to describe the problem compilation associated with obtrusive, repetitive thoughts and the physical manoeuvres instigated to eradicate, neutralize or prevent that thought content from occurring. The obsessive thoughts are recognized as belonging to, and being generated by, the self, and initially the behaviours may be resisted as senseless or unreasonable activities. Anxiety and tension created by resistance may be seen to be released only by the performance of stereotyped, ritualistic movements, which commonly include hand washing, touching, checking and counting procedures. The problem may be seen to begin in childhood, adolescence or early adult years.

Behavioural treatment has become the mainstay of psychological approaches to OCD. The vast majority of patients are managed as out-patients, often in groups. ⇒ Anxiety, Phobias.

OCCUPATIONAL HEALTH

Occupational health (syn. industrial hygiene) is the active and proactive management of health in the workplace. It includes all measures taken to preserve the individual's health while he or she is at work.

OCCUPATIONAL HEALTH NURSING

Occupational health nursing is the client care offered by nurses especially educated to deliver care in the workplace. It includes examination of the workplace for accident and illness risk, risk assessment, preventive teaching, pre-employment screening and assessment of new staff, on-going industry-specific screening (e.g. hearing tests) and maintaining records, as well as health promotion sessions and surgeries.

OCCUPATIONAL DISEASES

An occupational disease (syn. industrial disease) is one contracted by reason of occupational exposure to an industrial agent known to be hazardous (e.g. dust, fumes, chemicals, irradiation etc.), the notification of, safety precautions against and compensation for which are controlled by law.

These diseases include cancers (e.g. mesothelioma caused by exposure to asbestos), occupational asthma caused by inhalation of specific agents, industrial dermatitis, etc. Nowadays other conditions are recognized as being work related, such as stress, injuries related to moving and handling, hand–arm vibration syndrome and repetitive strain injury.

OCCUPATIONAL THERAPY

Occupational therapy (OT) relates to both the profession and the process used by occupational therapists to provide intervention.

Occupational therapists provide services to individuals who experience problems in occupational performance. They work with people of all ages in a variety of clinical and community settings. OT is founded on a set of assumptions that concern the importance of human occupations in maintaining health and well-being.

OT involves the active participation by the patient or client. Initially, using various techniques, the complex interactions between the individuals, their occupations and their environment are explored. On the basis of agreed goals and priorities, and through engagement in selected purposeful activities, skills are gained, knowledge is expanded and attitudes to self and others can be explored. Through adaptation and analysis of activities, and adaptation and analysis of environments, barriers to performance can be removed. By means of these processes individuals are enabled to do more of the things they both want and need to do in the course of their daily lives, in the environments that they occupy.

OLFACTION (SMELL)

Olfaction is the chemical sense of smell. ⇒ Nose and paranasal sinuses, Smell.

ONCOLOGY

Oncology is the scientific and medical study of tumours and their treatment. ⇒ Cancer, Cytotoxic chemotherapy, Radiotherapy.

OPIOIDS (OPIATES)

Opioids are a group of morphine-like drugs that produce the same effects as morphine and can be reversed by the antagonist naloxone. Opioid analgesics mimic the actions of naturally occurring endogenous opioid peptides and attach to the same receptor sites. They are widely used in the management of moderate-to-severe pain, such as postoperatively and in palliative care.

Opioids include morphine (the 'gold standard' analgesic), diamorphine, codeine, dihydrocodeine, pethidine, fentanyl, methadone, dextropropoxyphene, buprenorphine, tramadol, etc. Opioids are also used to control diarrhoea (e.g. codeine phosphate) and to suppress cough in terminal lung cancer (e.g. morphine). Various opioid drugs are subject to misuse. ⇒ Controlled drugs, Pain, Palliative care, Substance misuse.

OPIOID ANTAGONIST

Naloxone is a competitive antagonist to the opioid analgesics. A single dose can reverse opioid-induced respiratory depression, but a repeat dose or infusion may be needed, as most opioids have longer elimination half-lives than naloxone (i.e. opioid effects take longer to wear off than do those of the naloxone).

> **Practice application – side-effects of morphine**
> Many of the side-effects can be anticipated and nurses must ensure that appropriate drugs are prescribed, namely antiemetics for all patients, and laxatives when morphine is being used in palliative care. Patients who have morphine for acute pain must be monitored for respiratory depression (i.e. level of sedation and respiratory rate). Patients who have regular opioids in an acute setting must have an intravenous cannula *in situ* for the administration of

naloxone if required. ⇒ Defecation (laxatives), Oral (oral hygiene), Vomiting (antiemetic drugs).

The side-effects of morphine include:
- Sedation;
- Nausea and vomiting;
- Dry mouth;
- Constipation;
- Respiratory depression;
- Bradycardia;
- Postural hypotension;
- Euphoria;
- Confusion and hallucinations;
- Pruritus;
- Urinary retention.

ORAL

Oral means pertaining to the mouth.

ORAL ASSESSMENT

The nurse's role in the maintenance of oral hygiene involves the use of general observation skills and specific assessment tools. Although it has been recognized that much of the responsibility for the delivery of oral care in an institutional setting has devolved to the junior or untrained nurse, the initial and ongoing assessment is the responsibility of the registered practitioner. Specific assessment tools should aid this process. However, to date, these tools are not yet in common use and reliability is dependent upon the same nurse carrying out the assessment to reduce the subjective nature of the decision making about oral care. It is important to encourage the use of an objective assessment tool that is valid, reliable and practical to use on a day-to-day basis.

The content of the various oral assessment tools includes:
- Direct observation of areas of the oral cavity;
- Assessment of the functions of the mouth;
- Risk factors that have the potential to create oral problems.

All tools include scoring systems that indicate the severity of the patient's oral condition. *Table 32* demonstrates the common features of the various assessment tools presented in the literature.

In the assessment of different client groups it is important to remember that specific predisposing factors may put them at considerable risk of developing oral problems. For example, in older clients the ageing process leads to a decreased salivary flow. The use of an effective oral assessment tool is strongly advised to ensure the early detection of problems within vulnerable patient groups (Roberts 2000).

Many conditions, treatments and drugs can place the individual client at particular risk of developing oral problems. For example, drugs such as opioids cause xerostomia (dry mouth), and cytotoxic chemotherapy inhibits the renewal of the oral mucosa and causes oral mucositis (stomatitis, see below).

ORAL HYGIENE (MOUTH CARE)

Oral hygiene aims to help the person to maintain the cleanliness of his or her teeth or dentures and to encourage the flow of saliva to maintain a healthy oropharyngeal mucosa. It involves oral assessment (see above), ensuring adequate hydration (especially oral fluids), cleaning teeth, dentures and/or oral surfaces, lips creams and mouth washes.

Table 32 Common features of different oral assessment tools

Feature	Details
Observation of areas within mouth	Lips: colour, moisture, texture Tongue: colour, moisture, texture Gingiva: colour, moisture, haemorrhage, ulceration, oedema Teeth: shine, debris Palate: moisture, colour, ulceration
Functions within the mouth	Saliva: thin, watery, hypersalivation, scanty, absent, thick, ropy Voice: normal, deep, raspy, difficult or painful speech Swallow: normal, difficult, pain on swallowing fluids or solids, diminished or no gag reflex
Predisposing stressors	Mouth breathing Oxygen therapy Mechanical ventilation Restricted oral intake Chemotherapy or radiotherapy Drugs and concurrent disease
Subjective data from patients	Taste changes Pain profile

Oral hygiene may be required in the following situations:
- Any patient who has not eaten for a period of time or whose diet is restricted;
- Nausea and vomiting;
- Mouth breathing;
- During oxygen therapy, which dries the oral mucosa;
- During radiotherapy and chemotherapy;
- Patients with facial paralysis or muscle weakness, as the inability to masticate reduces the flow of saliva and causes food debris to be retained;
- Where patients are too weak to attend to their own oral hygiene;
- Unconsciousness;
- Lack of manual dexterity;
- Cognitive impairment such as dementia;
- Oral infections.

ORAL PROBLEMS

⇒ Fungi (candidiasis and/or candidosis), Taste (Practice application – taste alteration and appetite).

GINGIVITIS

Gingivitis is inflammation of the gingivae (gums).

GINGIVAL HYPERPLASIA

Gingival hyperplasia is overgrowth of gum tissue (e.g. as a side-effect associated with the antiepileptic drug phenytoin).

GLOSSITIS

Glossitis is inflammation of the tongue.

HALITOSIS

Foul-smelling breath is called halitosis.

ORAL CANCER

Oral cancers usually develop on the lateral borders of the tongue and the floor of the mouth. They are normally painless in the early stages, but may become painful as the tumour advances. They are also linked with heavy alcohol consumption, tobacco use and chewing of the betel nut. Risk factors include ill-fitting dentures, cheek chewing, etc. Oral tumours are treated by surgical excision and/or radio-therapy. Nurses are in a prime position to educate patients about the risks and to help them to reduce high-risk behaviours. Early detection is key to increasing the survival rate for these cancers. Leucoplakia (white patches) is often linked with heavy alcohol consumption and smoking – it is a premalignant condition.

PERIODONTITIS (PERIODONTAL DISEASE)

Periodontitis is an inflammatory disease of the periodontum, which results in the destruction of the periodontal ligament. The periodontum is the collective name given to the tissues that support a tooth and comprise the gingiva, periodontal ligament, cementum and surrounding alveolar bone.

STOMATITIS (ORAL MUCOSITIS)

Stomatitis is inflammation of the mouth. *Angular stomatitis* is fissuring in the corners of the mouth consequent to riboflavin deficiency. It is sometimes misapplied to:
• Superficial maceration and fissuring at the labial commisures in perlèche;
• Chronic fissuring at the site in older people with a loose lower lip or poorly fitting dentures.
In *aphthous stomatitis* crops of small ulcers recur in the mouth.

XEROSTOMIA

Xerostomia is dry mouth in which the saliva is thick and stringy or absent.

ORIENTATION

Orientation describes a state in which there is a clear awareness of one's position relative to the environment. In mental conditions orientation 'in space and time' means that the patient knows where he or she is and is aware of the passage of time (i.e. can give the correct date). Disorientation means the reverse.

REALITY ORIENTATION

Reality orientation is a form of therapy that is useful for withdrawn, confused and depressed patients: they are frequently reminded of their name, the time, place, date and so on. Reinforcement is provided by clocks, calendars and signs prominently displayed in the environment. ⇒ Confusion and delirium, Dementia.

ORTHOPAEDICS

The term orthopaedics gained popularity towards the end of the nineteenth century and, deriving from the Greek words *orthos* (straight) and *paedios* (child), was used to describe the management of a child with a physical abnormality. It is somewhat ironic, therefore, that of those who require musculoskeletal intervention at the beginning of the twenty-first century, perhaps the most significant proportion is the older adult population, a group that continues to grow as a proportion of the whole. Generally speaking, these days musculoskeletal conditions comprise a wide range of patient situations, such as an older woman with a fractured hip, a baby with developmental hip dysplasia, a teenager with muscular dystrophy or a footballer with a muscle strain.

As the specialty of orthopaedics is so vast it has been divided into several subdivisions within this book. ⇒ Amputation, Casts, External fixators, Fracture, Joint (joint diseases), Mobility (mobility aids), Musculoskeletal disorders, Orthotics, Prosthetics, Rheumatic disorders (rheumatoid arthritis), Traction.

However, the common surgical techniques are described in one place here in *Box 28*.

Box 28 Orthopaedic surgery: common techniques used in musculoskeletal surgery

Arthrodesis – surgical fusion of a joint;
Arthroplasty – remodelling of a joint, and often includes a prosthesis (an artificial part that is used to replace a damaged part);
Arthrotomy – surgical opening of a joint;
Fasciotomy – division of the fascia (connective tissue under the skin, and surrounding and separating muscles);
Meniscectomy – removal of the meniscus;
Osteotomy – surgical division of a bone;
Sequestrectomy – excision of dead bone (sequestrum);
Synovectomy – excision of synovial membrane, or its destruction by medical means using radiocolloids such as yttrium-90;
Tenosynovectomy – removal of a tendon sheath;
Tenotomy – surgical division of a tendon.

ORTHOTICS

In general terms, an orthosis is an external device used to correct, control or counteract the effect of an actual or developing deformity. Common types of orthosis the nurse may encounter in patients with musculoskeletal conditions include braces, callipers and splints. Such orthoses may be used to:

- Restrict movement postoperatively;
- Provide stability during mobilization of the paralysed limb;
- Compensate for dissimilarity of leg length (e.g. special footwear);
- Rest joints in a good position at night (*Fig. 135*).

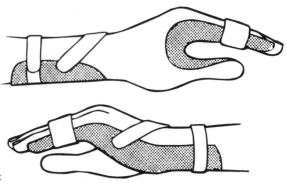

Fig 135 Resting splint

Practice application – care for clients wearing an orthosis
Education and support includes:
- How to use and care for the orthosis as appropriate;
- Exercise both in and out of the orthosis;
- Practical advice for the patient, family and nurses about the effects on and potential restrictions to the activities of clients that may result through wearing the orthosis (e.g. dressing, etc.);
- Checking skin condition on removal of the orthosis, as any orthosis that is too tight may cause undue pressure and sores, an outcome that may also result from weight gain – this check is a particularly vital in patients who have sensory impairment of the affected limb or body part;
- Psychological support – many clients may find that the altered body image that may result from the wearing of a new orthosis requires some period of adjustment, so stress the benefits of wearing the device, particularly so with an orthosis designed to enable increased function (provision of pictures or contact with similar patients may help to reduce anxiety);
- Report immediately any numbness or pins and needles that may indicate the onset of neurological impairment.

OVARIES

The female gonads or ovaries produce the cells destined to become ova (more properly called oocytes until penetration by a spermatozoon) and secrete the female sex hormones, oestrogens and progesterone, and small amounts of male androgens. The almond-shaped ovaries lie on the lateral pelvic walls, one on either side of the uterus, to which they are attached by ovarian ligaments. The follicles that contain oocytes are in the cortex or outer layer. The ovary varies in size during the ovarian cycle and contains follicles at different stages of maturation – primary, maturing, mature Graafian follicles and a structure known as the corpus luteum (yellow body) that forms after the ovum is released at ovulation. ⇒ Reproductive systems.

FEMALE SEX HORMONES

Oestrogens (oestradiol, oestrone and oestriol) are steroid hormones produced from cholesterol. They are secreted by the ovaries, the placenta and, in small amounts, the adrenal glands of both sexes. Oestrogens control reproductive function (oogenesis and follicle maturation), development of female secondary sexual characteristics and the pubertal growth spurt, and the growth and maintenance of reproductive organs. Oestrogens also have wider metabolic influences, such as that on blood lipids and calcium homeostasis, demonstrated by the increase in osteoporosis after the menopause. ⇒ Oestrogens.

Progesterone is another steroid hormone secreted by the ovary and placenta. It is the 'gestation hormone' that prepares for and maintains pregnancy.

OVARIAN CYCLE AND OVULATION

The maturation of oocytes occurs on a cyclical basis, commencing at puberty and continuing until the climacteric. The cycle of events that occurs in the ovaries is controlled by follicle-stimulating hormone (FSH) and luteinizing hormone (LH). FSH and LH are released cyclically from the pituitary gland in response to gonadotrophin-releasing hormone (GnRH) from the hypothalamus.

Normally, the ovarian cycle lasts for around 28 days, but it may vary between 21 and 35 days. The changes that occur in the ovary can be divided into two phases: follicular (days 1–14), which includes ovulation [release of the ovum (oocyte)], and luteal (days 14–28). Changes in cycle length are reflected in the follicular phase, as the luteal phase remains unchanged. ⇒ Gametogenesis (oogenesis), Menstrual cycle.

OVARIAN DISORDERS

OVARIAN CANCER

Ovarian cancer is the most common gynaecological cancer and predominantly affects women after the menopause. As the majority of women present with advanced disease the survival rates are extremely low.

Epithelial cancers account for nearly 90% of ovarian cancers, which are graded into three groups according to the level of cell differentiation. The classification of the stages of ovarian cancer is linked to the locality and extent of the disease, in a similar manner to that for cervical cancer.

The onset of the disease is insidious, with a lack of obvious symptoms. If a woman does experience symptoms, they are often vague and can include:
* Abnormal vaginal bleeding;
* Abdominal distension;
* Pressure symptoms on other pelvic organs, such as urinary frequency;
* Gastrointestinal symptoms;
* Abdominal ascites in advanced disease.

The vagueness of symptoms means the disease can be confused with other causes, such as 'middle-aged spread', irritable bowel or stress.

The management of ovarian cancer is complex and should only be carried out in a recognized gynaecological centre with a specialist multidisciplinary team who are experienced in providing care for women with this disease (Haward 1999). Management includes:
* Surgery – for histological diagnosis, tumour debulking prior to chemotherapy and to remove the uterus, tubes, ovaries and greater omentum;
* Chemotherapy (platinum-based, such as cisplatin or carboplatin with paclitaxel) – particularly in advanced disease for which surgery alone does not provide a cure;
* Palliative care services – palliative treatments are required to improve the quality of life, such as draining ascites or pleural effusions to alleviate acute abdominal distension or breathlessness.

⇒ Cancer, Cytotoxic chemotherapy, Radiotherapy, Screening and early detection, Tumour marker.

BENIGN OVARIAN TUMOURS

Benign growths on the ovary are usually cysts (follicular, corpus luteal or dermoid). These are often asymptomatic, but women can present with abdominal pain, particularly if the cyst has twisted (torsion).

Investigations may include a pelvic examination, ultrasound scan and a blood test for CA-125 (tumour marker for ovarian cancer) to exclude the risk of malignancy.

Follicular and corpus luteal cysts rarely require treatment, as they tend to resolve spontaneously. However, if it is thought that a cyst has twisted or ruptured, emergency surgery may be necessary to remove the cyst and control any bleeding, usually by laparotomy. Occasionally, if the cyst has become integral to the ovary, the latter may need to be removed (*oophorectomy*). A woman who presents with unexplained abdominal pain must have a urinary pregnancy test performed to exclude an ectopic pregnancy.

OOPHORITIS (OVARITIS)

Oophoritis is inflammation of an ovary.

Polycystic ovary syndrome

Polycystic ovary syndrome (PCOS), which is sometimes known as Stein–Leventhal syndrome, is a complex syndrome characterized by menstrual disorders (e.g. oligomenorrhoea), infertility, hirsutism, acne and sometimes obesity.

Women with PCOS have hormonal abnormalities – relatively high levels of LH and low levels of FSH; oestrogen levels are similar to those in the early part of the menstrual cycle and as a result women do not ovulate (anovulation). Also, abnormalities associated with androgen hormone (testosterone) production occur, and there is a reduced sensitivity to insulin, which raises insulin levels in the blood (hyperinsulinaemia).

Treatment is usually to relieve the symptoms and prevent long-term side-effects, such as type 2 diabetes mellitus. Clomifene may be used to induce ovulation in women being investigated for infertility. If amenorrhoea is a problem, the oral contraceptive pill can be given.

Surgical treatment to induce ovulation has been developed as a laparoscopic procedure whereby laser or diathermy is used to drill holes in the ovary (known as ovarian drilling).

Practice application – supporting women with PCOS

Women find this a particularly embarrassing condition, especially as the effects of androgen-hormone production can have a considerable impact on their physical appearance. Weight loss has been shown to improve symptoms and reduce hirsutism. Women may need information about and want to discuss ways to deal with unwanted body hair, particularly that on the face. Cosmetic therapies, such as depilatory treatments (e.g. creams or electrolysis), may be effective and are important in increasing a woman's self-esteem. She may need to attend hospital on a regular basis to assess the effectiveness of treatment and the nurse must be aware of how distressed the woman may become as she receives the results of investigations and the implications for her future fertility and lifestyle become a reality.

OXYGEN

Oxygen is a colourless, odourless, gaseous element that is necessary for life and supports combustion. It constitutes 20–21% of atmospheric air.

Oxygen is carried to the tissues by oxyhaemoglobin (haemoglobin saturated with oxygen). Each of the four haem groups of a haemoglobin molecule has a different affinity for oxygen, which produces a sigmoid-shaped *oxygen dissociation curve*. This indicates the ease with which the haem groups give up their oxygen to the tissues, which also depends on temperature, pH and carbon dioxide tension.

Oxygen delivery (DO_2) is the amount of oxygen delivered to the tissues, which depends on the cardiac output, haemoglobin level and haemoglobin saturation.

Oxygen consumption (VO_2) or oxygen uptake is the rate at which the tissues are able to remove oxygen from the blood.

An *oxygen debt* or *deficit* occurs when the metabolic demand for oxygen exceeds supply, such as during strenuous exercise. The resultant anaerobic utilization of fuel molecules leads to an accumulation of metabolites, including lactic acid (which accounts for aching muscles after exercise).

OXYGEN THERAPY

Oxygen is prescribed (like any other drug) in a variety of situations (e.g. during recovery from a general anaesthetic, severe acute asthma, etc.). It can be given in an emergency without a prescription. It is usually supplied via a piped system and occasionally in standard colour-coded cylinders (black with a white top) in which the gas is at a high pressure.

Oxygen is used to increase blood oxygenation by various means, including variable performance masks and nasal cannulae, fixed performance Venturi devices (*Fig. 136*), via a tracheostomy or endotracheal tube, and through the use of incubators, head or body–trunk boxes for babies and children.

As oxygen is very drying, humidification should be considered in patients with:
- Flow rates above 2 L/min;
- Respiratory infections;
- Tracheostomy;
- Nasal discomfort and/or dryness.

Several problems are associated with oxygen therapy (see Practice application).

Practice application – problems associated with oxygen therapy
- Mucosal drying can cause pain, discomfort and mucociliary dysfunction, which prevents warming and filtering of the air breathed into the lungs. Drying of the oral mucosa requires frequent drinks and oral hygiene.
- Dehydration of respiratory secretions and subsequent sputum retention.
- Difficulties with eating and drinking with face masks.
- Problems with communication, feelings of isolation, etc.
- Soreness from the mask, cannulae or fastening straps.
- Retention of carbon dioxide, because high percentages of oxygen can reduce the hypoxic respiratory drive in patients with type II respiratory failure;
- Fire is a risk (oxygen is combustible), and therefore patients need to be given advice on the dangers of smoking and exposure to naked flames (i.e. gas fires and cookers). Facial burns and death of patients who smoke when using oxygen have occurred.
- Toxicity can occur if high concentrations of oxygen (>60%) are given for more than 48 hours. Alveolar membrane damage results, progressing to acute respiratory distress syndrome in neonates; high oxygen concentrations can raise the PaO_2 abnormally high, which can cause the formation of fibrous tissue that damages the retina and results in permanent visual impairment or blindness (retinopathy of prematurity).

OXYGEN CONCENTRATOR

Patients who need long-term oxygen therapy (LTOT), for 15–16 hours per day in the community can use an oxygen concentrator. This is a device for removing nitrogen from the air to provide a high concentration of oxygen. The use of nasal cannulae allows the patient to eat and communicate.

OXYGEN SATURATION

Oxygen saturation is the percentage of oxygenated haemoglobin present in the blood.

PULSE OXIMETRY

A non-invasive procedure, pulse oximetry enables continuous transcutaneous measurement of oxygen saturation levels of haemoglobin (S_pO_2) using an oximeter. Sensors can be attached to the ear lobe, finger or nose (*Fig. 137*). Using this equipment reduces the need for repeated arterial blood gas analysis. S_pO_2 is the percentage of haemoglobin saturated with oxygen, which reflects arterial PaO_2 and is used to evaluate respiratory status, O_2 therapy and other interventions (e.g. suction, exercise or physiotherapy). Pulse oximetry is routinely used in many situations, including the perioperative period. For most patients the normal range

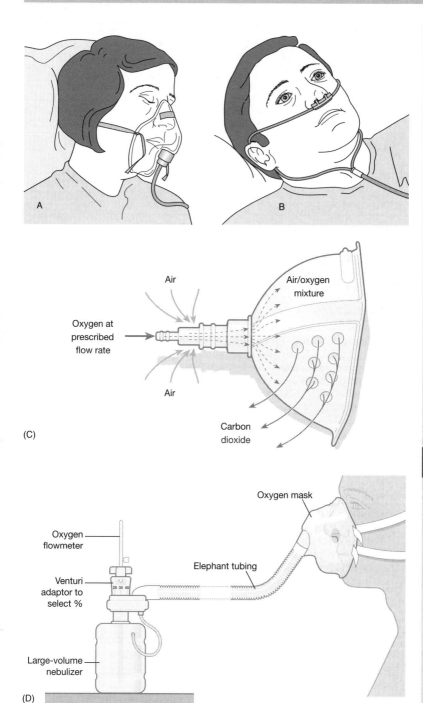

Fig 136 Oxygen delivery systems: (A) 'Hudson'-type mask, (B) nasal cannulae, (C) Venturi fixed-performance oxygen mask, (D) humidification of oxygen

O

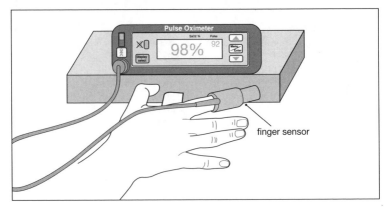

Fig 136 Pulse oximeter with finger sensor

is 95–98%. A sudden decrease or downwards trend requires evaluation, together with the vital signs and the patient's general condition. However, the results of oxygen saturation can be misleading in some situations and must be interpreted carefully (see Practice application). ⇒ Acid–base balance, Blood gases.

Practice application – factors that affect the accuracy of pulse oximetry
Although clearly useful, pulse oximetry has its limitations. It is unable to detect changes in carbon dioxide levels (Bateman and Leach 1998) and produces inaccurate readings at low oxygen saturation levels, so it may not be reliable in severe respiratory disease. Inaccurate readings may also result from a number of other factors, which include:
- Peripheral vasoconstriction;
- Anaemia;
- High bilirubin blood levels;
- Movement (i.e. shivering or seizures);
- Nail varnish and/or false nails;
- Blockage of the light detector in the oximeter;
- Dark skin;
- Intravenous dyes;
- Severe hypoxaemia;
- High levels of carboxyhaemoglobin caused by smoking;
- Exposure to carbon monoxide.

O

PAIN

Pain and its management is a vast topic of immense importance in nursing practice. It is only possible to provide an outline here and readers are directed to the Further reading suggestions. Pain may be acute (e.g. postoperatively) or chronic (e.g. back pain).

Pain is described as the distressing sensation felt when certain nerve endings (nociceptors) are stimulated. It is unique and subjective, consisting of the physiological sensation and the emotional response. Pain varies in intensity from mild to agonizing, but individual responses are influenced by factors such as knowledge about the cause, location, age, associated conditions, whether acute or chronic and pain tolerance.

The *pain threshold* is the lowest intensity at which a stimulus is felt as pain. It varies very little between individuals. Whereas *pain tolerance*, which is the greatest intensity of pain the individual is prepared to endure, varies considerably between individuals.

Phantom pain or *limb syndrome* is the sensation that a limb or part of the body is still attached to the body after it has been amputated. Phantom pain is experienced after amputation, as if it comes from the amputated limb or body part.

Referred pain is visceral pain perceived to be in sites distant from the injury (e.g. cardiac pain is referred to the arm or jaw). The explanation lies in the embryonic development of the central nervous system (CNS) and various tissues. For instance, diaphragmatic pain can be felt at the shoulder tip, for which one explanation is that both structures originate in the same area of the embryo. As the diaphragm descends it carries its original nerve supply with it. Since pain impulses from both areas enter the spinal cord at the same level, the brain is 'fooled' into believing that the pain originates at the shoulder tip (Melzack and Wall 1988).

PAIN ASSESSMENT

Assessment of pain is a vital part of the nurse's role. Nurses should take account of the biological, psychological, social and spiritual dimensions of pain. Most of the several pain-assessment tools include a longitudinal scale, at one end of which is 0 for 'no pain' and at the other 10 for 'the pain is as bad as it could possibly be'. The patient points to the number or description that equates with the current experience of pain. Some assessment tools include much more detail about the nature of the pain and are particularly useful in palliative care settings (*Fig. 138*). Several pain assessment tools have been developed for use with children of varying ages (e.g. the 'faces scale', in which the child points to the facial expression that corresponds to his or her pain experience).

The most reliable indicator of pain presence and severity is the patient's description. However, some patients cannot describe their own pain, for example:

• Infants or adults with poorly developed language skills;
• Patients with mental health problems or neurological disorders;
• Critically ill patients.

Under these circumstances, behavioural signs (e.g. crying) and physiological signs (e.g. tachycardia) can be used as indicators of pain. However, these signs are not accurate (e.g. the physiological signs may have causes other than pain) and provide no detailed information, but in the absence of self-reporting they may assist in detecting pain.

PAIN MANAGEMENT

Pain management involves a multidisciplinary approach, and in some healthcare settings there is a nurse specialist or a designated pain team. Holistic management

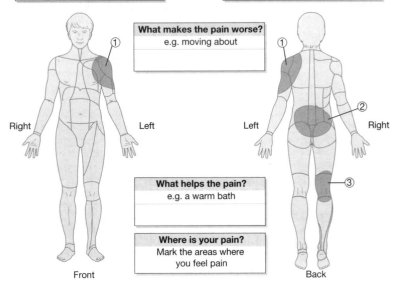

Fig 138 Pain-assessment tool

includes consideration of the physical, psychological, emotional, spiritual and social aspects of pain. It requires staff education, a structured approach, adequate information and education for patients, and regular assessment.

Management may include a variety of interventions selected to meet the needs of individual patients. Obviously, this depends on pain intensity and whether the pain is acute or chronic. They include:

- Information giving.
- Simple comfort measures that might include change in position, extra pillows, a warm bath, etc.
- Analgesics (which include local anaesthetics, nonsteroidal anti-inflammatory drugs and opioids) may be administered in a variety of ways, such as orally, inhalation (nitrous oxide in oxygen), transdermal, rectally, parenterally (intravenously, intramuscularly and subcutaneously) and by epidural analgesia. Patient-controlled analgesia (PCA) allows patients to self-administer analgesic drugs to achieve analgesia. PCA is used most commonly for intravenous demand dosing, but patient-controlled epidural analgesia (PCEA) is a developing service. ⇒ Anaesthesia, Nonsteroidal anti-inflammatory drugs, Opioids.

- Adjuvant analgesics (e.g. antidepressants).
- Nerve blocks.
- Spinal cord stimulation.
- Ablation techniques of the spinal cord where selected tracts are destroyed, etc.
- Transcutaneous electrical nerve stimulation (TENS).
- Physiotherapy.
- Complementary therapies for chronic pain (e.g. acupuncture).
- Simple relaxation techniques.
- Imagery.
- Biofeedback.
- Distraction.

Further reading

Brooker C and Nicol M (2003). *Nursing Adults. The Practice of Caring*, Ch 7. Edinburgh: Mosby.
Main C and Spanswick C (2000). *Pain Management. An Interdisciplinary Approach*. Edinburgh: Churchill Livingstone.

PALLIATIVE CARE

Palliative medicine and care is a recognized specialty in which the focus is to alleviate symptoms in people whose disease is not curable. Interventions may include surgical procedures (e.g. stent insertion to relieve jaundice, radiotherapy to relieve pain), chemotherapy and symptom control (e.g. drugs to manage pain or vomiting). According to the World Health Organization (WHO 1990), palliative care:

- Affirms life and regards dying as a normal process;
- Neither hastens nor postpones death;
- Provides relief from pain and other distressing physical symptoms;
- Integrates the psychological and spiritual aspects of care;
- Offers a support system to help patients live as actively as possible until death;
- Offers a support system to help families cope during patients' illnesses and in their bereavement.

Palliative care is not just about cancer, it is increasingly being provided for people who have any life-threatening illness, such as acquired immune deficiency syndrome (AIDS), chronic respiratory disease, etc.

Successful palliative care needs to be delivered within a multidisciplinary framework to provide the holistic care needed by patients and families. Care is both patient- and family-centred. It should be these groups, not the professionals, who decide the priorities. This can only be achieved by involving patients and families in the decision-making and care. It is therefore important that these parties have the information required for decision-making.

Effective palliative care should be undertaken in every area in which people might die (e.g. nursing or residential home, at home, hospital or hospice). To achieve this, there has been a gradual development of specialist healthcare professionals, including hospital and community clinical nurse specialists, doctors who specialize in palliative care and the education of general nurses through specialist courses.

Palliative care is appropriate from the moment it is clear that treatment is palliative until death. It involves the holistic care of patients and families, and keeps them informed, so that they might decide where to die. The number of people able to be nursed at home with their family and friends is increasing. Specialized care continues after the patient's death until the bereaved family members have started the recovery process. Palliative care offers a unique combination of support in hospices, hospitals, day centres and at home, each providing for the individual needs of the patient and family. ⇒ Bereavement, Grief, Opioids, Pain, Vomiting.

PANCREAS

The pancreas is a soft, yellowish, gland 12–15 cm long, which lies under the greater curvature of the stomach. It is divided into the head, body and tail (*Fig. 139*). The main pancreatic duct joins with the common bile duct at the hepatopancreatic ampulla (see *Fig. 22*).

As a mixed gland, the pancreas has both endocrine and exocrine function. It receives arterial blood from the mesenteric and splenic arteries, and venous blood returns to the general circulation by way of the hepatic portal vein and the liver.

The endocrine part of the pancreas consists of clusters of special cells called islets of Langerhans scattered throughout the pancreas. Within these islets are the α cells, which secrete the hormone glucagon, and the β cells, which secrete the hormone insulin. Together, insulin and glucagon are the main hormones responsible for the regulation of blood glucose. ⇒ Glucose.

In addition, other islet cells produce several substances, which include somatostatin [same substance as growth hormone inhibiting hormone (GHIH), produced by the hypothalamus].

The exocrine part of the pancreas produces alkaline pancreatic juice, which contains digestive enzymes. The main purpose of the pancreatic juice is to continue the digestive process started in the stomach. The high bicarbonate level in the fluid produces a pH of around 8, which raises the pH of the stomach contents as they enter the duodenum to a level that does not damage the duodenal mucosa. The pancreatic enzymes produced in active form are:

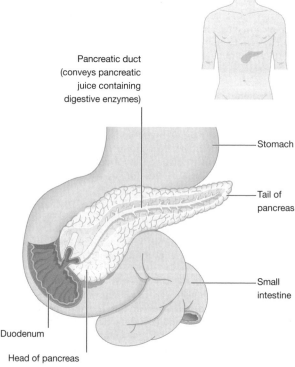

Pancreatic duct (conveys pancreatic juice containing digestive enzymes)

Stomach

Tail of pancreas

Small intestine

Duodenum

Head of pancreas

Fig 139 Position of the pancreas

- Lipases – fat digestion;
- Amylase – carbohydrate digestion.

The inactive protease proenzymes are:

- Trypsinogen;
- Chymotrypsinogen;
- Procarboxypeptidase.

The protease enzymes, once activated, are concerned with protein digestion. They are activated by the intestinal enzyme enterokinase (enteropeptidase). The proteases are released in inactive form as proenzymes, which are not activated until they reach the duodenum. This mechanism protects the pancreas from autodigestion, which causes pancreatitis.

PANCREATIC DISORDERS

⇒ Cystic fibrosis, Diabetes mellitus.

ISLET CELL TUMOURS

The rare islet cell tumours may be gastrin-secreting (gastrinoma, Zollinger–Ellison syndrome) or insulin-secreting (insulinoma), and arise in the islets of Langerhans.

PANCREATIC CANCER

Patients are only usually aware of pancreatic cancer once it has reached an advanced stage and the prognosis is very poor. It is an uncommon cancer and most occur in the head of the pancreas. The average age for patients with cancer of the head of pancreas is the late 60s.

The common presenting features include weight loss, anorexia and jaundice, pain, nausea and vomiting, diarrhoea, bloating and fatigue, sometimes with acute pancreatitis or diabetes.

Depending on the stage of the cancer, management may include:

- Symptom relief;
- Chemotherapy (first-line with gemcitabine for certain patients, 5-fluorouracil) with or without radiotherapy;
- Endoscopic placement of stents to relieve jaundice and pain;
- Anti-androgen drugs (e.g. flutamide);
- Surgery is an option. Choledochoduodenostomy is a palliative procedure to relieve jaundice and/or duodenal obstruction. ⇒ Biliary tract (*Box 2*). Whipple's procedure (pancreatoduodenectomy) involves a wide resection of the head of the pancreas and adjacent duodenum, including local lymph tissue, and usually includes a partial gastrectomy. This is radical surgery with an associated mortality rate of 1 in 10.

PANCREATITIS

Pancreatitis is inflammation of the pancreas, which may be acute or chronic.

Acute pancreatitis is characterized by upper abdominal pain, with raised serum levels of pancreatic enzymes. Most cases occur in association with gallstones or alcohol misuse, but other causes include trauma. This is a potentially serious and even life-threatening disorder, depending on the degree of inflammation of the gland. With mild inflammation, patients are able to recover quickly after treatment. If the inflammation is severe and persistent, damage to the pancreas becomes irreversible and the prognosis is much more serious.

Chronic pancreatitis is a progressive, inflammatory, destructive disease characterized by varying degrees of pancreatic insufficiency that persist even after the primary cause or factors have been removed. This results in decreased production of enzymes and bicarbonate and malabsorption of fats and proteins. Chronic alcohol misuse is the most frequent cause of the disease. Other causes include hyperparathyroidism, congenital abnormalities and pancreatic trauma.

Further reading

Brooker C and Nicol M (2003). *Nursing Adults. The Practice of Caring*, pp. 643–647. Edinburgh: Mosby.

PARALYSIS

Paralysis is complete or incomplete loss of nervous function (sensory or motor or both) to a part of the body. *Flaccid paralysis* mainly results from lower motor neuron (an anterior horn cell and its fibre) lesions (e.g. there is loss of muscle tone and tendon reflexes are absent). *Spastic paralysis* usually results from an upper motor neuron (the motor fibre within the central nervous system as far as its synapse with an anterior horn cell) lesion (e.g. stroke). Muscles affected by *spastic paralysis* are rigid and tendon reflexes are exaggerated.

The term paresis describes a partial or 'slight' paralysis or weakness of a limb.

TYPES OF PARALYSIS

⇒ Nervous system (cerebrovascular accident), Spinal problems (spinal injury).

HEMIPLEGIA AND HEMIPARESIS

Hemiplegia or hemiparesis is paralysis or weakness of one side of the body, usually resulting from a cerebrovascular accident that affects the opposite side of the brain.

MONOPLEGIA AND MONOPARESIS

Paralysis or weakness of only one limb is referred to as monoplegia (or monoparesis).

PARAPLEGIA

Paraplegia is paralysis of the lower limbs and trunk with motor and sensory loss. Depending on the level of the spinal lesion, it may include loss of bladder and bowel function. Causes include trauma (sporting injuries, road traffic accidents, falls) and diseases (e.g. tumours).

QUADRIPLEGIA OR TETRAPLEGIA

Paralysis of all four limbs and the trunk is referred to as quadriplegia or tetraplegia. Such paralysis is usually caused by spinal cord injury (see above for causes), especially in the area of the fifth to the seventh cervical vertebrae.

PARATHYROID GLANDS

The parathyroid glands are four small endocrine glands lying close to or embedded in the posterior surface of the thyroid gland. They secrete a single hormone, parathyroid hormone (PTH), also known as parathormone. PTH is vital in the regulation of calcium and phosphate homeostasis and is released when the ionized calcium level in the blood is low. It raises serum calcium and reduces phosphate levels by:

• Stimulating the reabsorption of calcium and phosphate from bone;
• Stimulating calcium reabsorption by the renal tubule while simultaneously inhibiting phosphate retention;
• Increasing calcium absorption in the bowel, which requires physiologically active vitamin D (1,25-dihydroxycholecalciferol).

PARATHYROID DISORDERS

HYPOPARATHYROIDISM

Hypoparathyroidism is the most common cause of chronic hypocalcaemia and is caused by a lack of PTH or a resistance to its action. It can be congenital, but the most likely cause in adults is damage after thyroid or laryngeal surgery. Insufficient calcium causes neuromuscular irritability, which gives rise to spasms (tetany) in the hands and feet (carpopedal spasm), paraesthesia in the face, fingers and toes and, occasionally, abdominal cramps. Treatment is with calcium and vitamin D supplementation. ⇒ Tetany.

HYPERPARATHYROIDISM

In hyperparathyroidism there is an excess of PTH. Therefore, most of the manifestations of hyperparathyroidism are related to hypercalcaemia. The causes include a single adenoma (most usual), hyperplasia, multiple adenomas or (rarely) cancer.

Most individuals with hyperparathyroidism have no symptoms or signs of hypercalcaemia. Those who do may have hypertension, malaise and fatigue, depression, constipation, anorexia, polydipsia, polyuria, renal colic, and joint and bone pains.

Parathyroidectomy (removal of a parathyroid gland) is undertaken for a single parathyroid adenoma, to leave the three normal parathyroid glands. In hyperplasia, three-and-a-half glands are removed. Bisphosphonates (e.g. pamidronate) may be prescribed for bone involvement, although the effects are not long term. Surgery is usually performed after symptom improvement.

Those who have only mild hypercalcaemia and no symptoms may be managed by a high fluid intake to reduce the risk of developing renal calculi.

PERCEPTION

Perception is the organization and interpretation of stimuli into meaningful knowledge.

ILLUSION

We are aware that, at times, perceptions may mislead or confuse the individual with ambiguities, via illusions. They occur both in health and in disturbances of somatic and psychosocial equilibrium in a variety of situations and circumstances.

Pareidolic images are one example of *sensory deception* that we may have experienced. A pareidolic image is a vivid perception of visual images in response to an indistinct stimulus. The image and the percept coexist, and the image is usually recognized as 'unreal'. The commonly quoted example is that of objects, faces or scenes 'seen' in the flames of a coal fire. The individual sees the coal, the flames and the image-fantasy within reality.

An *eidetic* image is vivid and is usually visual, although it may be auditory. It closely resembles actual perception and is very detailed in composition. It occurs mainly in children and may extend beyond adolescence in those who display an artistic ability or photographic memory. It may be referred to as a primary mental image and the individual is able to scan a visual display, even after the display has been removed. The image, while at times interfering with consequent stimuli, may be recalled with photographic accuracy, long after the event or experience.

Pareidolic and eidetic images are examples of an illusion, that is the *misinterpretation* of existing stimuli, and a relatively 'normal' phenomenon. A similar form of eidetic imagery may be seen to occur in individuals with a somatic disorder (e.g. tetany caused by hypocalcaemia). Systemic infections (particularly in the immature or ageing brain), hypoxia, hypercapnia, hypoglycaemia, thiamin deficiencies and postoperative states may also elicit the experience of imagery. ⇒ Hallucinations.

Penis

The penis, through which the spongy (penile) urethra runs, has a root embedded in the perineum and a body or shaft that terminates at the glans penis. The glans is normally covered with a loose double fold of skin known as the prepuce (foreskin). In some cultures removal of the prepuce, known as circumcision, is performed routinely, and in these cultures penile cancer (and cervical cancer) is extremely rare.

The penis consists of three columns of erectile tissue – a single corpus spongiosum and paired corpus cavernosum – that contain vascular spaces, connective tissue and involuntary muscle (*Fig. 140*). It is the corpora cavernosa that fill with blood from the pudendal artery during erection. ⇒ Reproductive systems.

PENILE PROBLEMS

Balanitis

Balanitis is inflammation of the glans penis and the prepuce.

Phimosis and paraphimosis

Phimosis refers to nonretractility of the prepuce of the penis and narrowing of the preputial ring, which results in difficulty in passing urine. Phimosis may be a congenital anomaly, but in adults it is associated more commonly with repeated episodes of infection, which, because of scarring, give rise to the preputial narrowing.

Paraphimosis occurs where there is a narrow preputial ring that can be pulled back behind the glans penis, but cannot be pulled forwards easily. If the prepuce cannot be returned to its normal position, circulation in the glans becomes constricted, with swelling and considerable pain and discomfort. Unresolved compression can result in gangrene of the glans penis. Paraphimosis can occur after catheterization and patient hygiene (see Practice application).

Medical and/or surgical management is by manual reduction with local anaesthetic (in some cases a light general anaesthesia), but if unsuccessful an emergency circumcision is required. Circumcision may be required for phimosis, paraphimosis and balanitis.

> **Practice application – preventing paraphimosis**
> The prepuce (foreskin) is retracted routinely to allow cleansing of the glans penis, which limits the chance of irritation and infection, but if the prepuce is not returned to its normal position after catheterization or during bed bathing, paraphimosis occurs easily. Nurses must ensure that self-caring patients, healthcare assistants and other carers are aware of the importance of repositioning the prepuce after retracting it to facilitate washing and drying of the glans penis.
>
> Nurses need to observe for signs of inflammation, such as redness or swelling, and report any difficulty in repositioning the prepuce. Note that a tight nonretractable prepuce is normal in boys younger than 2 years of age. Therefore attempts to retract the prepuce for washing before this age must be avoided.

Penile cancer

Cancer that affects the penis is usually squamous cell carcinoma. It is an uncommon cancer that occurs more usually in men over 60 years of age, but it can occur in young men.

There are various types of premalignant lesions (chronic red or pale whitish patches). The premalignant lesions found on the glans or prepuce grow locally beneath the prepuce, prior to invading the urethra and corpora cavernosa. Eventually, the cancer spreads into the perineum and pelvic cavity. Metastasis to the inguinal lymph nodes is slow. Blood-borne metastasis is rare, but may involve the lungs or liver.

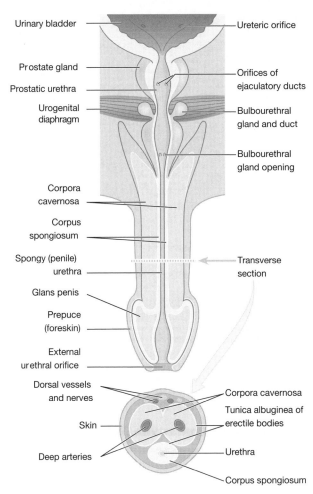

Fig 140 Structure of the penis (longitudinal and coronal)

The options for treatment are:
- Radiotherapy;
- Chemotherapy;
- Surgery – circumcision would normally be performed to avoid further irritation and to establish the extent of the premalignant or malignant lesions. Partial or total penectomy (amputation of the penis) is then required. Total penectomy requires excision of the scrotum and formation of some type of urostomy, and removal of lymph nodes may be required. Penectomy results in a profound change in body image in the patient. The patient and his partner need time to accept the diagnosis of cancer, its implications in terms of treatment and the long-term changes that will occur in his relationship. Involvement from the psychosexual counsellor and erectile dysfunction team assists the patient and partner. Reconstructive surgery of the penis is possible after a partial penectomy. Formation of a phallus in patients after a total penectomy is more difficult.

P

PERIOPERATIVE CARE

Perioperative care describes the entire surgical experience from pre-admission to discharge. The perioperative period is the source of a great deal of the anxiety and distress felt by the hospitalized person (see Practice application). Numerous studies have identified fears of the anaesthetic, loss of dignity, pain and simply losing control of the ability to function as major stressors for patients. It is imperative that the perioperative nurse has the knowledge, awareness and skills to act as patient advocate and ensure the safest, most dignified and most comfortable passage through this process. ⇒ Airway (airway maintenance during the perioperative period), Anaesthesia, Antiembolic, Asepsis (aseptic technique), Consent, informed consent, informed choice, Deep vein thrombosis, Discharge planning, Infection, Wounds and wound care.

Practice application – perioperative fears
The following list includes some of the common fears experienced by patients prior to anaesthesia and surgery:
• Being put to sleep and not waking up;
• Waking during surgery;
• Feeling pain while under the anaesthetic, yet unable to communicate;
• Pain postoperatively;
• Inappropriate behaviour while under the influence of anaesthetic;
• Talking and personal disclosures under anaesthetic;
• Postoperative nausea or vomiting;
• Diagnosis and outcome of surgery;
• Disfigurement and changes to normal body image;
• Loss of control and dependency on others;
• Fears of dying;
• Loss of dignity.

PERIPHERAL VASCULAR DISEASES

PERIPHERAL ARTERIAL DISEASE

Peripheral arterial disease (PAD) is usually caused by atheroma, and affects the arteries in the legs more often than those in the arms. The risk factors include age over 50 years, male gender, diabetes, smoking, hyperlipidaemia, obesity, hypertension, etc.

Signs and symptoms include:
• Peripheral pulses (e.g. dorsalis pedis, posterior tibial) are absent or very difficult to palpate;
• Intermittent claudication (discomfort or cramp in the lower limbs and buttocks) associated with exercise and relieved after resting;
• Pain at rest (severe PAD) in the toes and feet, which is worse at night – nocturnal rest pain is often relieved by hanging the foot off the side of the bed – and also worse in cold temperatures;
• Leg is cold and blanched, the skin is shiny and hairless and the calf muscles and toenails may atrophy;
• Gangrene of the toes in extreme cases;
• Loss of skin integrity and arterial ulcers.

Management includes:
• Risk factor modification through lifestyle changes (e.g. smoking cessation), and treatment of hypertension and diabetes;

- Pain relief;
- Aspirin or clopidogrel is used to reduce platelet aggregation;
- Exercise through a walking programme encourages the development of a collateral circulation;
- Advice about well-fitting shoes and to avoid trauma and tight-fitting socks and stockings to prevent further tissue damage (podiatry services may be required, particularly for those with diabetes);
- Revascularization – bypass surgery using a graft, embolectomy or percutaneous transluminal angioplasty with stent insertion.

Amputation may be the only option to reduce the pain, limited lifestyle and risk of acute infection and gangrene. ⇒ Amputation.

RAYNAUD'S PHENOMENON AND DISEASE

Raynaud's phenomenon is caused by intense vasospasm of the peripheral arteries. On exposure to cold, the fingers (and less commonly the toes) become initially pale and then cyanosed. Eventually, when blood flow returns, the digits become dusky, red and painful. Smoking clearly contributes to vasoconstriction and exacerbates the condition. Gangrene of the fingertips can occur in very severe cases.

The causes include drugs (e.g. β-blockers), vibration tools, exposure to cold, connective tissue diseases and stress. The condition is termed *Raynaud's disease* when it occurs in the absence of an obvious cause.

Treatment is aimed at reducing exposure to factors that trigger the arterial spasm (see Practice application). Those affected should stop smoking. Calcium-channel blockers, such as nifedipine, may be prescribed to reduce the arterial spasm. ⇒ Hand–arm vibration syndrome.

Practice application – information for coping with Raynaud's phenomenon
The fingers and toes should be protected from trauma and kept warm by wearing gloves and/or socks (thermal if needed). Smoking cessation is important. If patients are prescribed a calcium-channel blocker, such as nifedipine, they should be warned that side-effects include flushing, headaches, nausea and palpitations. If stress is a trigger, relaxation strategies should be taught and encouraged.

VARICOSE VEINS

Varicose veins are veins that have tortuous dilations. They are usually found in the superficial veins of the legs, and can lead to venous leg ulcers. The causes include trauma, deep vein thrombosis, pregnancy (hormone effects and increased pressure within the abdomen), abdominal tumours (increased abdominal pressure), long periods of standing, familial, and so on.

The valves in the veins become damaged and venous return is impaired. The blood is slowed and the veins dilate. The superficial veins bulge and appear as tortuous, purple vessels, with 'spider veins' visible under the skin. The legs become unsightly and patients may complain of a dull ache after a period of standing.

Treatment includes injecting a sclerosing agent into the veins or surgical removal of the varicose veins (e.g. vein stripping). This has a cosmetic advantage and also removes the aching and risk of venous ulcers developing. After the injection or surgery, support hosiery should be worn for about 6 weeks. Patients are advised to walk for 30 minutes twice daily, elevate the legs when sitting and avoid too much standing.

PERITONEUM

The peritoneum is the largest serous membrane in the body. The visceral peritoneum covers the organs of the abdomen, while the parietal peritoneum lines the abdominal wall (*Fig. 141*). The potential space between the two layers of the peritoneum (the peritoneal cavity) contains peritoneal fluid. There are four major divisions of the peritoneum in the body – the *greater omentum,* the *lesser omentum,* the *mesocolon* and the *mesentery.* These 'folds' of the peritoneum join certain parts of the digestive system together, such as the stomach and the large intestine in the case of the greater omentum. Other folds of the peritoneum anchor parts of the digestive system in the abdomen (e.g. the mesocolon holds the large intestine to the posterior abdominal wall while allowing it flexibility to expand and move as digested food passes along it). ⇒ Gastrointestinal tract.

PERITONITIS

Peritonitis is inflammation of the peritoneum, and it may be bacterial (e.g. from a perforated bowel) or be caused by the release of chemical irritants, such as bile, gastric acid or pancreatic enzymes. Peritonitis can result from a perforated organ, intestinal obstruction, visceral inflammation, penetrating abdominal wounds and blood-borne infections. It may be generalized or local with the formation of an abscess, e.g. pelvic or subphrenic (under the diaphragm).

> **Practice application – being alert to the signs and symptoms of peritonitis**
> Peritonitis is characterized by abdominal rigidity and pain, distension, rebound tenderness and altered bowel sounds. Patients have nausea and vomiting and dehydration occurs. The temperature is raised, the pulse rate increases and breathing is often rapid and shallow (as deep breaths exacerbate the pain). Untreated, the patient becomes hypovolaemic with electrolyte imbalances, and shock with hypotension and tachycardia develops.

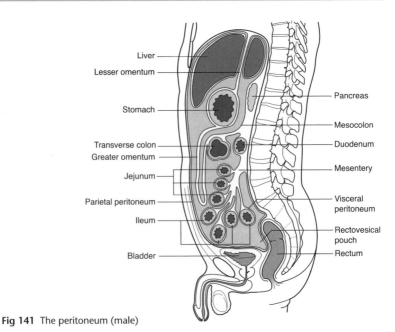

Fig 141 The peritoneum (male)

It is possible to develop peritonitis after surgery and the nurse must observe patients postoperatively for the development of this life-threatening condition. In addition to frequent and regular assessment of the general condition, such as abdominal rigidity and degree of pain, the nurse monitors temperature, pulse, respiration, blood pressure and fluid intake and output.

PERSISTENT VEGETATIVE STATE

Persistent vegetative state (PVS) describes a totally dependent state that occurs when the cerebral cortex is irreparably damaged (cortical brain death), but the brainstem, which controls vital functions, continues to function. The individual, who may appear to be awake, is unresponsive and unable to initiate any voluntary action (i.e. the higher senses are destroyed). This situation does not mean, however, that the patient's death is imminent. With feeding and skilled nursing management such an individual can exist for many years. It is difficult to class this as living, as this suggests a life of which one is aware. The fact remains that, unlike brainstem death, the life of these patients can be sustained. The ethicolegal issues that relate to sustaining life in PVS are complex in the extreme. There have been landmark cases in this area, such as the one in the UK that involved a young man in a PVS. In this case, a legal ruling to allow the medical team to stop enteral feeding was obtained, thus allowing him to die (Airedale NHS Trust v Bland [1993]1 All ER 821).

PERSONAL HYGIENE

Personal hygiene includes all those activities that have as their objective body cleanliness and appearance – they include washing, bathing, shaving for men as appropriate, care of eyes and vision aids, care of ears, care of hair, nails, teeth and gums, dealing with hygiene needs associated with toileting, indwelling catheter and during menstruation, as well as changes of clothing and bedding. ⇒ Infestations, Oral (oral hygiene).

Practice application – providing culturally sensitive personal hygiene care
Patients of some cultures may be entirely happy to wash in the bath, or under a shower, or from a bowl of water put by the bed. They may not like to remove underwear for surgical procedures, but are likely to comply with such a request from the nurse. However, patients who are Muslim may find such practices as washing from a bowl of water unacceptable, because running water is seen as essential for cleanliness before prayer and after urination or defecation. Nurses must learn to adapt their practices in this respect to allow patients to feel clean and comfortable. Patients who are Muslim distinguish between the 'clean' right hand and the 'dirty' left hand. The siting of intravenous infusions is therefore important.

Sikhs wear five identifying symbols, including the *kara*, a steel bangle that should not be removed, and *kaccha* (undershorts), which are intended to reinforce notions of sexual morality and modesty. *Kaccha* are never removed totally – the wearer changes *kaccha* by removing one leg from the old pair and putting it into the leg of a new pair before removing the old pair from the other leg. The garment is also worn when showering.

WASHING AND BATHING

Since maintaining the integrity of the skin is essential to prevent pressure ulcers, maintain dignity and promote self-esteem, bathing and skin care is an important part of nursing the vulnerable patient. The time spent meeting the hygiene needs of patients also provides opportunities to observe physical aspects, such as skin condition, respiration, etc., and to answer questions and deal with anxieties.

For the majority of people, a significant aspect of the sense of well-being and dignity is that they are clean and smart to their own standards.

Further reading

Jamieson E, McCall J and Whyte L (2002). *Clinical Nursing Practice*, Fourth Edition, pp. 25–37, 102–103, 151–152, 169–171, 225–234 and 341–349. Edinburgh: Churchill Livingstone.

PERSONALITY

In simplistic terms, personality is the various mental attitudes and characteristics that distinguish a person (the sum total of the person's mental make-up).

The study of personality is concerned with individual differences. However, it must be emphasized that, in spite of individual differences, people do not respond differently in all situations.

Some psychologists argue that personality and temperament are defined in similar ways (Eisenberg *et al.* 2000). However, trait theories associate differences in personality to the cognitive approaches used by individuals, such as thinking and feeling and how behaviour is influenced subsequently. The term temperament, though, refers to a person's emotional landscape, motor reaction and attention to personal management in response to subjective and external experiences.

Personality and temperament are linked intricately. For instance, individual differences in patients' responses to hospitalization, ill health and surgery can be observed in clinical practice. Responses to pain, terminal illness and mental health problems vary according to personality make up. An assessment of needs must therefore be tailored according to individual differences.

DISORDERS OF PERSONALITY AND BEHAVIOUR

Disorders of personality and behaviour consist of deeply ingrained and long-standing pervasive patterns of maladaptive behaviours and cognitions that constitute immature and inappropriate ways of problem solving or coping. Personality disorders are long lasting and a function of faulty or deviant personality development. The category contains a number of personality subgroups, including schizoid, dissocial and histrionic, and there is an overlap between individual personality subgroups. Personality disorders also includes disorders of sexual preference and habit, and impulse disorders such as pathological gambling.

Further reading

WHO (1992). ICD-10 (International Classification of Mental and Behavioural Disorders), Tenth Edition. Geneva: WHO.

PHARMACOKINETICS AND PHARMACODYNAMICS

Pharmacokinetics is the study of what the body does to a drug over time. It explores the processes of drug *absorption, distribution, metabolism* and *excretion*. Each of these processes occurs at a specific rate characteristic for a particular drug, and the overall action of the drug (be it therapeutic or toxic) is dependent on these processes.

A number of factors can affect the pharmacokinetics of a drug and so alter its effect on the body. For example, drug *absorption* is affected by the formulation of the drug (such as 'slow release', enteric coated), the gut contents and gut motility.

Drug *distribution* depends on blood flow to the tissues, on obstacles (such as the blood–brain barrier) that make it difficult for drugs to enter the central nervous system and on plasma protein binding.

Enzymes within the liver carry out drug *metabolism* and, as there is considerable genetic variation in hepatic enzymes, the ability to metabolize drugs can vary significantly from one person to another. The presence of other drugs can also affect the rate of metabolism, either speeding it up or slowing it down.

Drugs are mainly *excreted* (eliminated) by the kidneys and are affected by glomerular filtration rate particularly, which decreases with age and disease. Other routes for drug excretion are the hepatobiliary system (but usually reabsorption occurs in the intestine), the lungs and the body fluids (e.g. saliva, sweat and breast milk).

Pharmacodynamics is the study of how a drug acts in a living system and how it alters cell metabolism to have an effect. It is, perhaps, not surprising that many factors can influence the ability of drugs to have their therapeutic effect at the target tissue, given the precision of targeting required. As well as unpredictable idiosyncratic responses in individuals, various diseases may have pharmacodynamic effects. For example, in the nephrotic syndrome there is a reduced sensitivity to furosemide because of the abnormal influences of albumin in the kidney tubule lumen. Drug interactions can also have various pharmacodynamic effects. For example, in patients who take digoxin and diuretics, hypokalaemia caused by the diuresis may increase the cardiac effects of digoxin. Age also offers the potential for variation in the effects of drugs on tissues, because ageing tissues have altered sensitivity to drugs.

Drugs exert their effects by binding to molecules in body cells. The main target mechanisms for drugs is outlined in *Fig. 142*. ⇒ Agonist, Antagonist, Drug (adverse drug reactions, drug interaction), Polypharmacy.

ABSORPTION RATE CONSTANT

The absorption rate constant is the amount of drug absorbed in a unit of time.

ALPHA REDISTRIBUTION PHASE

Alpha redistribution phase describes the point after an intravenous injection at which blood concentrations of the drug start to fall below the peak levels achieved.

BETA PHASE

Beta phase describes the period that follows the alpha redistribution phase of drug administration, and is characterized by a slow decline in drug blood levels during its metabolism and excretion.

P

BIOAVAILABILITY

Bioavailability is the amount of drug that reaches the systemic circulation, and is related to the route of administration, absorption and any presystemic metabolism. Thus, if a drug is given intravenously, its bioavailability is 100%. However, drugs taken orally may be absorbed only partially from the gut into the blood because of interactions with food (e.g. tetracyclines are not absorbed effectively if taken with dairy products). Furthermore, drugs taken orally enter the hepatic portal circulation and are taken to the liver where they undergo *first-pass (presystemic) metabolism* (i.e. they are metabolized before entering the systemic circulation). The degree of metabolism is variable. For example, if glyceryl trinitrate is taken orally the hepatic enzymes metabolize it totally, so no active drug enters the systemic circulation and bioavailability is zero. For this reason glyceryl trinitrate is administered via the sublingual, buccal or transdermal route. (*Box 29* gives examples of drugs subject to first-pass metabolism). A smaller number of drugs are metabolized in the wall of the intestine.

a at receptors

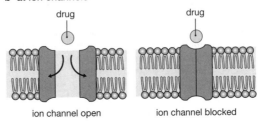

increased effect within
cell either directly or via
a regulatory G-protein

effect within cell blocked

b at ion channels

ion channel open   ion channel blocked

c on enzymes

- enzymes potentiated
  – active drug produced; reaction enhanced
- enzymes uninhibited – reaction decreased
- false substrate – abnormal metabolite produced;
  reaction decreased

d on cell membrane carriers

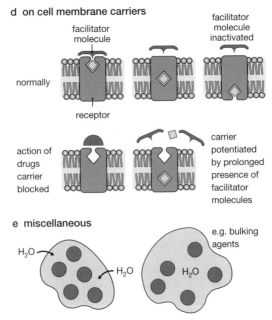

e miscellaneous

e.g. bulking
agents

Fig 142 Mechanisms of drug action

Box 29 Drugs subject to substantial first-pass metabolism
- Aspirin;
- Clomethiazole;
- Dextropropoxyphene;
- Glyceryl trinitrate;
- Imipramine;
- Isosorbide dinitrate;
- Morphine;
- Pethidine;
- Propanolol;
- Salbutamol;
- Verapamil.

CUMULATIVE ACTION

If the dose of a slowly excreted drug is repeated too frequently, an increasing action is obtained. This can be dangerous as, if the drug accumulates in the system, toxic symptoms may occur (e.g. with digoxin).

DRUG HALF-LIFE

Drug half-life is the time taken for the concentration of a drug in the plasma to fall by half the initial level.

EFFECTIVE DOSE

Effective dose is the amount of a drug that can be expected to cause a specific intensity of effect in individuals who receive the drug.

PRODRUG

Prodrugs are drugs administered in inactive forms that are activated within the body (e.g. by enzymes in the liver, in the brain or by bacteria in the bowel). They are used for a variety of reasons, which include:
- Overcoming gastrointestinal side-effects and damage, such as with the cytotoxic drug cyclophosphamide, which is activated in the liver only;
- The antiviral drug zidovudine is activated by the reverse transcriptase enzymes present in HIV-infected cells, and so it acts selectively;
- Oral L-dopa (given for parkinsonism) can be absorbed and passed through the blood–brain barrier, where it is converted into dopamine (whereas dopamine given parenterally acts upon the renal blood vessels and does not cross the blood–brain barrier).

THERAPEUTIC INDEX

The therapeutic index is an indicator of the difference between the drug dose that produces a therapeutic effect and the dose that causes toxic effects. It alerts the prescriber to the safety margin for a particular drug, but the therapeutic index varies between people, as we all process drugs in an individual way.

PHENYLKETONURIA

Phenylketonuria (PKU) is a metabolic disorder inherited as an autosomal recessive condition. The enzyme phenylalanine hydroxylase, which converts the amino acid phenylalanine into tyrosine, is absent or deficient. Toxic metabolites of phenylalanine, such as phenylketones derived from phenylpyruvate, accumulate in the blood and are excreted in the urine (PKU).

Untreated, PKU leads to individuals with severe learning disability and very fair hair and skin (because of the lack of tyrosine needed for the pigment melanin). A routine screening blood test during the first few days of life ensures early diagnosis and a treatment regimen that includes reducing phenylalanine intake and monitoring for toxic metabolites. The special dietary regimen is required until brain development is complete, but it is recommended when females with PKU plan to become pregnant. ⇒ Neonatal (neonatal checks).

PHOBIAS

Phobias represent a persistent and focused fear of a specific situation, event or object that evokes the autonomic anxiety response. There is a recognition of the unreasonable nature of the fear, but continued avoidance of the stimulus occurs, wherever feasible. Intense anxiety is elicited if exposure occurs, and an integral aspect of the phobia is often related to the possibility of humiliating oneself during such an exposure. Where the stimulus is commonly encountered within everyday life and living conditions, work, social routines and relationships may be impaired significantly.

Phobias include:
- Specific (simple) phobias, such as the common fears of spiders, heights, enclosed spaces, flying, thunder, and so on;
- Agoraphobia, which is defined in American Psychiatric Association's *Diagnostic and Statistical Manual* (Fourth Edition 1994, DSM-IV), as anxiety about being in places or situations from which escape is difficult or embarrassing, or in which help might not be available in the event of having a panic attack or panic-like symptoms;
- Social phobias, which are often characterized by fears of 'making a fool of oneself' and maybe associated fears of some inappropriate behaviour, not knowing what to say, being embarrassed about making eye contact, and fears of about being 'rejected'. The associated avoidance behaviour often leads to social isolation, which leads, in turn, to feeling dejected. Panic attacks and depression commonly accompany social phobia.

In simple phobias, contact or anticipated contact with the feared object or situation is feared above all, but in social phobia the key fear is frequently the perceived negative evaluation by others and its consequences. Generally, in simple phobia overt avoidance is the patient's main coping strategy, while in social phobia avoidance often involves a range of overt and subtle avoidances and props (i.e. alcohol) to cope with situations. ⇒ Anxiety, Disease (disease classification).

TREATMENT

Specialist treatment for phobias should be reserved for people whose problem causes serious life handicaps, such as being unable to travel to work on the train. In the majority of cases, simple exposure is the treatment of choice and produces very significant gains. The principles and practice of simple exposure must incorporate the following conditions:
- Planned and graded to the individual's most therapeutic pace;
- Regular and repeated;
- Engagement and proactive;
- Practised as homework;
- Of adequate duration to ensure a reduction of anxiety during exposure (see Practice application).

Some phobic problems may require far more graded exposure than others, which may take many more sessions of shorter duration over a longer period of time.

Some phobias are difficult to treat because exposure is not easily arranged (e.g. thunder and lightening, flying). Although simple exposure principles and practice are paramount, the application in many cases of agoraphobia is not straightforward. For instance, the patient may have numerous avoidance behaviours.

Practice application – simple exposure in spider phobia

It is possible for someone with a spider phobia to be exposed to live spiders gradually over a couple of sessions of 2–3 hours each. At first, the therapist exposes patients to small live spiders in a closed container several feet away, and then encourages them to continue with this exposure until their anxiety falls. At a pace acceptable to each patient, the therapist continues with exposure, graduating to open containers, until finally the patient is able to handle large, live spiders with little or no anxiety.

More often than not, patients require much less treatment than they anticipate, but (of course) effective treatment by a therapist is reinforced with home practice. The therapist should ask patients to record homework in a diary and report after a reasonable period.

PHYSIOTHERAPY

Traditionally, physiotherapy is treatment to ameliorate, restore and sometimes cure, using electrotherapy, manipulation and exercise therapy and rehabilitation, after injury or disease. Contemporarily, it also includes assessment and diagnosis, health education, health promotion and prevention of disabling conditions.

PITUITARY GLAND (SYN. HYPOPHYSIS CEREBRI)

The pituitary gland stimulates many other endocrine structures and metabolic processes. It is tiny, weighing only about 0.5 g, and comprises two separate structures, the anterior lobe (adenohypophysis) and the posterior lobe (neurohypophysis). The two lobes hang from the hypothalamus by a stalk that contains blood vessels and nerve fibres (*Fig. 143*). The pituitary gland sits in the pituitary (hypophyseal) fossa of the sphenoid bone. Its proximity to the optic chiasma means that pituitary tumours may cause visual problems if they press on the optic nerves.

ANTERIOR LOBE (ADENOHYPOPHYSIS)

Releasing and inhibiting hormones that travel in the portal system of blood vessels from the hypothalamus control the hormones produced by the anterior lobe of the pituitary gland. The six anterior pituitary hormones include four that stimulate other endocrine structures (trophic hormones; *Fig. 144*):
- Adrenocorticotrophic hormone (ACTH);
- Thyroid-stimulating hormone (TSH);
- Two gonadotrophins (acting on the ovaries or testes) – follicle-stimulating hormone (FSH) and luteinizing hormone (LH), known as interstitial cell stimulating hormone (ICSH) in males.

The other two act on other tissues:
- Growth hormone (GH);
- Prolactin (PRL).

In addition, the anterior lobe produces a precursor molecule (prohormone), which forms substances that include ACTH and beta-lipotrophin (LPH), which act on melanocytes (skin pigment cells).

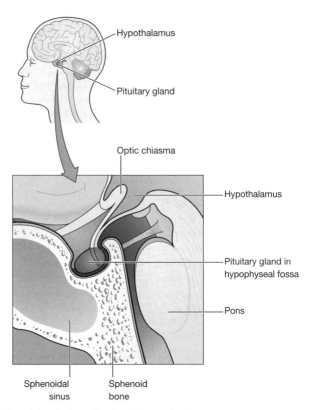

Fig 143 The position of the pituitary gland and its associated structures

P

POSTERIOR LOBE (NEUROHYPOPHYSIS)

The posterior lobe does not produce hormones, but it stores and secretes two – oxytocin and antidiuretic hormone [ADH, also called arginine vasopressin (AVP) or vasopressin]. These hormones are produced in the hypothalamus and travel in the nerve fibres of the stalk to the posterior lobe. Their release from the posterior pituitary gland is under neural control from the hypothalamus (*Fig. 144*).

Oxytocin is important in parturition and is also required for the 'let-down' (ejection) of milk during lactation.

ADH reduces diuresis (urine production) in the kidneys. It is released in response to an increase in plasma osmolality or a decrease in plasma volume. ADH causes some parts of the kidney tubules to become more permeable to water. Hence the kidney reabsorbs more water, less urine is produced and the plasma osmolality and volume return to normal. The release of ADH is regulated by a negative feedback mechanism – as plasma osmolality starts to fall and circulating blood volume is restored, the rate of ADH release is slowed. ADH release is important in maintaining fluid balance homeostasis. It also increases blood pressure by causing vasoconstriction, a pressor effect that accounts for its other name, vasopressin.

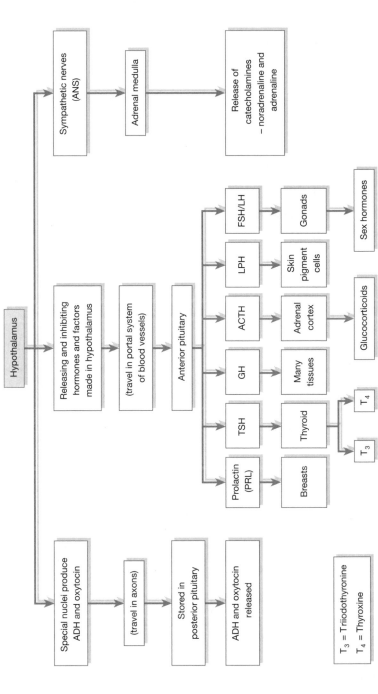

Fig 144 Hypothalamus and pituitary gland – hormones secreted and target cells

T_3 = Triiodothyronine
T_4 = Thyroxine

DISORDERS OF THE PITUITARY GLAND

⇒ Adrenal glands (Cushing's disease).

ACROMEGALY AND GIGANTISM

Acromegaly results from an excess of GH in an adult, almost always caused by an adenoma. It is characterized by enlargement of the hands, feet and face, cardio-vascular problems (e.g. enlarged heart, hypertension), insulin resistance and secondary diabetes, and local signs, such as visual field defects caused by pressure on the optic chiasma.

Gigantism is abnormal growth, especially in height (in excess of 7 feet, 2.2 m), caused by excess GH in childhood prior to fusion of the epiphyses. It is almost always caused by a pituitary tumour.

Treatment for both includes surgical removal, octreotide (analogue of GH-inhibitory hormone) or radiotherapy.

Lack of GH in children results in short stature (see below, dwarfism).

HYPERPROLACTINAEMIA

Hyperprolactinaemia is an elevation in circulating PRL levels, sometimes caused by stress; if pathological it results in galactorrhoea, menstrual irregularity and sub-fertility. In men erectile dysfunction, gynaecomastia (male breast development) and loss of muscle mass can be caused. It may result from dopamine antagonists (such as metoclopramide), large, often nonfunctioning pituitary tumours or pro-lactinomas.

Treatment is with dopamine-receptor stimulants (such as bromocriptine), surgical removal or radiotherapy. ⇒ Infertility.

HYPOPITUITARISM

Hypopituitarism is pituitary gland insufficiency, especially of the anterior lobe. If all six anterior lobe hormones are affected it is termed panhypopituitarism.

The absence of gonadotrophins leads to failure of ovulation, uterine atrophy and amenorrhoea in women, and loss of libido and pubic and axillary hair in both sexes. Lack of ACTH and thyrotrophin (TSH) may result in lack of energy, pallor, fine dry skin, cold intolerance and sometimes hypoglycaemia. It usually results from a tumour of or involving the pituitary gland or hypothalamus, but in other cases the cause is unknown. It occasionally arises from postpartum infarction of the pituitary gland.

Treatment depends on the underlying cause and may include surgical removal of tumours or hormone replacement.

DWARFISM

Pituitary dwarfism (*Lorain–Lévi syndrome*) is caused by a severe deficiency of GH and possibly other hormones in childhood, and results from genetic abnormality or a tumour. The individual is of small stature, but is well proportioned and mental development is normal. Puberty is delayed.

Frölich's syndrome is panhypopituitarism, but the main features are associated with lack of GH, FSH and LH. In children there is diminished growth, lack of sexual development, obesity with female fat distribution and problems with mental development. In adults there is obesity and sterility. It may be caused by a tumour in the anterior pituitary and/or hypothalamus, but most are idiopathic.

DIABETES INSIPIDUS

Diabetes insipidus is caused by disordered water homeostasis. It may be *cranial* through deficiency of ADH (AVP), either idiopathic or from trauma, tumour or inflammation that affects the posterior pituitary function, or it may be *nephrogenic* because of renal tubular resistance to AVP action. Treatment is with desmopressin (analogue of ADH), which can be taken intranasally, by subcutaneous or intramuscular injection or by mouth.

Placebo, placebo effect

A placebo is a harmless substance given as medicine. In a randomized placebo-controlled trial, an inert substance, identical in appearance with the material being tested, is used. When neither the researcher nor the patient knows which is which, the term 'double blind trial' is used. A *placebo effect* is a therapeutic one that occurs after the administration of a placebo, or some nondrug intervention (e.g. information in advance of surgery may reduce the need for pain relieving drugs).

Planning

Planning is regarded as the second phase of the nursing process. After identification of the patient's actual and potential problems with everyday living activities, the patient participates in setting-appropriate goals to be achieved by the selected nursing interventions. A date is set to evaluate whether or not the goals have been achieved. $\Rightarrow$ Goals (goal-setting), Integrated care pathway.

Platelets

Platelets are disc-shaped cellular fragments that have an important role in haemostasis, and are also known as thrombocytes. *Platelet plug* formation is one of the four overlapping stages of haemostasis. Platelets adhere and aggregate at the site of blood vessel damage and form a temporary plug to close the defect. The platelets release substances, such as adenosine diphosphate (ADP), thromboxanes and 5-hydroxytryptamine, which cause further aggregation and vasoconstriction. $\Rightarrow$ Blood (*Box 3*), Haemostasis.

DISORDERS OF PLATELETS

Thrombocythaemia

In thrombocythaemia there is an increase in circulating blood platelets, which can encourage clotting within blood vessels. $\Rightarrow$ Myeloproliferative disorders.

Thrombocytopenia

In thrombocytopenia a reduction in the number of platelets in the blood can result in spontaneous bruising and prolonged bleeding after injury. Spontaneous bleeding tends to occur when the platelet count falls below $10 \times 10^9/L$. Causes include idiopathic [idiopathic thrombocytopenic purpura (ITP)], drugs [e.g. nonsteroidal anti-inflammatory drugs (NSAIDs), heparin, etc.], infections, bone marrow malignancy and radiation.

Thrombocytopenia is most often caused by inadequate platelet production or increased platelet destruction. Inadequate platelet production may be secondary to conditions such as myelodysplasia or aplastic anaemia. It can also result from bone marrow infiltration by malignant cells, as in acute leukaemia, lymphoma and myeloma. Treatments for these conditions can also inhibit platelet production by suppressing bone marrow activity.

Increased platelet destruction is often immunological in nature and may be secondary to autoimmune conditions, such as systemic lupus erythematosus. There may, however, be no obvious underlying cause, as in chronic ITP. $\Rightarrow$ Bone (myelodysplasia, multiple myeloma), Erythrocyte (anaemia).

The aim of the treatment is to preserve platelets by reducing the number of circulating antibodies. Measures include:

- Short-term use of intravenous immunoglobulin therapies;
- High-dose prednisolone;
- Splenectomy;
- Immunosuppressant medications (e.g. azathioprine, ciclosporin and cyclophosphamide).

Practice application – thrombocytopenia, observing for bleeding

Patients should be encouraged to report bleeding gums, nosebleeds or the presence of bruising or petechiae. Urinalysis and testing for faecal occult blood can also indicate the presence of bleeding. Severe haemorrhage can happen spontaneously and may be life-threatening if it occurs in sites such as the brain or gastrointestinal tract. An intracranial bleed may be suspected if there is a rapid change in consciousness, agitation or confusion, or collapse. In such instances, urgent medical attention is required.

Any patient with thrombocytopenia who is actively bleeding must have vital signs checked frequently to detect early signs of hypovolaemic shock. Intravenous fluid and blood or platelet transfusion may be indicated.

THROMBOCYTOSIS

Thrombocytosis is an increase in the number of platelets in the blood. It can arise in a reaction to infection, bleeding, inflammation or malignancy, or as part of thrombocythaemia and other myeloproliferative disorders.

PLAY

Play is the spontaneous or planned activities vital to normal social, physical, emotional and intellectual development during childhood.

Play is vitally important in the life of a sick child. Play in hospital aims to inform children about the unusual situation in which they find themselves and thereby allay fears and increase confidence. It also provides a much-needed link with home and normality. Using play preoperatively, or prior to other frightening procedures (e.g. blood test), goes a long way in helping children to express their real feelings. The functions of play are illustrated in *Fig. 145*. ⇒ Injection (Practice application – needle phobia).

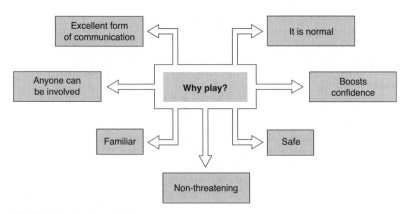

Fig 145 The functions of play

TYPES OF PLAY

Play in hospital can be based on the work of Sylva (1993) who describes two main categories of play – normative and therapeutic.

The purpose of *normative* play is to establish norms and rules. This sort of play, which children use most often, engages others, including friends and siblings, and uses the toys around the child. Normative play helps to bring familiarity to an unfamiliar situation, such as that experienced in hospital. Normative play is undertaken voluntarily and it is pleasurable. Very rarely does it have any goals and the child is in control. In a safe, relaxed and inviting environment, children can feel able to carry out their play.

Therapeutic play, the second category described by Sylva, is structured by adults and followed through by the child. Its purpose is to help the child to achieve 'emotional and physical well-being' by means of various activities, so as to achieve therapeutic ends. Through play, a child is given the opportunity to overcome fears and anxieties by bringing unconscious feelings to the surface. This play also incorporates desensitization.

Practice application – using puppets to help children to talk about their illness

Puppets allow children to talk about their illness through the third person, and are very simple and quick to create (e.g. draw a face on your finger and bring the child into the conversation). A 3-year-old child with cancer was able to express her feelings of anger with ease when encouraged to do so with a finger puppet. She talked to the puppet about the horrible taste of the medicine in her mouth and how cold it felt when it went into her tummy.

PLAY AND THE WAY FORWARDS

Siblings often experience feelings of abandonment, guilt, loss and uncertainty. Introducing play that includes siblings goes a long way to encourage harmony within the family during an unfamiliar experience of hospitalization.

Play specialists are now employed on most children's wards and hospices. The introduction of a team member who works regular hours and is responsible for creating a safe, fun and nonthreatening environment gives the child some normality in an abnormal situation. The ability to create an environment in which play occurs naturally is the best gift offered to sick children and their families.

The children's nurse who is able to understand the importance and value of play adds a vital component to her or his nursing skills, not only in the ward, but also *en route* to the theatre, in the anaesthetic room and in all other areas where children are nursed.

Further reading

Huband S and Trigg E (2000). *Practices in Children's Nursing. Guidelines for Hospital and Community*, pp. 329–334. Edinburgh: Churchill Livingstone.

POLYPHARMACY

Polypharmacy is the administration of multiple medications to an individual client, with the implication that more drugs are being given than is justified clinically. This phenomenon is frequently seen in older people and commonly involves the 'prescribing cascade', in which a drug is prescribed that causes a side-effect, another drug is then prescribed to combat the side-effect, but this drug causes further side-effects, and so on. Polypharmacy often also involves the use of duplicate medications in the same drug category, prescription of drugs with no apparent indication or that are contraindicated for use among older people, the use of inappropriate dosages and concurrent use of interacting medications. The problem is also augmented by use of over-the-counter medications, including complementary therapies. When discussing medications with a patient it is important to identify the drugs they are taking and the sources. Discontinuation of all or most of the drugs usually results in improvement of the patient's clinical condition.

POSTMORTEM

Postmortem (after death) usually implies dissection of the body during a postmortem examination. ⇒ Death.

POSTREGISTRATION EDUCATION AND PRACTICE

For all nurses, health visitors and midwives to maintain their registered status with the Nursing and Midwifery Council (NMC) they have to:
- Complete a notification of practice form at the point of re-registration every 3 years and/or when their area of professional practice changes to one in which they will use a different qualification that needs to be registered;
- Undertake a minimum of 5 days or 35 hours of learning that is relevant to their practice; ⇒ Continuing professional development (CPD)
- Work in some capacity by virtue of their nursing qualifications for a minimum of 750 hours (100 days) during the most recent 5 years, or have done an approved *return to practice* course;
- Keep a personal professional profile of their learning (see below);
- Comply with any request by the NMC to audit how the requirements have been met.

The NMC emphasizes that the CPD requirement for postregistration education and practice (PREP) can be achieved in a number of ways, and it is up to the individual practitioner to decide what is most appropriate for their CPD. For example, reading journal articles, conducting literature searches, visiting other units, ward teaching sessions, study days, conferences or seminars, shadowing other professionals and undertaking courses.

The NMC stresses that this is not purely undertaking an activity that fulfils the nurse's PREP needs, but it is a demonstration, through the nurse's profile and reflective practice, as to how the nurse's learning has affected his or her practice and therefore benefited patient and client care. ⇒ Reflection and reflective practice.

PERSONAL PROFESSIONAL PROFILE

A personal professional profile is a record of professional and career development. The intention is that an individual develops a profile that indicates their own development, and that grows and develops as the individual gains more experience, expertise and knowledge. Therefore, a personal professional profile illustrates career development, CPD and life-long learning. Clearly, this profile can also be used for a variety of needs, including the potential to demonstrate higher levels of practice.

It therefore appears logical that individuals begin to develop a personal professional profile at the point of registration, and indeed earlier. However, it must be based on regular reflection and recording of learning from experiences, as well as on structured learning opportunities. ⇒ Profiles and portfolios.

Further reading

Nursing and Midwifery Council (2002). *The PREP Handbook*. London: NMC.

POVERTY

⇒ Inequalities in health.

P-QRS-T COMPLEX

⇒ Electrocardiogram.

PRECEPTORSHIP

It has been recognized that newly qualified registered nurses require practical supervision and support for the first 6–12 months after registration, and so a *preceptor* should be assigned to the *probationer* nurse.

The key elements of preceptorship are to provide the newly qualified nurse with a role model, education about practice issues and feedback on performance. The purpose of preceptorship is to assist in the transition from student to registered nurse and to help the new nurse gain confidence and expertise in the new role. ⇒ Mentorship.

PREGNANCY

Pregnancy is being with child (i.e. gestation from previous menstrual period to parturition, normally 40 weeks or 280 days), and is divided into three periods, or trimesters, each lasting 3 months. A pregnancy of 40 weeks is said to be at term.

LABOUR (SYN. PARTURITION)

Labour is the act of giving birth to a child. There are three stages:
- First stage is from the onset of contractions until there is full dilation of the cervical os;
- Second stage lasts from full dilation of the cervical os until the baby is delivered;
- Third stage is until the placenta and membranes are expelled with control of bleeding.

Induced labour is one that has been initiated with drugs and/or artificial rupture of the fetal membranes. It may be performed for a variety of reasons, including eclampsia. *Precipitate labour* is a very rapid labour in which the baby is born after very few contractions. *Premature or preterm labour* is one that occurs before term, usually taken to be before the 37th week of pregnancy. ⇒ Conception and fertilization (Practice application – preconception care), Early pregnancy problems (ectopic pregnancy, miscarriage), Preterm and/or premature infants.

A discussion of all the problems associated with pregnancy is beyond the scope of this book. However, because hypertension is the medical condition encountered most commonly in pregnancy, a brief discussion is given here. The placenta is generally considered to be the primary cause of hypertensive disorders of pregnancy, as following birth the disease regresses. Hypertensive disorders are serious and can lead to maternal death.

CHRONIC HYPERTENSION

Chronic hypertension is known hypertension before pregnancy or a rise in blood pressure >140/90 mmHg before 20 weeks' gestation, and persisting for 6 weeks after delivery.

GESTATIONAL HYPERTENSION

Gestational hypertension is the development of hypertension without other signs of pre-eclampsia. It is diagnosed when, after resting, the woman's blood pressure rises above 140/90 mmHg on at least two occasions no more than a week apart after the 20th week of pregnancy in a woman known to be normotensive. Hypertension that is diagnosed for the first time in pregnancy and that does not resolve postpartum is also classified as gestational hypertension.

PRE-ECLAMPSIA

Pre-eclampsia is diagnosed on the basis of hypertension with proteinuria, when proteinuria is measured as >1+ on a dipstick or >0.3 g/L of protein in a random clean-catch specimen or an excretion of 0.3 g protein per 24 hours. In the absence of proteinuria, pre-eclampsia is suspected when hypertension is accompanied by symptoms such as headache, blurred vision, abdominal and/or epigastric pain, or altered biochemistry, specifically low platelet counts and abnormal liver enzyme levels (see *Table 28*). These signs and symptoms, together with blood pressure >160 mmHg systolic or >110 mmHg diastolic and proteinuria of 2+ or 3+ on a dipstick, represent the more severe form of the disease.

ECLAMPSIA

Eclampsia is defined as the new onset of convulsions during pregnancy or post-partum, unrelated to other cerebral pathologies, in a woman with pre-eclampsia.

HELLP SYNDROME

HELLP is a syndrome characterized by haemolysis (H), elevated liver enzymes (EL) and low platelet count (LP). It is generally thought to represent a variant of the pre-eclampsia–eclampsia syndrome. HELLP is associated with significant maternal and perinatal morbidity and mortality. In women it can lead to disseminated intravascular coagulation (DIC), rupture of the liver, pulmonary oedema and renal failure. Babies of affected women tend to be small for gestational age.

Further reading

Fraser D and Cooper M (2003). *Myles Textbook for Midwives*, Fourteenth Edition, Ch 20. Edinburgh: Churchill Livingstone.

PRESSURE POINTS

⇒ Haemorrhage.

PRESSURE ULCERS (SYN. PRESSURE SORES, DECUBITUS ULCER)

The prevention, early recognition of risk through assessment and effective treatment of pressure ulcers is an important part of nursing practice. The European Pressure Ulcer Advisory Panel (1999a) defines a pressure ulcer as an area of localized damage to the skin and underlying tissue caused by pressure, shear, friction or a combination of these factors (*Fig. 146*). ⇒ Tissue viability, Wounds and wound care.

A pressure ulcer can develop on any area of the body subjected to pressure sufficient to compress the capillaries and disrupt the microcirculation (i.e. *pressure areas*). It usually occurs where tissues are compressed between a bone and a hard surface (e.g. trolley, bed, chair, splint, cast, etc.) or where two skin surfaces are in contact. Pressure areas include the elbows, heels, ankles, hips, sacrum, spine, shoulders, head, buttocks and under the breasts.

Pressure ulcers develop when any area of the body is subjected to unrelieved pressure that leads to tissue hypoxia, ischaemia and necrosis with inflammation and ulcer formation. Shearing forces also disrupt the microcirculation when they

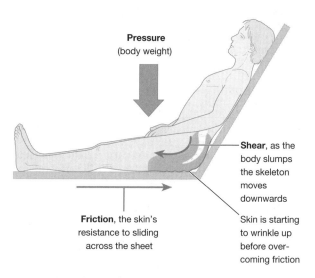

Fig 146 The relationship between pressure, shear and friction. The shaded area around the patient's buttocks is the area of highest risk – combined forces of pressure, shear and friction compress and stretch the tissue between the bone and surface

cause the skin layers to move against one another, such as a person slipping down the bed or being dragged instead of being moved correctly. Shearing injury damages the deeper tissues and can result in an extensive pressure ulcer. Friction from continual rubbing leads to blisters, abrasions and superficial pressure ulcers, and is exacerbated by the presence of moisture, such as sweat or urine (*Fig. 147*).

P

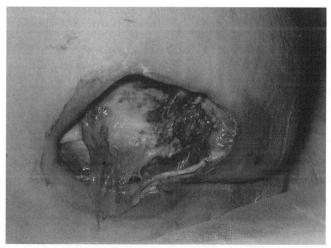

Fig 147 A pressure ulcer showing signs of damage to the surrounding skin

RISK ASSESSMENT – PRESSURE ULCERS

Although the true causes of tissue damage are pressure, shear and friction, other factors (known as intrinsic risk factors) determine an individual's susceptibility to these external forces. Factors that increase an individual's risk include any concurrent disease process that affects either the blood supply (e.g. cardiac failure) or the ability of the blood to provide adequate oxygen and nutrition to the tissues (e.g. lung disease and malabsorption syndrome). A variety of intrinsic factors are thought to predispose to pressure ulcer development and those more frequently described include general medical condition, skin condition, immobility, nutritional status and incontinence (European Pressure Ulcer Advisory Panel 1999b).

To prevent the development of pressure ulcers, it is therefore important to identify those who are at increased risk of tissue damage. The most common way to do this is to use a pressure ulcer risk assessment tool.

Pressure ulcer risk assessment tools

A range of risk assessment tools is available to help identify individuals at risk of developing pressure ulcers. Only one assessment tool is outlined here and readers are directed to the Further reading suggestions for more detailed information.

Risk assessment tools, such as that developed in the UK by Waterlow in the 1980s, are more comprehensive than earlier risk scales and include six main criteria:
- Build and weight for height;
- Continence;
- Skin type and visual risk areas;
- Mobility;
- Sex, age and appetite;
- Special risks, such as tissue malnutrition, neurological deficit, major surgery or trauma and medication.

The Waterlow Score (Waterlow 1985) also suggests risk bands of 'at risk', 'high risk' and 'very high risk'.

Many clinical areas now routinely use these tools to assist in the decision-making process, particularly to allocate specialist equipment, but also to plan general care. Many criticisms have been levelled at the tools, but remember that they are used to support and not replace the clinical decision-making process. The accuracy of the tools may be improved by ensuring that they are appropriate to the patient group and that all those who use the tools receive adequate educational preparation and support.

As the patient's condition may change, regular reassessments are necessary. There is no defined time interval, but recent guidance from the European Pressure Ulcer Advisory Panel (EPUAP) suggests that assessment should be ongoing, with the frequency of reassessment dependent upon changes in the patient's overall condition (European Pressure Ulcer Advisory Panel 1999b). This ensures that if the patient's level of risk increases, adequate preventive action is taken, and also that if the level of risk reduces, the preventive strategies are altered accordingly. Thus resources are utilized effectively, with the associated benefits for both patients and funding.

CLASSIFICATION OF PRESSURE DAMAGE

Should pressure damage occur, it is important to be able to quantify the extent of the damage, both to ensure adequate and accurate record-keeping and to improve communication between all the healthcare professionals involved in the patient's care. As with the risk assessment tools, a variety of classification or grading tools may be used to describe the degree of tissue damage. There is little agreement between these tools (e.g. whether to include or exclude transient reddening of the skin as pressure damage). Grades described range from 0 to 5 with some tools, and from 1 to 4 with others.

The grade of damage described usually refers to the layers of skin involved. EPUAP suggest the use of a four-grade classification tool (European Pressure Ulcer Advisory Panel 1999a; see *Box 30*).

Box 30 European Pressure Ulcer Advisory Panel (EPUAP) four-grade classification tool

Grade 1 – nonblanchable erythema of intact skin. Discolouration of the skin, warmth, oedema, induration or hardness may also be used as indicators, particularly in individuals with darker skin.

Grade 2 – partial-thickness skin loss that involves the epidermis or dermis, or both. The ulcer is superficial and presents clinically as an abrasion or blister.

Grade 3 – full-thickness skin loss that involves damage to, or necrosis of, subcutaneous tissue, which may extend down to, but not through, underlying fascia.

Grade 4 – extensive destruction, tissue necrosis or damage to muscle, bone or supporting structures with or without full-thickness skin loss.

Practice application – pressure ulcer prevention

The main points are (European Pressure Ulcer Advisory Panel 1999b):
- Identify 'at risk' individuals who need prevention and the specific factors that place them at risk;
- Maintain and improve tissue tolerance to pressure so as to prevent injury;
- Protect against the adverse effects of external mechanical forces – pressure, friction and shear;
- Use educational programmes to improve the outcome for patients at risk of pressure damage.

Further reading

Brooker C and Nicol M (2003). *Nursing Adults. The Practice of Caring*, pp. 187–193. Edinburgh: Mosby.
Morison MJ (2001). *The Prevention and Treatment of Pressure Ulcers*. Edinburgh: Mosby.
National Institute for Clinical Excellence (2003). *Pressure Ulcers: Prevention and Pressure-Relieving Devices*. Understanding NICE guidance – information for people at risk of pressure ulcers, their carers, and the public. NICE Guideline. Online at http://www.nice.org.uk

PRETERM AND/OR PREMATURE INFANTS

A preterm (premature) baby is one born after 24 weeks, but before 37 weeks gestation.

The term *low birthweight* is used to indicate a weight of 2.5 kg or less at birth, whether or not gestation was below 37 weeks.

Small for gestational age babies are those who weigh less than expected for a given gestational age. They are either constitutionally small or suffer from growth restriction. ⇒ Neonatal (neonatal respiratory distress syndrome, neonatal unit and neonatal intensive care unit).

PHYSICAL CHARACTERISTICS OF PRETERM INFANTS

Preterm babies have a number of distinct characteristics at various gestational ages, which include:

- Small and appear thin or scrawny because they have very little subcutaneous fat;
- Large head in proportion to the body;
- The skin is bright pink and often translucent (depends on degree of immaturity), smooth and shiny, with blood vessels clearly visible;
- Fine lanugo body hair (depends on gestational age), but head hair is sparse and fine;
- Ear cartilage is soft, and the soles and palms have few creases and look smooth;
- Bones of the skull and ribs feel soft;
- In male babies the testes are not descended;
- Female babies have a prominent labia and clitoris;
- Inactive and listless;
- The extremities maintain extension and stay in any position in which they are placed;
- Reflex activity is only partially developed – sucking is absent, weak or ineffectual; swallow, gag and cough reflexes are absent or diminished; and other neurological signs are absent or diminished.

Physiologically immature, preterm babies are unable to maintain body temperature, have limited ability to excrete solutes in the urine and have increased susceptibility to infection. A pliable thorax, immature lung tissue and immature respiratory regulatory centre lead to periodic breathing, hypoventilation and frequent periods of apnoea. Preterm babies are more susceptible to hyperbilirubinaemia and hypoglycaemia, and they are more vulnerable to fluid and electrolyte imbalance.

Following immediate resuscitation after delivery, preterm babies need some degree of support of physiological functions, depending on gestational age and condition. Supportive measures include:

- Oxygen therapy, assisted ventilation;
- Conservation of body heat, the use of incubators or warming units;
- Intravenous fluids to provide hydration, electrolytes and nutrition until enteral, breast or bottle feeding is possible;
- Pain relief as appropriate;
- Careful monitoring.

⇒ Haemolytic disease of the newborn, Learning disability, Necrosis (necrotizing enterocolitis), Oxygen (oxygen therapy).

PRIMARY HEALTHCARE

Primary healthcare is provided outside of the hospital sector to individuals and families in their own homes or in the community. The World Health Organization's declaration at Alma Ata in 1978 stated that such care should be acceptable, accessible, involve community participation and be available at a cost all families could afford. Most contacts that people have with health services are through primary care.

PRIMARY HEALTHCARE TEAM

An interdependent multiprofessional group of individuals, the primary healthcare team share a common purpose and responsibility, and each member clearly understands his or her own role, and those of other team members, in offering an effective service. The professionals involved may include community nurses, community mental health nurses, counsellors, general practitioners, health visitors, midwives, occupational therapists, physiotherapists, podiatrists, practice nurses, speech and language therapists, etc. ⇒ Community (community nurse, community mental health teams).

PRIMARY NURSING

Primary nursing is a professional model of practice, based on a belief in the thera-peutic value of the nurse–patient relationship. A qualified nurse (primary nurse) is responsible and accountable for the assessment, planning and implementation of all the nursing care of particular patients or group of patients for the entire duration of their stay in a particular care setting. The nurse is supported in this role by an asso-ciate nurse who cares for the patients while the primary nurse is absent, according to the nursing plan drawn up by the primary nurse. Other nurses, including students and healthcare assistants, may also provide care for the patients, but this is always under the supervision and co-ordination of the primary nurse. Primary nursing is not the same as named nursing – it is simply one form of named nursing, although probably the most highly developed form. ⇒ Named nurse, Team nursing.

PROFESSIONAL SELF-REGULATION

For most professions, self- (as opposed to externally imposed) regulation was a hard-won battle and passionately argued as serving the public good. 'Self' can refer to the individual or the profession as a whole through the statutory regulatory body [e.g. Nursing and Midwifery Council (NMC) and the Health Professions Council (HPC), which regulates professions such as physiotherapy]. Maintaining an active self-regulatory process is part of the duty of every practitioner and must be under-stood properly and re-negotiated regularly to maintain the special relationship that has been developed over time with the public.

Regulation is the means by which order, consistency and control are brought to a profession. The goal of an effective regulatory system should be to protect the public. Regulation in its widest sense refers to all the standards set in relation to a profession – not merely those that relate to professional conduct, competence or discipline. It should encompass the education standards that lead to registra-tion, standards for registration itself, standards for maintaining registration and standards for the removal or limitation of registration. The register, therefore, is at the heart of the process as an instrument of public protection.

Self-regulation is an accountability-based system, which carries with it spe-cific responsibilities. Such responsibilities are frequently set out in codes of con-duct or behaviour (e.g. the code of conduct produced by the NMC, which applies to all registered nurses, midwives and specialist community public health nurses).

Self-regulation activities include self- and peer-review, clinical supervision, sys-tematic practice development, professional audit and portfolio development, etc. ⇒ Accountability, Code of Professional Conduct, Competence and competencies, Council for the Regulation of Healthcare Professionals, Fitness for practice, Nursing and Midwifery Council.

PROFILES AND PORTFOLIOS

The terms profile and portfolio are often used interchangeably. Strictly speaking, the term portfolio should be used when referring to a wider ranging collection of evidence about learning, which might include personal and professional inter-ests. A profile is much more specific – a selection of evidence for a specific pur-pose. For example, the personal professional profile that nurses are required by the Nursing and Midwifery Council to keep to meet their re-registration require-ments. ⇒ Postregistration education and practice.

It is important that when an individual is required to keep a profile or portfo-lio the purpose is clear and that the expectations about content and style, for exam-ple, are unambiguous. Generally speaking, whichever term is used, there are common characteristics. Profiles and portfolios:

P

- Value experience as a source of learning;
- Provide a storehouse of evidence of experience, learning and achievements;
- Encourage personal and professional development.

PROSTATE

In the male, the prostate is a firm structure that lies immediately below the bladder neck and completely encircles the upper section of the male urethra (prostatic urethra). The prostate is a fibromuscular glandular organ that normally has two capsules, an outer layer of fibrous tissue and a thin inner fibrous sheath. Both encapsulate the prostatic glandular tissue (*Fig. 148*).

The prostatic secretion consists of a thin, slightly acidic, milky fluid that contains enzymes, including fibrinolysin and acid phosphatase; it is also rich in calcium and citrates. It forms 30% of the volume of semen. Prostatic secretion is thought to stimulate the motility of the spermatozoa, coagulate the fluid from the seminal vesicles and go some way towards neutralizing the prevailing vaginal acidity and influencing the motility of spermatozoa. ⇒ Reproductive systems, Urinary system.

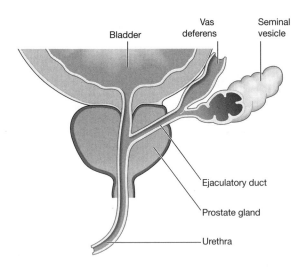

Fig 148 Section of the prostate gland and associated reproductive structures on one side

PROSTATIC DISORDERS

PROSTATE CANCER, PROSTATE SPECIFIC ANTIGEN

With over 24 700 new cases each year, prostate cancer is the most common cancer to affect men in the UK (Cancer Research UK 2003). Prostate cancer predominantly affects those aged over 60 years. Men of African descent have a higher risk of developing prostate cancer. There may be a genetic predisposition, and men with a first-degree relative with prostate cancer diagnosed at a young age are at higher risk. Men exposed to radiation, such as at work, may be at increased risk.

The presentation has many features in common with benign prostatic hyperplasia (BPH), and includes:

- Dysuria;
- Cystitis or prostatitis;
- Frequency and nocturia;
- Urgency;
- Hesitancy starting, poor stream and dribbling;
- Haematuria or bloody semen;
- Acute retention may also be a feature.

Symptoms associated with metastatic spread to the bones include weight loss, anorexia, anaemia and bone pain, such as backache. Advanced disease may present with signs of uraemia caused by the cancer obstructing the ureters.

The investigations are outlined in *Box 31*.

Box 31 Investigations for prostate cancer

Investigations for prostate cancer include:

- Rectal examination to assess size, shape and tenderness of prostate;
- Transrectal or transperineal biopsy of the prostate for histological examination;
- Serologic assessment of renal function, acid phosphatase and prostate specific antigen levels (PSA) – PSA is a protein secreted by prostatic tissue that acts as a tumour marker for prostate cancer, and its presence in the blood forms the basis for a screening test (however, conditions other than cancer can cause an increase in PSA);
- Urodynamic studies;
- Prostate and renal ultrasound;
- Radiograph (X-ray) of the pelvis or lumbar spine to detect bony metastases;
- Radioisotope scans for possible bone involvement.

The management of prostate cancer depends on the type, stage and extent of the cancer, and the health and general wishes of the patient. Management options include:

- Watchful waiting – prostate cancer can be slow growing and for some patients, a 'wait and see' approach may be appropriate. Regular follow-up and serial estimation of PSA levels are required.
- Surgery – radical prostatectomy. Transurethral resection of the prostate (TURP) may be undertaken in advanced prostatic cancer to relieve urinary outflow obstruction.
- Radiotherapy.
- Hormonal therapy – androgen suppression can be achieved surgically by bilateral orchidectomy (removal of the testes) or by the use of drugs that include gonadorelin analogues (e.g. goserelin) and anti-androgen drugs (e.g. flutamide).
- Chemotherapy (e.g. fluorouracil).

Benign prostatic hyperplasia

Benign prostatic hyperplasia (BPH) causes prostatic enlargement through the growth of new cells. It occurs most often in males over 60 years of age. The cause is unclear. BPH distorts the prostatic urethra and obstructs bladder outflow.

Clinical presentation includes:

- Frequency of micturition;
- Nocturia;
- Poor stream;
- Delay or difficulty in initiating urination;
- Post-urination dribbling;

- Overflow incontinence secondary to acute urinary retention.

Blood sampling for PSA may be undertaken if cancer is suspected (see above).

Treatment is dependent on the clinical presentation of the patient. In acute retention, relief of pain and outflow obstruction are priorities. Suprapubic catheterization through the abdominal wall is required if urethral catheterization is not possible. Treatment options include:

- TURP is usually undertaken, but open prostatectomy may be required if the prostate is too large to be resected transurethrally;
- Open prostatectomy – retropubic (via a suprapubic incision), transvesical (through the bladder) or via a perineal approach;
- Anti-androgen (against testosterone) drugs, such as finasteride, may be used in some cases to reduce the size of the prostate to improve urine flow rate.

Practice application – information for patients having transurethral resection of the prostate

Patients need a full explanation of the operative procedure and the requirement for bladder irrigation via a urethral catheter in the postoperative period (*Fig. 149*). They should be forewarned that the initial urine drainage will be bloodstained. The urologist will have explained the potential risks associated with TURP, and as part of the preoperative preparation nurses must ensure that patients understand the risk (albeit very small) of incontinence, erectile dysfunction and disordered ejaculation associated with this procedure. The consequences could have significant implications for quality of life and psychosexual relationships postoperatively. Patients should also be encouraged to perform pelvic floor exercises, both pre- and postoperatively. These exercises help them to overcome postoperative urine dribbling.

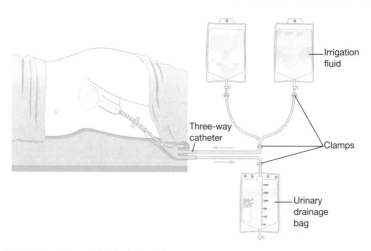

Fig 149 Continuous bladder irrigation

PROSTATISM

Prostatism is a term used to describe the symptom complex associated with bladder outflow obstruction (see BPH above).

PROSTATITIS

Prostatitis is inflammation of the prostate.

Further reading

Brooker C and Nicol M (2003). *Nursing Adults. The Practice of Caring*, pp. 696–701. Edinburgh: Mosby.

PROSTHETICS

Prosthetics is the specialty that deals with prostheses. A prosthesis is an artificial substitute for a missing or dysfunctional body part. Prostheses include an artificial eye, intraocular lens, hearing aids, cochlear implant, removable dental prosthesis (dentures), cardiac pacemaker, heart valve, breast implant after mastectomy or for cosmetic reasons, artificial limb, joint replacements, penile implant to replace the corpus cavernosum used for erectile dysfunction, and so on. ⇒ Amputation.

PROTEIN

Proteins, highly complex nitrogenous compounds, are found in all animal and vegetable tissues. They are built up of amino acids and are essential for the growth and repair of the body. Those from animal sources are of high biological value, as they contain the essential amino acids. Those from vegetable sources contain not all, but some of the essential amino acids. Proteins are hydrolysed in the body to produce amino acids, which are then used to build up new body proteins.

Protein produces 17 kJ/g (4 kcal/g), but protein is not normally used as an energy source in health. ⇒ Amino acids, Gastrointestinal tract (*Table 19*), Macronutrients, Malnutrition (protein-energy malnutrition).

PROTEUS SPP.

Proteus spp. are part of the large group of coliform micro-organisms. They are Gram-negative bacilli (rods) and can survive in either aerobic or anaerobic environments under a wide range of different temperatures. Found in warm, moist environments, they are commensals of the intestinal tract. They often colonize sites in which normal defence mechanisms are breached, such as intravenous cannulae, urinary catheters (causing encrustation) and endotracheal or tracheostomy tubes. They can cause severe infections of the urinary tract, wounds, respiratory system, etc., especially in seriously ill, immunocompromised individuals and neonates.

PROTOCOLS AND POLICIES

The use of national protocols (also called clinical guidelines) is increasing as nurses seek to base their care on sound evidence. The Cochrane Library offers systematic reviews of a range of topics to provide practitioners with a sound evidence base for their practice. Government organizations, such as the National Institute for Clinical Excellence (NICE), US Centers for Disease Control and Prevention (CDC), etc., produce clear guidance for clinicians about which treatments work best for which patients. In addition, the government sets national standards through National Service Frameworks, which detail how services can best be organized to cater for particular patient groups (e.g. diabetics, older adults), and indicate the standards that services have to meet. These standards are monitored by the Commission for Healthcare Audit and Inspection (CHAI; the Healthcare Commission) and annual national surveys of patient and user experience.

Other evidence-based guidance includes the Royal College of Nursing Clinical Guidelines and those formulated by the Scottish Intercollegiate Guidelines Network (SIGN), etc.

Policies and protocols are important because they make a statement about the way in which the employer expects a particular activity to be performed. For example, there is a policy for dealing with patients' property and a policy for handling complaints. There are also policies for clinical activities (e.g. moving and handling, infection control and intravenous therapy), which detail how these activities should be performed, who should perform them, etc. Failure to follow the employer's policy may mean that the employer refuses to accept responsibility for the nurse's actions in the event of a complaint. This responsibility that an employer bears for any omission or error of their employees is called vicarious liability. The principle of vicarious liability means that the employer is responsible for all the actions of its employees that are carried out in the 'course of employment' (i.e. following local protocols and policies). Protocols and policies authorize employees to work in certain ways and thus it is important that nurses be familiar with these in their area of practice. ⇒ Commission for Healthcare Audit and Inspection, Evidence-based practice, Health economics, National Institute for Clinical Excellence, National Service Frameworks.

PROTOZOA

Protozoa are unicellular microscopic animals. They are usually harmless, but may be pathogenic.

PROTOZOAL DISEASES

Protozoal diseases in humans can be classified into three broad groups, those in the blood (e.g. malaria, trypanosomiasis), the gut (e.g. giardiasis, amoebiasis, cryptosporidiosis, cyclosporiasis) and the tissues (e.g. toxoplasmosis, leishmaniasis). ⇒ Dysentery (amoebic dysentery), Malaria.

CRYPTOSPORIDIOSIS

Cryptosporidiosis is an infection caused by *Cryptosporidium pavum*. The organisms are present in the faeces of both domestic and farm animals, and transmission to humans occurs through contaminated water and food. Infection may be symptomless or result in profuse watery diarrhoea. Immunocompromised individuals, such as those with human immunodeficiency virus (HIV) disease, may be seriously affected.

CYCLOSPORIASIS

Cyclosporiasis is caused by *Cyclospora cayetanensis*. It has been reported particularly from Nepal, the Indian subcontinent and South America. Infection is caused by ingestion of contaminated water. There is acute diarrhoea and abdominal cramps, and the disease is more severe in immunosuppressed individuals. Treatment, if necessary, is with co-trimoxazole.

GIARDIASIS (SYN. LAMBLIASIS)

Giardiasis is an infection with the flagellate *Giardia intestinalis* (*G. lamblia*) that occurs world-wide, but is common in the tropics. Infection usually occurs by ingesting contaminated water. It particularly affects children in endemic areas, tourists and immunocompromised individuals, and it causes diarrhoea, abdominal pain, anorexia, nausea and vomiting. Treatment is with metronidazole, tinidazole or mepacrine hydrochloride.

LEISHMANIASIS

Leishmaniasis is a group of diseases caused by protozoa of the genus *Leishmania*, spread by sandflies. It may take the form of a generalized visceral infection, kala-azar (caused by *L. donovani*) or a purely cutaneous infection, known in the

Old World as oriental sore (caused by *L. major, L. tropica* or *L. aethiopica*). In South America, cutaneous leishmaniasis may remain confined to the skin or metastasize to the nose and mouth (caused by *L. mexicana, L. amazonensis* and *L. brasiliensis*).

Treatment is with sodium stibogluconate, amphotericin and pentamidine isetionate.

Microsporidiosis

Intestinal microsporidiosis causes diarrhoea in people with acquired immune deficiency syndrome (AIDS). The causative organisms are *Enterocytozoon bieneusi* or *Encephalitozoon intestalis*. Treatment is with albendazole.

Toxoplasmosis

Toxoplasmosis is a world-wide infection caused by *Toxoplasma gondii*. The definitive host is the domestic cat, and other felines and rodents are intermediate hosts. It can cause serious infections in humans and other mammals (e.g. sheep). Infected animals contaminate the environment with faeces that contain cysts.

Human infection occurs through environmental contact (e.g. gardening, playing and cleaning cat litter trays), by contacting infected animals or by eating undercooked meat. Most infections are symptomless or may cause mild illness with tiredness and myalgia. There is serious disease in immunosuppressed individuals (e.g. AIDS patients), who develop encephalitis and eye involvement. It is possible to be infected from a donated organ during transplant surgery.

Primary toxoplasmosis during pregnancy can lead to disease transmission, via the placenta, to the fetus. This is extremely serious and can lead to stillbirth or an infant with problems such as microcephaly or hydrocephaly, convulsions or liver damage, thrombocytopenia and purpura, or eye involvement. Infants who survive may have learning disability and develop encephalitis, liver cirrhosis and blindness.

Most infections resolve spontaneously. Patients for whom treatment is essential include infants, the immunosuppressed and those with eye involvement. Drugs used in various combinations include pyrimethamine, sulfadiazine, clarithromycin and clindamycin. Spiramycin may be used during pregnancy to reduce the risk of placental transmission.

Trichomoniasis

Trichomoniasis is caused by motile protozoan parasites of the genus *Trichomonas* (e.g. *T. vaginalis*, which causes vaginitis in females and urethral infection in males). ⇒ Sexually transmitted and acquired infection.

Trypanosomiasis

Trypanosomiasis is caused by parasitic protozoa of the genus *Trypanosoma*. In Africa, where the disease is called *sleeping sickness*, these include *Tr. brucei rhodesiense* or *Tr. brucei gambiense*. Both are transmitted by the bite of infected tsetse flies. Their life cycle alternates between blood-sucking arthropods, such as the tsetse fly, and vertebrate hosts. In South America, trypanosomiasis is also known as Chagas' disease and is caused by *T. cruzi*, which is transmitted by bugs.

The disease caused by *T. brucei gambiense* is usually chronic. Central nervous system (CNS) involvement causes headache, confusion, insomnia, daytime sleepiness and eventual coma and death. Infection with *T. brucei rhodesiense* is more acute, with myocarditis, hepatitis, pleural effusion and CNS involvement that leads to coma, tremors and death.

Treatment is complex and requires specialist input.

PRURITUS

Pruritus is intense itching, and repeated scratching can lead to secondary infection. It may occur as a manifestation of a particular skin disease. Generalized pruritus may be a symptom of systemic disease (as in infection), renal failure, diabetes, jaundice, thyroid disease, allergy and malignancy, such as in Hodgkin's disease and other lymphomas. ⇒ Anorectal problems (pruritus ani), Infestations (head lice), Jaundice, Vulva (pruritus vulvae).

PSEUDOMONAS SPP.

Pseudomonas are aerobic, environmental bacteria (Gram negative bacilli) commonly found in soil and water, but sometimes they colonize the intestines. The main pathogenic species is *Ps. Aeruginosa*, which takes advantage of damaged host defences to establish infection in burns, wounds and the urinary tract, and consequently it has become a major cause of hospital-acquired infection. It produces blue–green exudate or pus, which has a characteristic musty odour. *Pseudomonas* is sometimes found in the bowel of healthy people, but rapidly colonizes the bowel of hospital patients. Many infections caused by *Pseudomonas* are acquired from the patients' own intestinal colonization, although cross-infection on equipment and the hands of staff may occur. Strains of *Pseudomonas* resistant to aminoglycoside antibiotics may cause outbreaks of infection that are difficult to treat, especially in intensive care or burns units.

It can cause superinfection, whereby the normal commensals have been destroyed by broad-spectrum antibiotics. ⇒ Superinfection.

PSYCHIATRY

Psychiatry is the branch of medicine that addresses the diagnosis, treatment and prevention of mental illness. ⇒ Anxiety, Attention-deficit hyperactivity disorder, Autism, Child and adolescent mental health, Commission for Healthcare Audit and Inspection, Community (community mental health teams), Dementia, Disorders of mood, Eating disorders, Mental health, Obsessive–compulsive disorder, Phobias, Schizophrenia, Somatization, Suicide and deliberate self-harm.

PSYCHOLOGY

Psychology is a social science that seeks to understand and explain human mental processes and behaviour, and their developmental aspects. The subject matter of psychology includes how human beings think, behave and experience the world. Within the psychological literature are found a number of themes that represent different ways to interpret mental processing and behaviour. These are summarized in *Table 33*. ⇒ Behaviour, Behaviourism, Cognition, Mental defence mechanisms.

PSYCHOLOGIST

A psychologist is a person who specializes in the study and/or practice of psychology. A *clinical psychologist* is a suitably qualified person who provides professional services to people within a healthcare setting. They are able to assess patients and treat a wide range of emotional and mental health problems, often as part of a multidisciplinary team.

Educational psychologists have specialist knowledge of the emotional and cognitive development of children. They work within the education service where they assess the cognitive, emotions and behaviour of individual children, and advise teachers and parents or carers about management strategies to minimize specific difficulties (e.g. behavioural problems).

Table 33 Psychological themes

Theme	Examples of areas of psychological study	Examples of relevance to clinical practice
Absolute and negotiated knowledge	Positivist and interpretative research	Evidence-based practice and reflective practice
Commonalities and differences between people	Idiographic and nomothetic ways to explore human similarities and individuality	National Service Frameworks (to standardize clinical practice) and individualized assessment to inform holistic care planning
Autonomy and constraining factors	Theories to explain stress and coping	Responding to, and coping with, stressful situations
Consciousness and unconsciousness	Theories to explain memory	Making clinical assessments based on patient histories

Further reading

Kenworthy N, Snowley G and Gilling C (2002). *Common Foundation Studies in Nursing*, Third Edition, pp. 198–210. Edinburgh: Churchill Livingstone.

PSYCHOSEXUAL

Psychosexual describes the mental aspects of sexuality. ⇒ Sexuality.

PSYCHOSEXUAL DEVELOPMENT

According to Freud's theory, development occurs through five stages (oral, anal, phallic, latent and genital). Each stage is characterized by a different area of pleasurable stimulation. For example, the oral stage is characterized by the child's sensual interest in the mouth and lips, especially suckling. Psychosexual development encompasses all the processes whereby the individual reaches maturity in sexual behaviour (e.g. establishment of gender identity and role).

PSYCHOSIS

A psychosis is a major mental health disorder in which individuals lack insight into their condition. The term psychotic is used to group disorders characterized by a lack of contact with reality (e.g. by hallucinations or delusions). ⇒ Delusions, Disorders of mood (psychotic depression), Hallucinations, Schizophrenia.

PSYCHOTHERAPY

Psychotherapy describes a wide range of techniques used in the treatment of emotional and psychological problems by individual or group interaction. The usual method is by talking, but many other approaches exist. In *Group psychotherapy* or *group therapy*, a therapist enables and encourages people to understand and analyse their own problems and those of other group members. ⇒ Behaviour (behaviour therapy), Cognition (cognitive behavioural therapy, cognitive restructuring).

PSYCHODRAMA

Psychodrama is a group psychotherapy technique whereby patients act out past experiences by adopting roles in spontaneous dramatic performances. Group discussion aims to give the patients a greater insight into themselves, the problems presented and possible strategies to deal with them.

PULMONARY EMBOLISM

A pulmonary embolism (PE) is an embolus that occurs in the pulmonary arterial system, most commonly as a result of deep vein thrombosis (DVT) in the leg or pelvic veins. Preventing PE obviously depends on the prophylactic measures put in place to prevent DVT – these include deep breathing and foot exercises, early mobilization, anti-embolic stockings and the administration of heparin for at-risk groups.

A DVT may break off and travel in the veins and through the right side of the heart into the pulmonary circulation, where it causes a PE that leads to infarction (death of tissue) of lung tissue. Pulmonary emboli may be massive, acute, small-to-medium size or chronic multiple microemboli, and are estimated to cause some 30 000 deaths every year in the UK.

Nurses involved in the management of patients with DVT should be alert to the possibility of the patient having a PE. Vital signs of heart rate, blood pressure, temperature and respiration should be recorded every 4 hours to detect early signs of PE. Dependent on the type of PE, patients develop chest pain (often pleuritic), dyspnoea, pyrexia and haemoptysis (coughing up blood). A massive PE leads to sudden and severe dyspnoea and chest pain, cyanosis, tachycardia, hypotension, syncope and oliguria.

Treatment includes urgent resuscitation as appropriate (such as cardiopulmonary resuscitation), oxygen, pain relief, anticoagulation or thrombolytic drugs. Surgical intervention may be indicated occasionally. It may be an embolectomy (removal of the embolus) or a procedure that modifies the venous system to prevent recurrent emboli reaching the pulmonary circulation. ⇒ Advanced life support, Anticoagulants, Basic life support, Circulation, Deep vein thrombosis.

PULMONARY HYPERTENSION

Pulmonary hypertension is raised blood pressure within the pulmonary circulation, caused by increased resistance to blood flow within the pulmonary vessels. It may be primary (genetic), or secondary from chronic lung disease or chronic pulmonary embolism.

PULMONARY OEDEMA

Pulmonary oedema is fluid within the alveoli. The lungs are 'waterlogged' and gas exchange is reduced, such as in cardiogenic shock, left ventricular failure, mitral stenosis or fluid excess associated with intravenous fluids and in renal failure.

P

Practice application – signs and symptoms of pulmonary oedema in chronic left-sided heart failure
There is:
- Pulmonary congestion;
- Persistent coughing (pink-tinged, frothy secretions in extreme cases);
- Breathlessness (dyspnoea), more likely during exercise or on lying down;
- Nocturnal breathlessness and coughing.

Pulmonary oedema is managed with diuretics, such as furosemide, usually orally, but they can be given intravenously in acute situations. ⇒ Coronary heart disease (heart failure).

PULMONARY ARTERY FLOTATION CATHETER

In the critically ill, the central venous pressure (CVP) is an inadequate guide to circulating volume and cardiac filling pressures, particularly for the left side of the heart, and in such circumstances it may be necessary to gain a more accurate understanding of the left-sided pressures. A pulmonary artery flotation catheter (PAFC) is a specialized balloon-tipped catheter that is 'floated' from the central veins, through the right ventricle of the heart and into the pulmonary artery (*Fig. 150*). It enables the measurement of pulmonary artery pressure, pulmonary artery occlusion pressure and cardiac output.

Pulmonary artery occlusion pressure (PAOP), also known as *pulmonary artery wedge pressure* (PAWP), is the pressure in the left atrium measured by inflating a balloon on the tip of a PAFC, thereby temporarily occluding the pulmonary artery. ⇒ Circulation.

PAFCs can be modified to allow measurement of the cardiac output. A cold solution is injected into the right atrium and the subsequent decrease in temperature is measured in the pulmonary artery, which allows the cardiac output to be calculated. The PAFC can also be used to calculate a number of other variables, including:

• Systemic vascular resistance (SVR) – this relates to the resistance (afterload) being offered to the left ventricle by the systemic circulation;
• Oxygen delivery and oxygen consumption – it is important to know if sufficient levels of oxygen are being delivered to the tissues, but, equally importantly, whether the tissues are utilizing that oxygen effectively (oxygen delivery and consumption, respectively). ⇒ Oxygen.

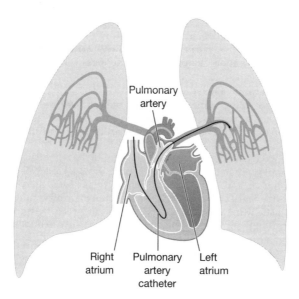

Pulmonary
artery

Right   Pulmonary   Left
atrium   artery   atrium
             catheter

Fig 150 Pulmonary artery flotation catheter

PULSE

The pulse is the rhythmic expansion and recoil of the elastic arteries caused by the ejection of blood as the left ventricle contracts. It can be palpated where an artery near the body surface can be pressed against a firm surface, such as bone. It is palpated customarily in the radial artery at the wrist. There are, however, other sites at which the pulse may be palpated, including the temporal, carotid, brachial, ulnar, femoral, popliteal, posterior tibial and dorsalis pedis pulses. The location of these pulses is illustrated in *Fig. 94* (pressure points for arresting haemorrhage). The choice of pulse is determined by factors such as age (the apex beat of the heart is used in babies aged under 6 months), accessibility and specific purpose (e.g. the dorsalis pedis and posterior tibial pulses are palpated in patients with peripheral arterial disease).

CHARACTERISTICS OF THE PULSE

When palpating the pulse the characteristics noted are rate, rhythm, volume and force or strength.

The *pulse rate* is the number of beats per minute (bpm). It is about 130 bpm in the newborn infant, which reduces during childhood until adulthood, at which it is 60–100 bpm at rest. *Tachycardia* is a rapid pulse rate and can result from exercise, pain, fear, anger, etc. A rapid pulse can occur in fever, blood loss, anaemia, heart disease, etc. A slow pulse is called *bradycardia*, and may occur in very fit athletes, but can result from certain drugs, raised intracranial pressure, heart disease, etc.

The *pulse rhythm* is its regularity – and can be regular or irregular. If the pulse is regular it is sufficient to count for 30 seconds and double the result, but if the pulse is irregular it should be counted for the full minute. It should be noted whether any irregularity occurs on a regular basis or is itself irregular.

The *pulse volume* is the amplitude of expansion of the arterial wall during the passage of the wave. It might be described as expansive or bounding, normal, difficult to palpate, thready or weak.

Pulse force or tension is its strength, estimated by the force needed to obliterate it by pressure of the finger.

A *pulse deficit* describes a difference between the rate of the heart and a peripheral pulse (counted at the wrist). It can be associated with arrhythmias, such as atrial fibrillation (see Practice application). ⇒ Heart (disorders of electrical conduction).

Practice application – apex–radial pulses

Simultaneous recording of the apex (using a stethoscope) and radial pulses may be necessary in patients with cardiac arrhythmias (e.g. atrial fibrillation), those receiving medication to improve heart action (e.g. digoxin) and those with peripheral arterial disease.

One nurse holds the stethoscope over the apex of the heart (located in the fifth intercostal space in the mid-clavicular line, *Fig. 151*) to locate the heart beat. Using the same watch and starting at exactly the same time, the other nurse counts the radial pulse rate. Both nurses count for a full minute because the pulse is usually irregular if apex–radial recordings have been requested. The two recordings are charted using different colours (e.g. red for apex and black for radial pulse). Any differences between the two recordings are reported and recorded in the nursing records.

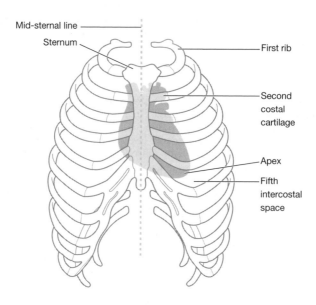

Mid-sternal line

Sternum

First rib

Second costal cartilage

Apex

Fifth intercostal space

Fig 151 Position of the apex of the heart

PUPILLARY RESPONSE (REFLEX)

The pupil response is controlled by two cranial nerves – optic (II) and oculomotor (III). When assessing pupil response the nurse should assess the size, shape and reaction to light of both pupils and record the findings on the chart (Woodward 1997b; see Practice application).

There is usually space on a neurological observation chart to record pupillary responses. This is not part of the Glasgow coma scale and does not assess consciousness. It does, however, assist in identifying the location of an expanding mass lesion and is a later sign of increasing intracranial pressure (ICP), after deterioration in level of consciousness.

ABNORMAL FINDINGS AND WHAT THEY MAY INDICATE

A pupil that is becoming oval, enlarging or losing the ability to react to light may indicate a rising ICP. This often occurs before a pupil becomes fixed and dilated, although this process can be rapid and the intermediate stages can be missed. ⇒ Head injury (brain shifts and 'coning').

An expanding lesion in the right cerebral hemisphere causes herniation of part of the temporal lobe through the tentorium, so that the right oculomotor nerve becomes compressed. This results in loss of the ability to constrict the pupil in response to light, so the pupil becomes fixed and dilated. If the pressure is unrelieved and continues to increase, the oculomotor nerve on the opposite side also becomes compressed and the contralateral pupil to the side of the lesion becomes fixed and dilated.

Pinpoint pupils may result from the administration of narcotics, including codeine phosphate. Codeine is often used as an analgesic within neurosciences as it does not mask neurological signs; however, it does still have an effect on pupil constriction.

Practice application – assessing pupillary response

Explain to the patient what you are going to do and why.

Examine each eye separately, moving a bright pen-torch from the outer aspect of the eye towards the pupil, watching the pupil into which the light is being shone; then remove the light source. The pupil should constrict briskly and then dilate to its usual size immediately on removal of the light source, known as the *direct light reflex*. Repeat the above procedure, shining the light into the same eye as before, but this time watch the reaction of the opposite (contralateral) pupil. This pupil should respond in exactly the same way as the other one simultaneously, called the *consensual light reflex*. Repeat this procedure exactly, shining the light into the second pupil. Normally, both pupils are equal in size and react briskly to light, both directly and consensually (*Fig. 152*).

The response from each is documented separately. The size (in millimetres) is measured and the printed scale of pupil sizes on the chart used to estimate the size of each pupil. Note the shape of each pupil (normally round).

It may be necessary to darken the environment to see a pupil constricting, especially in a darkly coloured iris or if the room is particularly brightly lit. It is easier to see if a larger pupil reacts or not.

A brisk constriction to light is recorded with a plus (+) sign on the chart, while an unreactive pupil is documented with a minus (–) sign. Pupil size is recorded on the chart using the pupil scale (mm).

Any abnormal findings are reported.

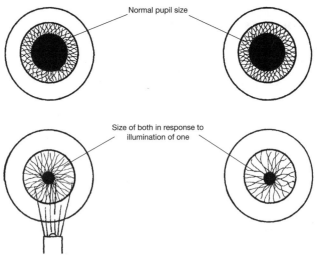

Normal pupil size

Size of both in response to illumination of one

Fig 152 Normal pupil responses. Light on one eye causes constriction of both pupils – direct and consensual reflex

QUALITY ASSURANCE

Quality assurance is the systematic monitoring and evaluation of agreed levels of service provision, followed by modifications in the light of the evaluation and or audit. It has both clinical and managerial inputs, involves audit and usually applies to all aspects of a healthcare service. ⇒ Audit, Benchmarking, Clinical governance, Commission for Healthcare Audit and Inspection, Evidence-based practice, Health economics, National Institute for Clinical Excellence.

Practice application – quality-of-life scales

Quality-of-life scales are measures of the factors that allow individuals to cope successfully with every aspect of life and challenges encountered. Quality of life is a conceptual or operational measurement commonly used in the chronic disease setting as a means to assess the impact of treatment on the person. Conceptual measurements include well-being, quality of survival, human values and satisfaction of needs, while operational measures record a person's ability to independently fulfil the tasks of daily living (Montazeri *et al*. 1996). One major critique of quality-of-life scales is that they seek to obtain quantitative (statistical) data about an aspect of life that is fundamentally subjective and qualitative, and individual patients may attribute different meanings to their responses. Only the patients can make valid assessments of their quality of life, so they are required to complete questionnaires themselves, unless they are not in a position to do so because of their physical or psychological condition. It is notable that the outcome of any assessment of the patient's quality of life is dependent upon how they feel and what life circumstances are affecting them at that time. These aspects may not be related directly to the chronic condition and its treatment, and therefore it is important to seek qualitative data to inform nursing interventions.

Q

RACISM

Racism is an opinion of particular groups that is founded on race alone. It results in negative stereotyping, prejudice and discrimination. Racism may be overt, whereby individuals are subjected to oppressive acts, or covert, whereby a climate of institutional racism permits one section of society to oppress and subordinate other groups. ⇒ Discrimination, Equality, Ethnicity, Fair and antidiscriminatory practice.

RADIATION AND RADIOACTIVITY

Radiation is the emanation of radiant energy in the form of electromagnetic waves, such as gamma, infrared, ultraviolet and X-rays, and visible light rays. Subatomic particles, such as neutrons or electrons, may also be radiated. Radiation may be nonionizing or ionizing and has many diagnostic and therapeutic uses. *Ionizing radiation* destabilizes an atom to form an ion. Examples include gamma rays, X-rays and particle radiation. It has the ability to cause tissue damage. *Radiation sickness* is the tissue damage caused by exposure to ionizing radiation. It leads to diarrhoea, vomiting, anorexia and bone marrow failure.

An unstable atomic nucleus that emits charged particles as it disintegrates is described as exhibiting radioactivity (i.e. being radioactive).

RADIOISOTOPE (SYN. RADIONUCLIDE)

Radioisotopes are forms of an element that have the same atomic number but different mass numbers and so exhibit the property of spontaneous nuclear disintegration [e.g. radioactive iodine (^{131}I)]. When taken orally, inhaled or given by injection, the disintegration can be traced by a Geigercounter. A radioisotope scan is a pictorial representation of the amount and distribution of radioactive isotope present in a particular organ – it is a diagnostic tool. Radioisotopes are also used in the treatment of disease.

HALF-LIFE AND RADIOACTIVE DECAY

Radioactive decay describes the spontaneous disintegration of radioactive atoms within a radioactive substance. *Half-life* ($t^1/_2$) is the amount of time taken for the radioactivity of a radioactive substance to decay by half the initial value. The half-life is a constant for each radioactive isotope (e.g. iodine-131 is 8 days). *Biological half-life* is the time taken by the body to eliminate 50% of the dose of any substance by normal biological processes and the *effective half-life* is the time taken for a combination of radioactive decay and biological processes to reduce radioactivity by 50%.

RADIOGRAPHY

Radiography is the use of X-rays:
- To create images of the body from which medical diagnosis can be made (diagnostic radiography) – a *radiograph* is a photographic image formed by exposure to X-rays, and is the correct term for the commonly used term 'X-ray';
- To treat a person suffering from a (malignant) disease, according to a medically prescribed regimen (therapeutic radiography). ⇒ Radiotherapy.

RADIOGRAPHER

There are two distinct professional disciplines within radiography, diagnostic and therapeutic. Radiographers are registered health professionals qualified in the use of ionizing radiation and other techniques, either in diagnostic imaging or radiotherapy.

RADIOLOGY

Radiology is the study of the diagnosis of disease by using X-rays and other allied imaging techniques.

RADIOLOGIST

A radiologist is a medical specialist in diagnosis by using X-rays and other allied imaging techniques. Some radiologists use imaging techniques to help them to carry out interventions.

A *radiation oncologist* is a medical specialist in the treatment of disease using X-rays and other forms of radiation.

RADIOTHERAPY

Radiotherapy is the use of ionizing radiation in the treatment of proliferative disease, especially cancer, and certain nonmalignant diseases. It may be used alone, but is commonly used as an adjunct to surgery, chemotherapy or hormone therapy and other treatment modalities with either a curative intent or as a palliative treatment to alleviate symptoms of advanced disease. The ionizing radiation disrupts deoxyribonucleic acid (DNA) synthesis, so that cellular replication is prevented, although several cell divisions may need to take place before cell death ultimately occurs.

The radiation may be applied by external beam methods (teletherapy) through the use of linear accelerators that emit megavoltage radiation to treat deeply seated tumours, and of lower energy units (e.g. orthovoltage or kilovoltage units) for more superficial lesions. Treatment commonly takes a few minutes each day, extended over several weeks. Other radiotherapeutic modalities include the use of sealed and unsealed radiation sources (brachytherapy). This is the delivery of radiation close to the tumour source, via a radioactive source placed into the body (i.e. the Selectron therapy for gynaecological cancers). In systemic therapy, radioactive isotopes are administered orally or intravenously and are preferentially taken up by the target tissue.

The main aims of radiotherapy are to apply a homogeneous tumouricidal dose to a precisely localized area of the body, to avoid as much normal tissue as possible without compromising the outcome to treatment and to avoid any critical structures (e.g. spinal cord or kidney) that may be sensitive to radiation. Although radiation is unable to discriminate between normal and malignant tissues, there is a differential effect and cancer cells are more sensitive to the effects of treatment. Healthy cells that surround the tumour are affected during treatment, so localized toxicity can develop (see Practice application). ⇒ Cancer, Cell (cell cycle).

R

Practice application – toxicity and side-effects associated with radiotherapy

The action of radiotherapy within the G_2 and M phases of the cell cycle means that the side-effects of treatment commonly present in rapidly dividing tissues (e.g. the mouth, bowel and the skin). Notably, the toxicities associated with radiotherapy are localized to the site of the treatment. Early toxicities that commonly present (dependent upon the target treatment area) while treatment is ongoing include mucositis, diarrhoea, proctitis (sore rectal area), cystitis, localized redness of the skin and alopecia. The degree of toxicity is dose-dependent. The administration of radiation treatment is associated with the development of a range of late effects, which manifest after the treatment. These include radiation pneumonitis and the development of secondary cancers many years after.

RANGE OF MOVEMENTS

⇒ Exercise, Mobility (range of movement).

RAYNAUD'S PHENOMENON AND DISEASE

⇒ Peripheral vascular diseases.

RECORD KEEPING AND DOCUMENTATION

Accurate record keeping and careful documentation is an essential part of nursing practice. The Nursing and Midwifery Council (NMC) *Guidelines for Records and Record Keeping* (NMC 2002b, 7) state that 'good record keeping helps to protect the welfare of patients and clients'.

High-quality record keeping helps nurses give skilled and safe care wherever they are working. Registered nurses and midwives have a legal and professional duty of care. According to the NMC *Guidelines* (NMC 2002b, 9–10) a nurse's record keeping and documentation should demonstrate:
- 'a full account of your assessment and the care planned and provided';
- 'relevant information about the condition of the patient or client at any given time and the measures you have taken to respond to their needs';
- 'evidence that you have understood and honoured your duty of care, that you have taken all reasonable steps to care for the patient or client and that any actions or omissions on your part have not compromised their safety in any way';
- 'a record of any arrangement you have made for the continuing care of a patient or client'.

Investigations into complaints about care look at and use the patient and client documents and records as evidence, so high-quality record keeping is essential. The employer, the NMC, a court of law or the Health Service Commissioner may investigate the complaint. A court of law tends to assume that if care has not been recorded, it has not been done.

GUIDELINES FOR DOCUMENTATION AND RECORD KEEPING

The basic guidelines for good practice in documentation and record keeping apply equally to written records and to computer-held records. The NMC (2002b, 8) states that patient and client records should:
- 'be factual, consistent and accurate';
- 'be written as soon as possible after an event has occurred, providing current information on the care and condition of the patient or client';
- 'be written clearly and in such a manner that the text cannot be erased';
- 'be written in such a way that any alterations or additions are dated, timed and signed in such a way that the original entry can still be read clearly';
- 'be accurately dated, timed and signed, with the signature printed alongside the first entry';
- 'not include abbreviations, jargon, meaningless phrases, irrelevant speculation and offensive subjective statements';
- 'readable on any photocopies'.

The NMC (2002b, 8–9) goes on to say that records should:
- 'be written, wherever possible, with the involvement of patient, client or their carer';
- 'be written in terms that the patient or client can understand';
- 'be consecutive';
- 'identify problems that have arisen and the action taken to rectify them';

- 'provide clear evidence of the care planned, the decisions made, the care given and the information shared'.

⇒ Access to health data, Data [Data Protection Acts (1994, 1998)], Malpractice, Negligence.

REFERENCING AND CITATION SYSTEMS

The previous work, upon which any study is built (or sometimes is attempting to replace) needs to be *referenced*, so the reader knows from where the evidence derives, and can locate the original if required.

There are several forms of referencing, but most are based on two types, Harvard and Vancouver. Each academic journal or textbook is likely to have a house style, such as that used in this book, and these are usually just variants from either of these two systems. Increasingly, material on the Internet, especially the Web, may be referenced.

The order of items depends on the reference style used (e.g. Harvard has the date immediately after the author). In the Harvard style, papers are cited in the text using the author and date, and the reference list is given in alphabetical order (A to Z). In Vancouver citation is by number, and the reference list is in order of citation appearance.

Thus, a sentence using the Harvard system might be: 'The Department of Health (DoH) has issued several documents which support clinical governance and clinical guidelines (Mann 1996, Department of Health 1999)'. The references would then be listed as:

Department of Health (1999). *Steps Towards Clinical Governance*. London: Department of Health.
Mann T (1996). *Clinical Guidelines: Using Clinical Guidelines to Improve Patient Care within the NHS*. Leeds: NHS Executive.

In the Vancouver system the same sentence would be: 'The Department of Health (DoH) has issued several documents which support clinical governance and clinical guidelines.[1,2]' The references would then be listed as:

1. Mann T. *Clinical Guidelines: Using Clinical Guidelines to Improve Patient Care within the NHS*. 1996. Leeds: NHS Executive.
2. Department of Health. *Steps Towards Clinical Governance*. 1999. London: Department of Health.

There are many places with information on how to reference articles from the Web, either articles placed on the Web, but available on paper, or those available only on the Web. The important points are that the type of medium could be the Web, not simply paper publications, and that the date you access such a Web-based article should be given on the grounds that Web-based material could evolve over time, and the accession date is thus the equivalent of the edition in a book.

REFLECTION AND REFLECTIVE PRACTICE

Reflection is an important process that enables people to consider experiences and their actions in response to a given situation. It requires the ability to analyse and evaluate events. Reflection needs to take place at a conscious level to allow us to make decisions about our learning. It is only by consciously considering our thoughts and ideas that we are able to evaluate them and make choices about what we should do next (Boud *et al.* 1985).

Reflection on all learning experiences (e.g. lectures, etc.) is a good idea, but it is most powerful in helping students gain the maximum benefit from their clinical placements. Despite their supernumerary status, nursing students are expected to, and indeed should, become involved in providing care for patients and helping to 'get the work done'. It is in this way that they learn the art and science of nursing, by observing and learning from expert nurses and, under their supervision, developing their own skills. Reflection helps nurses to look back at their experiences and determine what they have learnt, what knowledge they were applying and what they do not understand. This helps nurses to identify learning needs that will enable them to perform better in the future. ⇒ Code of Professional Conduct, Evidence-based practice, Postregistration education and practice, Profiles and portfolios.

USING A MODEL OF REFLECTION

Using a framework for reflection can help nurses examine what happened and how they felt about it, and help them to think through what they might do differently if a similar situation were to arise again. It also helps to identify what knowledge they need to learn to be able to deal with such situations. Several models or frameworks for reflection are available [e.g. Boud *et al.* (1985), Johns (1996) and Gibbs (1988), *Fig. 153*]. It is important to choose a model that is easy to use and develop the habit to regularly reflect on experience. This enables any negative emotions to be dealt with in a more positive and objective way, and enables the nurse to learn from the experience. It is a good idea to reflect on positive experiences as well as on negative ones, as they are equally good sources of learning.

> **Practice application – keeping a reflective journal and reflective writing**
> Writing a reflective journal (diary) can really help you to learn from experience. Also, looking back over the journal can help you to see just how much you have learnt over time. To learn from the experience and be able to deal with similar situations in the future, it is important not to be too hard on yourself when reflecting, but to focus on what happened and why. It is vital to ensure that no patient or client could be identified from the entries in your journal or from articles, essays and assignments.

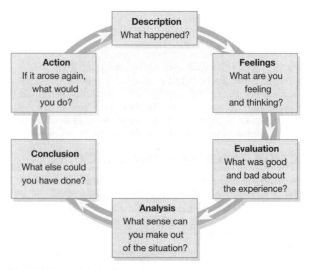

Fig 153 Gibbs' (1988) model of reflection

It is only by reflecting on a situation that you are truly able to learn from it in a positive way and to use the experience to develop your professional knowledge and skill. When writing down such an incident, work through what happened and try to think about what you have learnt from a particular experience. That is the key to development as a professional.

Reflection and reflective writing are important for all nurses because lifelong learning is not just about fulfilling PREP requirements and the competency required by the *Code of Professional Conduct* – there is also an ethical dimension. It is unethical to provide care that is neither reflective (i.e. has not benefited from previous experience and formal learning opportunities) nor evidence-based.

REFRACTIVE ERRORS

⇒ Vision (refractive errors).

REHABILITATION

In attempts to identify both its aim and purpose, definitions of rehabilitation have been proposed by numerous authors. Common identifiable threads appear to exist across these definitions (e.g. problem solving). The key characteristics involved in the aims and expectations of rehabilitation are outlined in *Box 32*.

Box 32 Characteristics of rehabilitation
- Reduction of disability and handicap;
- Independence;
- Empowerment;
- Problem solving;
- Client centred;
- Holistic approach;
- Educational process.

REHABILITATION MODELS

The key criteria for appraising or developing an appropriate model are that it is:
- Comprehensive;
- Relevant to and focused on the needs of the client;
- Client friendly;
- Rehabilitation-team friendly;
- A framework for practice and service development;

MODELS BASED ON DISABILITY MEASURE

Methods commonly used to measure the extent of disability include the Functional Independence Measure (FIM) and the Barthel index. These methods involve the rating of various self-care activities (such as eating, grooming, bathing, dressing and toileting) that may be used as a basis for rehabilitation. These reinforce the approach that disability and rehabilitation may often be thought of in terms of the individual being able or unable to perform various physical or mental activities.

HANDICAP-BASED MODEL

The assessment of handicap is based on dimensions of societal functioning. The WHO (1980) proposed six such dimensions – physical independence, mobility, occupation, social integration, economic self-sufficiency and orientation (*Fig. 154*).

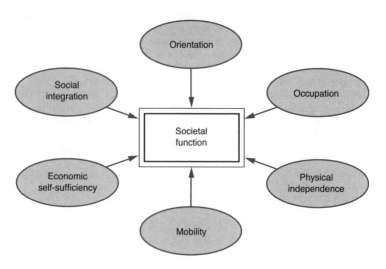

Fig 154 The six dimensions of societal functioning

AREAS OF NEED MODEL

A programme of rehabilitation based on a model with 11 areas of need. The under-pinning principle is to ensure that the rehabilitation team addresses all the relevant aspects within the life of the individual, so that goals planned within these areas are comprehensive and relevant to the individual.

The 11 areas of need are:
- Physical well-being;
- Accommodation;
- Mobility;
- Psychological well-being;
- Finance;
- Functional independence;
- Sexuality;
- Social reintegration;
- Family support;
- Self-care and independence;
- Communication.

Further reading

Smith M (1999). *Rehabilitation in Adult Nursing Practice.* Edinburgh: Churchill Livingstone.

RELAXATION

Relaxation techniques are used in the control of symptoms of stress. Although this is a reactive measure, these techniques are sometimes used to prevent a stressful period in an individual's life from developing into a crisis. Relaxation techniques can be used in specific situations, such as part of pain or symptom management, for tension headaches or prior to a frightening procedure in children.

The various methods include meditation, progressive muscle relaxation (see Practice application), massage (with or without aromatherapy oils) and biofeedback.
⇒ Complementary medicine and therapy (biofeedback, massage, relaxation, yoga).

Practice application – progressive muscle relaxation
Individuals are asked to contract and then relax one muscle group at a time, to compare the difference and to remember the feeling of relaxation. This usually takes place with the person lying in a quiet room, with relaxing music playing in the background. Each major muscle group is addressed in turn, leading to an overall reduction in muscle tone. Relaxed muscles are incompatible with feelings of tension, so progressive muscle relaxation thereby results in the individual feeling relaxed. A trained therapist usually leads the initial relaxation sessions. This is necessary because some patients may react to the feelings of relaxation with panic as they feel a loss of control, while others may require additional instruction. Relaxation requires practice and patients are often given an audiotape to use at home. However, while the therapy can provide relief from the physical symptoms of stress, it does not address the causes. Therefore, it is usually used as a supplement to other interventions that focus on managing stressors.

RENAL FAILURE

Renal failure may be acute or chronic. In either case, loss of normal renal function results in an inability to maintain fluid, electrolyte and acid–base homeostasis. Where there is chronic renal failure, additional sequelae to functional derangements of the kidney develop over time. Symptoms that arise from loss of renal function are referred to collectively as the *uraemic syndrome*. Renal physiology and renal disorders are covered in a separate entry. ⇒ Urinary system (urinary disorders).

ACUTE RENAL FAILURE

Acute renal failure (ARF) is defined as a sudden loss of renal function that is potentially reversible. The causes of ARF may be classified as pre-renal, renal and post-renal:
• Pre-renal causes are principally those that reduce kidney perfusion with blood, which results in hypoxic damage, such as the loss of circulatory volume or alteration to cardiac output;
• Renal causes include damage to the renal parenchyma by nephrotoxins, diseases such as glomerulonephritis or hypoxia resulting from prolonged and uncorrected underperfusion of the kidney – acute tubular necrosis (ATN) is a term commonly associated with ARF;
• Post-renal causes (obstructive) include stricture, renal calculi, prostatic hyperplasia, etc.
The treatment of ARF involves:
• Restoration of kidney perfusion pressures through restoration of effective vascular volume;
• Minimizing further renal injury by elimination of iatrogenic (prescribed drugs) and toxins;
• Specific treatment for the cause of renal failure;
• Instigation of dialytic support (see below), if this is required to assist the management of fluid, electrolyte and acid–base disturbances.

CHRONIC RENAL FAILURE

Chronic renal failure (CRF) is the chronic irreversible loss of renal function. A patient with CRF may or may not need renal replacement with dialytic therapy, but in end-stage renal failure (ESRF), failure to replace the renal function results in death.
Any condition that disrupts the normal structure and function of the kidney may eventually lead to CRF. Important causes include reflux nephropathy, adult

polycystic kidney disease, glomerulonephritis, tubulointerstitial disease and diabetes, etc. ⇒ Urinary system (urinary disorders).

RENAL REPLACEMENT THERAPIES

The term renal replacement therapy is used to describe the dialytic therapies (haemodialysis, haemofiltration, peritoneal dialysis) and renal transplantation. Dialysis cannot replace normal renal function fully, but offers at best a means to palliate some of the symptoms. Effective dialysis therapy must be accompanied by dietary and pharmacological interventions, which require considerable patient compliance.

Further reading

Brooker C and Nicol M (2003). *Nursing Adults. The Practice of Caring*, pp. 685–696. Edinburgh: Mosby.

REPETITIVE STRAIN INJURY

⇒ Occupational health (occupational diseases).

REPRODUCTIVE SYSTEMS

The basic structures and functions of the female and male reproductive systems are outlined here. However, in view of the importance and complexity of reproduction and sexual health issues, further detailed information is provided in separate entries and readers are directed to the suggested cross-references. ⇒ Abortion, Cervix, Climacteric, Conception and fertilization, Gametogenesis (oogenesis, spermatogenesis and spermiogenesis), Family planning, Infections of female reproductive tract, Infertility, Menstrual cycle, Ovaries, Penis, Prostate, Sexuality (*Box 36* – sexual dysfunction), Sexually transmitted and acquired infections, Testes, Uterus and vagina, Vulva.

FEMALE

The female reproductive system can be divided into two parts:
• Internal genitalia (*Fig. 155A*), which comprises the ovaries, uterine (fallopian) tubes, uterus and vagina;
• Structures of the external genitalia (pudendum; *Fig. 155B*).
The female reproductive system has a complex role:
• Produces ova or oocytes (female gametes or germ cells) in a process known as oogenesis;
• Provides the site for insemination and fertilization by a sperm;
• Hormone production – oestrogens and progesterone;
• Provides an environment suitable for the nurture and development of the fetus.

MALE

The male reproductive tract consists of the testes, scrotum, vas deferens (ductus deferens), ejaculatory ducts, prostate, urethra, penis, and their accessory ducts and glands, and an extensive venous and nerve plexus (*Fig. 156*).

The testes produce sperm (spermatozoa, i.e. spermatogenesis) and hormones. The scrotum, ducts, glands (seminal vesicles, prostate, bulbourethral or Cowper's glands) and the penis are termed the accessory reproductive organs, since they assist the passage and delivery of sperm to the female reproductive tract.

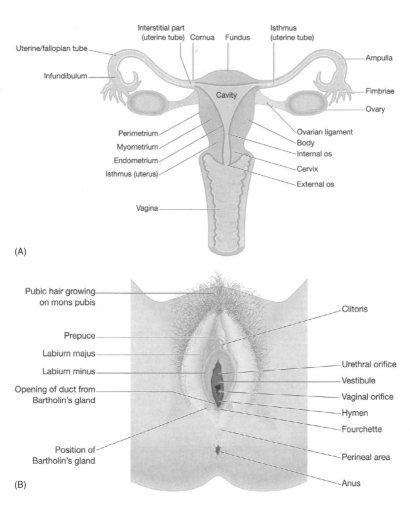

Fig 155 Female reproductive structures: (A) internal (anterior view), (B) external genitalia

RESEARCH

Research is the purposeful, systematic and rigorous collection of data, which are analysed and interpreted to gain new knowledge. Its purpose is to produce organized scientific knowledge.

In nursing we use both *quantitative* (deductive) and *qualitative* (inductive) research methods. In quantitative research the variables to be collected are defined, and then translated into numerical values. The data are analysed either to describe the data (descriptive statistics) or to test whether there are relationships between the data (inferential statistics). In qualitative research, typically it is not clear which data are relevant, so to predefine the data to collect makes little sense. Qualitative research tends to use smaller samples, but collect more data on each subject, typically by observing them or interviewing them.

In either case one needs a research question or a hypothesis. A research question is a concise statement of what the research is attempting to find out. A hypothesis

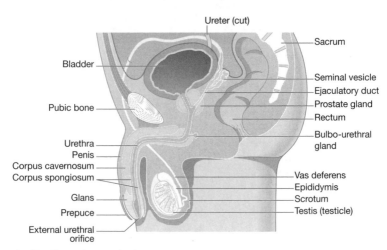

Fig 156 The male reproductive structures

is a statement that is testable, such that one may state the hypothesis to be accepted (true) or rejected (false). A hypothesis is needed in all cases where inferential statistics are used, otherwise a research question is required. Typically, the null hypothesis is used, which means that there is no difference between two groups, or no correlation between two variables, etc.

Concrete examples:

- A researcher wants to know the level of training for healthcare assistants (HCAs). A questionnaire is sent to a random sample of HCAs, with tick box items to determine the types of training they have had. The data are summarized in tables and charts to describe the situation – this is descriptive quantitative research.
- Researchers want to determine if female HCAs are more or less likely to receive professional training. Their hypothesis is that there is no difference between the two genders. They apply a statistical test, and decide that the null hypothesis is not rejected (i.e. there appears to be little or no difference between the genders). This is inferential quantitative research.
- A researcher wants to discover how HCAs feel about their professional development. A series of interviews with HCAs is arranged in which the researcher asks a set of questions, tapes the responses and develops themes from the transcripts. This is qualitative research.

Research is a huge subject area and readers are directed to the Further reading suggestions. However, basic definitions of some research terms are provided in *Box 33.* ⇒ Evidence-based practice, Literature searching and review, Referencing and citation systems, Statistics.

Box 33 Research terms

Case-control study – retrospective study that compares outcomes for a group with a particular condition with those of a control group without the condition.
Case study – research study that examines data from one case, or a small group of cases.
Cohort study – research study that investigates a population that shares a common feature, such as year of birth.
Comparative study – study that compares two populations.

Confounding factors – outside factors, apart from the variables already taken into account, that distort the results of research.

Control group – group that is not exposed to the independent variable, such as a particular nursing intervention or drug.

Cross-over study – study participants experience both the experimental agent and the placebo one after another.

Ecological study – research study in which a group of people (e.g. towns, etc.) is the observation unit.

Experimental group – the group exposed to the independent variable (the experimental agent or intervention).

Focus groups – research method whereby data are obtained by interviewing people in small interacting groups.

Grounded theory – research in which a hypothesis is derived from the data obtained.

Interviewing (in-depth, taped) – technique used, in qualitative research, to obtain information from the participants.

Likert scale – a scale used in questionnaire surveys whereby the participants are asked to indicate their level of agreement of a particular statement: strongly agree, agree, unsure, disagree and strongly disagree.

Longitudinal study – research study that collects data on more than one occasion (e.g. may study a cohort of people over many years).

Meta-analysis – a statistical summary of several research studies using complex quantitative analysis of the primary data.

Null hypothesis – a statement that asserts there is no difference between the factors being studied (i.e. no relationship between the dependent and independent variables). A null hypothesis is also known as a statistical hypothesis of no difference.

Observational study – research in which the researcher observes, listens and records the events of interest. *Participant observational study* is one in which the researcher takes part and has a role.

Pilot study – an initial smaller scale study used prior to the main research project to assess feasibility and to highlight deficiencies in the methodology.

Prospective study – research that collects data in the future, moving forward in time.

Random sampling – selection process whereby every individual in the population has an equal chance of being selected.

Randomized controlled trial (RCT) – research using two or more randomly selected groups (experimental and control). It produces a high level of evidence for practice.

Reliability – a measure of how repeatable the captured data are (i.e. if a researcher does this experiment again will the same outcome be obtained, or if the researcher interviews the same person twice will the answers be similar on both occasions?).

Research method – the various ways in which data are collected (e.g. observation, postal survey, interviews, using records, etc.).

Retrospective study – research that collects data from the past, moving backwards in time.

Survey – a data collection method. It may be postal questionnaire, telephone, face-to-face interview or via the Internet.

Triangulation – a term used to describe the use of a multi-method approach and/or data source to study a given research problem.

Type I and type II errors – in research, a type I error (alpha error) is rejecting a true null hypothesis, and a type II error (beta error) is not rejecting a null hypothesis that is false.

R

Validity – indicates the degree to which a method or test measures what it intends to measure. Validity refers to whether the appropriate data are being measured, recorded, observed or assessed.

Variables – any factor or circumstance that is part of the study. A *confounding variable* is one that affects the conditions of the independent variables unequally. A *dependent variable* is one that depends on the experimental conditions. An *independent variable* describes the variable conditions of an experimental situation (e.g. experimental or control). *Random variables* are background factors (e.g. noise) that may affect any conditions of the independent variable conditions equally.

ETHICS COMMITTEES

Ethics committees are bodies set up by Health authorities, NHS trusts, universities, etc., to consider proposals for research projects. The statutory committees, such as the Local Research Ethics Committees (LRECs), reviews, monitors and controls research that involves human subjects within healthcare. Any health research carried out must be submitted to the LREC committee within the area it is to be carried out. For situations in which research covers different geographical areas, a Multi-centre Research Ethics Committee (MREC) should be consulted. Funding bodies usually require the approval of the relevant ethics committee prior to the award of a grant.

The Central Office for Research Ethics Committees (COREC) co-ordinates the development of LRECs and MRECs for the NHS in England. COREC also manages the MRECs in England. Regional Offices of Research Ethics Committees (ORECs) supervise the work of the LRECs. Other organizations fulfil the same functions in Northern Ireland, Scotland and Wales.

Further reading and resources

Central Office for Research Ethics Committees (COREC) – http://www.corec.org.uk
Kenworthy N, Snowley G and Gilling C (2002). *Common Foundation Studies in Nursing*, Third Edition, Ch 12. Edinburgh: Churchill Livingstone.
Royal College of Nursing Research Advisory Group (1993). *Ethics Related to Research in Nursing*. London: Scutari.

RESPIRATORY SYSTEM

The respiratory system comprises the upper and lower airways and the thoracic cage (*Fig. 157*). The upper airway, which has a protective role, includes the nose, mouth, nasopharynx, oropharynx, laryngopharynx and larynx. The nasopharynx filters, warms and moistens the air before it enters the lungs, and so protects the lung from exposure to micro-organisms, toxic gases and particulates larger than 10 μm in diameter. Any particles that are deposited in the airways are propelled upwards, towards the oropharynx, by the mucociliary system. The mucus traps the particles and the cilia (microscopic hair-like projections) sweep the mucus upwards so that it can be expectorated. Ciliary movement can be impaired by tobacco smoke, pollution and excessive mucus production. The larynx protects the lower airways by closing during swallowing, and so prevents food entering them. It is also responsible for initiating the cough reflex, as it is sensitive to particles that cause irritation.

The lower airways include the trachea, bronchi, lungs, bronchioles (conducting air passages) and alveoli (small grape-like sacs that extend from alveolar ducts) responsible for the passage of gases between the lungs and the bloodstream. These structures work in combination with the thoracic cage, which includes the ribs, sternum and vertebrae, in the exchange of gases in the lungs.

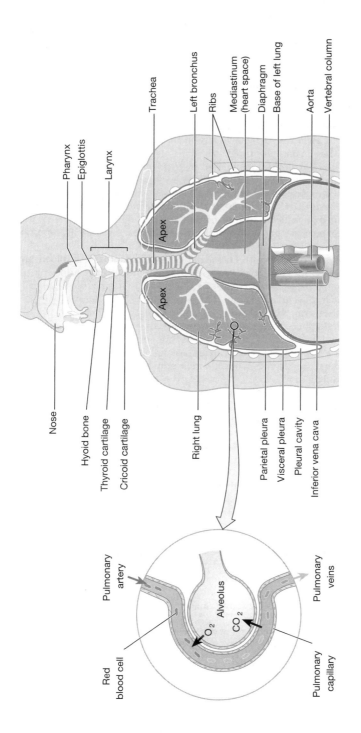

Fig 157 The respiratory system

R

The main function of the respiratory system is the transfer of gases, principally oxygen and carbon dioxide. It also has an important role in maintaining acid–base balance. Some words associated with respiration and oxygenation are defined in *Box 34*. ⇒ Acid–base balance.

Box 34 Respiratory terms

Apnoea – a transitory cessation of breathing, as seen in Cheyne–Stokes respiration.

Cheyne–Stokes respiration – cyclical waxing and waning of breathing, characterized at one extreme by deep fast breaths and at the other by apnoea. It generally has an ominous prognosis.

Cyanosis – a bluish tinge manifested by hypoxic tissue, observed most frequently under the nails, lips and skin. It always results from lack of oxygen, for which the causes are legion. *Central cyanosis* is blueness seen on the warm surfaces, such as the oral mucosa and tongue. *Peripheral cyanosis* is blueness of the limb extremities, the nose and the ear lobes.

Dyspnoea (breathlessness) – difficulty in, or laboured, breathing (see Practice application).

Haemoptysis – coughing up of blood or blood-stained mucus. The blood may be bright red, frothy and pink, dark red or have a 'rusty' appearance.

Hypercapnia (hypercarbia) – raised CO_2 tension in arterial blood, usually caused by hypoventilation.

Hyperpnoea – rapid deep breathing, panting, gasping.

Hyperventilation – overbreathing (an increased respiratory rate) may occur during anxiety attacks, in salicylate poisoning or head injury, or passively as part of a technique of general anaesthesia in intensive care. ⇒ Tetany.

Hypocapnia – reduced CO_2 tension in arterial blood, usually produced by hyperventilation.

Hypopnoea – shallow and slow respirations.

Hypoventilation – diminished breathing or underventilation.

Hypoxaemia – reduced oxygen in arterial blood, shown by decreased PaO_2 and reduced saturation.

Hypoxia – reduced oxygen level in the tissues.

Kussmaul's respiration – deep sighing respiration typical of diabetic ketoacidosis.

Orthopnoea – breathlessness that occurs when the person lies flat. It occurs because this position results in the redistribution of blood, which leads to an increased central and pulmonary blood volume and fluid accumulation in the lungs.

Paradoxical respiration – associated with injuries that result in the ribs on one side being fractured in two places, such as in flail chest. The injured side of the chest moves in (deflates) on inspiration and vice versa.

Sputum – the mucus and other material expectorated (coughed up) from the lower respiratory tract.

Stridor – a harsh breathing sound caused by turbulent airflow through constricted air passages.

Tachypnoea – abnormal frequency of respiration.

Wheezing – a whistling or rasping breathing sound, associated with the bronchospasm of asthma and other conditions.

⇒ Blood gases, Pulmonary oedema.

RESPIRATORY ASSESSMENT

Respiratory assessment involves the following:
- Respiratory rate – breaths/min (normal for newborn is 35, for 1–11 months it is 30, for 2 years it is 25, for 8 years it is 20, and for adults it is 12–20).
- Breathing rhythm and depth.
- Use of accessory muscles in neck and shoulders.
- Chest movement – is it symmetrical?
- Skin colour – is there cyanosis? The patient's skin should be observed for blueness of the lips, tongue and oral mucosa, as this indicates the presence of central cyanosis caused by hypoxaemia. In patients with dark skin, it may not be possible to see changes in lip colour and therefore the oral mucosa and tongue should always be examined.
- Oxygen saturation. ⇒ Oxygen (pulse oximetry).
- Smoking history.
- Triggers (e.g. exercise).
- Peak expiratory flow rate (PEFR; peak flow), see below.
- Cough (productive/dry).
- Sputum – colour (white, green–yellow, blood-stained), viscosity, odour and amount (see Practice application).
- Chest tightness and/or wheeze.
- Chest pain, ache and/or soreness.
- Mental state – confusion and disorientation may be a sign of severe hypoxia – drowsiness may indicate hypercapnia.
- Fluid retention and/or presence of oedema.
- Finger clubbing (seen in chronic tissue hypoxia).
- Temperature, blood pressure and pulse.

The impact of breathlessness on activities of living must also be assessed:
- Identify deficits;
- Mobility;
- Communicating;
- Nutrition.

Psychosocial impacts also need to be assessed:
- The patient's perceptions and concerns;
- Housing;
- Community support.

Practice application – care of patients producing sputum
Patients who are producing (expectorating) sputum require:
- A sputum pot with a lid (swallowing sputum may cause nausea). Expectorating into a tissue can increase the risk of cross-infection, as tissues are often re-used and left lying around.
- Tissues to allow patients to wipe excess secretions from their mouth and nose.
- Mouthwash and/or mouth care, as sputum often tastes foul.
- Encouragement with fluid intake, as dehydration increases the viscosity of the sputum.

R

RESPIRATORY FUNCTION TESTS

Respiratory function tests aid in the diagnosis of and monitoring progress of respiratory disease. These include spirometry to measure FEV_1 (forced expiratory volume in one second), and FVC (forced vital capacity), and in more specialized laboratories measurements of total lung volume and gas transfer factor are made.

RESPIRATORY DISORDERS

The most common causes of respiratory disease are smoking, allergens and trigger factors, genetics, micro-organisms and poverty. Tobacco smoke, which contains nicotine, tar, carbon monoxide and 4000 chemicals, is currently the leading cause of respiratory ill health and premature death. In susceptible individuals, smoking may cause lung cancer, chronic bronchitis, emphysema, recurrent infection, etc.

Some respiratory disorders are outlined below. Further information can be found in separate entries and also in the suggestions for Further reading. ⇒ Cystic fibrosis, Influenza, Oxygen (oxygen therapy), Systemic inflammatory response syndrome, Tuberculosis.

RESPIRATORY FAILURE

As a result of respiratory disease, the mechanics of breathing can be impaired, which leads to respiratory failure (i.e. the inability to maintain adequate oxygenation and adequate carbon dioxide elimination). There are two types of respiratory failure:
- Type I respiratory failure, in which an oxygenation problem results in hypoxaemia;
- Type II respiratory failure, in which a ventilatory problem results in hypoxaemia and hypercapnia.

Treatment options include:
- Type I respiratory failure – oxygen therapy and noninvasive continuous positive airway pressure (CPAP) via a mask;
- Type II respiratory failure – oxygen therapy, respiratory stimulants (e.g. doxapram), noninvasive positive pressure ventilation (NIPPV), invasive mechanical ventilation [intermittent positive pressure ventilation (IPPV)]. To provide invasive mechanical ventilation, patients must be intubated with an endotracheal tube or tracheostomy tube.

ACUTE BRONCHITIS

Acute bronchitis as an isolated incident is usually a primary viral infection that occurs in children as a complication of the common cold, influenza, whooping cough, measles, etc. Secondary infection occurs with bacteria, commonly *Streptococcus pneumoniae* or *Haemophilus influenzae*. Acute bronchitis in adults is usually an acute exacerbation of chronic bronchitis precipitated by a viral infection, but sometimes by a sudden increase in atmospheric pollution.

ACUTE RESPIRATORY DISTRESS SYNDROME

Acute respiratory distress syndrome (ARDS) is characterized by difficulty in breathing, poor oxygenation, stiff lungs and typical changes on a chest radiograph, following a recognized cause of acute lung injury. Analysis of arterial blood gases reveals a fall in PaO_2 and eventually an increased $PaCO_2$ and a fall in pH. ARDS can be part of multiple organ dysfunction syndrome. Patients require increasing inspired oxygen and then either noninvasive ventilation via a nasal or facial mask, such as CPAP or NIPPV support, or invasive mechanical ventilation (see above).

ASTHMA

Asthma is a chronic inflammatory condition that results in narrowing of the airways caused by inflammation and bronchoconstriction. It is characterized by paroxysmal dyspnoea, inspiratory wheezing, nonproductive cough and chest tightness.

Treatment is based on bronchodilators (inhaled β_2 agonists, e.g. short-acting salbutamol, long-acting salmeterol), which act as 'relievers' and corticosteroids, which act as 'preventers' (e.g. inhaled beclometasone or oral prednisolone). Other drugs include leukotriene receptor antagonists (e.g. montelukast, etc.). ⇒ Corticosteroids.

The measurement of PEFR is an integral part of the self-management of asthma; it is also used in acute asthma to monitor responses to treatment (Fig. 158).

Acute severe asthma is a severe life-threatening asthma attack. Typically, there is respiratory distress, reduced PEFR, cyanosis (central), tachycardia, sweating, an unproductive cough, exhaustion and severe hypoxia. It is a medical emergency that requires immediate treatment with high-concentration oxygen, intravenous access, systemic corticosteroids and inhaled β_2 agonists. Some patients may need ventilation.

CHRONIC OBSTRUCTIVE PULMONARY DISEASE

Chronic obstructive pulmonary disease (COPD) is a group of obstructive lung diseases in which airway resistance is increased with impaired airflow (e.g. pulmonary emphysema and chronic bronchitis). *Chronic bronchitis* is defined as a cough productive of sputum for at least 3 months consecutively in 2 years consecutively. The bronchial mucus-secreting glands are hypertrophied with an increase in goblet cells and loss of ciliated cells because of irritation from tobacco smoke or atmospheric pollutants. *Pulmonary emphysema* is an overdistension and subsequent destruction of alveoli and reduced gas exchange in the lungs. It is also associated with tobacco smoking.

The FEV_1 is <80% and the FEV_1:FVC ratio is <70%. COPD is usually seen as a long-term sequelae of smoking. Genetic factors include α_1-antitrypsin deficiency and, more recently, family clustering studies suggest other genetic susceptibility factors. COPD is characterized by dyspnoea, wheeze, cough and poor gaseous exchange.

Management includes smoking cessation, annual influenza vaccination, pneumococcal vaccination, nebulized bronchodilators (β_2 agonists or muscarinic antagonists), corticosteroids, prompt treatment of chest infection, oxygen therapy (often for many hours a day) and rehabilitation. ⇒ Oxygen (oxygen concentrator).

LUNG (BRONCHIAL) CANCER

Lung cancer may be caused by a *nonsmall cell carcinoma* (NSCLC), which is the most common type of lung cancer (around 80%), or an *oat cell carcinoma* (around 20%). Smoking is the most important factor in its aetiology, but passive smoking, environmental pollution and exposure to carcinogens (e.g. asbestos) are implicated. Exposure to asbestos leads to the development of mesothelioma, a rare lung cancer.

The presentation of primary lung cancer may be with cough, haemoptysis, recurrent pneumonia, increasing breathlessness or weight loss, or it may be an incidental finding on chest radiography. Therapy may include surgery, chemotherapy and/or radiotherapy, depending on the type and stage. Lung cancer can metastasize to the lymph nodes, brain, liver, etc.

The prognosis is generally poor because the cancer is often at an advanced stage at presentation.

PNEUMONIA

Pneumonia is an acute infection of the lungs by an invading micro-organism (bacteria, viruses, fungi) associated with new pulmonary shadowing on a chest radiograph. Pneumonia can be divided into community-acquired, hospital-acquired (nosocomial) and that associated with profound immunosuppression.

The type of pneumonia is determined by the causative organism [e.g. pneumococcal pneumonia, streptococcal pneumonia and *Pneumocystis carinii* pneumonia (PCP)].

1. Fit disposable mouthpiece to peak flow meter

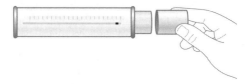

2. Ensure patient stands up or sits upright and holds peak flow meter horizontally without restricting movement of the marker. Ensure the marker is at the bottom of the scale

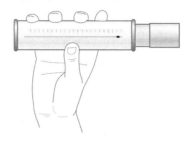

3. Ask patient to breathe in deeply, seal lips around mouthpiece and breathe out as quickly as possible

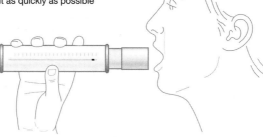

R

4. Repeat steps 2 and 3 twice more. Choose and record the highest of the three readings

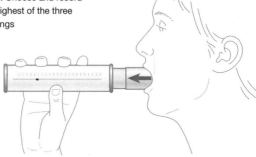

Fig 158 Measuring peak expiratory flow rate (PEFR) using a peak flow meter

Pneumonia can occur in previously healthy people, although there is a higher incidence among people with predisposing factors, including:
- Impaired respiratory defences (e.g. reduced cough reflex or tracheostomy);
- Old age;
- Underlying respiratory disease (e.g. asthma, COPD, etc.);
- Secondary to influenza;
- Immunodeficiency [e.g. human immunodeficiency virus (HIV) and/or acquired autoimmune disease (AIDS), or chemotherapy];
- Aspiration of vomit (aspiration pneumonia) or associated with chronic diseases, such as hepatic and renal disease, and alcohol misuse.

The presentation includes:
- Cough – often nonproductive with bacterial pneumonia, but with subsequently increased production of mucopurulent yellow and/or green sputum;
- Pleuritic chest pain;
- Pyrexia;
- Anorexia;
- Low oxygen levels.

Treatment is with the appropriate antimicrobial drugs (e.g. antibiotics for bacterial pneumonia). Initially, a broad-spectrum antibiotic, such as amoxicillin or erythromycin, is used until sputum microbiological results are available. The choice of the oral or intravenous route depends on the severity of presenting features.

A vaccine, effective against pneumococcal pneumonia, is available and is recommended for high-risk groups, such as older people and those with underlying respiratory disease. The vaccine is a single 'one-off' injection, although in immunocompromised patients and those who have undergone splenectomy a booster is recommended every 5 years. ⇒ Influenza (Practice application – flu vaccination).

The needs of the patient with pneumonia are determined by the causative factors and symptoms. To assist with sputum clearance, the patient needs to be encouraged to expectorate the sputum through coughing (see Practice application). Chest physiotherapy will also be initiated to assist with airway clearance and usually consists of postural drainage, percussion and breathing control.

Positioning the breathless patient is important (see Practice application).

Practice application – positioning the breathless patient
Being breathless can be extremely frightening for patients. Nurses can help a great deal by ensuring that the patient is in the best possible position. Positioning the patient in an upright position supported by pillows (in bed or a chair) or leaning over a bed table alleviates breathlessness by allowing effective lung expansion (*Fig. 159*).

Pneumothorax and haemothorax

Pneumothorax is air or gas in the pleural cavity that separates the visceral from the parietal pleura, so lung tissue is compressed. Blood in the pleural cavity is termed *haemothorax*. Pneumothorax occurs spontaneously when an over-dilated pulmonary air sac ruptures, which allows communication between respiratory passages and the pleural cavity. It is associated with many lung diseases, including asthma, bronchial cancer, COPD, congenital cysts, tuberculosis, trauma and positive pressure ventilation. Management involves the insertion of a cannula into the chest and connecting it to either a nonreturn valve or an underwater-seal drainage system.

Tension pneumothorax is a valve-like wound or tear in the lung that allows air to enter the pleural cavity with each inspiration, but not to escape on expiration, and thus progressively increases intrathoracic pressure and constitutes an acute medical emergency. Signs are of hyperinflation, midline shift and increasing respiratory distress.

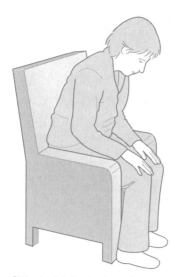

Sitting in chair leaning forward

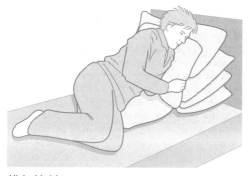

High side lying

R

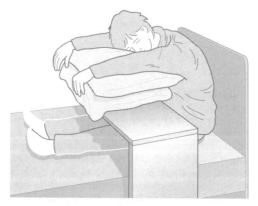

Upright positioning in bed leaning forward
onto pillows or bedside table with pillows

Fig 159 Positioning the breathless patient

Severe acute respiratory syndrome

Severe acute respiratory syndrome (SARS) is an atypical pneumonia caused by the SARS coronavirus (SARS CoV). It emerged, as a new infection, in South East Asia to cause a world-wide outbreak during 2003. It is characterized by pyrexia, dyspnoea, cough and changes on chest radiography (pneumonia or ARDS).

There is neither specific treatment nor an effective vaccine. Deaths from SARS are more likely to occur in those over 65 years of age and in those with pre-existing disease.

Further reading and resource

Brooker C and Nicol M (2003). *Nursing Adults. The Practice of Caring*, Ch 20. Edinburgh: Mosby.

Health Protection Agency – http://www.hpa.org.uk

Resuscitation

Resuscitation is the restoration to life of a person who is collapsed or apparently dead. The term is commonly used in the context of cardiac arrest and the basic and advanced life-support measures used to restart breathing and circulation. However, resuscitation can also include the measures required in critical situations, such as intravenous fluids to restore an adequate circulating blood volume. ⇒ Advanced life support, Basic life support, Cardiac arrest (cardiopulmonary resuscitation).

Rheumatic disorders

The rheumatic disorders are a diverse group of diseases that affect connective tissue, joints and bones. They include inflammatory joint disease (e.g. rheumatoid arthritis, septic arthritis and gout), connective tissue disorders, osteoarthritis, nonarticular and/or soft tissue rheumatism. ⇒ Joint (joint diseases – osteoarthritis, septic arthritis, gout), Systemic lupus erythematosus.

RHEUMATOID ARTHRITIS

Rheumatoid arthritis (RA) is a disease of unknown aetiology, characterized by polyarthritis that usually affects, firstly, the smaller peripheral joints, before it extends to involve larger joints accompanied by general ill health and results, eventually, in varying degrees of joint destruction and deformity with associated muscle wasting. It is not just a disease of joints, and most body systems can be affected (e.g. lungs). Many rheumatologists therefore prefer the term 'rheumatoid disease'. There is some question of it being an autoimmune process. *Rheumatoid factors* are autoantibodies found in the blood of most people with RA. It is not yet known whether they are the cause of, or the result of, arthritis.

Common presenting features of RA include pain (arthralgia) and stiffness of the affected joints, which result in mobility problems and reduced function in the sufferer. Usually the pain and stiffness are more severe early in the day. There may be low-grade pyrexia, often with general malaise and anorexia, all of which further compromise the person's ability and desire to function at full capacity. They also contribute to secondary complications (e.g. pressure ulcer development). Additionally, involvement of the nonarticular connective tissues may be present, which results in degenerative lesions (e.g. in muscles, tendons and blood vessels). These, again, may have an impact on the functional abilities of the client.

Management

Usually, management involves drug therapy:

- Nonsteroidal anti-inflammatory drugs (NSAIDs), simple painkillers;
- Disease-modifying anti-rheumatic drugs (DMARDs), such as sulfasalazine, methotrexate, hydroxychloroquine, penicillamine and parenteral gold salts;
- Other drugs that modify the immune system may be used (e.g. azathioprine and ciclosporin) and selective immunosuppressants (e.g. etanercept and infliximab);
- Corticosteroids.

Specialist physiotherapy (exercise, heat, the use of splints) and traction may be used to prevent or treat deformity, and facilitate pain relief and rest. Occupational therapy, environment modification and the provision of mobility aids are required in some cases.

Surgical options for the patient with RA include tenosynovectomy, surgical repair of a ruptured tendon, synovectomy, arthroplasty, arthrotomy or arthrodesis. ⇒ Orthopaedics (*Box 28*).

JUVENILE CHRONIC ARTHRITIS

Juvenile chronic arthritis (JCA) is a form of inflammatory arthritis that occurs in children. There are varying degrees of inflammation in the joints, with loss of articular cartilage and premature ossification of the epiphyseal growing plates. Management includes relief of pain and inflammation with warmth and drugs (e.g. NSAIDs), attention to nutrition and general well-being, adequate rest (both general and for specific joints with splints), good positioning and posture with expert physiotherapy.

RICKETTSIA

Rickettsia are small parasitic Gram-negative micro-organisms that have similarities with both viruses and bacteria. Like viruses, they are obligate intracellular parasites. Rickettsia are intestinal parasites of arthropods such as fleas, lice, mites and ticks; infection is usually conveyed to humans through the skin from the excreta of arthropods, but the saliva of some biting vectors is also infected. They cause various types of the typhus group and Rocky Mountain spotted fever.

RICKETTSIAL FEVERS

Rickettsial fevers are a group of rickettsial diseases that include epidemic typhus caused by *Rickettsia prowazekii* (louse-borne), endemic typhus caused by *R. typhi* (flea-borne), scrub typhus (mite-borne) caused by *R. tsutsugamushi* and Rocky Mountain spotted fever caused by *R. rickettsii* (from tick bites). The diseases are associated with overcrowding and poor hygiene conditions (e.g. after natural disasters, in refugee camps).

Q (Query) fever is caused by *Coxiella burnetii*, a rickettsial-like micro-organism. It is carried by ticks among animals, including cattle and sheep. Transmission to humans is airborne through aerosols from animal placentae and contaminated dust. Unpasteurized milk is another source of infection.

RIBONUCLEIC ACID

⇒ Nucleic acids.

RISK

Risk is a potential hazard. *Attributable risk* describes the disease rate in people exposed to the risk factor minus the occurrence in unexposed people. *Relative* risk is the ratio of disease rate in exposed people to those who have not been exposed. It is related to the *odds ratio*, which is the odds (as in betting) of disease occurring in an exposed person divided by the odds of the disease occurring in an unexposed person.

RISK ASSESSMENT AND MANAGEMENT

A risk assessment is a structured and methodical assessment of risk carried out for a particular area of activity (e.g. moving and handling patients in the operating theatre). This assessment then enables decisions to be made about problems, both actual and potential. Decisions may be based upon a number of criteria, such as placing people at risk, which may then be sub-divided into patients, staff and others. Other criteria may be the frequency of the problem, and whether incidents are likely to cause major injury or contribute to cumulative strain.

Managing risk in healthcare settings involves identification of the risk, analysis of the risk and controlling the risk:

- Identifying the risk is a data-gathering exercise to establish the kinds of risks likely to occur, and to make judgements about their frequency.
- Analysing the risk is a complex process that involves understanding the risks identified, and examining them within a framework of incidence, causes and impact on the organization. A range of management tools (e.g. flowcharts, pathway charts and cause-and-effect diagrams) is available to analyse the material gathered.
- Controlling the risk has two phases. Phase one involves introducing a range of focused activities, which may include physical safety features (e.g. handrails) or organizational controls in the form of protocols or guidelines. Phase two is to decide whether the NHS Trust retains the responsibility for the risk (i.e. will it deal with the financial consequences of any mishaps, or will it seek to transfer the risk to some form of insurance).

R

SALICYLATES

Salicylates are salts of salicylic acid, such as aspirin. They have anti-inflammatory, analgesic and antipyretic properties. ⇒ Nonsteroidal anti-inflammatory drugs.

> **Practice application – Reye's syndrome and aspirin**
> Reye's syndrome, 'wet brain and fatty liver', was described in 1963. There is cerebral oedema and diffuse fatty infiltration of the liver and other organs, including the kidney. The age range of recorded cases is 2 months to 15 years. It presents with vomiting, hypoglycaemia and disturbed consciousness, jaundice being conspicuous. There is an association with salicylate administration and chicken pox.
>
> The association with Reye's syndrome means aspirin should not be given to children under 16 years of age. There are conditions, however (e.g. Kawasaki disease – systemic vasculitis), in which the use of aspirin is specifically indicated.

SALMONELLA

Salmonella belong to a genus of Gram-negative bacilli. They are parasitic in many animals and humans, in whom they are often pathogenic. Some species, such as *S. typhi* and *S. paratyphi*, are host-specific so infect humans only, in whom they cause the enteric fevers (see below). Others, such as *S. typhimurium*, may infect a wide range of host species, usually through contaminated foods. *S. enteritidis* is a motile bacterium, widely distributed in domestic animals, particularly poultry, and in wild animals (e.g. rodents) and sporadic in humans as a cause of food poisoning. ⇒ Food problems (food poisoning), Gastrointestinal tract (gastroenteritis).

ENTERIC FEVERS

Enteric fevers include typhoid and paratyphoid, individual features of which are outlined below. Treatment of the enteric fevers is with antibiotics (e.g. ciprofloxacin, co-trimoxazole, amoxicillin and chloramphenicol).

TYPHOID

Typhoid is caused by the bacterium *S. typhi*, transmitted by contaminated food, milk or water. Contamination occurs directly by sewage, and indirectly by flies or faulty personal hygiene. It is commonly associated with a lack of clean water and poor sanitation, but outbreaks occur in other areas, usually through food contamination by asymptomatic carriers. The average incubation period is 10–14 days. There is bacteraemia and inflammation of small bowel lymphoid tissue (Peyer's patches), which ulcerates and may perforate or bleed. The onset is characterized by a 'stepladder' rise in temperature, slow pulse, headache, drowsiness and cough. Later there is a 'rose-red' spot rash on the abdomen, splenomegaly and typical 'pea-soup' diarrhoea with abdominal tenderness, delirium and bronchitis. Immunization is available for those who travel to areas where typhoid is endemic; however, it is not a substitute for careful hygiene measures.

PARATYPHOID

Paratyphoid is caused by the bacterium *S. paratyphi* A and B, which usually originates from animals. Transmission is by the faecal–oral route and humans may become infected by direct contact with animals, such as poultry, or indirectly via contaminated food, water or milk. Food may become contaminated by food handlers, who are carriers. Paratyphoid tends to be less severe and of shorter duration than typhoid fever. The presentation includes fever, headaches, myalgia, acute enteritis with vomiting and diarrhoea and a rash. Intestinal complications are less common than with typhoid.

SCARLATINA

⇒ Communicable diseases (scarlet fever).

SCHIZOPHRENIA

Schizophrenia is an umbrella term to cover a number of different conditions that share common clinical features. It is the most severe and enduring of the functional illnesses – only one-third of patients make a complete recovery. Schizophrenia causes very significant levels of distress and in many cases lifelong handicap for the sufferer. Furthermore, schizophrenia also produces a considerable burden on both carers and the healthcare system.

Schizophrenia is one of the major diagnostic categories of mental illness and the diagnosis relies on the presence of key ('first rank') symptoms. These are any one of (a) to (d) or any two of (e) to (h), listed below, for 1 month or more on most days and not caused by organic brain disease, alcohol or drug intoxication.

(a) Thought echo, insertion, withdrawal or broadcasting;
(b) Delusions of control, influence or passivity, clearly referred to body or limb movements or specific thoughts, actions or sensations, delusional perception;
(c) Third person auditory hallucinations, either running commentary on actions or discussing the client among themselves;
(d) Persistent delusions that are culturally inappropriate and completely impossible;
(e) Persistent hallucinations when accompanied by fleeting or half-formed delusions without clear affective content, or by persistent overvalued ideas or when occurring every day for weeks or months on end;
(f) Breaks or interpolations in the train of thought, incoherence, irrelevant speech or neologisms;
(g) Catatonic behaviour;
(h) Negative symptoms of apathy, paucity of speech and blunting or incongruity of affect, usually resulting in social withdrawal, not caused by depression or neuroleptic medication.

Symptoms can be grouped as positive and negative. Positive symptoms include hallucinations and delusions or hearing voices and/or having strange thoughts. Negative symptoms include social withdrawal and lack of energy or motivation. The negative symptoms are harder to recognize, and they are often ascribed to reasons other than the illness, such as personality, laziness or unwanted effects of medication.

Until very recently medication was the first and generally only treatment of choice. Despite the introduction of new 'atypical antipsychotics (neuroleptics)', the drugs generally produce a range of unwanted and unpleasant side-effects. The atypical antipsychotics used to treat people with newly diagnosed schizophrenia include amisulpride, olanzapine, quetiapine, risperidone and zotepine. Although drugs remove positive symptoms, they do so entirely only in a minority of cases. Most people continue to have a level of residual symptoms and the user movement has been actively campaigning for alternative treatments. New forms of treatment include social-skills training, and cognitive behavioural and psychosocial interventions. Helping clients and their carers understand the illness and its symptoms and enabling them to develop practical solutions to the problems that the illness brings have proved very effective. The stress vulnerability model (Zubin and Spring 1977) is a useful one for considering the illness. This model suggests that we all have a different level of vulnerability to a mental health problem. If we become sufficiently stressed we can cross the vulnerability threshold and become mentally unwell. Therefore, educating people who have schizophrenia and their families to be alert to stress levels and learn strategies to moderate stress helps to reduce the impact of the illness. ⇒ Antipsychotics, Expressed emotion, Mental health.

SCIATICA

⇒ Musculoskeletal disorders (back problems and back pain).

SCREENING AND EARLY DETECTION

Screening is a preventive measure used to identify potential or incipient disease at an early stage, when it may be treated more easily. It is carried out in a variety of settings, including primary care, the workplace, hospitals, clinics for antenatal care, and well babies, well men and well women clinics. Screening checks include mammography, cervical cytology, blood pressure checks, checks for diabetes mellitus, faecal occult blood, prostatic specific antigen test for prostate cancer, ultrasound and blood tests during pregnancy, urine examination to detect bladder cancers associated with some industrial processes, etc.

The screening process can cause anxiety even when no abnormality is found (negative result). ⇒ Breast (breast cancer), Cancer, Cervix (cancer of the cervix), Fetus (fetal assessment and screening), Gastrointestinal tract (colorectal cancer), Gynaecological examination (cervical cytology), Prostate (prostate cancer).

SENSITIVITY AND SPECIFICITY

Screening tests should have both *sensitivity* and *specificity*. High sensitivity is the ability to detect abnormality (i.e. in all those with the disease), and high specificity is having a high level of accuracy where the results are confirmed as positive or negative (i.e. only detect those with the disease).

False negatives occur if the test has low sensitivity (i.e. it does not detect all abnormal cases). The higher the sensitivity, the fewer are the false-negative results.

False positives occur if a test has low specificity (i.e. it detects the disease in cases where it is not present). The higher the specificity, the fewer are the false-positive results.

SEIZURE

A seizure occurs when cerebral neurons fire (i.e. generate impulses) abnormally. A seizure can be regarded as an electrical disturbance in the brain. The word 'fit' is not useful because seizures may not resemble the 'classic fit' of convulsions and loss of consciousness – seizure is a more suitable term. Seizures may or may not show clinical manifestations. Seizures may be caused by several triggers [e.g. hyperventilation, alcohol (particularly withdrawal), flickering light stimulation, exhaustion, intercurrent infection, recreational drug misuse, sleep deprivation and migraine], as well as those causes that occur in people diagnosed with epilepsy and other disorders (*Box 35*).

Convulsions are involuntary contractions of muscles that result from abnormal cerebral stimulation. They occur with or without loss of consciousness. *Clonic convulsions* are associated with muscle contraction and relaxation, with violent jerky movements of the face and limbs, incontinence of urine and tongue biting.

Tonic convulsions are characterized by sudden contraction of the muscles that leads to sustained rigidity. The person may be cyanosed with loss of consciousness. In *tonic–clonic convulsions* the person becomes rigid (tonic), falls to the ground and jerks all over (clonic). ⇒ Febrile (febrile seizure), Nervous system (epilepsy), Tetany.

Box 35 Some causes of seizures
- Brain tumour;
- Epilepsy, idiopathic and secondary;
- High body temperature (febrile seizure);
- Meningitis;
- Metabolic disorders, such as severe hypoglycaemia;
- Stroke;
- Traumatic brain injury.

Practice application – care during and after a seizure
As patients with epilepsy may have very individual problems and seizure types, the management is based on an individual assessment of needs. However, some general points include:
- Stay calm and reassure onlookers.
- Do not put anything in the person's mouth.
- Protect patients from harm (e.g. by moving furniture, or moving them away from hazards or using a pillow to protect their heads during convulsions).
- After the convulsion is over, place patients in the recovery position until they regain consciousness.
- If the seizure occurs in the community, do not call an ambulance immediately. Patients should be asked if they have had a fit before; if it is a regular occurrence, they can usually return to everyday activities, but are advised to consult their doctor. If it is a first seizure, they convulse for more than 3–5 minutes or they do not regain consciousness within 10 minutes, an ambulance should be called. If they progress to continuous seizures (status epilepticus), medical help is required.
- Patients should be observed carefully during the seizure (e.g. noting whether the seizure is focal or generalized).
- Within healthcare settings, patients may be given anti-epileptic drugs. However, during a seizure patients must not receive any medication by mouth – drugs may be administered rectally, or by intramuscular or intravenous injection.
- After the seizure has ended, patients should be allowed to rest. Patients who have been incontinent of urine need assistance and/or facilities to wash and change their clothing.
- Stay with patients until they are recovered fully, as they may show unusual behaviour of which they are not aware. This is called automatism.
- It may be necessary to monitor consciousness and blood pressure, pulse and respiration after the seizure.
- Explain to the person who has had a seizure what has happened.

Sensory

Sensory is pertaining to sensation, the consciousness of a feeling that results from nerve impulses from the sensory organs and structures that reach the brain. Sensory (afferent) nerves convey impulses from the peripheral receptors in the sensory organs and structures to the brain and spinal cord. The sensory cortex is the region of the cerebral cortex at which sensory inputs are received. The main area is posterior to the central sulcus in the parietal lobes in both cerebral hemispheres. ⇒ Ear, Eye, Hearing, Nose and paranasal sinuses, Smell, Taste, Touch, Vision.

Practice application – sensory reduction and/or overload in critical care
Any critical illness is frightening for patients and causes stress, and the critical care environment is likely to cause stress for their family as well.

Alteration in sensory perception can occur for a number of reasons, including both a reduction in and an overload of sensory inputs. It is important that patients be given personal space and time, yet not be left isolated for long periods. This highlights the needs to plan the care and management for patients over a 24-hour period and not just over the course of one shift. Co-ordination of activities is required to ensure that patients are allowed to rest without procedures and other interventions for periods of the day, and wherever possible a normal day–night pattern should be created (e.g. having a break from enteral feeding for a period during the night).

Touch, as opposed to the clinical contact made through nursing or medical interventions, and speech – reminding patients of the date, time and where they are – are extremely important, even if they are unable to respond. Critical care environments can be noisy, because of the number of people and amount of equipment, and all efforts should be made to minimize this. The presence of personal items and/or the use of favourite music can help to relax the patient and provide comfort. Constant light can also be problematic and, although the care of critically ill patients must continue throughout the 24-hour period, the reduction of activity, noise and light at night to enable sleep is important. Sleep deprivation and alterations in sensory perception can lead to tiredness, confusion, disorientation, hallucinations and delirium.

SEPTIC SHOCK

Septic shock is shock that occurs as a result of an overwhelming inflammatory response to infection. ⇒ Shock, Systemic inflammatory response syndrome.

SEPTICAEMIA

Septicaemia is the multiplication of bacteria in the bloodstream that causes infection (e.g. meningococcal septicaemia). ⇒ Group C meningococcal disease, Systemic inflammatory response syndrome.

SEVERE ACUTE RESPIRATORY SYNDROME

⇒ Respiratory system.

SEXISM

Sexism is a belief that members of one sex are superior to members of the other, and thereby have advantages over them. It leads to discrimination and can act as a limiting factor (e.g. in educational and professional development, and/or access to healthcare).

SEXUAL ABUSE

⇒ Abuse.

SEXUALITY

To define sexuality is not an easy task. Sexual activity, including feelings, thoughts and actions, is central to such a definition, and the concepts of masculinity and femininity are also significant. Writers who have grappled with the nature of sexuality have often included these ideas, but the need to take a broad view has been emphasized. Obviously, there is much more to sexuality than sexual intercourse – it can be considered as being the sum of the physical, functional and psychological attributes that are expressed by one's gender identity and sexual behaviour, whether or not related to the sex organs or to procreation.

There is no simple answer, but in the literature the following common elements appear:

- Sex;
- Sexual orientation;
- Gender and associated roles;
- Relationships;
- Self-image;
- Self-esteem;
- Human attraction;
- Love.

This list attempts to expand on the concept of sexuality, but it is not definitive. As sexuality is a social construct and is open to change and interpretation, complete and accurate definitions cannot exist. From the above list it is clear that the elements in themselves are complex and difficult to define. Also, they are surrounded by notions of normality – what is right and what is wrong. In coming to an understanding of sexuality, we must take into account its changing nature and the social and historical forces that shape it. ⇒ Psychosexual (psychosexual development).

The expression of sexuality changes as people progress through their life span. It includes the many ways in which a person expresses gender to other people by clothes, hairstyle, perfume, jewellery and toilet articles used, make-up worn, behaviour and attitude to, and behaviour with, members of the opposite sex and those of the same sex.

PROBLEMS RELATED TO SEXUALITY

SEXUALITY AS A PRIMARY PROBLEM

Primary problems with sexuality include:

- Difficulties with sexual activities or relationships (see *Box 36*);
- Unfulfilling sexual activity;
- Antisocial or inappropriate sexual behaviour;
- Fertility problems;
- Contraceptive difficulties. ⇒ Family planning, Infertility.

These kinds of problems usually require the input of a specialist nurse. In some cases clients raise the problems with 'generic' nurses (e.g. practice nurses, health visitors or community mental health nurses). It is important for these staff to be aware of the specialist services available (e.g. sex therapists, psychosexual counsellors, fertility clinics and family planning clinics).

S

Box 36 Sexual dysfunction

Sexual dysfunction can cause major problems between couples, so what starts as a small incident can develop into something more serious, and cause considerable discord and distress.

Anorgasmia – failure to achieve orgasm, more often experienced by females than males.

Changes in libido (sexual drive and urge) – loss of interest in sexual activity can be a feature of many conditions (e.g. during cancer treatment, depression).

Dyspareunia – painful or difficult coitus experienced by women. It may be superficial at the introduction of the penis, or deep due to the penis causing pressure at the vaginal vault. Causes include vaginal dryness during and after the climacteric, perineal tear or episiotomy, pelvic pathology, such as fibroids or endometriosis, etc.

Erectile dysfunction (ED), previously known as impotence – ED is a common complaint thought to have an annual incidence in men from 15 to 20%. It can be defined as the inability of the man to gain an erection of sufficient quality for intercourse. Causes may be psychogenic (e.g. stress, relationship difficulties) or organic (e.g. diabetes mellitus, spinal injury, anti-hypertensive drugs, etc.).

Rapid ejaculation – premature or rapid ejaculation is a common male sexual problem. The complaint is often ascribed to anxiety, in which ejaculation and orgasm occur before the person wishes because of a lack of control during sexual activity. Ejaculation occurs with minimal sexual stimulation before, during or very soon after penetration.

Vaginismus – contraction of the vaginal muscles occurs when the penis is introduced and makes intercourse impossible or painful. In extreme cases there may be contraction of the thigh muscles. Vaginismus can also occur when a doctor or nurse attempts to examine a woman vaginally.

SEXUALITY PROBLEMS SECONDARY TO OTHER HEALTH CONDITIONS

Many diseases, illnesses and health conditions can affect an individual's sexuality (*Table 34*). Sexuality is a complex blend of physical, psychological and social factors. It is not always possible to identify the cause-and-effect relationship between illness and sexuality problems.

A number of medications have potential side-effects on sexual activity – thiazide diuretics, calcium antagonists and antidepressants can result in ED; corticosteroids can cause weight gain and abnormal hair growth; alcohol, nicotine and recreational drugs are known to contribute to ED.

SEXUALITY AND NORMAL DEVELOPMENTAL CHANGES

People can experience difficulties in managing and coming to terms with normal developmental changes. Nurses have an important role in helping individuals to understand these changes and also in offering support and practical advice on how these changes can be managed (e.g. changes during puberty and adolescence).

Further reading

Brooker C and Nicol M (2003). *Nursing Adults. The Practice of Caring*, pp. 752–757. Edinburgh: Mosby.

SEXUALLY TRANSMITTED AND ACQUIRED INFECTION

Sexually transmitted infections (STIs), now increasingly known as sexually acquired infections (SAIs), are an ancient and common problem. Risk factors for STIs include young, single individuals, and people who have multiple sexual partners, who do not use barrier contraceptives and who live in metropolitan areas. The numbers of all episodes of STIs continues to increase in the UK.

Any sexual act that involves exposure to, or transfer of, bodily fluids carries a risk. Using a condom, whether for vaginal, anal or oral sex, dramatically reduces the chances of problems, although it does not remove the chances altogether. The condom should be worn throughout the sexual encounter (i.e. before penetration), and using alternative methods of contraception, such as the diaphragm, may not be as effective.

Table 34 Sexuality-related problems sometimes associated the certain types of health problems

Type of health condition	Sexuality-related problems
Musculoskeletal	Sexual activity Body image Work and leisure activities Dressing and hygiene
Cardiovascular and respiratory conditions	Energy levels Breathing Body image Emotional state Male and female sexual response
Neurological conditions	Sensations Movement and co-ordination Male and female sexual response Libido
Endocrine and hormonal conditions	Libido Male and female sexual response Body image Growth and development Onset of puberty
Skin conditions	Body image Sensations Emotional state
Genitourinary conditions	Male and female sexual response Body image Libido Choice of clothing
Mental health problems	Self-concept Body image Libido Male and female sexual response Work and leisure activities Interpersonal relationships
Learning disabilities	Relationship skills Emotional state Work and leisure activities Vulnerability to sexual abuse Self-concept

S

Intercourse is often a spontaneous event, and therefore both partners should be responsible for their sexual health; this may be achieved by both having condoms in their possession and acknowledging the effects of alcohol on inhibition.

Sexual health centres maintain a policy of confidentiality that often allows previously hidden sexual expression from the patient or client.

Often contact tracing is required to limit the spread of the disease, managed by anonymous cards that are sent to request attendance at the nearest sexual health clinic. These cards record a 'code number' that indicates which treatment is required. Health advisors attached to sexual health clinics organize contact tracing.

The common STIs are outlined below. ⇒ Acquired immune deficiency syndrome, Herpesviruses and herpes, Human immunodeficiency virus, Infections of female reproductive tract, Infertility, Liver (hepatitis).

GENITAL WARTS

External anogenital warts are caused by various types of human papillomavirus (HPV) and are very common. HPV is passed by close physical contact, which is almost always through genital contact, although warts in the oral cavity are not uncommon. The HPV attacks the tissues of the cervix, vagina, vulva, penis, anal cavity and oral cavity. The cauliflower-like warts appear as pink or whitish lumps, either singly or in groups.

Patients should always be tested for other STIs. Treatment is aimed at removing visible warts, since it is impossible to eradicate the virus. The treatment options include solutions and creams that contain podophyllin, or its major active constituent podophyllotoxin, or cryotherapy. ⇒ Human papilloma virus.

CANDIDIASIS AND CANDIDOSIS (VAGINAL THRUSH)

The causative organism is usually *Candida albicans*, and most women have an episode in their lifetime. The vagina can be considered an ideal environment for the growth of this infection, since semen, menstrual blood, pregnancy and feminine hygiene products can all change vaginal pH. These changes in pH create an imbalance that predisposes to the development of thrush. Additional risk factors include diabetes mellitus, thyroid disease, iron deficiency, oral contraceptive, antibiotic therapy and immunodeficiency.

Transmission can be by sexual contact. Men are more likely to acquire the infection during sexual activity, whereas women acquire it as a result of their predisposing factors.

Signs and symptoms include intense pruritus, vaginal soreness, white patches on the vulva and/or vagina, sometimes dysuria, creamy white vaginal discharge and balanitis in men, although these signs are nonspecific.

Antifungal drugs, such as clotrimazole, miconazole and nystatin, are commonly used as creams and pessaries in the management of this condition. Systemic treatment may be necessary if symptoms persist. Sexual partners with symptoms should also be treated, as they may cause re-infection.

Some patients prefer to use many traditional and alternative therapies (e.g. oral garlic and dietary changes). ⇒ Fungi (candidiasis and/or candidosis).

S

TRICHOMONIASIS

Trichomonas vaginalis (a protozoon) causes trichomoniasis, and in adults is exclusively a sexually acquired disease. It is a very common STI (the protozoon that causes disease lives as a parasite in the genital tract) that affects the vagina and urethra.

The signs and symptoms include profuse vaginal discharge (offensive, yellow, thin, frothy and irritating), dysuria, vulval soreness and lower abdominal pain, although men can remain asymptomatic. It can be difficult to diagnose in men because of the lack of distinct symptoms and, although there are difficulties, it is vital to trace contacts.

Treatment options include the antibiotic metronidazole, given to both partners over 5 days. This should be taken with food – alcohol and sexual activity should be avoided during the treatment programme.

CHLAMYDIA

Chlamydia is caused by the bacterium *Chlamydia trachomatis*. It is particularly common in young, sexually active women (16–24 years). Chlamydia is a serious disease and has a number of complications, so early detection and treatment are important.

Many patients with chlamydia are asymptomatic. However, women may present with postcoital or intermenstrual bleeding, purulent vaginal discharge, lower abdominal pain or proctitis. Men may have urethral discharge, dysuria, testicular pain or proctitis.

Testing for chlamydia now involves tests to detect chlamydial DNA in urine, vaginal, cervical and vulval swabs. A national screening service for chlamydial infection operates in England. Chlamydia can cause epididymitis in men, and in women it leads to pelvic inflammatory disease (PID), endometritis, salpingitis, tubal damage and chronic pelvic pain. PID increases the risk of ectopic pregnancy and infertility.

Treatment is with antibiotics. Doxycycline can be used, provided the patient is not at risk of pregnancy and is not breastfeeding. Alternative treatment can be with erythromycin. Partner notification must be discussed with patients.

Autoinoculation from the genital tract can cause conjunctivitis in adults. Chlamydial conjunctivitis and pneumonia in infants can result from infection during birth. Lymphogranuloma venereum is caused by different subgroups of *C. trachomatis*.

GENITAL HERPES

Genital herpes is a highly contagious viral disease transmitted through close physical or sexual contact and is caused by the herpes simplex virus (HSV). There are two types of HSV, both of which infect the skin and mucous membranes:
* HSV-1, which usually causes cold sores;
* HSV-2, which infects the genital areas.
⇒ Herpesviruses and herpes.
Blisters that contain clear fluid occur. Prior to the formation of these blisters, however, the skin often becomes 'tingly' or more sensitive. In addition to the signs described above, patients may complain of fever, joint and/or muscle pain and cystitis.

There is no cure for HSV – once infected the individual always carries the virus. It lies dormant around nerve roots, but in the presence of a weakened immune system, the virus reactivates. Patients should be given advice about mild painkillers (e.g. paracetamol), resting and taking extra fluids during the systemic disturbance associated with the primary infection. Treatment with aciclovir may help to prevent the formation of blisters. The blisters should be kept dry and clean.

Since transmission of HSV is through close contact, a barrier (condom) method of contraception should be used. Even though there are no blisters or ulcers visible, the virus can be passed on during sexual intercourse, oral sex (from a cold sore to the genitals) and via the vulva when giving birth (this does not include caesarean section).

GONORRHOEA

Gonorrhoea is caused by the bacterium *Neisseria gonorrhoeae*, which infects the mucosa of the genital tract, rectum and oropharynx. The infection is always transmitted by sexual contact (however, eye infections can occur in infants during birth, and gonococcal vulvovaginitis in young girls can result from sexual abuse).

The signs and symptoms of gonorrhoea depend on the site of infection, but include urethritis (causes dysuria and purulent discharge), cervicitis (causes vaginal discharge), proctitis with discharge and pharyngitis. However, many patients, especially women with uncomplicated infection, are asymptomatic.

Complications of gonorrhoea include abscess formation, epididymitis, prostatitis and urethral strictures in men. Women may develop endometritis, ovarian abscesses, salpingitis and infertility, and bartholinitis.

Treatment options include single-dose antibiotics, such as intramuscular procaine benzylpenicillin with probenecid, oral amoxicillin with probenecid, or oral ciprofloxacin if the micro-organisms is penicillin resistant.

Single-dose treatment is useful the in appropriate circumstances, as it overcomes problems of noncompliance. Patients are asked to abstain from sexual activity until a second test confirms that treatment has been effective. The opportunity should be taken to advise patients about the use of condoms to prevent the spread of STIs. Contact tracing with partner notification must be discussed with patients.

SYPHILIS

Syphilis is caused by the spirochaete bacterium *Treponema pallidum*. In adults it is spread through close sexual contact. *Congenital syphilis* occurs by vertical transmission from mother to fetus. The affected infant may exhibit the characteristic features, which include a generalized rash, lymphadenopathy and hepatitis.

Acquired syphilis has two main stages – early and late (but some authorities describe four stages – primary, secondary, latent and tertiary):

- Early stage is characterized by a primary lesion (chancre) at the site of entry into the body, which heals within about 1 month, and may be followed by a generalized illness (secondary syphilis) characterized by a skin rash, fever, generalized lymph node enlargement and mucosal ulcers (snail track);
- Late stage (occurs many years after the infection) shows skin or visceral lesions (gumma), neurosyphilis (tabes dorsalis and general paralysis of the insane) or cardiovascular syphilis (e.g. aortic aneurysm).

In many individuals there may be no clinical signs of syphilis (latent syphilis).

Diagnosis may be made from the presence of the micro-organism in exudate obtained from the ulcer (chancre), or by serological tests to detect the presence of antibodies.

Treatment depends on the disease stage – intramuscular procaine benzylpenicillin, or oral erythromycin if allergic to penicillin, or oral doxycycline and oxytetracycline are used. Patients who take penicillin should be warned about the possibility of a Jarisch–Herxheimer reaction (fever, chills, nausea, muscle pain, dizziness and headache). Patients should also abstain from sexual activity during antibiotic treatment and continue to use a barrier method (i.e. condoms), at least until blood tests show that the infection has passed.

SHARPS

Many procedures in a healthcare setting involve the use of needles or other devices capable of puncturing the skin (e.g. scalpels, cannulae, administration sets, broken ampoules, razor blades, stitch cutters, lancets, etc.). An injury from a needle or other device contaminated with blood or other body fluids poses a high risk of exposure to blood-borne viruses [e.g. hepatitis viruses and human immunodeficiency virus (HIV)] to healthcare workers and so special care must be taken when using and disposing of sharps. All sharps must be discarded into special yellow sharps bins, which are rigid, puncture resistant and leak proof (*Fig. 160*). They have a special opening designed to allow sharps to be dropped easily into the container, but not to allow items to spill out should the container topple over. Sharps bins must not be filled more than three-quarters full, and once closed they cannot be reopened.

Used needles must never be re-sheathed and should not be separated from the syringe. If this is unavoidable, a sharps bin with a needle-removing facility on top

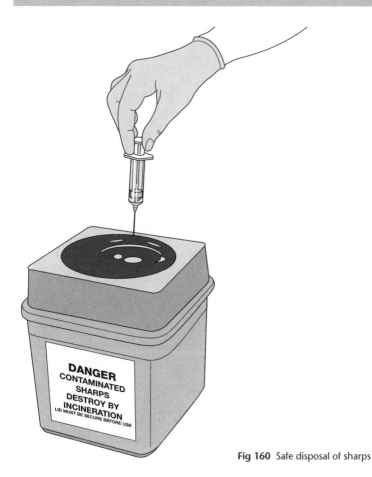

Fig 160 Safe disposal of sharps

should be used so that the needle is not handled. The safe disposal of needles and other sharps is always the responsibility of the person who uses them. Sharps should not be left for anyone else to clear away. Where possible, the sharps bin should be taken to the place where the sharps are used, as this allows immediate disposal after use. If this is not possible, a rigid tray or receiver should be used to contain the sharps until they can be tipped safely, without further handling, into the sharps bin. Items must not be pushed into to an already full container, as this may result in injury.

NEEDLE-STICK INJURIES – PREVENTION

Most injuries are preventable. The risk of needle-stick injuries should be minimized by implementing procedures for the safe handling and disposal of sharps (see above). Staff training and education are vital and should include the possible risks, and the procedures for safe handling and in the event of a sharps injury (see Practice application). Risk assessments should be undertaken wherever 'sharps' are in use, in conjunction with regular clinical audits to identify where practice could be improved. The use of sharps should be avoided whenever possible and staff should wear gloves and ensure that they cover all nonintact skin with occlusive dressing. ⇒ Human immunodeficiency virus, Infection (universal and/or standard precautions), Liver (hepatitis).

Practice application – management of needle-stick injuries and other exposures to blood or body fluids
- Wash off splashes on the skin with warm soapy water.
- If the skin has been punctured or broken, encourage bleeding by milking outwards while washing under warm running water (not by pressing or sucking the wound).
- Splashes into the eye, nose or mouth should be washed out with large amounts of water – sterile water for the eye if available.
- The incident must be recorded and the source of contamination (i.e. name of the patient if known, type of fluid, the injury and how it occurred) should be recorded for legal reasons and reported in line with local policy.
- A risk assessment must be undertaken by either the occupational health department or a clinical virologist without delay, in accordance with local Trust policy.
- The risk assessment determines whether exposure to a blood-borne pathogen has been likely, and if the source is known this makes it easier. The need for antiretroviral therapy is based on the risk assessment and should be taken within 1 hour of the injury. Therefore speed is of the essence and expert advice should be sought without delay. Post-exposure prophylaxis should be considered whenever there has been exposure to material that is known or suspected to be infected with HIV. Local policies must be based on the Department of Health's comprehensive guidelines (see Further reading) and risk assessment after an incident. Given the potentially serious health risks that follow exposure to blood-borne pathogens and the lack of vaccination programmes for both hepatitis C and HIV, the prevention of inoculation injuries is of great importance.

Further reading

Department of Health (1998). *Guidance for Clinical Health Care Workers: Protection against Blood Borne Viruses*. Recommendations of the expert advisory group on AIDS and the advisory group on hepatitis. London: HMSO.

SHIFT WORK

⇒ Biorhythm.

SHOCK

Shock is an inadequate or inappropriately distributed tissue perfusion that results in generalized cellular hypoxia. There are a number of causes of shock, but the final effect is always to reduce the ability of the cells to acquire or possibly utilize oxygen adequately. ⇒ Systemic inflammatory response syndrome.

HYPOVOLAEMIC SHOCK

Hypovolaemic shock is caused by the loss of circulating blood volume. The loss can be either external (as in haemorrhage or burns) or internal (as in plasma loss through altered permeability of the blood vessels or leakage into body cavities, such as the peritoneum).

CARDIOGENIC SHOCK

Cardiogenic shock is caused by failure of the heart to pump an adequate volume of blood through the circulation. The cardiac output is low and there is peripheral vasoconstriction. Vasoconstriction increases resistance to blood flow and increases the ventricular workload, and so adds to the cardiac failure. A degenerative spiral ensues unless intervention occurs.

Causes of cardiogenic shock include acute myocardial infarction, valvular disease, arrhythmias and cardiomyopathies or myocarditis.

DISTRIBUTIVE SHOCK

Distributive shock is caused by abnormalities of peripheral circulation (i.e. inappropriate vasodilatation of the capillary beds) that increase the capacity of the system. Hypovolaemia occurs because the same volume of blood is distributed through an enlarged system. Causes of distributive shock are anaphylaxis and sepsis.

In *anaphylaxis*, a normal inflammatory response becomes life-threatening when it is grossly exaggerated and produces generalized inflammatory responses. Inflammatory mediators, particularly histamine, greatly increase the capillary permeability with an immediate loss of intravascular fluid into the interstitial space. ⇒ Allergy.

Septic shock manifests as hypotension (systolic blood pressure <90 mmHg or reduced by more than 40 mmHg from baseline without other cause), which is associated with infection and is unresponsive to fluid resuscitation. There are also indications of organ hypoperfusion, such as low urine output. The cause of the hypotension is peripheral vasodilatation, which is induced by the systemic inflammatory response to the infection and, later, to fluid losses as a result of alterations in capillary permeability. ⇒ Infections of female reproductive tract (toxic shock syndrome).

OBSTRUCTIVE SHOCK

Obstructive shock is caused by a central mechanical impediment (such as a pulmonary embolus) to the flow of blood around the circulation. It causes increased resistance to blood flow and thus increased cardiac workload and produces hypotension, although central venous pressure is increased.

SPINAL SHOCK

Transection of the spinal cord causes temporary loss or depression of spinal reflex activity below the level of the lesion. This results in loss of peripheral sympathetic tone (the neural signals that maintain the level of constriction of the capillaries), diminished venous return and venous pooling. Reflexes return in time, but those that derive directly from the area of injury may not.

NEUROGENIC SHOCK

Neurogenic shock is caused by sudden cessation of sympathetic impulses from the central nervous system to the peripheral vascular system. The result is similar to that of spinal shock, as loss of sympathetic tone and diminished venous return occurs because of the venous pooling of blood. However, this is usually short-lived.

The sympathetic nerve blockade produced by local anaesthetic agents (e.g. lidocaine) used for epidural anaesthesia can promote profound hypotension.

SIGN LANGUAGE

Sign language is a form of nonverbal language that uses the hands and upper body to make signs, whereby people with hearing impairment, and sometimes those with a learning disability, can communicate with each other and with family members and friends. When a person who relies on the use of sign language needs to see a health professional or is admitted to hospital, special arrangements should

be made to ensure that a person skilled in using sign language is available.
There are different types of signing and sign languages, including:

- British Sign Language (BSL) – a sign language used by people with pro-found hearing impairment in the UK. It has an individual grammatical structure and idioms. It does not have the same grammatical structure as English and is the *first language* of many users, who may not read or write standard English. Other nations, for example, the USA, have their own sign language.
- Finger spelling – a form of communication used by people with hearing impairment, and can be used in conjunction with BSL.
- Sign Supported English (SSE) – SSE uses English grammar, but often makes use of BSL signs.
- Makaton – a form of sign language (more basic than BSL) particularly useful for people with some forms of learning disability.

Resources

Royal National Institute for Deaf and Hard of Hearing People – http://www.rnid.org.uk

SKELETON

The skeleton forms the bony framework of the body, and supports and protects the soft tissues and organs, acts as levers for movement and provides an attachment for muscles. In addition, some bone marrow is concerned with haemopoiesis. Adults have just over 200 bones (including the middle ear ossicles). The skeleton is divided into two parts – axial and appendicular (*Fig. 161*). The *axial skeleton*, which is the longitudinal axis of the body, consists of the skull, spine, sternum, ribs and hyoid bone. The *appendicular skeleton* is formed from the pectoral (shoulder) girdle (scapula, clavicle), upper limbs (humerus, radius, ulna, carpals, metacarpals, phalanges), pelvic (hip) girdle and lower limbs (femur, patella, tibia, fibula, tarsals, metatarsals, phalanges). ⇒ Bone, Fracture, Haemopoiesis.

SKIN

The skin has two layers, the superficial epidermis and the dermis (true skin), which are attached to the subcutaneous (below the skin) layer of hypodermis and fatty tissue (*Fig. 162A*). The skin appendages consist of the pilosebaceous unit, sweat and nails. The skin has several functions:

- Protection – physical/chemical/biological barrier; ⇒ Defence mechanisms;
- Sensation;
- Thermoregulation;
- Metabolism – synthesis of vitamin D;
- Excretion (small role);
- Absorption of substances (e.g. some drugs);
- Storage of water and energy.

A healthy intact skin is therefore vital to physiological homeostasis. The skin also has a role in nonverbal communication, in terms of the emotions (e.g. blushing) and clues to age and health status.

The epidermis has several layers of stratified epithelium through which cells progress, losing water and protein as they go. The epidermis contains several special cell types – keratinocytes (produce keratin and contain lipids), corneocytes (contain natural moisturizing factor), immune cells and melanocytes (pigment cells).

The epidermis has five layers (*Fig. 162B*). If the stratum corneum is imagined as a wall, the corneocytes are the bricks, held together by the lamellar lipids as the mortar. The lipid barrier helps the corneocytes to retain water. The swollen corneocytes

Fig 161 Skeleton (axial = shaded, appendicular = unshaded): (A) front view

(**B**)

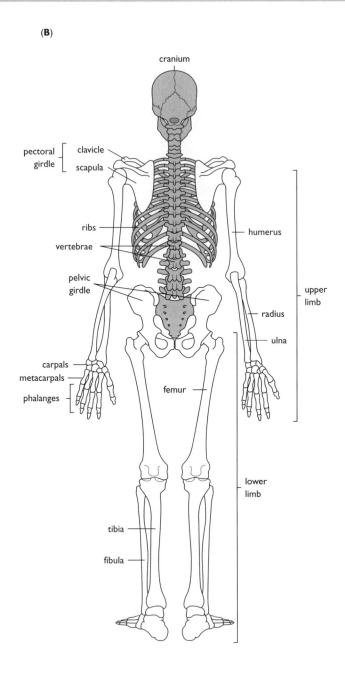

Fig 161 (*cont.*) Skeleton (axial = shaded, appendicular = unshaded): (B) back view

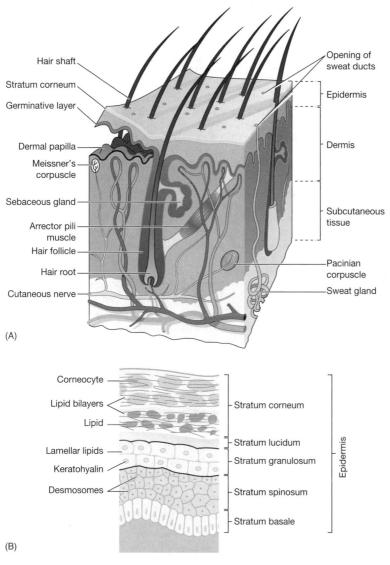

Fig 162 (A) The skin showing the main structures, (B) detail of the epidermis

prevent cracks forming between them. Renewal occurs as the stratum corneum, which is continually shed (desquamation or exfoliation), is replaced by new cells formed in the stratum basale of the germinative layer. The new cells migrate through the layers over a period of around 35 days. The cells undergo several changes as they migrate upwards, which include the addition of keratin (keratinization). As a result, the stratum corneum comprises dead cells that contain keratin. Renewal is most rapid during childhood; it stabilizes in adult life and declines with advancing age.

Micro-organisms present in exfoliated epidermal cells pose a potential infection risk in a surgical area, as they can be transferred to wounds when the dust is disturbed.

PILOSEBACEOUS UNIT

A pilosebaceous unit comprises a hair, its follicle and the associated sebaceous gland (*Fig. 162A*).

Hair protects the skin, has a minimal role in thermoregulation and is used in the expression of sexuality. It is formed from keratinized cells and comprises a growing region (bulb) at the base of the follicle, a root and the shaft visible above the surface of the epidermis. Each hair follicle is associated with an involuntary muscle (the arrector pili) controlled by sympathetic nerve fibres, which causes the hair to stand more erect, giving 'gooseflesh' when cold or frightened.

Sebaceous glands secrete sebum, a fatty substance that contains cholesterol and other lipids. Sebum waterproofs the skin and helps to keep hair and skin supple and resistant to cracking. It may have some bactericidal and/or fungicidal properties. The activity declines in older people, which renders the skin more prone to dryness and damage and reinforces the view that older people need particular care to maintain skin integrity (see Practice application).

Sweat glands are of two types. *Eccrine sweat glands* produce watery sweat that exits via a sweat duct to empty on to the skin surface through pores. The principal function of eccrine sweat glands is thermoregulation. *Apocrine sweat glands* are located in the external genitalia, groin, axillae and areola. These glands do not become active until puberty, when they start to produce thicker sweat that, when subjected to bacterial action, has a distinctive musky odour. ⇒ Defence mechanisms, Hair, Nail, Pressure ulcers, Wounds and wound care.

Practice application – maintaining healthy skin
- Use of medicated bath oils and soap substitutes suitable for the patient's skin. Remember that some products can make the bath and shower slippery.
- Bathing and/or showering daily is recommended, but the time in the water should be restricted to 10–15 minutes.
- The temperature of the bath water should be tepid or equal to body temperature.
- Careful drying – the skin should be gently patted dry with no heavy rubbing.
- Topical emollient (moisturizer that stays in the skin) should be applied lightly to the skin using smooth strokes (following the direction of the hairs) so that the skin glistens. Personal preference can guide the choice of emollient, but nurses should always ask patients about any allergies. On exposed areas (e.g. the face, neck and hands) the application may need to be more frequent, especially for those who do 'wet work', such as nursing. Drying the hands thoroughly after washing is vital.

MANIFESTATIONS OF SKIN PROBLEMS

Some common skin lesions are illustrated in *Fig. 163*, and information about describing lesions by configuration and distribution is provided in *Table 35*.

SKIN DISORDERS (SELECTED)

⇒ Infestations, Latex sensitivity, Pruritus.

Acne

Acne is a condition in which the pilosebaceous glands are overstimulated by circulating androgens and the excessive sebum is trapped by a plug of keratin. Skin bacteria then colonize the glands and convert the trapped sebum into irritant fatty acids responsible for the swelling and inflammation (pustules) that follow.

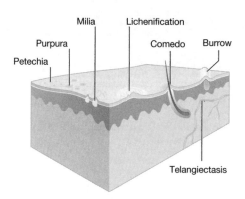

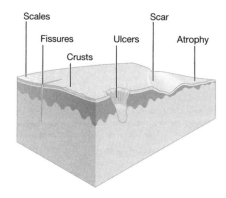

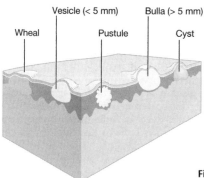

Fig 163 Common skin lesions

Treatments include azelaic acid (topical), minocycline (systemic), clindamycin (topical), retinoids (local and systemic) and anti-androgen medication.

BLISTERING DISORDERS

A blister is a fluid-filled lesion in the skin. A lesion less than 5 mm diameter is termed a vesicle, and one greater than 5 mm diameter a bulla. Multiple bullae may suggest pemphigoid or pemphigus, but occur sometimes in other diseases of the skin (e.g. in impetigo, dermatitis herpetiformis, etc.).

Table 35 Describing lesions by configuration and distribution[a]

Type of lesion	Pattern and distribution
Annular	Shaped like a ring
Asymmetrical	Unilateral distribution of lesions
Confluent	Lesions merge
Diffuse	Lesions are spread widely over different parts of the body
Discrete	Lesions are separate from others
Generalized	Widespread distribution
Grouped	Lesions in clusters
Gyrate	Ring spiral shape
Iris lesion	Concentric rings
Linear	Lesions in a line
Localized	Lesions in limited, well-defined areas
Nummular or discoid	Shaped like a coin
Polymorphous	Lesions display variable forms
Punctate	Marked by the points or dots
Serpiginous	Snake-like
Solitary	Single lesion
Satellite	Single lesion situated close to a larger group
Symmetrical	Bilateral distribution of lesions
Zosteriform	Distribution of lesions is band-like along a dermatome [area of skin innervated by sensory nerve (afferent) fibres from the cutaneous branches of a particular spinal nerve]

[a]Configuration is the arrangement or pattern of lesions in relation to other lesions, whereas distribution is the arrangement of lesions over an area of skin.

Pemphigoid is a bullous eruption, usually in the latter half of life, of autoimmune cause. Histological examination of a blister differentiates it from pemphigus. It is treated by systemic corticosteroids.

Pemphigus vulgaris is a bullous disease, mostly of middle-age, of autoimmune aetiology. Blister formation occurs in the epidermis, with resulting secondary infection and rupture, so that large raw areas develop. Bullae develop also on mucous membranes. The condition is treated by systemic corticosteroids and immuno-suppressive drugs.

DERMATITIS

Dermatitis is inflammation of the skin. *Contact dermatitis* is an exogenous dermatitis (eczema) that may be irritant or allergic in aetiology. Irritant substances, such as detergents, solvents and abrasives, may be encountered occupationally or at home. Nappy dermatitis is another form of irritant contact dermatitis caused by ammonia (in urine) and faeces. Allergic dermatitis results from a delayed hypersensitivity reaction to various substances, including nickel, latex, cosmetics and sticking plaster.

Dermatitis herpetiformis (syn. hydroa) is an intensely itchy skin eruption of unknown cause, most commonly characterized by papules and vesicles that remit and relapse. It is associated with coeliac disease.

ECZEMA

Eczema is an inflammatory skin reaction. In *atopic eczema* the aetiology is unclear, but immunological factors are the cause in many cases. Atopic individuals who have a genetic predisposition to asthma and hay fever also develop eczema. Environmental or lifestyle triggers include house mite dust, stress, change in temperature, etc.

Acute atopic eczema may begin with erythema (redness), itching, oedema, papules, vesicles, excoriation, exudating lesions, crusting or scaling. In chronic forms the skin becomes thickened.

The management includes:
- Topical therapies – corticosteroids, immunosuppressants, soap substitutes, bath oils;
- Systemic therapies – antibiotics, antihistamines to aid sleep, immunosuppressants.

Some authorities limit the word 'eczema' to cases with internal (endogenous) causes, while those caused by external (exogenous) contact factors are called dermatitis. The skin of patients with eczema may be colonized or infected with *Staphylococcus aureus*.

Atopic eczema can become infected with herpes simplex virus (HSV-I). Patients feel very unwell, and are given antiviral drugs, often intravenously.

IMPETIGO

Impetigo is an inflammatory, pustular skin disease usually caused by *Staphylococcus,* occasionally by *Streptococcus*. Impetigo contagiosa is a highly contagious form of impetigo, most common on the face and scalp, characterized by vesicles that become pustules and then honey-coloured crusts.

INTERTRIGO

Intertrigo is a superficial inflammation that occurs in moist skin folds (e.g. under the breasts). Skin folds must be kept clean and dry.

LICHEN PLANUS

Lichen planus is a skin disorder characterized by an eruption of unknown cause that shows purple, angulated, shiny, flat-topped papules.

SKIN CANCER

Malignant melanoma is a malignant cutaneous mole or freckle (usually), and is the most dangerous of all skin cancers. Related to overexposure to ultraviolet radiation (sunburn), it is most common in fair skinned, blond and red-haired people. It is characterized by change in the colour, shape and size of a mole or with bleeding or itching in a mole. The prognosis depends on Breslow thickness; staging involves lymph node status with sentinel node biopsy (SNB) now becoming an integral part along with computed tomography (CT) scan. Surgery is the only curative treatment, with chemotherapy and radiotherapy being of limited effectiveness.

Basal cell cancer (BCC) or rodent ulcer is the most common skin cancer. It is commonly associated with prolonged sun exposure over many years, such as in individuals who work outside (e.g. builders) or those with light skins who live near the equator. Although BCC can cause extensive local damage, it almost never metastasizes. Treatment is by wide surgical excision.

Squamous cell carcinoma is an invasive cancer that, if left, may metastasize. Treatment may be by wide excision. Radiotherapy may be used in older or frail patients.

S

PSORIASIS

Psoriasis is a genetically determined chronic skin disease in which erythematous scaly plaques characteristically occur on the elbows, knees and scalp. Keratinization is abnormal. There are several different types – guttae, erythrodermic and pustular.

Topical therapy includes:
- Soap substitute, bath oils (choice includes coal-tar additives);
- Emollients;
- Corticosteroids (mild-to-moderate potency only);
- Mild-to-moderate potency corticosteroids and coal-tar solution;
- Salicylic acid used with emollients;
- Coal tar (shampoos, bath oils, creams and ointments);
- Dithranol – application must be precise to prevent the burning of normal skin, and because it stains whatever it touches;
- Vitamin D;
- Vitamin A;
- Phototherapy (UV radiation).

Systemic therapies may be used where other therapies fail, and include:
- Methotrexate (cytotoxic drug);
- Ciclosporin (immunosuppressant drug).

ROSACEA

Rosacea is a skin disease that shows on flush areas of the face. In areas affected, chronic dilation of the superficial capillaries and hypertrophy of the sebaceous follicles occurs, often complicated by a papulopustular eruption.

TINEA (SYN. RINGWORM)

Tinea is a fungal infection of the skin, hair or nails caused by a variety of dermatophytes (related genera of fungi) – *Trichophyton*, *Epidermophyton* and *Microsporum*. It is usually named for the area of the body affected [i.e. *tinea barbae*, the beard area; *tinea capitis*, the head; *tinea corporis* (circinata), the body; *tinea cruris* (dhobie itch), the groin; tinea pedis, ringworm of the foot (athlete's foot); and *tinea unguium*, ringworm that affects the nails]. Treatment of tinea is with topical antifungal creams, such as clotrimazole. Systemic treatment is required for tinea that affects the head, nails and more generalized skin infections (e.g. itraconazole).

Further reading

Brooker C and Nicol M (2003). *Nursing Adults. The Practice of Caring*, Ch 28. Edinburgh: Mosby.

SLEEP

Sleep is a naturally altered state of consciousness that usually occurs in humans in a 24-hour biological rhythm. ⇒ Biorhythm.

STAGES OF SLEEP AND THE SLEEP CYCLE

Sleep consists of five main stages, four of nonrapid eye movement (NREM), or orthodox sleep, and one of rapid eye movement (REM), or paradoxical sleep. The five stages are as follows:
- Stage 1 – the person becomes drowsy and begins to fall asleep, breathing slows and becomes regular;
- Stage 2 – the person is now asleep, although sleeping lightly so an unusual sound will disturb and arouse the subject quite easily, but breathing is regular and slow;

- Stage 3 – the beginning of slow wave sleep, so the person is more deeply asleep and more difficult to arouse;
- Stage 4 – this is the stage of deepest sleep during which the person is most difficult to arouse, and sleepwalking and enuresis (bedwetting) may occur during this stage of sleep;
- REM sleep – this stage is characterized by rapid eye movement and the person sleeps more lightly. It is the stage of sleep in which dreaming is thought to occur. In many people this stage is characterized by sleep paralysis, and they are unable to move.

People move in and out of these various stages throughout the night, or period of sleep, depending on how long they have been asleep. Sleep begins with stage 1 and, once established, progresses through stages 2, 3 and 4; there is then a sudden shift to stage 2 followed by a period of REM sleep, a process that usually takes about 90–100 minutes (an ultradian rhythm). The pattern then repeats, but as the night progresses, less time is spent in stages 3 and 4 and more time is spent in REM sleep. Therefore, the early part of the night is more important for sleep stages 3 and 4 and the latter part of the night is more important for REM sleep.

Several factors known to affect sleep patterns are age (*Table 36*), culture, individuality, gender, body mass, genetic make-up and physical activity.

Patients who are unable to sleep or who can only doze for short periods may not be acquiring the amount of sleep they need for health or healing.

Sleep deprivation is a cumulative condition that arises when there is interference with a person's established rhythm of paradoxical sleep. It can result in slurred rambling speech, irritability, disorientation, slowed reaction time, malaise, progressing to illusions, delusions, paranoia and hyperactivity. ⇒ Sensory (Practice application – sensory reduction and/or overload in critical care).

Table 36 How sleep patterns alter with age

	Age (years)		
	3	25	75
Amount of sleep in 24 h	13 h	8 h	5 h
Pattern of sleep	Night sleep and daytime naps	Night sleep only	Night sleep and daytime naps

SMELL (OLFACTION)

A sense of smell is important for protection – many harmful agents have a characteristic odour (e.g. rotten food or fire). In many species odours are vital to recognize individuals and in reproductive behaviour. Human behaviour is also influenced by odours from chemicals, called pheromones, contained within sweat and other body secretions.

Humans have the ability to recognize thousands of odours and it is proposed that all odours are made up from seven primary odour classes (*musky, floral, pepperminty, camphorous, pungent, ethereal* and *putrid*), but larger numbers of 30 to 50 have been suggested. A strong link between smell, appetite and taste exists – appetite increases and food tastes better if it also smells good.

Specialized chemoreceptor cells are found within the olfactory epithelium that forms part of the mucous membrane lining the roof of the nasal cavity (*Fig. 164*). The receptors respond to minute amounts of chemical vapours that enter the nose during inspiration; the concentration of chemical in contact with the receptor is

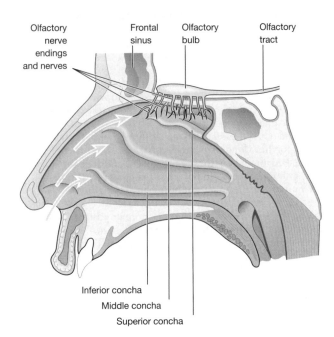

Fig 164 Nose showing the olfactory nerve endings

greatly enhanced by sniffing. Cilia that project from each olfactory receptor increase the surface area for contact with the odour molecule, which dissolves in mucus prior to contact.

Axons from the olfactory receptors form the fibres of the olfactory nerves (first cranial nerves), which pass through the cribriform plate of the ethmoid bone prior to synapsing in the olfactory bulbs. Olfactory tracts transmit impulses to the olfactory cortex in the temporal lobes of each cerebral hemisphere for interpretation and to areas of the limbic system concerned with the emotional aspects of smell. A specific odour may stimulate memories (e.g. the typical 'hospital smell' may remind you of a relative who died in hospital when you were a child).

When an individual is continuously exposed to an odour, perception of the odour decreases and ceases within a few minutes. This is known as *adaptation*. Loss of perception only affects that specific odour. ⇒ Taste.

ABNORMALITIES OF OLFACTION

Abnormalities of olfaction include hyposmia (reduced sense of smell) or anosmia (complete loss of smell). The causes include inflammation of the nasal mucosa (commonly associated with the common cold) or disease or injury that affects the brain (e.g. head injury).

SOCIAL SERVICES

Social Services are provided by local authorities (local government) in the UK (e.g. Norfolk County Council provides services for the people who live in the county of Norfolk). Social service departments have a statutory responsibility to provide care for groups that include:

- Children and young people (e.g. child protection);
- People with disabilities, including sensory impairments;
- People who have problems with alcohol and drugs;
- Older people;
- People with mental health problems.

Care and support is provided in the person's own home or in small community-based care units. People who need these services have a named qualified social worker to co-ordinate and monitor the care package. The care package may include help with personal care, day centres, respite care and home modifications, such as bath rails and a stair lift.

Joint working between health and social care professionals is vital for effective care planning and delivery. This is especially so in discharge planning, and in the community where there is considerable overlap between the work of health and social care professionals. In many areas, such as mental health and children, health and social services have formed a single Social Services & NHS Trust that aims to provide high-quality care. In addition to the collaboration between the NHS and local government, there is considerable input from the independent sector (particularly in the provision of nursing home and residential home places) and voluntary agencies. ⇒ Commission for Social Care Inspection.

SOCIAL DEPRIVATION MEASUREMENT

⇒ Care and/or case manager, Inequalities in health (deprivation indices).

SOCIAL FUNCTIONING

Social functioning describes the everyday activities and abilities that enable social interaction, interpersonal relationships and independent living. Social functioning ability may be affected severely by mental health problems, such as depression and schizophrenia.

SOCIAL FUNCTIONING SCALE

Social Functioning Scale (SFS) is used to assess aspects of day-to-day social functioning that are affected adversely by clients' mental health difficulties. It covers seven main areas of social functioning, such as social engagement, interpersonal behaviour, independence in living skills (competence and performance). The scale can provide a guide to goals and interventions, as well as measure progress and outcome.

SOMATIZATION

Physical symptoms without organic pathology have been referred to by a variety of labels, such as medically unexplained symptoms, hypochondriasis and somatization. Various terminology is used to describe such events, including psychosomatic symptoms, hysteria and/or conversion disorder and functional illness.

Patients present with somatic symptoms without obvious organic pathology in every specialism within the health service, such as abdominal pain with intermittent diarrhoea and constipation (irritable bowel syndrome) and chronic fatigue syndrome (CFS). Patients who experience real physical symptoms without a clear-cut organic pathology are usually distressed at not being able to control the symptom and have varying degrees of disability that stops them from carrying out everyday activities. In addition, many of these patients believe they are physically ill. ⇒ Illness behaviour.

S

SOMATOFORM DISORDERS

For the sake of clarity, the ICD-10 (WHO 1992) defines seven categories of *somatoform* disorders (somatization disorder, undifferentiated somatoform disorder, hypochondriacal disorder, somatoform autonomic dysfunction, persistent somatoform pain disorder, other somatoform disorders and somatoform disorder unspecified). All have overlapping criteria and, in clinical practice, it is often difficult to differentiate between them. Neurasthenia, which overlaps with CFS, is placed under the other somatoform disorders category, but has things in common with the somatoform disorders.

For each disorder, a description is provided of the main clinical features. In contrast to DSM-IV, which is more specific, some degree of flexibility is apparent.

Two of the more common somatizing disorders are described here.

Hypochondriasis

Hypochondriasis is an example of a somatoform disorder that most people are familiar with. It is a persistent preoccupation with the idea of having one or more serious physical disorders. Patients experience persistent somatic complaints and, even though numerous investigations reveal no physical abnormality, the preoccupation persists. There is an inability to accept the advice and reassurance of doctors that no physical abnormality underlies the symptoms.

Somatization disorder

Somatization disorder is characterized by multiple, recurrent and frequently changing physical symptoms that have been present for many years. Most patients have a long and complicated history of contact with both primary and secondary care, during which many negative investigations and, in severe cases, fruitless operations have been carried out. Symptoms may occur in any system of the body, but gastrointestinal symptoms and abnormal skin sensations are common. The course of the disorder is chronic and fluctuating and is associated with marked disability that affects all aspects of a person's life.

CHRONIC FATIGUE SYNDROME

CFS is categorized in ICD-10 under neurasthenia. The illness has attracted a variety of other labels, including *myalgic encephalomyelitis* (ME) and *post-infectious fatigue syndrome*. Given that the term CFS does not imply any specific aetiology, it is the preferred term. The condition is characterized by physical and mental fatigue, provoked by minimal exertion, that results in marked disability and is associated with a myriad of other symptoms.

Specimen collection

Nurses are responsible for obtaining many different types of specimens from patients (e.g. urine for microbiological examination, blood for electrolyte estimation, etc.). Specimens may be required to make or confirm a diagnosis, screen for disease or monitor the progress of a disease and the efficacy of treatment. The quality of the results obtained from a specimen sent to the laboratory depends on the way it was obtained, how it was stored, the information provided to the scientific staff and how the specimen was transported to the laboratory.

Practice application – general principles: specimen collection
- Use the correct sampling technique – make sure that the specimen contains only micro-organisms from the site under investigation. Ensure that the correct material is collected (do not collect saliva when sputum is required).

- Make sure that enough material is collected (e.g. if possible, collect pus from a wound rather than a wound swab).
- Except in an emergency, specimens for microbiology should be obtained before antibiotics are started.
- The correct container must be used (e.g. examination for certain micro-organisms requires a specific transport medium).
- Ensure that the specimen is labelled correctly and that the request card information is correct and complete. Always use a unique identification, such as the patient's hospital number.
- Provide sufficient information on the request form (e.g. the signs and symptoms, the time the specimen was collected and, in the case of micro-biological examinations, any antibiotic therapy).
- Arrange for the specimen to be taken to the laboratory without delay – try to arrange for specimens to be collected just prior to a routine 'pick-up' time.
- Ensure safety by making sure that specimens are in leak-proof containers and that the request form is separate (in a double bag). Appropriate *bio-hazard* labels are affixed to the specimens in cases where they may contain dangerous pathogens (e.g. blood-borne viruses).
- Remember to check that the results are available when expected and that the medical team are informed.

SPEECH

Speech involves the processes of breathing, phonation, articulation, resonance and rhythm. Prosody is a descriptive term for the phonological features of speech, including rate, stress, rhythm, loudness and pitch.

SPEECH-AND-LANGUAGE THERAPIST OR THERAPY

Speech-and-language therapists (SLTs) are the health professionals responsible for the assessment, diagnosis and treatment of speech and language disorders in children and adults. They are known as *speech pathologists* in the USA and Australia.

SLTs aim to assist the millions of individuals (children and adults) with difficulties in communication. These individuals may be dysfluent (stammer), have a hearing impairment, have language difficulties (including problems with vocabulary and grammar and the social use of language), have problems producing the correct sounds for speech so that they are difficult to understand, or have difficulties with their voice. SLTs also work with people who have dysphagia (difficulties swallowing). SLTs can provide other members of the multidisciplinary team with advice on how to achieve optimum communication with a person who has difficulty in communicating. SLTs also provide alternative and augmentative communication systems for individuals who require them. ⇒ Hearing (hearing impairment), Swallowing and problems with swallowing.

SPEECH PATHOLOGY

The various speech pathologies include stammering, stuttering, slurring, and explosive and staccato speech. Aphasia, dysarthria and dysphasia may be part of another disorder, such as stroke or head injury. ⇒ Dyslexia.

APHASIA

Aphasia is a disorder of language that follows brain damage, primarily because of impairment to the linguistic system. The term does not include disorders in language comprehension or expression that primarily result from mental disorders (including psychosis, dementia and confusion) or to hearing impairment or muscle weakness. There are several classification systems, but the most commonly used terms are *expressive aphasia* and *receptive aphasia*, although patients may exhibit difficulties in both language expression and comprehension.

Expressive aphasia is characterized by difficulty in language production. Word-finding difficulties and problems in producing sentence structures may occur. Whereas receptive aphasia is characterized by problems in language comprehension, and occurs with varying degrees of severity. *Anomia* is a difficulty in word finding that occurs in many aphasic patients. It is most often demonstrated in naming tasks, but also evident by the use of circumlocutions in spontaneous speech samples (see Practice application - dysphasia).

APHONIA AND DYSPHONIA

Aphonia and dysphonia are loss or disorder, respectively, of voice from organic, neurological, behavioural or psychogenic causes.

DYSARTHRIA

Dysarthria is a speech disorder that results from a disturbance in muscular control of the speech mechanism caused by damage to the central and/or peripheral nervous system. The loss of muscular control may involve weakness, slowness and/or inco-ordination. Disturbance may involve respiration, phonation, articulation, resonance and prosody. *Anarthria* is a severe form of dysarthria caused by a loss of ability to produce the motor movements for speech.

Practice application – dysphasia

Sometimes called aphasia, dysphasia is a disorder of language, not a disorder of intellect. It occurs most commonly after a left-sided stroke, but can occur after a head injury or neurosurgery. Dysphasia can affect a person's ability to understand language and also to use language to express themselves (see aphasia above). People with dysphasia vary greatly in their profiles of skills and difficulties, so it is important that detailed, individual consideration be given to their difficulties. Understanding language includes both understanding what is said and what is written. Likewise, expressing oneself includes both verbal expression and written expression. A discrepancy between the level of understanding and expression of language is common. Most often, individuals with dysphasia have impairments both in comprehension and in expression, although the degree of impairment in each may vary.

Assessment and treatment of dysphasia requires a detailed understanding of language and the breakdown of language. SLTs can provide therapy to assist individuals and their carers to improve their communication. Rehabilitation may take many months. Dysphasia has a considerable impact on many aspects of life, such as work and leisure activities, and also on relationships. People with dysphasia can become very withdrawn and isolated if they do not receive sufficient support.

SPINAL PROBLEMS

Some spinal problems are discussed here – curvature, cord compression and trauma. Patients with spinal cord disorders often require care in a specialist setting, such as a spinal injuries unit, and hence only an outline of spinal trauma is provided. ⇒ Moving and handling, Musculoskeletal disorders (back problems and back pain), Nervous system, Skeleton.

SPINAL CURVATURE

Abnormal spinal curvature can be congenital or acquired. Apart from causing pain and loss of mobility, this can lead to respiratory problems by reducing chest expansion.

KYPHOSIS

Kyphosis is characterized by an increased convexity of the thoracic spine as viewed from the side – the shoulders are rounded with a 'humpback'. It is particularly associated with osteoporosis, but can be caused by rickets or tuberculosis of the spine.

LORDOSIS

Lordosis is an abnormal forwards curve of the lumbar spine.

SCOLIOSIS

Scoliosis is lateral curvature of the spine, a common abnormality of childhood, especially females. The causes include congenital malformation, poliomyelitis, skeletal dysplasias, unequal leg length, etc.

Scoliosis may occur with both lordosis and kyphosis.

SPINAL CORD COMPRESSION

Spinal cord compression (SCC) is extremely serious and can occur over time, but may present acutely. Metastatic malignant SCC is a common oncology emergency. Early detection is vital to start treatment before irreversible nerve damage occurs.

SCC has a number of causes, including vertebral [the most common (e.g. metastatic cancers, trauma – see below – and prolapsed intervertebral disc)] or spinal cord and meningeal causes (e.g. tumour or infection).

Over 95% of people with SCC present with back pain, which may be localized or may radiate. Other symptoms include weakness, pins and needles, sensory loss, and bowel and bladder dysfunction.

Prompt treatment with radiotherapy, supported with corticosteroids to reduce inflammation, is the key to maintaining function. Active intervention may be required to assist patients to manage the loss of function. The potential for rehabilitation is dependent upon the level of function that the individual has at presentation and the response to treatment. Nurses have a vital role to play in educating patients about the signs of SCC so that prompt investigation and treatment can be initiated at an early stage for neurological function, and therefore quality of life, to be preserved.

SPINAL INJURY

Spinal injury occurs when the spinal cord is damaged or severed. As the main motor and sensory pathways to and from the body use the spinal cord as a communication trunk, any damage interferes with functions below the level of the damage.

Spinal injuries occur most commonly as a result of accidents (e.g. road traffic accidents and sporting injuries, such as those incurred in a rugby scrum or diving in shallow water). Falling downstairs is also a common cause, as landing on the head can flex the neck and damage the spinal cord.

A high spinal injury results in the loss of limb and trunk movement and feeling (quadriplegia or tetraplegia if all four limbs are affected). Respiration may also be affected, which necessitates respiratory support. A low spinal injury may affect movement and feeling in the legs (paraplegia), loss of bowel and bladder control and, in men, erectile dysfunction.

Patients with spinal injuries are usually transferred to a specialist unit for treatment. They often require emergency surgery to decompress the spinal cord and stabilize bony injury. This is a very delicate procedure, as moving and transferring patients with spinal injury can cause further damage to the cord, and currently damage cannot be reversed once it has occurred.

For this reason, moving patients before the spine has been stabilized is a very skilled procedure that involves several people who maintain the spine in supported alignment at all times. The movement is co-ordinated and careful so that further damage is not caused during the procedure (log-rolling). Once the spine is stable, patients may be mobilized. They may have a plaster jacket applied or wear a brace support. Traction is used sometimes if the break is very high in the cervical spine.

After surgery, patients may require many months to recover and undergo rehabilitation. The rehabilitation covers all aspects of care, but the actual need is based on a holistic assessment that involves a multidisciplinary team of nurses, doctors and therapists. For example, patients with low spinal damage may be able to use a wheelchair unaided and return to work, whereas those with a high spinal injury may be unable to breathe unaided and require respiratory support. The latter group requires considerably more rehabilitation input to achieve some independence and autonomy for patients.

SPIRITUAL ISSUES

Spiritual issues are all-important in caring for those who face life-threatening illness, death, chronic illness, grief and distress. It is vital not to mistake religious issues for spiritual ones. Religion provides a framework for some of our spiritual beliefs, but seldom encompasses the wholeness of our values. In an increasingly secular society, spiritual rather than religious values inform and support more and more of us as we search for meaning and face our own and others' deaths.

We are all individuals and need to have our spiritual and religious needs assessed and solutions to our specific needs explored. For those who are members of certain religious groups, the needs may be specific. You will be able to find a guide to the religious care of patients who belong to various faiths from hospital chaplains and religious and spiritual leaders in the community. However, never assume that because your patient belongs to a particular faith you know what his or her needs are – you only know these when you have explored the issues with the patient.

Spiritual assessment is often regarded as being difficult. The North American Nursing Diagnosis Association (NANDA) is very helpful in giving both definition (spiritual distress and risk for spiritual distress) and direction to our exploration of patient needs (see Further reading). ⇒ Culture, Death (Practice application – end of life; meeting spiritual, religious and cultural needs), Holistic health and care.

Further reading

Neuberger J (1994). Caring for Dying People of Different Faiths, Second Edition. London: Mosby.

North American Nursing Diagnosis Association (2001). *Nursing Diagnosis: Definitions and Classification 2001–2002*. Philadelphia: NANDA.

SPLEEN

The spleen is formed by reticular and lymphatic tissue and is the largest lymph organ. It lies in the left hypochondriac region of the abdominal cavity between the fundus of the stomach and the diaphragm. It is enclosed in a capsule that dips into the organ, to form *trabeculae*. The cellular material, which consists of lymphocytes and macrophages, is called *splenic pulp*, and it lies between the trabeculae. *Red pulp* is the part suffused with blood and *white pulp* consists of areas of lymphatic tissue in which sleeves of lymphocytes and macrophages form around blood vessels (*Fig. 165*).

The structures that enter and leave the spleen at the hilum are the splenic artery, splenic vein (a branch of the hepatic portal vein), lymph vessels (efferent only) and nerves. Blood that passes through the spleen flows in sinuses with distinct pores between the endothelial cells, which allow it to come into close association with splenic pulp. ⇒ Lymphatic system.

The functions of the spleen include:

- Phagocytosis of old and abnormal erythrocytes, leucocytes, platelets and microbes;
- Erythropoiesis – an important site of fetal blood-cell production, and in adults in times of great need;
- Storage of blood – the spleen contains up to 350 mL of blood and, in response to sympathetic stimulation, can rapidly return a large part of this volume to the circulation (e.g. in haemorrhage);
- Immune response – the spleen contains T- and B-cells. ⇒ Defence mechanisms.

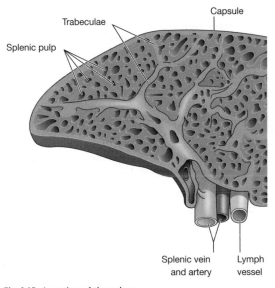

Fig 165 A section of the spleen

Practice application – splenectomy

It may necessary for the spleen to be removed (splenectomy) in a variety of situations, which include:

- Beta thalassaemia;
- Sickle cell disease;
- Idiopathic thrombocytopenic purpura;
- Ruptured spleen, such as after trauma.

Following a splenectomy, patients are at higher risk of severe and over-whelming infections and so they may be given prophylactic antibiotics. They should be advised to have the influenza, pneumococcal and meningococcal vaccines, in addition to any vaccines that form part of a routine programme.

S

SPUTUM

Sputum is the mucus and other material expectorated (coughed up) from the lower respiratory system. ⇒ Respiratory system (Practice application – care of patients producing sputum).

STAPHYLOCOCCUS

A genus of bacteria, the staphylococci, are Gram-positive cocci that occur in clusters. Some staphylococci are commensal on the skin and may be found in the nasopharynx, axillae and perineum of some individuals. Staphylococcal infections include boils, impetigo, wound infection, endocarditis, pneumonia, osteomyelitis, toxic shock syndrome and septicaemia. Staphylococci are an important cause of hospital-acquired infection (nosocomial infection). The genus includes the major pathogen *S. aureus*, which produces the enzyme coagulase, and some strains produce a powerful exotoxin, while others are methicillin resistant (see Practice application). *S. epidermidis* is a skin commensal that does not produce coagulase. It causes wound infection and is increasingly responsible for infection involving prosthetic valves, intravascular devices and peritoneal dialysis catheters. Treatment is difficult because the organism possesses a natural resistance to many antibiotics.

> **Practice application – methicillin-resistant *Staphylococcus aureus* (MRSA)**
> Strains of *S. aureus* are resistant to most antibiotics, including methicillin (not used clinically) and flucloxacillin. MRSA causes serious and sometimes fatal infections in hospitals, and patients with the micro-organism are encountered increasingly in community settings. Treatment involves vancomycin or teicoplanin, or various combinations of rifampicin, sodium fusidate and ciprofloxacin. Topical mupirocin is used to eliminate nasal or skin carriage. Infection-control measures, such as strict adherence to hand-washing policies, proper environmental cleaning and isolation or patient cohorting, are vital in the control of MRSA. In addition, the appropriate use of antibiotics is a vital strategy to prevent the emergence of antibiotic-resistant strains. Recently, a case of vancomycin-resistant *S. aureus* (VRSA) was reported in the USA, which restricts still further the drugs available to treat *S. aureus*.

STATISTICS

Statistics is the scientific study of numerical data collection and their analysis and evaluation. *Descriptive statistics* describe or summarize the observations of a sample. Whereas *inferential (inductive) statistics* use the observations of a sample to make a prediction about other samples (i.e. makes generalizations from the sample).

Brief definitions of some statistical terms are provided here.

TYPES OF DATA

Data can described as being categorical (nominal or ordinal), interval or ratio.

Categorical data can be categorized (e.g. hair colour). *Nominal data* are categorical data for which the classes have no particular value or order, such as road names or colours, whereas *ordinal data* are categorical data that can be ordered or ranked (e.g. general condition – good, fair or bad – or size in general terms, as in 'smaller than').

Interval data are measurement data with a numerical value (e.g. temperature) that has an arbitrary zero. The intervals between successive values are the same (e.g. a 1° increase from 38° to 39° is exactly the same as that from 39° to 40°).

Ratio data are measurement data with a numerical score (e.g. height) that has an absolute zero of 0. They are interval data with an absolute zero.

Frequency describes the number of times (frequency) a particular value occurs.

CENTRAL TENDENCY STATISTIC (AVERAGES)

Central tendency statistic describe the tendency for observations to centre around a specific value rather than across the entire range. They are the mean, median and mode (*Fig. 166A*). The *mean* is the average. Arithmetic mean is the figure arrived at by dividing the sum of a set of values by the number of items in the set. The *median* is the midway or middle value in a set of scores when placed in increasing order. The *mode* is the most frequent (common) value in a series of scores.

CONFIDENCE INTERVAL

In statistics, the confidence interval is a level (e.g. 95%) that indicates the level of confidence that the test result, such as a mean, will occur within a specified range.

SAMPLING DISTRIBUTION

A normal distribution curve is one in which when scores are plotted they form a symmetrical bell-shaped curve that has the mean, median and mode in the centre (*Fig. 166B*). *Skewed distribution* describes any distribution of scores in which a greater number of values are on one side of the mean than the other (i.e. not symmetrical).

Sampling distribution becomes more normal, the more samples that are taken (*central limit theorem*).

NONPARAMETRIC AND PARAMETRIC TESTS

Any statistical test makes some assumptions about the data. *Parametric tests* (e.g. unrelated t-test) assume the data are distributed normally. However, not all data

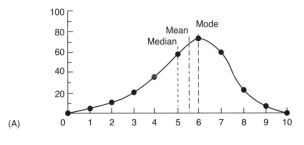

(A)

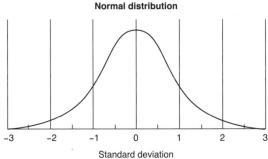

(B)

Fig 166 (A) Central tendency statistic – mean, median and mode, (B) normal distribution

are distributed normally; when they are not, these tests should not be applied (in most cases), but an equivalent *nonparametric test* (e.g. Mann–Whitney U test), which does not assume a normal distribution, is preferred.

Parametric tests are more powerful than nonparametric tests, and if the data support them, parametric tests are preferred.

P VALUE

In all inferential statistics a *P* value is given. This is the probability that the results found have occurred by chance alone. It is measured on a scale of 0 to 1, so a *P* value of 0.05 means 5% (one in 20) chance, and $P = 0.01$ means a 1% (one in a 100) chance. A common error is to assume a high *P* value means the result is significant – a low value shows significance. So the probability that a test result occurs by chance is the *P* value. Lower case *p* is used for proportions.

It is always possible that the apparent relationships between data came about by chance, so the *P* value is always above zero. The interpretation of the *P* value is dependent upon:

* α value – the significance at which a test result is said to be significant, which by convention is typically 0.05;
* 1-tailed or 2-tailed test – a test in which results in one direction only are of interest (e.g. a positive correlation rather than a positive or negative one) is one-tailed, whereas a test in which results in either direction are of interest (e.g. a positive correlation or a negative one) is two-tailed.

STANDARD DEVIATION AND STANDARD ERROR

Standard deviation (SD) is a measure of dispersion of scores around the mean value. It is the square root of *variance* (the distribution range of a set of results around the mean).

Standard error (SE) is the standard deviation of a sampling distribution of means.

Further reading

Gunn C (2001). *Using Maths in Health Sciences*, pp. 3–69. Edinburgh: Churchill Livingstone.

STIGMA

⇒ Labelling and stigma.

STOMA

A stoma is a mouth – any opening (e.g. opening of the bowel or ureters on to the abdominal surface, etc.). ⇒ Gastrointestinal tract (colorectal cancer, diverticular disease, inflammatory bowel disease), Urinary system (bladder cancer).

COLOSTOMY

A colostomy is a surgically established fistula between the colon and the surface of the abdomen – a type of stoma that discharges faeces. A colostomy may be temporary, such as after perforation of the bowel in diverticular disease, or permanent in some surgical procedures for colorectal cancer.

ILEAL CONDUIT (URETEROSTOMY OR ILEOURETEROSTOMY)

An ileal conduit is transplantation of the lower ends of the ureters from the urinary bladder to an isolated loop of small bowel (ileal bladder) which, in turn, is made to open on the abdominal wall (ileal conduit; *Fig. 167*). Ileal conduit is

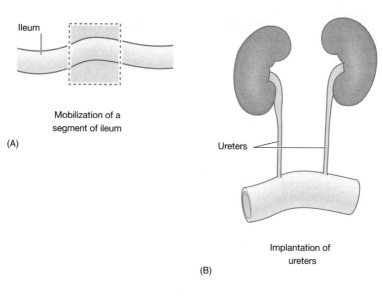

Ileum

Mobilization of a
segment of ileum

(A)

Ureters

Implantation of
ureters

(B)

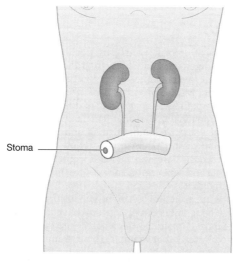

Stoma

Stoma opens on to
(C)   anterior abdominal wall

Fig 167 Ileal conduit

performed with total cystectomy (removal of urinary bladder) for bladder cancer.
As an alternative, some patients may have a continent internal urinary pouch.

Bowel is mobilized and used to create a reservoir for urine. The ureters are joined
to this reservoir. The pouch is externalized for access with a surgically created one-
way valve that opens onto the skin. The reservoir is drained of urine by catheterization through the one-way valve.

S

Practice application – postoperative observation, ileal conduit

After formation of an ileal conduit, the stoma should be observed for size, shape, colour and the presence or absence of oedema. Ureteric stents may have been inserted during the operation to maintain patency of the ureters while the ureteric anastomoses are healing. Stents may be seen to protrude through the opening of the stoma. The presence of these should be noted in both the nursing documentation and the record of the surgical procedure in the hospital notes.

The newly formed stoma should be moist and red. Stomal oedema is expected in the early postoperative period. Changes in the colour of the stoma (e.g. if it becomes dusky red, cyanotic or pale) indicate vascular insufficiency. If you note these, check that the flange or baseplate around the stoma is not constricting it. Document (in the nursing or multidisciplinary notes) the change in appearance, and verbally report this to the senior ward nurse and surgical team.

ILEOSTOMY

A surgically made fistula between the ileum and the anterior abdominal wall; a type of stoma that discharges liquid faecal matter. It is usually permanent when the whole of the large bowel (panproctocolectomy) has to be removed (e.g. in severe inflammatory bowel disease).

*S*TREPTOCOCCUS

A genus of bacteria, the streptococci are Gram-positive cocci that often occur in chains. They have varying haemolytic ability (α, β and nonhaemolytic) and some types produce powerful toxins. Some streptococci are commensal in the intestinal tract (*S. faecalis*) and respiratory tract (*S. viridans*). The commensal streptococci, together with the pathogens *S. pyogenes* and *S. pneumoniae*, cause serious infections, which include tonsillitis, scarlet fever, otitis media, erysipelas, endocarditis, wound infections, pneumonia, meningitis and urinary infection. Glomerulonephritis and rheumatic fever may follow some streptococcal infections. Group B streptococcus, an intestinal and vaginal commensal, may cause meningitis, pneumonia and septicaemia in neonates infected by bacteria present in the maternal genital tract.

Lancefield's groups are a subdivision of the genus *Streptococcus* on the basis of antigenic structure. The members of each group have a characteristic capsular polysaccharide. The most dangerous streptococci of epidemiological importance to humans belong to Group A. For example, some strains of group A *S. pyogenes* can cause necrotizing fasciitis. ⇒ Necrosis (necrotizing fasciitis).

*S*TRESS

Selye (1984) argues that stress is the response of an organism to any demand made upon it. Stress is generally associated with negative effects on health, but a certain amount of stress is necessary for survival. Stress can be described as being either *distress* that is viewed as a negative event (with long-term effects on health when it becomes chronic) or *eustress* that accompanies pleasurable excitement and euphoria and is viewed more positively.

Stressors are the factors that initiate stress responses. They may be structural and/or physical, physiological, psychological and sociocultural, and include pain, hunger, cold, blood loss, overwork, a life crisis (e.g. divorce), poor housing, etc.

PHYSIOLOGICAL RESPONSES – THE GENERAL ADAPTATION SYNDROME

The physiological responses to stress were described by Selye (1984) in the triphasic General Adaptation Syndrome (GAS; *Fig. 168*).

On exposure to the stressor, the limbic system in the brain stimulates the hypothalamus, which causes the autonomic nervous system (ANS) to initiate the initial physiological responses – the alarm and resistance reactions.

The immediate physiological response to stress is the *alarm reaction*. Its function is to prepare the body for defensive action to counter the stressor. Before an impending stressful event, a paradoxical fear may be generated with activation of the parasympathetic division of the ANS, which leads to urgency and frequency of urination and defecation. In an emergency situation, however, the fight-or-flight response is invoked. This occurs through the dominant sympathetic division of the ANS and the increased secretion of adrenaline (epinephrine) and noradrenaline (norepinephrine) by the adrenal medulla. The *fight-or-flight response* (*Table 37*), prepares the body for intense physical action either to fight against or to escape from the object of stress.

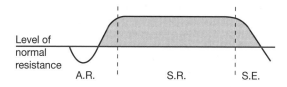

Fig 168 The general adaptation syndrome (adapted from Selye 1984). AR, alarm reaction; SR, stage of resistance; SE, stage of exhaustion

Table 37 Physiological changes associated with the fight-or-flight response

System	Effect
Circulatory system	Increased heart rate and force contraction Increased blood pressure Peripheral vasoconstriction
Respiratory system	Increase in respiration rate Dilation of bronchi
Liver	Increased conversion of glycogen into glucose
Eyes	Pupil dilation
Digestive system	All secretions within the digestive tract diminished or stopped Decreased peristaltic activity
Skeletal muscles	Increased tension
Skin	Sweat gland activation Erection of body hair by pilomotor contraction

S

The alarm reaction is followed by the *resistance reaction*, which is stimulated by hypothalamic hormones and continues for as long as the stressor threatens. The resistance reaction provides energy to sustain the stress response and protects the body by compensating for any damage that occurs during the alarm reaction. There is increased secretion of cortisol (a glucocorticoid) by the adrenal cortex.

The final reaction to stress, according to Selye (1984), is the *exhaustion stage*. This occurs after prolonged excessive distress and, if continued, leads to illness and eventually death. Thus, the repeated instigation of GAS, as occurs in stressful environments from which there is no escape, has negative health consequences. ⇒ Adrenal glands, Corticosteroids.

PSYCHOLOGICAL RESPONSES

Psychological responses to stress vary according to the level of threat from the stressor. Eustress stimulation is accompanied by feelings of well-being and increased alertness, a confident posture and positive outlook (Selye 1984, Sutherland and Cooper 1990). As eustress becomes distress, however, the feelings of well-being are replaced by those of losing control and being overwhelmed. Individuals become restless, demanding and sometimes aggressive. Indeed, within stressful departments such as accident and emergency, patients or relatives may act out their distress by behaving aggressively. Consequently, defusing aggression focuses on addressing those factors that contribute towards the distress being experienced.

Continued exposure to distress makes individuals unable to concentrate and problem solving becomes impossible. They drift undirected between tasks. Interpersonal relationships deteriorate, further worsening their difficulties, and individuals become locked into a stress cycle.

Some individuals adopt mental defence mechanisms to cope with psychological distress. In the short term, the use of mental defence mechanisms is a healthy response as they help individuals to survive the period immediately after exposure to distress. Mental defence mechanisms do not alter the cause of distress, however, but simply create an illusion. Consequently, they involve a degree of self-deception and the individual remains vulnerable to the stressor. Prolonged use of mental defence mechanisms is therefore unhealthy. ⇒ Mental defence mechanisms.

BURNOUT

Burnout describes a state that results from exposure to stressors. The stressors are often chronic and work-related, but burnout may occur after exposure to an acute stressor and may also result from stressful family roles, such as caring for a relative, or a combination of these. Health professionals are at particular risk of burnout because of their prolonged contact with ill people. It has been described as emotional exhaustion, isolation, being hardened towards others and an inability to deal positively with problems. The adverse effects can be divided into physical, emotional, intellectual, social and spiritual, and may include ineffective coping strategies, anxiety, insomnia, inability to make decisions, appetite and weight changes, extreme tiredness, apathy, lack of motivation, relationship difficulties and misuse of alcohol and drugs.

The symptoms of long-term burnout are outlined in *Table 38*.

POST-TRAUMATIC STRESS DISORDER

Post-traumatic stress disorder (PTSD) is characterized by anxiety (with nightmares, irritability, poor memory and concentration, headaches, flashbacks and depression) that may occur after involvement in any traumatic situation such as serious road accidents, crimes (e.g. rape), fire, explosion, war, natural disasters, etc. The condition may affect the professionals involved, the victims and people who witness the event.

Table 38 Symptoms of long-term burnout

Area affected	Symptoms
Physical	Lack of energy and persistent feeling of fatigue, which often lead to a lack of exercise and poor nutrition
Intellectual	Loss of problem-solving and cognitive abilities Lack of creativity and interest in hobbies
Emotional	Feelings of helplessness and depression Over-investment in work to the exclusion of other interests
Social	Inability to share problems with others; withdrawal from others May act aggressively towards those whom they feel threatened by
Spiritual	Individuals feel unfulfilled, cheated, resentful and cynical

STRESS MANAGEMENT

Stress management is complex and may involve various combinations of the following:
- Pharmacological methods (e.g. anxiolytics, antidepressants);
- Complementary herbal remedies (e.g. valarian);
- Nonpharmacological methods (e.g. diet, exercise, counselling, clinical supervision, group therapy, relaxation).

Readers are directed to Further reading for a fuller account. ⇒ Antidepressants, Anxiety (anxiolytics), Clinical supervision, Complementary medicine and therapy, Counselling, Relaxation.

Further reading

Brooker C and Nicol M (2003). *Nursing Adults. The Practice of Caring*, Ch 6. Edinburgh: Mosby.

SUBSTANCE MISUSE

An all-inclusive term that describes the misuse of alcohol, drugs (including solvents) and tobacco to the point where health and/or social functioning is affected adversely.

Drugs involved may be over-the-counter, prescribed or obtained illegally. Groups of drugs involved include amphetamines, barbiturates, benzodiazepines, cannabis, cocaine, heroin (diamorphine), morphine, hallucinogens, solvents, etc.

Drugs used as an adjunct in the management of opioid dependence include buprenorphine and methadone.

ASSESSMENT TOOLS

The Case Managers Rating Scale (CMRS) is used in the assessment of substance misuse. It contains a five-point scale, with each point operationally defined in terms of levels of substance misuse and their biopsychosocial consequences.

The Leeds Dependence Questionnaire (LDQ) is designed to detect and rate the severity of illicit substance misuse. It contains 10 items rated on a four-point scale. ⇒ Alcohol, Controlled drugs.

SUDDEN INFANT DEATH SYNDROME

Sudden infant death syndrome (SIDS), also known as cot death, is the unexpected sudden death of an infant, usually overnight while sleeping in a cot, but it may occur in other situations. It is the most common mode of death in infants between the ages of 1 month and 1 year, with neither clinical nor postmortem findings being adequate to account for the death. Overheating, sleeping in the prone position, respiratory illness and infection, and being in an environment where people smoke, have all been implicated as risk factors. Cigarette smoking in pregnancy increases the risk of babies dying from SIDS (Blair *et al*. 1996).

> **Practice application – preventing SIDS**
> Parents and carers are recommended to put babies to sleep on their backs, at the foot of the cot to prevent them wriggling under bedclothes, not to over-heat the room, not to smoke in the same room and to seek advice from a health professional if the baby seems unwell (*Fig. 169*).

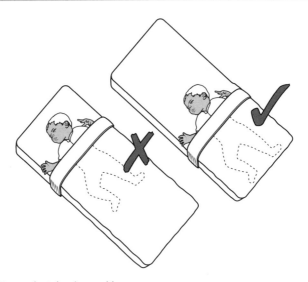

Fig 169 Feet-to-foot sleeping position

SUICIDE AND DELIBERATE SELF-HARM

During 2001 the suicide rate in England was 10.1 per 100 000 population for men and 2.8 per 100 000 population for women (Department of Health 2003). Mental illness is a feature most commonly associated with suicide, particularly affec-tive–depressive disorder with symptoms of hopelessness.

Suicide, in which death is intentionally self-inflicted, must be distinguished care-fully from a range of behaviours variously referred to as *parasuicide, deliberate self-harm* (DSH) and *attempted suicide*. The term parasuicide covers any nonfatal acts that involve deliberate self-injury, such as cutting or a drugs overdose. This includes acts that were intended to be fatal as well as those (e.g. self-poisoning) for which the motives are often ambivalent, and self-injury (e.g. cutting), which usually has no fatal intention and to which the notion of 'suicide' is not pertinent.

In practice, however, it is usual to use the term DSH to refer to the whole range of nonfatal self-harming behaviours.

Although suicidal and self-harming behaviours are extremely varied and individual, there are clear differences between people who complete suicide and people who engage in DSH. *Completed suicide* usually involves males. Men over 75 years of age are at greatest risk, although this rate has been rapidly increasing for younger men. DSH has, in the past, usually involved females (although the gender gap is closing) and mainly involves younger people.

Self-harming behaviour of all kinds is a major public health issue. Each death from suicide (and those recorded as undetermined deaths) represents both an individual tragedy and a loss to society, while the destructive ripples often spread out from the suicide to affect families and other 'survivors' economically, psychologically and spiritually.

In recent years, a disturbing rise has occurred in the number of young people who kill themselves, especially young men of age 15–24 years, for whom suicide has become the second leading cause of death behind road traffic deaths. Along with these deaths are very large numbers of people (perhaps as many as 142 000) who are admitted annually to emergency departments because they have harmed themselves nonfatally (Hawton *et al.* 1997). Most of these involve self-poisoning. These numbers are less than the actual total of people who harm themselves, since they may not attend hospital afterwards.

Table 39 presents a number of individual attributes that have been shown to correlate with suicide. These factors have an accumulative effect and their presence should raise the index of concern among staff.

Further reading

Thompson T and Mathias P (2000). *Lyttle's Mental Health and Disorder*, Third Edition, Ch 17. Edinburgh: Baillière Tindal.

Table 39 Suicide risk factors

Variable	Risk categories
Age	Generally increases with age, but also: young men young Asian females
Gender	More common in men than women
Physical health	Chronic life-threatening illness Chronic pain
Psychological health	Low self-esteem Depression Feelings of hopelessness Experience of significant loss Unrelenting and distressing delusions and/or hallucinations Command hallucinations Impulsiveness
Social health	Social isolation with poor social supports Conflict with supportive others Social upheaval (e.g. divorce, accommodation changes)
History	Suicide attempt in previous 12 months

S

SUPERINFECTION

Superinfection is an infection that follows the destruction of normal flora by treatment with broad-spectrum antibiotics. This allows other micro-organisms, such as *Clostridium difficile, Pseudomonas, Klebsiella,* staphylococci and yeasts (e.g. *Candida albicans*) to flourish in the bowel without competition from micro-organisms of the normal flora. The tetracyclines, cephalosporins and clindamycin can cause superinfection. ⇒ *Clostridium*, Infection.

SURGERY

Surgery is performed for different reasons and with varying degrees of urgency. With the advent and continual refinement of minimally invasive endoscopic techniques, many surgical procedures are diagnostic in nature. The use of a fibreoptic endoscope in the visualization of gastrointestinal, genitourinary and respiratory tracts and bony joints is commonplace. Surgery may also be considered as curative, ablative (amputation or excision of a body part or tissue) or reparative, whereby the identified or diagnosed source of a problem is excised, repaired, refashioned or reconstructed to promote the patient's quality of life.

The timing of intervention may differ according to the identified level of urgency. Surgery may be elective (preferably performed at a time of optimum benefit to the patient) or it may be an urgent or emergency procedure to save life, preserve function or reduce the risk of longer term complications or disability.

Surgery in all its forms may take place in a variety of settings, from the general practitioner surgery and outpatient clinic to the community hospital and larger specialist surgical centres. However, whenever and wherever surgery is performed, the nursing and medical management in the perioperative process always have the same goal: to provide the safest, most effective and efficient service for the patient. ⇒ Day-care surgery, Discharge planning, Perioperative care.

PATIENT POSITIONING

On arrival in the operating theatre, patients are placed in a position appropriate to the need for surgical access and anaesthetic integrity (*Fig. 170*). The likely access indications for specific positions are outlined in *Box 37*.

Box 37 Table positions and indications
- Supine (most commonly used general position) – abdominal, cardiac, thoracic.
- Prone – cervical spine, back, rectal area, dorsal aspects of extremities.
- Trendelenburg – varicose veins, pelvic surgery.
- Reverse Trendelenburg – head and neck, shoulder.
- Lithotomy – perineal, vaginal, endoscopic urological.
- Lateral – upper chest, kidney and ureter.
- Jack-knife – spinal, pilonidal sinus procedure, haemorrhoidectomy.

SWALLOWING AND PROBLEMS WITH SWALLOWING

Swallowing is divided into three phases (sometimes described as four):
- Oral phase – during which food is placed in the mouth and chewed and prepared for swallowing. This is a voluntary phase because the person may decide to stop and spit out the food at any time during this phase.
- Pharyngeal phase – during which there are movements of the tongue and pharyngeal muscles. It is involuntary and cannot be stopped at will,

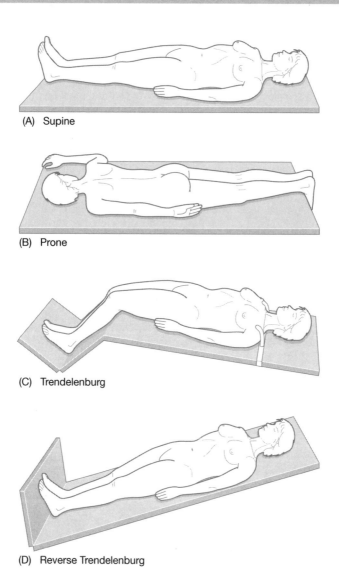

(A) Supine

(B) Prone

(C) Trendelenburg

(D) Reverse Trendelenburg

Fig 170 Table positions commonly used in surgery: (A) supine, (B) prone, (C) Trendelenburg, (D) reverse Trendelenburg

S

although reflexes such as the cough reflex may 'reverse' the action. Food may become stuck in the pharynx, which in turn may lead to aspiration and potential choking or pneumonia.
- Oesophageal phase – during which the food or fluid moves down the oesophagus to the stomach. Patients may complain of the sensation of a foreign body in the oesophagus. There may be regurgitation while lying down. Solid food is more difficult to swallow than fluids when a disorder of the oesophagus is present.

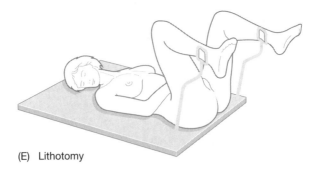

(E) Lithotomy

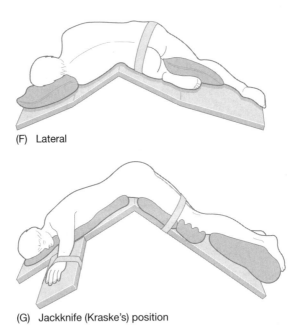

(F) Lateral

(G) Jackknife (Kraske's) position

Fig 170 Table positions commonly used in surgery (*cont.*): (E) lithotomy, (F) lateral, (G) jack-knife (Kraske's) position

DYSPHAGIA

Dysphagia is a disorder of swallowing. Difficulty in swallowing can occur in many different conditions, which include stroke, multiple sclerosis, Parkinson's disease and motor neuron disease, and sometimes follows head injury, cerebral palsy, dementia, head and neck cancer and oesophageal disorders. A person can experience difficulty swallowing fluids and / or foods and the degree of difficulty can range from mild to severe. Assessment and management of dysphagia is best conducted by a multidisciplinary team, including a speech-and-language thera-pist. The composition of the team is determined by the needs of the patient, the medical condition that underlies the swallowing problem and the clinical setting. The signs and symptoms that may indicate a swallowing problem include:

- Excessive coughing and choking;
- Excess mucus secretion and a wet and gurgly voice;
- Drooling;
- Pocketing of food in the cheeks;
- Loss of nasal resonance;
- Nasal regurgitation of food or drink;
- Chest infections;
- Weight loss;
- Failure to thrive;
- Aversion to eating;
- Oral sensitivity and drooling;
- Prolonged swallowing time and time taken to eat a meal;
- Avoidance of certain types of foods.

Practice application – assessment of swallowing
Food, fluid and air for respiration share a common pathway in the pharynx. This means that poor swallowing may result in inhalation of food or fluid, which can lead to chronic or acute chest infection, or even death by asphyx-iation. For this reason the safety of the swallowing process is of crucial impor-tance in all patients.

The muscles and nerves of swallowing are essentially the same as those used for speech. This means that patients with a language or speech problem, such as dysarthria, are likely to have (but not necessarily) dysphagia as well. Thus the first clue that a patient may have dysphagia is a language or speech problem. Many hospitals and care homes have a swallowing assessment pro-tocol that leads the assessor through a series of questions and activities, including swallowing increasing amounts of clear water (which is less likely to cause problems if it is inhaled). If the patient fails the test (or the nurse is unsure of the safety of oral feeding for any other reason), referral to a speech-and-language therapist or other experienced professional for a full swal-lowing assessment is required before oral feeding can be commenced.

Further reading

Brooker C and Nicol M (2003). *Nursing Adults. The Practice of Caring*, pp. 212–213. Edinburgh: Mosby.

SYSTÈME INTERNATIONAL D'UNITÉS

Système international d'unités (SI units) is a system of measurement that com-prises seven *base units* and is used for scientific, technical and medical purposes in most countries.

Each unit has its own symbol and is expressed as a decimal multiple or sub-multiple of the base unit by using the appropriate prefix (e.g. millimetre is one thousandth of a metre). The base units are:

- metre (m) – length;
- kilogram (kg) – mass;
- Kelvin (°K) – temperature;
- second (s) – time;
- mole (mol) – amount of substance;
- ampere (A) – electric current;

- candela (cd) – luminous intensity.

Various *derived units*, such as the pascal (Pa), becquerel (Bq), etc., are obtained by dividing or multiplying any two or more of the seven base units.

SYSTEMIC INFLAMMATORY RESPONSE SYNDROME (MULTIPLE ORGAN DYSFUNCTION SYNDROME)

Systemic inflammatory response syndrome (SIRS) and multiple organ dysfunction syndrome (MODS) frequently coexist in critically ill patients and are conditions commonly seen in intensive care units. Previously, septic shock, sepsis or septicaemia were the terms used to describe the clinical scenario of pyrexia, tachycardia, tachypnoea and deranged white cell count. It was then discovered that a number of other factors (i.e. in the complete absence of infection) could also precipitate the same clinical features, including trauma, reduced perfusion, major burns and pancreatitis. This resulted in the adoption of the term SIRS. Regardless of the cause, SIRS results in a response of the inflammatory system that is unnatural, in that it is exaggerated and not localized, and causes widespread physiological derangement and damage.

MODS describes the alteration of organ function significant enough to require intervention to maintain body function and stability. MODS may be a result of SIRS or may follow a direct insult (it was previously known as multiple organ failure or multisystem organ failure). The physiological damage is an accumulative result of the inflammatory response, mediator, toxin and enzyme production, reduced perfusion and reduced oxygen delivery to the cells.

Organ systems commonly affected are the lungs [as in acute respiratory distress syndrome (ARDS), for which mechanical ventilation is usually required], the kidneys (as in acute tubular necrosis, for which haemofiltration is required) and the cardiovascular system for which fluids and inotrope drugs are needed.

Other organ systems can also be affected:
- Central nervous system with confusion, encephalopathy and neuropathy;
- Coagulation system, as shown by disseminated intravascular coagulation (DIC);
- Gastrointestinal system with pancreatitis, reduced motility and ulceration;
- Hepatobiliary system with liver dysfunction and acalculous cholecystitis.
⇒ Haemostasis (disseminated intravascular coagulation) , Renal failure, Respiratory system (acute respiratory distress syndrome).

SYSTEMIC LUPUS ERYTHEMATOSUS

Systemic lupus erythematosus (SLE) is a connective tissue disease in which autoantibodies cause effects in many parts of the body (e.g. sun-exposed skin, joints, kidneys, lungs, heart and blood vessels). The aetiology is multifactorial, with genetic, immunological, environmental (sunlight, drugs) and possibly infective elements. The presentation depends on the areas affected, but may include pyrexia, alopecia, skin changes with a typically butterfly-shaped facial rash, pleurisy, alveolitis, pericarditis, arthritis and renal damage. It occurs most commonly in younger women. Management may include corticosteroids, immunosuppressant drugs, plasma exchange and system-specific treatment as required.

S

TASTE (GUSTATION)

Being able to taste enhances appetite and our enjoyment of food. The sense of taste triggers salivation and the secretion of gastric juice. It also has a protective function (e.g. when foul-tasting food is eaten, reflex gagging or vomiting may be induced). Taste helps to ensure that we eat a variety of foods that provide a balanced intake of minerals, vitamins and other nutrients.

Taste buds contain sensory receptors (chemoreceptors) found in the papillae of the tongue and widely distributed in the epithelia of the tongue, soft palate, pharynx and epiglottis. They consist of small sensory nerve endings of the facial, glossopharyngeal and vagus nerves (cranial nerves VII, IX and X). Some of the cells have hair-like microvilli on their free border, which project towards tiny pores in the epithelium (*Fig. 171*). The sensory receptors are stimulated by chemicals that enter the pores dissolved in saliva. Nerve impulses are generated and conducted along the three cranial nerves before synapsing in the medulla and thalamus. Their final destination is the *taste area* in the parietal lobe of the cerebral cortex, where taste is perceived.

PHYSIOLOGY OF TASTE

Four fundamental sensations of taste have been described – sweet, sour, bitter and salt. This is probably an oversimplification because perception varies widely (e.g. some people are particularly sensitive to certain bitter tastes and avoid bitter foods such as olives) and many 'tastes' cannot be classified easily. However, some tastes consistently stimulate taste buds in specific parts of the tongue:

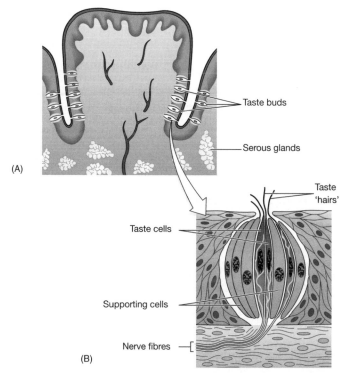

(A)

Taste buds

Serous glands

Taste 'hairs'

Taste cells

Supporting cells

Nerve fibres

(B)

Fig 171 Structure of taste buds: (A) section of a papilla, (B) taste bud – greatly magnified

- Sweet and salty, mainly at the tip;
- Sour, at the sides;
- Bitter, at the back.

⇒ Fluid balance and body fluids (fluid replacement), Oral (oral hygiene), Smell.

Practice application – taste alteration (dysgeusia) and appetite

The sense of taste changes with normal ageing – a gradual loss of taste receptors, starting in midlife, accounts for the diminished sense of taste in older people. This may account for the common complaint voiced by older people that 'modern food' has no taste and contributes to a reduction in appetite. Nurses can encourage food intake by ascertaining preferences and making suggestions about stronger flavours and aromas, seasoning and interesting textures.

Dehydration, which leads to a dry mouth (substances can be 'tasted' only when they are in solution), and oral infections (e.g. candidiasis) both reduce taste sensations. Nurses should ensure adequate hydration, oral hygiene and dental health.

The sense of taste is linked closely with that of olfaction, and so taste (and hence appetite) can be impaired if an upper respiratory tract infection affects the olfactory receptors in the nose.

Disturbances in taste can occur as part of a disease state, including the aura experienced by some people with epilepsy who perceive a strange taste immediately before a seizure. Taste sensation may also change in some malignant conditions and with chemotherapy and drugs such as morphine, baclofen (a muscle relaxant), etc. Patients with liver disease may also complain of altered taste.

T-CELLS

⇒ Defence mechanisms.

TEAM NURSING

Team nursing is a method of care delivery designed to provide maximum continuity of patient-centred care. A small team of nurses, working together, but led by one registered nurse, is responsible and accountable for the assessment, planning and implementation of the care of a particular group of patients for the length of time they require care in a particular setting. Team care differs from patient allocation or primary nursing in that it is based on the belief that a small group of nurses working together can give better care than if each works individually, using the skills of all the team members to the benefit of each patient, but retaining continuity of care. Effective verbal and written communication between the team members is vital. ⇒ Named nurse, Primary nursing.

TEETH

The teeth are embedded in the alveoli or sockets of the alveolar ridges of the mandible and the maxilla. Each individual has two sets, or *dentitions*, the *temporary* or *deciduous teeth* and the *permanent teeth*.

There are 20 temporary teeth, 10 in each jaw. They begin to erupt when the child is about 6 months old, and should all be present after 24 months (*Fig. 172A*). The permanent teeth begin to replace the deciduous teeth in the sixth year of age and this dentition, which consists of 32 teeth, is usually complete by the 24th year (*Fig. 172B*).

(A)

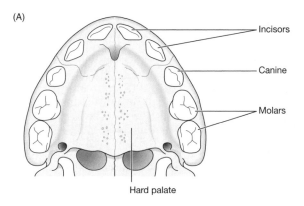

(B)

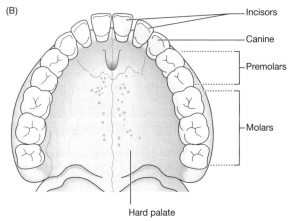

Fig 172 (A) Upper jaw deciduous teeth – viewed from below; (B) upper jaw permanent teeth – viewed from below

FUNCTIONS OF THE TEETH

The *incisor* and *canine* teeth are the cutting teeth and are used to bite off pieces of food, whereas the *premolar* and *molar* teeth, with broad, flat surfaces, are used to grind or chew food.

STRUCTURE OF A TOOTH

Although the shapes of the different teeth vary, the structure is the same and consists of (*Fig. 173*):
• *Crown* – the part that protrudes from the gum;
• *Root* – the part embedded in the bone;
• *Neck* – the slightly narrowed region where the crown merges with the root.
A tooth is composed largely of dentine with enamel that covers the crown and cement (cementum) that covers the root surface. The pulp occupies the cavity at the core of the crown (pulp chamber) and the channel running along the length of the root (root canal). The tooth is secured in its socket by the periodontal ligament and the cement. Blood vessels and nerves pass to the tooth through a small foramen at the apex of each root. ⇒ Oral (oral hygiene, periodontitis).

T

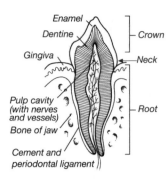

Enamel

Dentine — Crown

Gingiva — Neck

Pulp cavity
(with nerves — Root
and vessels)

Bone of jaw

Cement and
periodontal ligament

Fig 173 A section through a tooth

TESTES

The testes (singular: testis) are each suspended by a spermatic cord within the scrotum on the exterior of the male body. The spermatic cord, which passes through the inguinal canal, encloses blood vessels, lymphatics, nerves that supply the testes and the vas deferens. Sperm production and survival are dependent on a constant temperature of around 4–7°C less than 'core' body temperature – hence the position of the testes in the scrotum.

The testes are covered by the tunica vaginalis (a double membrane) and the fibrous tunica albuginea. The testes produce spermatozoa (spermatogenesis, see *Fig. 89*) and hormones.

Sperm develop in the tubules in association with Sertoli cells, whereas androgen hormones are made between the tubules in the Leydig cells (interstitial cells). A barrier that develops at puberty, called the blood–testis barrier, separates these two compartments. This barrier prevents spermatozoa from escaping into the systemic and lymphatic circulation, where they would cause an immune response.

Sperm enter the epididymis (coiled tubule on the back of the testis), where they mature for approximately 20 days. At ejaculation, the epididymis contracts, which forces the motile sperm into the vas deferens.

TESTICULAR HORMONE PRODUCTION

The main testicular androgen is testosterone, a steroid hormone formed in the Leydig cells. Testosterone is responsible for initiating maturation of the reproductive organs, secondary sexual characteristics, such as deepening of the voice, etc. In addition, testosterone exerts widespread anabolic (growth-promoting) effects. ⇒ Gametogenesis (spermatogenesis and spermiogenesis), Reproductive systems.

TESTICULAR DISORDERS

TESTICULAR CANCER

Testicular cancer is relatively rare, but it is the most common cancer in young men under 35 years of age. It is one of the most curable solid tumours. Early detection of testicular cancer is vital, and all men should be taught how to examine their testes (see Practice application). The testes contain several types of cells, each of which may develop into one or more types of cancer.

Testicular cancer is more common in developed countries, and is associated with an undescended testis (see below). It is rare before puberty and commonly occurs in the mid-20s.

Presentation is usually with a lump or painless swelling in one testis. Men may have a dull ache or heavy sensation in the lower abdomen, anal or scrotal area. Other signs and symptoms include back pain or gynaecomastia (breast development).

The treatment modalities include:

- Surgery – *orchidectomy* (removal of a testis), either partial or total;
- Chemotherapy – commonly BEP, a combination of bleomycin, etoposide and cisplatin (platinum-based);
- Radiotherapy.

These treatment modalities can be used alone or in combination, depending on the type of tumour and its stage. ⇒ Cancer, Cytotoxic chemotherapy, Radiotherapy, Screening and early detection, Tumour marker.

Practice application – education for testicular self-examination (TSE)

- It is easiest to examine your testes after a warm bath or shower (scrotum relaxed).
- Support your scrotum in the palm of one hand, and note the size and weight of your testes to help you to detect any changes in the future. It is normal for one testis to hang slightly lower than does the other.
- Examine each testis in more detail by rolling it between your fingers and thumb. Press firmly but gently to feel for any lumps, swellings or changes in firmness (*Fig. 174*).
- Don't worry if you find the epididymis, a tube that carries sperm to the penis. This can be felt at the top and back of each testis.
- Examine yourself about once every month or two. It is also important not to become obsessed with self-examination – remember testicular cancer is uncommon. However, if you do find anything unusual, don't wait for it to disappear or start throbbing – see your doctor as soon as possible.

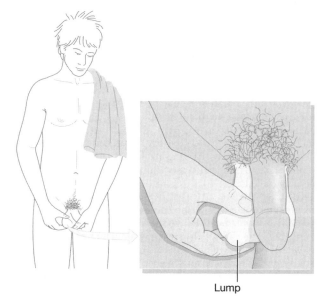

Lump

Fig 174 Testicular self-examination

EPIDIDYMITIS

Epididymitis is inflammation of the epididymis, usually acute inflammation and pain. It is a bacterial infection and the micro-organisms responsible are usually *Escherichia coli* or *Chlamydia trachomatis*. It is important to differentiate between epididymitis and torsion, given the urgent surgical management of the latter.

HYDROCELE

A hydrocele is a swelling caused by accumulation of serous fluid between the tunica vaginalis and tunica albuginea of the testis or in the spermatic cord.

ORCHITIS

Orchitis is inflammation of the testis – viral infection, particularly mumps can cause swollen, painful testes.

TORSION OF TESTIS

Torsion is the rotation of the testis on the spermatic cord. The blood supply is disrupted, which can result in ischaemia and testicular infarction. Urgent surgery to untwist the testis is undertaken.

UNDESCENDED TESTIS (CRYPTORCHISM)

An undescended testis is one that has failed to migrate to the correct position in the scrotum. The complications of undescended testes are torsion, infertility and cancer.

Treatment is surgical mobilization by *orchiopexy* (i.e. mobilization of the testis into the scrotum). If an undescended testis is found in an adult male, an orchidectomy is required, given the risk of developing cancer.

VARICOCELE

Varicocele is a dilatation of the veins that lead from the testis.

TETANY

Tetany is a condition of muscular hyperexcitability in which mild stimuli produce cramps and painful spasms in the hands and feet (carpopedal spasm). In children there may be laryngeal spasm. Tetany is caused by a reduction in ionized calcium levels in the blood (hypocalcaemia), for example as a result of alkalosis or hypoparathyroidism. Causes include:
- Hypoparathyroidism;
- Damage to or removal of the parathyroid glands during thyroid surgery;
- Radioactive iodine used to treat thyroid disease;
- Deficiency of calcium or vitamin D;
- Chronic renal failure when there is excessive loss of calcium in the urine;
- Hyperventilation (excess CO_2 is lost causing alkalosis);
- Excessive ingestion of alkali indigestion medicines or persistent vomiting that leads to metabolic alkalosis.

Treatment depends on the cause:
- Intravenous calcium gluconate when tetany occurs after thyroid surgery;
- Calcium and vitamin D supplements in hypoparathyroidism;
- Re-inhaling expired CO_2 using a paper bag in hyperventilation associated with panic attacks. Note that patients with life-threatening chest problems (e.g. tension pneumothorax) may be mistaken for someone having a panic attack, and therefore physical causes of hyperventilation must be excluded beforehand.

CHVOSTEK'S SIGN

Chvostek's sign is excessive twitching of the face on tapping the facial nerve, a sign of tetany.

TROUSSEAU'S SIGN

Trousseau's sign is a test for latent tetany. Spasm of the forearm muscle is observed within 3–4 minutes of inflating a cuff on the upper arm to a pressure greater than systolic blood pressure.

THERMOREGULATION

Thermoregulation involves the homeostatic mechanisms that maintain body temperature within a normal range. This is achieved by maintaining a balance between heat produced in the body and heat lost. ⇒ Body temperature, Homeostasis (negative feedback mechanisms).

HEAT PRODUCTION

Some of the energy released in the cells during metabolic activity is in the form of heat and the most active organs, chemically and physically, produce the most heat. The principal organs involved are:
* Contraction of skeletal muscles and shivering;
* Liver produces heat as a metabolic by-product;
* Heat is produced during peristalsis and in the chemical reactions of digestion.

HEAT LOSS

Most of the heat loss from the body occurs through the skin (*Fig. 175*). Small amounts are lost in expired air, urine and faeces.

Heat loss through the skin is affected by the difference between body and environmental temperatures, the amount of the body surface exposed to the air and the type of clothes worn. Control is achieved mainly by thermoreceptors in the hypothalamus.

MECHANISMS OF HEAT LOSS

Heat is lost through the *evaporation* of sweat from the skin, by *radiation* of heat from exposed skin, and by *conduction*, as clothes and other objects in contact with the skin take up heat. In *convection*, air passing over the exposed parts of the body is heated and rises, cool air replaces it and convection currents are set up. Heat is also lost from the clothes by convection.

These mechanisms involve the activity of the sweat glands and vasodilatation of vessels in the skin, which brings more blood to the skin surface for heat loss by radiation, conduction and convection. ⇒ Skin.

THROMBOCYTOPENIA

⇒ Platelets.

THROMBOSIS

Thrombosis is any unwanted intravascular formation of a blood clot (or *thrombus*). *Thromboembolic* describes the phenomenon whereby a thrombus detaches itself and is carried to another part of the body in the blood stream to block a blood vessel there. ⇒ Coronary heart disease (myocardial infarction), Deep vein thrombosis, Embolism, Haemostasis, Nervous system (cerebrovascular accident), Pulmonary embolism.

T

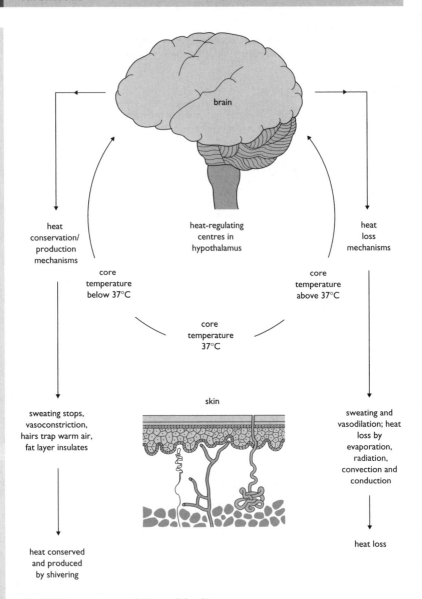

Fig 175 Temperature regulation and the skin

THROMBOLYTIC THERAPY

Thrombolytic therapy is the attempted removal of preformed intravascular fibrin occlusions using fibrinolytic drugs, such as alteplase and streptokinase. It is used in a variety of conditions, including myocardial infarction, deep vein thrombosis, pulmonary embolism, some types of stroke, acute arterial embolism, etc.

Practice application – thrombolytic therapy after acute myocardial infarction
Reperfusion of the myocardium should be attempted as soon as possible
through the administration of thrombolytics. Ideally, they should be given
within 1 hour of the onset of pain (Department of Health 2000b), but may be
of benefit within 12 hours. Thrombolysis is started either as pre-hospital delivery with reteplase or tenecteplase, or in hospital where an appropriate choice
is made from streptokinase, alteplase, reteplase or tenecteplase (NICE 2002).
Streptokinase is the most widely used thrombolytic in the UK. The prescribed
dose should be given intravenously over 1 hour. Streptokinase is a protein
extracted from streptococcal strains and antibody production occurs. Repeat
use within 1 year is therefore contraindicated. Tissue plasminogen activator
(tPA) is an alternative thrombolytic agent and ideally should be given over
90 minutes and accompanied by an intravenous infusion of heparin. Reteplase
can be administered over a much shorter period (two bolus doses, 30 minutes apart).

THYMUS GLAND

The thymus gland lies in the upper part of the mediastinum behind the sternum
and extends upwards into the root of the neck (*Fig. 176*). It grows until the individual reaches puberty, when it begins to atrophy.

The thymus consists of two lobes joined by areolar tissue. The lobes are divided
into lobules that consist of an irregular branching framework of epithelial cells
and lymphocytes.

The thymus gland 'processes' lymphocytes to produce mature T-cells that can
distinguish 'self' tissue from foreign tissue. The maturation of the thymus and
other lymphoid tissue is stimulated by *thymosin*, a hormone secreted by the epithelial cells of the thymus gland. The effectiveness of the T-cell response to antigens
declines with increasing age. ⇒ Defence mechanisms.

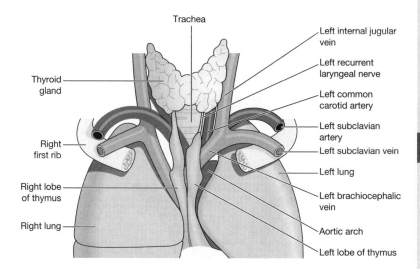

Fig 176 The thymus gland in the adult, and related structures

MYASTHENIA GRAVIS

Myasthenia gravis is an autoimmune disorder in which an antibody reduces the efficiency of transmission between the motor neuron and muscle. The antibody blocks receptor sites at the neuromuscular junctions and prevents the normal action of acetylcholine and nerve impulse transmission. In most cases there is thymic hyperplasia or a thyoma. It is characterized by marked fatigue that affects the voluntary muscles, especially after exercise. Other muscles involved include those of the eye and shoulder girdle, and those required to speak, swallow, chew and breath.

THYROID GLAND

The thyroid gland is situated in the neck in front of the larynx and trachea. It is a highly vascular, butterfly-shaped gland. It consists of two lobes (joined by an isthmus), one on either side of the trachea (*Fig. 177*).

The gland is composed of follicles that secrete and store colloid, a thick sticky protein material. Between the follicles are the parafollicular cells, also called C-cells.

THYROID HORMONES

The thyroid synthesizes and secretes three hormones. Two are metabolic hormones, *thyroxine* (T_4) and *triiodothyronine* (T_3), which are synthesized as large precursor molecules called *thyroglobulin*, the major constituent of colloid. The release of T_3 and T_4 into the blood is regulated by *thyroid-stimulating hormone* (TSH) from the anterior pituitary.

The level of secretion of TSH depends on the plasma levels of T_3 and T_4, because these hormones affect the sensitivity of the anterior pituitary to *thyroid-releasing hormone* (TRH). Increased levels of T_3 and T_4 decrease TSH secretion, and vice versa. When the supply of iodine is deficient, excess TSH is secreted and there is enlargement of the gland (see Disorders below).

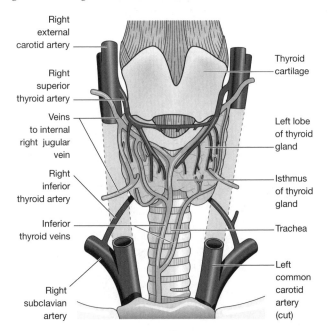

Fig 177 The position of the thyroid gland and its associated structures

T_3 and T_4 affect most cells of the body by:
- Increasing the basal metabolic rate and heat production;
- Regulating metabolism of carbohydrates, proteins and fats.

T_3 and T_4 are essential for normal growth and development, especially of the skeleton and nervous system.

Calcitonin is secreted by the parafollicular or C-cells in the thyroid gland. It acts on bone and the kidneys to reduce the blood calcium level when this is raised. It reduces the reabsorption of calcium from bones and inhibits reabsorption of calcium by the renal tubules. It opposes the effects parathormone (PTH). $\Rightarrow$ Parathyroid glands.

DISORDERS OF THE THYROID GLAND

HYPERTHYROIDISM

Hyperthyroidism (thyrotoxicosis) is a condition caused by excessive production of T_3 and T_4 (usually through Graves' disease, but also by multiple or solitary toxic nodules) and results classically in anxiety, tachycardia, sweating, increased appetite with weight loss and a fine tremor of the outstretched hands; it is much more common in women than in men. Treatment of Graves' disease is with antithyroid drugs, such as carbimazole and beta-blockers for severe cardiac symptoms. If drugs are not successful partial thyroidectomy is undertaken or radioactive iodine used. Toxic nodules are treated with radioactive iodine or surgery.

HYPOTHYROIDISM

Hypothyroidism encompasses conditions caused by low circulating levels of one or both T_3 and T_4. Hypothyroidism is much more common in women than in men and may be:
- Associated with goitre, such as autoimmune thyroiditis, lack of iodine or as a drug side-effect (e.g. with lithium);
- Caused by spontaneous atrophy;
- After surgical treatment for hyperthyroidism.

Some individuals have a subclinical form, and in others it may be transient. It results in a decreased metabolic rate and may be characterized by any of fatigue, bradycardia, angina, aches and pains, carpal tunnel syndrome, low temperature and cold intolerance, weight gain, constipation, hair and skin changes (dry coarse skin), puffy face, anaemia, hoarseness, slow speech, menorrhagia and depression. Treatment is with replacement levothyroxine sodium.

Congenital hypothyroidism can be detected (by routine blood testing) soon after birth and treated successfully with levothyroxine sodium. Untreated, it leads to impaired mental and physical development. It is recognized by the presence of coarse facies and protruding tongue. The term cretinism was used previously. $\Rightarrow$ Neonatal (neonatal checks).

THYROID CANCER

Thyroid cancer can be primary or secondary. Although thyroid cancer is the most common endocrine cancer, it is a rare malignancy. Treatment is by partial or total thyroidectomy, followed as necessary by the use of radioactive iodine. Replacement thyroid hormone therapy is required postoperatively.

TISSUE VIABILITY

The term 'tissue viability' refers literally to the preservation of healthy tissues. It is a phrase that was first defined in the early 1990s to refer to the prevention and management of patients with skin damage, including those who have acute and chronic wounds. Tissue viability services have developed over the past 20 years as a result of technological advances in wound management. These services tend to concentrate on the management of patients with chronic, nonhealing wounds, such as pressure ulcers and leg ulcers. Specialist wound-care units have emerged in the UK and offer patients a comprehensive range of support services and the combined expertise of a wide range of health professionals. ⇒ Burn injuries, Leg ulcers, Pressure ulcers, Wounds and wound care.

TONSILS

The tonsils are small aggregations of noncapsulated lymphoid tissue located around the pharynx. Forming part of the body's defences, they contain macrophages and B- and T-lymphocytes. There are *lingual tonsils* under the tongue, *nasopharyngeal tonsils* located on the posterior wall of the nasopharynx (called *adenoids* when enlarged) and the *palatine tonsils*, found in the oropharynx. The tonsils provide defence against micro-organisms entering the respiratory tact. The lymphoid tissue circle that surrounds the pharynx is known as *Waldeyer's ring.* ⇒ Lymphatic system.

DISORDERS OF THE TONSILS

TONSILLITIS

Tonsillitis (inflammation) usually results from bacterial infection, which may be secondary to a viral infection.

Modes of presentation include sore throat, dysphagia, pyrexia, earache and general malaise. The tonsils are enlarged and red bilaterally, sometimes with pus discharging from the tonsillar crypts. Cervical lymph nodes may be enlarged and tender.

Management consists of analgesics and antibiotics, and possibly tonsillectomy (removal of the tonsillar tissue bilaterally). The main indication for tonsillectomy is recurrent tonsillitis (four or more attacks per year for at least 18 months), which causes disruption to work or study. Other indications include chronic infection, unilateral enlargement (possibly indicating malignancy), peritonsillar abscess and very large tonsils that cause dysphagia or sleep problems.

> **Practice application – observing for haemorrhage after tonsillectomy**
> Haemorrhage (reactionary or secondary) is the main risk after tonsillectomy. In the postoperative period patients must be observed closely for evidence of haemorrhage, leakage, spitting blood from the mouth, excessive swallowing or vomiting blood. Blood pressure and pulse should be monitored regularly (hypotension and / or tachycardia could indicate hypovolaemia).

PERITONSILLAR ABSCESS

Peritonsillar abscess (or *quinsy*) is a collection of pus around the tonsil. It may follow tonsillitis as inflammation spreads from the tonsil to the surrounding tissue and forms an abscess.

Symptoms include severe sore throat, pyrexia, dysphagia, otalgia and possibly trismus (difficulty opening the mouth) and voice changes. There is tonsillar enlargement and inflammation with displacement of the tonsil towards the midline.

Management includes:
- Aspiration or incision and drainage of the abscess under local anaesthesia;
- Airway observation is essential, as oedema could lead to airway obstruction, which is important both prior to drainage and afterwards, as swelling may persist for several days;
- Intravenous antibiotics;

- Intravenous fluids to correct fluid imbalance;
- Psychological support;
- Analgesics;
- Regular oral hygiene;
- Oral fluids;
- Suitable diet – cool, soft foods are more likely to be tolerated.

TOUCH (SENSATION)

Touch, one of the senses, is:
- The ability to feel objects and to distinguish their various characteristics – the tactile sense;
- The ability to perceive pressure when it is exerted on the skin, which contains specialized sensory nerve endings sensitive to tactile stimuli or mucosa of the body. ⇒ Complementary medicine and therapy (therapeutic touch).

Box 38 gives some sensations related to touch.

Box 38 – Types of touch sensations

Anaesthesia – loss of sensation. ⇒ Anaesthesia.
Analgesia – loss of sensation of pain without loss of touch.
Hyperaesthesia – excessive sensitiveness of a part.
Hyperalgesia – excessive sensibility to pain.
Hypoaesthesia – diminished sensitiveness of a part.
Paraesthesia – any abnormality of sensation, such as tingling ('pins and needles') or loss of peripheral sensation (anaesthesia) associated with spinal disease or peripheral nerve disease or damage.

TOXIC SHOCK SYNDROME

⇒ Infections of the female reproductive tract (Toxic shock syndrome).

TRACHEOSTOMY

A tracheostomy is an opening in the trachea, to establish a safe airway with the insertion of a tube (*Fig. 178*). It may be temporary or permanent (after a laryngectomy). Tracheostomy can be performed surgically or percutaneously by inserting a guide wire into the trachea and dilating the tract until it is wide enough for the tracheostomy tube.

The reasons for performing a temporary tracheostomy include:
- To bypass an upper airway obstruction;
- To enable long-term mechanical ventilation;
- To facilitate tracheobronchial suction;
- To prevent aspiration of secretions.

There are many types of tracheostomy tube. If the tracheostomy is permanent and self-care is anticipated, the manual dexterity and ability of the patient must be considered. Tubes are generally constructed from metal or flexible synthetic materials. Most synthetic tubes have an inflatable cuff that creates an air-tight seal between tube and trachea (*Fig. 178*). This arrangement prevents the aspiration of secretions into the lungs and facilitates mechanical ventilation.

Where possible, nurses must provide patients with information about what to expect after the tracheostomy, such as suction and communication problems. In some emergency situations, there is little opportunity for preoperative explanations.

The specific care priorities after a tracheostomy include airway maintenance and preventing chest infection, suction, humidification, care of the tube and wound (see

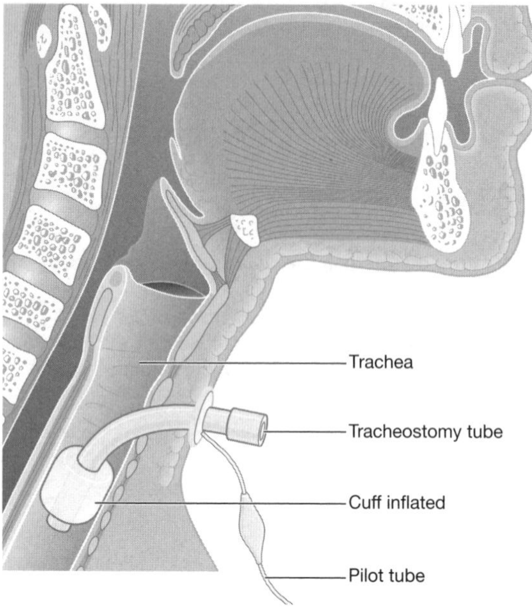

Fig 178 Cuffed tracheostomy tube in place (tapes not shown)

Practice application), effective communication, altered body image and patient education for self-care (permanent tracheostomy). For a detailed discussion of these major issues readers are directed to Further reading. ⇒ Larynx (cancer of the larynx).

Practice application – care of tracheostomy tube and wound

The tapes that secure the tracheostomy tube in position are changed whenever they become soiled. While one person holds the tube in position, the old tapes are cut and removed one at a time. If the tube has an inflatable cuff, care must be taken to avoid cutting the pilot tube when cutting the tapes. Two nurses are required to ensure that the tube is not dislodged. New tape is threaded through the hole in the flange and tied securely onto the flange. The tapes are then tied securely around the patient's neck, but the nurse should check that the tapes are not too tight or causing skin soreness. The tapes may be threaded through a foam tube for comfort.

Depending on the type of tube used, the inner tube should be removed and cleaned according to local protocols.

The area around the tracheostomy may be left exposed or dressed with an absorbent 'keyhole' dressing, which is changed whenever soiling occurs. The area must be cleaned with sterile saline as required and any crusts should be removed carefully.

Further reading

Brooker C and Nicol M (2003). *Nursing Adults. The Practice of Caring*, pp. 584–586. Edinburgh: Mosby.

Harkin H (1998). Tracheostomy management. *Nurs Times* **94**(21): 56–58.

Nicol M, Bavin C, Bedford-Turner S, Cronin P and Rawlings-Anderson K (2004). *Essential Nursing Skills*, Second Edition. Edinburgh: Mosby.

TRACTION

Traction is a steady pull exerted on a body part. It is generally used to counteract the potential or actual problems caused by the pull of muscles on a damaged bone or joint. The purpose of traction may comprise any one or more of the following:
• To maintain or achieve correct alignment of injured bone;
• To prevent the development or deformity, or reduce existing deformity;
• To immobilize a damaged joint;
• To relieve pain through attaining normal anatomical alignment and reduce muscle spasm around the injury site;
• Occasionally, to protect underlying tissues and structures. An obvious example is cervical traction to protect the spinal cord.
Clearly, the type of traction utilized is dependent on the particular condition and age of the patient.

METHODS OF APPLYING TRACTION

To apply traction a satisfactory grip must be obtained on a part of the patient's body. This may be achieved through the skin or bone:
• Manual traction is applied by hand as, for example, when reducing a fracture.
• Skin traction is the application of the traction force over a large area of skin, and the force is then transmitted via the soft tissues to the bone (*Fig. 179A*). Two common ways to apply this traction are the adhesive or nonadhesive forms.
• Skeletal traction is the application of the traction force directly to a bone, commonly through metal pins or wires.

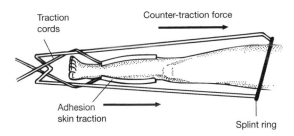

(A)   Fixed skin traction using a Thomas' splint.

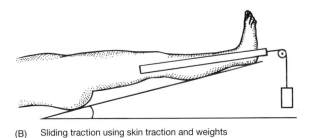

(B)   Sliding traction using skin traction and weights

Fig 179 (A) Fixed skin traction using a Thomas' splint, (B) sliding traction using skin traction and weights

COUNTER-TRACTION

In any traction set-up, the whole body tends to be pulled in the direction of the traction force if counter-traction is not present. Counter-traction is achieved using one of two main ways:

- Fixed traction is the application of counter-traction acting through an appliance that obtains purchase on a part of the body. To apply a force against a fixed point on the body, an appliance such as a Thomas' splint is used (*Fig. 179A*). Traction cords are tied to the distal end of the splint and the counter-traction force passes along the side bars to the ring. The grip on the leg is achieved by adhesive skin traction.
- Sliding or balanced traction makes use of the weight of all or part of the body (influenced by gravity) to supply counter-traction; for instance, the bed is tilted so that the patient tends to 'slide' or move in the opposite direction to that of the traction force. In reality, the pull of gravity should equal that of the traction so that the two are 'balanced' and hence the patient remains stationary. The traction force is produced by weights and may be applied through a cord passing over a pulley (*Fig. 179B*).

Further reading

Davis PS (1994). *Nursing the Orthopaedic Patient*, pp. 105–110. Edinburgh: Churchill Livingstone.

TRANSCULTURAL NURSING

In multicultural societies, a nurse's knowledge of such factors as the customs and perceptions of health, ill-health, pain, hygiene, dress, diet, birth, circumcision, contraception, menstruation, marriage, religion and death can alert him or her to the actual or potential health needs or problems of individual clients. ⇒ Culture, Personal hygiene (see Practice application).

Further reading

Kenworthy N, Snowley G and Gilling C (2002). *Common Foundation Studies in Nursing*, Third Edition, Ch 5. Edinburgh: Churchill Livingstone.

TRIAGE

The term 'triage' is derived from the French word *trier*, meaning 'to sort'.

Nurse triage is not merely a way to allocate a category rating to a patient, although pressures on emergency departments to speed up the flow of patients present a difficult task. Decisions have to be made quickly and acted upon. Triage encompasses assessment, prioritization of need, first aid, the initiation of relevant investigations and the provision of health promotion.

Skills include effective communication, objectivity and the ability to make rapid clinical decisions to achieve the best care for every patient.

Many departments have a designated triage area that provides some privacy from the rest of the waiting area. However, a difficult balance has to be struck between the preservation of dignity, and visibility and access to and from the triage nurse.

TRIAGE STANDARDS

The triage nurse is faced with the difficult task of identifying the sickest patients, while providing a service for the large numbers of people whose problems may not be serious, yet who suffer long waits.

A standard triage scale (Crouch and Marrow 1996) was designed to provide five categories of urgency to indicate the appropriate waiting times for patients – immediate resuscitation (red), very urgent (orange), urgent (yellow), standard (green) and nonurgent (blue).

Triage is a dynamic process. The condition of patients may change and their needs alter. People in pain require special attention and pain relief must therefore be seen as a high priority, which can be altered when the person is more comfortable.

TUBERCULOSIS

Tuberculosis (TB) is a chronic granulomatous infection caused by *Mycobacterium tuberculosis* (human type), an acid-fast bacillus (AFB). Other types include *M. bovis* (cattle) and atypical mycobacteria [e.g. *M. avium intracellulare* (MAI) and *M. kansasii*].

TB is a notifiable disease. It affects the lungs mainly, as it is transmitted by inhalation of infected droplets of sputum coughed up by someone with active TB. However, other parts of the body (extrapulmonary) can be affected, with the bacterium entering the bloodstream through the lymphatic system. The most common forms of extrapulmonary disease are lymphadenopathy, pleural effusion, pericardial TB, miliary TB and TB meningitis.

Protection against TB is with the Bacille–Calmette–Guérin (BCG). BCG is a live attenuated strain of *M. bovis* that has lost its power to cause TB (pathogenicity), but retains its antigenic function; it is the base of a vaccine used for immunization against TB.

Most people infected with *M. tuberculosis* do not develop active disease, as the body's immune system makes the bacterium dormant. Soon after the *primary infection* enters the lung, the inflammatory response occurs and a calcified lesion is left. The primary infection remains dormant, but may be reactivated (*post-primary infection*) if the immune system is weakened, which results in active TB.

The risk factors for developing active TB are associated with the immune system weakening and exposure to infectious TB. They include:
- Immunodeficiency [i.e. human immune deficiency virus (HIV) and acquired immune deficiency syndrome (AIDS)];
- Immunosuppression with corticosteroids, chemotherapy, etc.;
- Close contact with someone newly diagnosed with infectious TB;
- Homelessness, particularly those with a history of alcohol misuse and malnutrition;
- Older adults, particularly those resident in long-term care facilities;
- Chronic respiratory disease (e.g. bronchiectasis and cystic fibrosis).

TB is characterized by systemic effects, such as fever, night sweats and weight loss, plus those dependent upon the site (e.g. cough and haemoptysis in pulmonary disease, haematuria in renal TB, etc.). Diagnosis is made on clinical signs, chest radiographs (X-rays), skin tests (see Practice application) and the presence of AFB in sputum, urine, etc. ⇒ Mycobacterium.

T

Practice application – tuberculin skin test

A tuberculin skin test (e.g. Heaf test) is used to detect past or present TB infection. It is a multiple skin puncture test with tuberculin purified protein derivative (PPD) using a special Heaf device (gun), also used for routine screening before BCG immunization. The inflammatory reaction grade (0–4) is read after 3–7 days. A positive Heaf test when there has been no BCG vaccination, or a grade 3 or 4 Heaf when BCG vaccination has taken place, gives rise to suspicion of active TB, although this alone is not sufficient to diagnose the disease.

TREATMENT OF PULMONARY TUBERCULOSIS

Currently, first-line treatment for TB consists of a 6-month regimen of rifampicin, isoniazid, pyrazinamide and ethambutol or streptomycin for 2 months, and then rifampicin and isoniazid for a further 4 months. The fourth drug, ethambutol or streptomycin, can be omitted when patients have a low risk of developing resistance to isoniazid.

MULTI-DRUG RESISTANT TUBERCULOSIS

Pulmonary TB is a treatable condition, but if the initial therapy is inadequate or the course of treatment is not completed, multi-drug resistant tuberculosis (MDR-TB) can develop. The reasons for this are:
- Inadequate treatment;
- Failure to complete course of antibiotics;
- Asymptomatic after 2–4 weeks of treatment, and so patients believe they no longer need the medication;
- Lack of knowledge and understanding of TB and its treatment;
- Inability to access healthcare, which is prevalent among the homeless and minority ethnic groups, if there are language problems.

TUMOUR

A tumour is a swelling, a mass of abnormal tissue that resembles the normal tissues in structure, but that fulfils no useful function and grows at the expense of the body. *Benign* (simple or innocent) tumours are encapsulated, do not infiltrate adjacent tissue or cause metastases and are unlikely to recur if removed. Whereas *malignant* ('cancers') tumours are not encapsulated, infiltrate adjacent tissue and cause metastases. ⇒ Cancer, Cytotoxic chemotherapy, Radiotherapy, Screening and early detection.

TUMOUR LYSIS SYNDROME

Cytotoxic chemotherapy can have a very rapid effect on tumour cells, which can cause problems in patients with large, bulky tumours. As the cancer cells die, they release substances into the bloodstream that can be highly toxic and lead to hyperkalaemia, hypocalcaemia, hyperuricaemia and hyperphosphataemia. This condition is called *tumour lysis syndrome* (TLS). TLS tends to occur during the first few days of treatment and can result in renal failure through the crystallization of uric acid in the renal tubules, acidosis and cardiac and respiratory failure (see Practice application).

> **Practice application – preventing tumour lysis syndrome**
> TLS can be prevented by the administration of allopurinol before and during cytotoxic treatment and by maintaining a good diuresis. Patients should therefore be encouraged to drink 2–3 L of fluid daily. People with bulky tumours or a high tumour burden require intravenous fluids prior to and during treatment. Sodium bicarbonate may also be given to reduce acidosis. An accurate measure of fluid balance is essential to monitor renal function and to assess adequate fluid intake.

TUMOUR MARKER

A tumour marker is a chemical detected in the serum that may be associated with a specific cancer, or sometimes with nonmalignant diseases. They may be used to monitor disease progress and efficacy of treatment, but are of limited use for population screening. Tumour markers (*Table 40*) include alpha-fetoprotein (AFP), Ca-125, carcinoembryonic antigen (CEA), human chorionic gonadotrophin (hCG) and prostate specific antigen (PSA).

Table 40 Serum tumour markers

Cancer	marker
Testicular (germ cell)	Alpha-fetoprotein (AFP) β-human chorionic gonadotrophin (β-hCG)
Choriocarcinoma	β-hCG
Ovary	Ca-125
Prostate	Prostate specific antigen (PSA)
Hepatocellular carcinoma	AFP
Colorectal	Carcinoembryonic antigen (CEA)

TYPHOID AND PARATYPHOID

⇒ *Salmonella* (enteric fevers).

T

UNIPOLAR DISORDER

⇒ Disorders of mood.

URINARY SYSTEM

The normal urinary tract (system) comprises two kidneys, two ureters, a bladder and a urethra (*Fig. 180*). Essentially, the functions of the kidney are to preserve fluid and solute homeostasis. The lower urinary tract provides a conduit for the urine to pass from the body. ⇒ Micturition.

The kidney has an outer cortex that forms a pale red–brown layer under the capsule. Below the cortex is the darker medulla, which contains the cone-shaped striations called renal pyramids. At the apex of each pyramid a papilla opens into a minor calyx, which communicates with the major calyces and funnel-shaped renal pelvis, which distends to receive urine.

The kidney receives around 25% of the cardiac output via the renal artery. Most of this blood is not to supply renal tissue *per se*, but rather to be processed by the functional unit of the kidney, the nephron. A high volume of blood supply to the kidneys is thus required to maintain glomerular filtration rates (GFRs) and to supply oxygen to active cells.

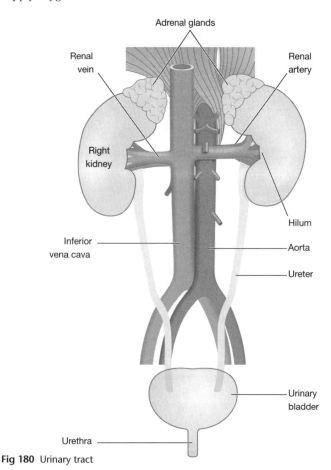

Fig 180 Urinary tract

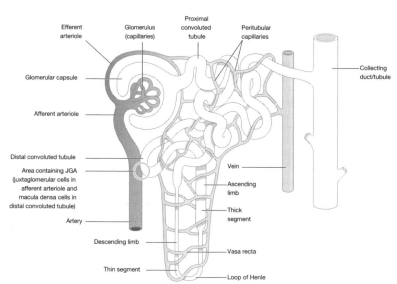

Fig 181 A nephron (diagrammatic)

Each kidney contains about one million microscopic nephrons. A nephron comprises a renal tubule and the glomerulus, a knot of capillaries, which lies within the invaginated blind end of the tubule. The tubule, which is lined with cuboidal epithelium, is divided into the glomerular (Bowman's) capsule, which encloses the glomerulus, the proximal convoluted tubule (PCT), the loop of Henle, the distal convoluted tubule (DCT) and the collecting ducts and/or tubules that drain urine from several nephrons (*Fig. 181*).

Homeostasis is achieved through the production of urine by three processes that occur in the nephrons of the kidney: *filtration, reabsorption* and *secretion*. In addition to fluid and solute balance, the kidneys normally make important contributions to homeostasis in other physiological systems within the body, as summarized in *Box 39*.

Box 39
Important contributions of the kidneys to homeostasis in physiological systems within the body
Water balance:
• Preservation of intracellular environment;
• Preservation of extracellular fluid (ECF) volume;
• Contribution to the control of blood pressure.
Solute balance:
• Preservation of intracellular and extracellular solute concentrations.
Excretion of end products of metabolism:
• Maintenance of the internal environment;
• Elimination of toxic substances.
Acid–base balance:
• Preservation and maintenance of buffers (e.g., sodium bicarbonate);
• Excretion of acids that cannot be converted into carbon dioxide for excretion by the lungs.
Production of erythropoietin:
• Maintenance of erythrocyte numbers.

Calcium and phosphate balance:
- Maintenance of ionized calcium balance in the ECF;
- Preservation of compounded calcium balance in the ECF;
- Preservation of calcium and phosphate balance in the skeleton.

RENAL FUNCTION TESTS

A series of tests that include routine urine testing (*Box 40*), urine concentration tests, haemoglobin level, serum urea and electrolytes, coagulation studies and serum creatinine (reference range 60–120 mol/L, depending on weight and age) to estimate GFR. ⇒ Micturition, *Box 22* Disorders of micturition.

Box 40
Urinalysis (observation and dipstick test) – abnormal findings
Colour (pale straw colour to deep amber) – abnormal colour may indicate the presence of red blood cells and/or abnormal substances (e.g., bilirubin), and drug or food residue excretion.
Clarity and/or deposits (clear, possibly some mucus) – opacity may indicate the presence of white cells, pus and/or protein.
Odour (faintly aromatic, ammonia on standing, some food residues produce odours) – abnormal 'fishy' odour may indicate infection. The presence of abnormal substances, such as ketones, may affect the odour.
Specific gravity (1.002–1.035) – inability to concentrate or dilute urine, or the presence of abnormal substances (e.g., glucose).
pH (4.5–8.0) – inability to produce acid or alkaline urine, urinary tract infection (UTI) or prolonged vomiting.
Protein (normally negative) – protein in the urine is an indication of glomerular and/or tubular damage, viral illness and UTI.
Glucose (normally negative) – glucose loss associated with inadequately controlled diabetes; may appear in pregnancy.
Ketones (normally negative) – ketonuria is an indication of inadequately controlled diabetes, starvation or excessive or prolonged vomiting.
Blood (normally negative) – haematuria is associated with damage to the nephron and surrounding structures. Urinary causes of frank haematuria include UTI, renal calculi, tumours and trauma.
Leucocytes (none to 4) – presence may indicate infection or nephritis.
Bilirubin (normally negative) – biliary obstruction and hepatocellular disease.
Urobilinogen (normally present) – absent in biliary obstruction. Excessive amounts present in haemolytic disease.

URINARY DISORDERS

Some urinary disorders are outlined below. Further information can be found in separate entries and also in the suggestion for Further reading. ⇒ Catheters and urinary catheterization; Continence; Incontinence; Prostate; Renal failure.

Various renal and urinary surgical procedures, along with some investigations, are outlined in *Box 41*.

Box 41
Renal and urinary surgery and selected investigations
Cystectomy – partial or total removal of the urinary bladder; total cystectomy necessitates urinary diversion.
Cystodiathermy – the application of a cauterizing electrical current to the walls of the urinary bladder through a cystoscope, or by open operation.
Cystography – radiographic examination of the urinary bladder, after it has been filled with a contrast medium.
Cystometry – the study of pressure changes within the urinary bladder under various conditions; used in the study of voiding disorders.
Cystoplasty – surgical repair or augmentation of the urinary bladder.
Cystoscopy – endoscopic examination of the internal surface of the urinary bladder.
Cystostomy (vesicostomy) – an operation whereby a fistulous opening is made into the urinary bladder via the abdominal wall.
Cystotomy – incision into the urinary bladder via the abdominal wall.
Cystourethrogram – radiographic examination of the urinary bladder and urethra. *Micturating cystourethrogram* is a dynamic radiograph performed during micturition, often to assess the degree of ureteric reflux.
Nephrectomy – removal of a kidney.
Nephrolithotomy – removal of a stone from the kidney by an incision through the kidney substance. *Percutaneous nephrolithotomy* is a minimally invasive technique in which the kidney pelvis is punctured using radiographic control. A guide wire is inserted, through which the stone is removed using a nephroscope.
Nephroscopy – an endoscopic examination of kidney tissue.
Nephrostomy – a surgically established fistula from the pelvis of the kidney to the body surface.
Nephroureterectomy – removal of the kidney, along with a part of or the whole of the ureter.
Pyelolithotomy — the operation to remove a stone from the renal pelvis.
Pyeloplasty – a reconstructive operation on the kidney pelvis.
Pyelostomy – surgical formation of an opening into the kidney pelvis.
Ureterectomy – excision of a ureter.
Ureterolithotomy – removal of a stone from the ureter.
Ureterostomy, urostomy – the formation of a permanent fistula through which the ureter discharges urine, such as an ileal conduit.
Urodynamics – the method used to study bladder function (*see above*, cystometry).
Urography (pyelography) – radiographic visualization of the renal pelvis and ureter by injection of a contrast medium. The medium may be injected intravenously, in which case it is excreted by the kidney (intravenous urography), or it may be injected directly into the renal pelvis or ureter by way of a fine catheter introduced through a cystoscope (retrograde or ascending urography).

DIABETIC NEPHROPATHY

Diabetic nephropathy is the renal (kidney) disease associated with diabetes mellitus. It is a common cause of end-stage renal failure (ESRF) worldwide. Diabetic nephropathy is characterized by disruption to the normal structure of small blood vessels (microvasculature).

GLOMERULONEPHRITIS

Glomerulonephritis is an autoimmune disease and is associated with an immune injury to the glomerulus and surrounding structures. Some types of glomerulonephritis are associated with rapid deterioration in renal function to ESRF. Commonly, patients with glomerulonephritis present with acute renal failure. Hypertension may be a feature of presentation.

Medical management can include:

- Dialysis, primarily to manage fluid, electrolyte and acid–base imbalances;
- Correction of anaemia;
- Immunosuppressive drugs (e.g., corticosteroids), plasma exchange to reduce circulating antibody titres;
- Control of hypertension.

NEPHROLITHIASIS (RENAL CALCULI)

Nephrolithiasis (renal calculi) is the formation of stones within the kidney. Stones may be found within the renal tubules or renal pelvis, ureters and bladder. There are a number of different types of renal stones and they can range in size from small to large *staghorn* calculi that can obstruct the collecting system (*Fig. 182*).

The clinical presentation depends on the site of the calculus, and the presence of infection and/or urinary tract obstruction. Ureteric colic is associated classically with renal calculi. The severe flank (loin) pain generated frequently has a sudden onset and then gradually intensifies. Pain may radiate to the groin, testes or labia majora. Stones <5 mm in diameter can be passed spontaneously with adequate hydration. Larger stones usually require intervention for removal. Calculi that are sufficiently large to obstruct the urinary tract may present as acute renal failure.

The treatment of calculi that obstruct the ureter involves elimination of the obstruction, pain relief and treatment of infection with antibiotics. Upper urinary tract obstruction can be treated with percutaneous nephrostomy tubes. Urologic interventions to remove renal stones include:

- Disintegration of stones using a number of techniques, including shock-wave lithotripsy; ⇒ Extracorporeal (extracorporeal shock-wave lithotripsy);
- A large stone may require open surgical removal.

NEPHROTIC SYNDROME

Nephrotic syndrome is a manifestation of glomerular damage and is characterized by proteinuria, hypoalbuminaemia (low level of albumin in the blood) and

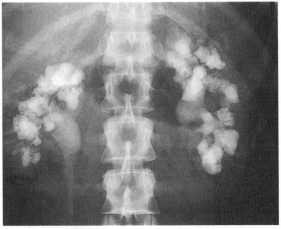

Fig 182 Bilateral staghorn calculus shown on an intravenous urogram (pyelogram)

gross oedema. It is a sequel to glomerulonephritis. The medical management centres on reducing proteinuria and controlling oedema, blood pressure and other associated physiological disruptions.

POLYCYSTIC KIDNEY DISEASE

Adult polycystic kidney disease (APKD) is an inherited multisystem disease characterized by multiple cyst formation in the kidneys and other body sites. As the cysts enlarge normal renal tissue is compressed and progressive deterioration in renal function occurs.

No curative treatment is available for APKD and management involves the surveillance of renal function with symptom control and dialysis, or renal transplantation if ESRF develops.

REFLUX NEPHROPATHY (CHRONIC PYELONEPHRITIS)

The principal predisposing cause of reflux nephropathy is incompetence of the one-way valve system where the ureters enter the bladder. The faulty valve allows urine to reflux up the ureter – vesicoureteric reflux (VUR). Additionally, there is stasis of urine in the bladder. This predisposes to infection, and persistent reflux of infected urine up the ureters results in damage to the renal parenchyma (renal tissue). The defect is present in infants and young children, and confirmed bacteriuria (bacteria in the urine) in the young should be investigated thoroughly. Early detection and treatment can minimize or prevent renal damage in later life. Prompt treatment of infection and low-dose prophylactic antibiotic therapy are the mainstays of management. Surgical re-implantation of one or both ureters to form a competent valve may be undertaken.

RENAL TRAUMA

Traumatic damage to the kidneys and urinary tract is associated with blunt trauma (e.g., road traffic accident or assault), deceleration trauma (e.g., fall from a height) or penetrating injury (e.g., stab wound). Minor injuries are usually treated conservatively, if the patient is haemodynamically stable. Major injuries warrant surgical exploration, repair if possible and nephrectomy if repair is impossible.

URINARY CANCER

Tumours may affect renal cells and the transitional epithelium (urothelium) that lines the urinary tract from the renal pelvis to the urethra.

Renal cancers

Malignant renal tumours are more common in males and rarely seen before the fourth decade. In the presence of unilateral disease and an acceptable level of function in the other kidney, the affected kidney is removed. Partial nephrectomy may be undertaken if there is abnormal renal function in the other kidney. Primarily, chemotherapy is used to control metastatic spread. Nephroureterectomy is undertaken for renal pelvis and ureteric tumours.

Nephroblastoma (Wilms' tumour) is the most common abdominal tumour of childhood, and one that usually affects the kidneys. It is usually diagnosed during the preschool period. Prognosis is uncertain and depends on the stage of the tumour and child's age at diagnosis and treatment (radiotherapy, surgical removal and chemotherapy).

U

Bladder cancer

Bladder cancer occurs most commonly between the ages of 60 and 70 years – men are affected more often than women are. Early-stage superficial tumours have an excellent prognosis. Presenting features include intermittent and painless haematuria, dysuria, urinary frequency and urgency, as well as prostatism in men. Flank pain may be a feature of advanced disease or may indicate ureteral obstruction.

The major risk factor for bladder cancer is tobacco smoking. Other factors include chronic bladder inflammation, exposure to industrial chemicals (e.g., aniline) and certain drugs (e.g., cyclophosphamide).

Treatment of superficial bladder tumours includes diathermy and transurethral resection of the tumour. Intravesical (into the bladder) chemotherapy and regular check cystoscopies are adjunctive therapies.

Treatment for invasive bladder tumours includes:
- Transurethral resection;
- Partial cystectomy;
- Total (radical) cystectomy with urinary diversion (e.g., ileal conduit) and removal of regional lymph nodes; $\Rightarrow$ Stoma (ileal conduit);
- Radiotherapy;
- Palliative therapy.

U RINARY TRACT INFECTION

Urinary tract infections (UTIs) include cystitis (inflammation of the bladder, usually bacterial) and acute pyelonephritis (infection within the substance of the kidney, often derived either from the urine or from the blood; *see above*, reflux nephropathy). UTIs are more common in women than in men. The micro-organisms most commonly associated with UTIs are bowel flora, such as *Escherichia coli*. In young women, *Staphylococcus epidermidis* and *S. saprophyticus* are the causative organisms. Commensal micro-organisms usually gain access to the urinary tract by the ascending transurethral route, although other routes exist, such as bloodborne micro-organisms.

The development of a UTI can be summarized as follows:
- Entry of bacteria – the perineum and periurethral area are heavily colonized with bacteria. Females have short urethras and the transfer of bacteria transurethrally may be spontaneous or facilitated by sexual intercourse or catheterization. The relatively long urethra in males provides some degree of protection against transurethral bacterial transfer, although, as in females, catheterization is a potential source of transfer.
- Multiplication of bacteria in the bladder – normally urine in the bladder is sterile because of the mucosal defence mechanisms and the 'flushing' effect that normal bladder voiding has. Urinary stasis and incomplete bladder emptying are contributory factors to the development of UTIs.

Some patients have bacteria in their urine without symptoms – *asymptomatic bacteriuria*. This is the presence of $\geq$100 000/mL of the same bacterial species in two or more consecutive midstream specimens of urine (MSSUs), without symptoms. Asymptomatic bacteriuria is treated with antibiotics in pregnant women, in patients with diabetes and/or abnormal urinary tracts and in immunocompromised individuals to prevent ascending infection.

Commonly, individuals with cystitis report:
- Frequency and dysuria (painful micturition);
- Urine has a 'fishy' odour;
- Haematuria;
- Suprapubic pain;
- Strangury (constant painful urge to micturate).

Note that changes in behaviour, such as confusion in older people, may indicate UTI.

Symptoms such as fever, loin pain and nausea and/or vomiting suggest infection that has ascended via the ureters into the renal pelvis and the kidneys to cause acute pyelonephritis.

A urine specimen (MSSU) is obtained for microscopy, culture and sensitivity. In patients with recurrent UTI, or for whom post-treatment urinalysis remains abnormal, urodynamic studies may be indicated to exclude abnormality of the lower urinary tract. In children, this is mandatory after a proved first episode of bacteriuria. A micturating cystogram is indicated in adults to investigate abnormal bladder voiding.

Treatment of uncomplicated cystitis is with antibiotic therapy (e.g., amoxicillin, nitrofurantoin, cefalexin or trimethoprim). This may be either a 3-day regimen or a single-dose treatment.

Acute pyelonephritis is also treated with antibiotics on an outpatient basis, unless the clinical condition of the individual warrants hospitalization for intravenous fluids and antibiotics, and pain relief.

Patients should be given advice about avoiding UTI (see Practice Application).

Further reading

Brooker C and Nicol M (2003). *Nursing Adults. The Practice of Caring*, Ch 25. Edinburgh: Mosby.

Practice application – avoiding UTI
- Use different towels for the genital and anal regions;
- Pass urine after sexual intercourse;
- Maintain hydration at >3 L/day (the majority being water);
- Pass urine frequently during the day;
- Pass urine just before going to bed;
- Avoid the use of potentially irritant toiletries;
- Reduce intake of caffeine and alcohol;
- Consider taking cranberry juice. However, care should be taken when providing this advice, as increased urinary acidity can diminish the effectiveness of concurrent antibiotic therapy;
- Seek advice from a health professional if symptoms of UTI occur.

UTERUS AND VAGINA

The uterus is a hollow pear-shaped muscular organ in the pelvic cavity. It has three parts, the top or fundus, the body and the cervix. It connects bilaterally with the uterine tubes and opens inferiorly into the vagina (*see Fig 155A*).

Normally, the uterus is anteverted (inclined forwards) and anteflexed (bent forwards) over the bladder (*Fig. 183*). It has three layers:
- The perimetrium (serous layer);
- The myometrium, a thick layer of interlocking smooth muscle fibres;
- The endometrium, a mucosal lining of highly vascular glandular epithelium that, during the reproductive years, is influenced by the cyclical secretion of hormones.

The uterus receives the fertilized ovum, provides the environment for implantation and fetal development and expels the fetus through the vagina.

The vagina is the muscular, membranous passage that extends from the cervix uteri to the vulva. The front wall is about 7.5 cm long and is close to the urethra and bladder, and the posterior wall, which is longer at 9 cm, has contact with the rectum and rectovaginal pouch. The vagina runs up and backwards at an angle of 45°. The mucosa is arranged in rugae (folds) that allow for distension. During the reproductive years, the vagina is acidic (pH 4.0–4.5) because of the lactic acid produced by bacteria (*Lactobacillus* species) of the normal body flora. The lactic acid helps to

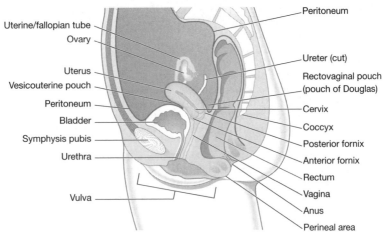

Peritoneum

Uterine/fallopian tube

Ovary

Ureter (cut)

Uterus

Rectovaginal pouch
(pouch of Douglas)

Vesicouterine pouch

Peritoneum

Cervix

Bladder

Coccyx

Symphysis pubis

Posterior fornix

Urethra

Anterior fornix

Rectum

Vagina

Vulva

Anus

Perineal area

Fig 183 Female reproductive structures (mid-sagittal section)

protect the vagina against many pathogenic micro-organisms. ⇒ Cervix; Early pregnancy problems; Gynaecological examination; Infections of female reproductive tract; Menstrual cycle (*Box 20* – Disorders of menstruation); Reproductive systems.

UTERINE AND VAGINAL DISORDERS

The common surgical procedures undertaken are outlined in *Box 42*.

Box 42
Surgical procedures – uterus, uterine tubes and vagina
Colpectomy – excision of the vagina.
Colpohysterectomy – *see below* hysterectomy, vaginal.
Colpoperineorrhaphy – repair of vaginal injury and deficient perineum.
Colporrhaphy or vaginal repair – surgical repair of the vagina. An anterior colporrhaphy repairs a cystocele and a posterior colporrhaphy (also called *colpoperineorrhaphy*) repairs a rectocele.
Colposuspension – surgery to alleviate genuine stress incontinence. In Burch colposuspension the vagina is suspended from the iliopectineal ligament.
Colpotomy – incision of the vaginal wall. A posterior colpotomy drains an abscess in the pouch of Douglas through the vagina.
Dilation and curettage (D&C) – dilating the uterine cervix to obtain an endometrial sample by curettage.
Endometrial ablation – endoscopic, transcervical destruction of the endometrium, usually using some form of heat, such as laser.
Hysterectomy – surgical removal of the uterus. *Abdominal hysterectomy* is effected via a lower abdominal incision. This may be a *total abdominal hysterectomy* (TAH) with removal of the uterine body and cervix. The ovaries and tubes may also be removed [*bilateral salpingo-oophorectomy* (BSO)] or the cervix left *in situ* [*subtotal abdominal hysterectomy* (STAH)]. A *vaginal hysterectomy* is carried out through the vagina. In *Wertheim's hysterectomy*, a radical and extensive operation performed for cervical cancer, the uterus, cervix, upper vagina, uterine tubes, ovaries and regional lymph nodes are removed.

U

Hysteroscopy – the passage of a small-diameter telescope through the cervix to visualize the uterine cavity. The procedure is also used for treatments such as transcervical resection of the endometrium.
Hysterotomy – incision of the uterus to remove a pregnancy. The word is usually reserved for a method of late abortion.
Manchester operation – anterior colporrhaphy, amputation of part of the cervix and posterior colpoperineorrhaphy, performed for uterovaginal prolapse.
Myomectomy – enucleation of fibroid(s).
Perineorrhaphy – repair of a torn perineum.
Salpingectomy – excision of a uterine tube.
Salpingostomy – operation performed to restore tubal patency.
Ventrosuspension – fixation of a displaced uterus to the anterior abdominal wall.

ENDOMETRIAL CANCER

Endometrial cancer is the second most common gynaecological cancer and treatment, if begun in the early stages, has a high success rate. Postmenopausal women are most at risk and the majority of cases present in women of age 65–75 years.
Other risk factors include:

• Obesity;
• Late menopause;
• Smoking;
• Oestrogen – only hormone replacement therapy (HRT) in women with an intact uterus;
• Parity – less than a third of cases are childless.

The woman usually presents with vaginal bleeding, which may be sporadic or show only as light spotting and so may be ignored in the first instance. However, vaginal bleeding is not normal for postmenopausal women – those with it should be encouraged to seek medical advice. Other causes of postmenopausal bleeding (PMB) include cervical or endometrial polyps and atrophic vaginitis (see below). Any woman who presents with PMB must be investigated urgently to exclude cancer.
Surgical treatment is usually recommended for both endometrial hyperplasia and cancer. The planned management is usually a total abdominal hysterectomy and bilateral salpingo-oophorectomy. For more advanced cancers, a course of radiotherapy may be prescribed postoperatively.

ENDOMETRIOSIS

Endometriosis is the presence of functional endometrium in abnormal sites (e.g., myometrium, uterine tubes, ovary, peritoneum, etc.). The presentation depends on the site, but includes pain, dyspareunia, etc. Treatment is symptomatic and, as the condition is oestrogen-dependent, treatment aims to reduce oestrogen secretion or oppose its action. This includes progestogens, combined oral contraceptive pill and danazol (anti-oestrogen and androgenic). Surgery is undertaken laparoscopically and aims to destroy the lesions.

DYSFUNCTIONAL UTERINE BLEEDING

Dysfunctional uterine bleeding is excessive uterine bleeding for which no organic cause is found. It is possibly caused by an abnormal function of the control mechanisms of the menstrual cycle. It is important to exclude an organic lesion.

FIBROIDS

Fibroids (leiomyomata) are benign oestrogen-dependent tumours that develop in the myometrium (uterine muscle layer). Fibroids can cause menorrhagia, because

U

Table 41 Most common types of uterovaginal prolapse

Type	Area affected	Description
First degree	Uterus	Uterus descends from the normal position into the vagina
Second degree	Uterus	Uterus descends from the normal position to outside the vulva; cervix becomes ulcerated
Third degree	Uterus	Complete prolapse of uterus outside the body – also known as complete procidentia
Cystocele	Uterus, anterior vaginal wall and bladder	Uterus prolapses, but stays in the pelvis; bladder prolapses (herniates) into the vagina through anterior vaginal wall (*Fig. 184A*)
Urethrocele	Uterus, anterior vaginal wall and urethra	Uterus prolapses, but stays in the pelvis; urethra herniates through anterior vaginal wall
Rectocele	Uterus, posterior vaginal wall and rectum	Uterus prolapses, but stays in the pelvis; rectum prolapses (herniates) into the vagina through posterior vaginal wall (see *Fig. 184B*)
Enterocele	Uterus, posterior vaginal wall and pouch of Douglas	Uterus prolapses, but stays in the pelvis; pouch of Douglas (peritoneal pouch behind uterus) herniates through the posterior vaginal wall; small bowel may also descend

of the increase in surface area of the endometrial cavity, and increased period pain because the uterine contractions squeeze against them. Fibroids are thought to occur in up to 20% of women over 35 years of age and, because they are oestrogen-dependent, decrease in size after the menopause.

Fibroids may be asymptomatic and women can be unaware of having them. However, fibroids can be detected on ultrasound scan and on examination – the uterus may feel enlarged.

Treatment may be conservative if the fibroids are small and asymptomatic. Gonadotrophin-releasing hormone (GnRH) analogues may be used to reduce the size and vascularity of the fibroids. Surgical options include myomectomy, resection via hysteroscopy or laparoscopy, fibroid embolization or hysterectomy (see *Box 42*).

UTEROVAGINAL PROLAPSE

Uterovaginal prolapse, in which there is prolapse of the uterus or vaginal walls (Table 4), is an extremely common disorder. The true incidence is not known as many women cope with the symptoms and do not seek medical help, often because of embarrassment.

This disorder, which is also known as uterine displacement, occurs when the muscles become lax and are unable to support the pelvic organs in their anatomically correct position. This often happens after the menopause and with the loss of oestrogenic effects on the pelvic muscles and other tissues. It can be caused by:

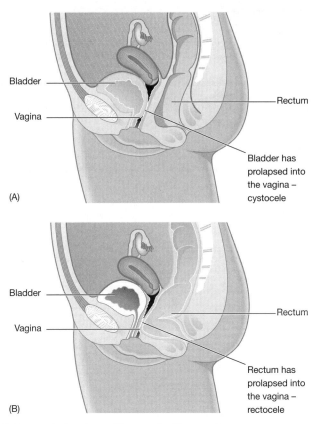

Bladder

Vagina

Rectum

Bladder has
prolapsed into
the vagina –
cystocele

(A)

Bladder

Vagina

Rectum

Rectum has
prolapsed into
the vagina –
rectocele

(B)

Fig 184 Uterovaginal prolapse: (A) cystocele, (B) rectocele

• Pregnancy and childbirth;
• Chronic cough, obesity, heavy work and/or lifting.
The types of uterovaginal prolapse are described in *Table 41* (*Fig. 184*).

Women commonly describe a feeling of 'something coming down' when they have a prolapse. The close proximity to the bladder and bowel (*see Fig. 183*) may result in stress incontinence, frequency of micturition or difficulty in passing urine or stool.

Treatment depends on the severity of symptoms, the health status of the patient and whether the woman has completed her family or not.

A ring pessary made of smooth plastic can be inserted into the vagina and sits at the top, to support the uterus. If tolerated, this can be an excellent solution and needs replacing at intervals of 6 months.

Surgical treatment includes making an incision into the vaginal wall and inserting sutures into the fascia to provide additional support to the pelvic structures. Support of the bladder involves repair of the anterior vaginal wall, known as anterior colporrhaphy or repair. Support of the rectum involves repair of the posterior vaginal wall, known as colpoperineorrhaphy or posterior repair. Hysterectomy via the vaginal route is usually undertaken for a uterine prolapse.

U

Atrophic vaginitis

Atrophic vaginitis results from a lack of oestrogen, which causes the vaginal tissue to be friable and fragile. It occurs in postmenopausal women, and produces a thin bloodstained discharge. It is essential that cancer of the endometrium be excluded as the cause of PMB.

Topical vaginal creams, pessaries and/or rings that contain oestrogen may be used in the short term to improve the vaginal epithelium. Women with an intact uterus who use vaginal oestrogen in the longer term need oral progestogen to prevent endometrial hyperplasia.

Further reading

Brooker C and Nicol M (2003). *Nursing Adults. The Practice of Caring*, Ch 25. Edinburgh: Mosby.

Valsalva's Manoeuvre

Valsalva's manoeuvre is the maximum intrathoracic pressure achieved by forced expiration against a closed glottis. It occurs in such activities as lifting heavy objects, changing position and during defecation: the glottis narrows simultaneously with contraction of the abdominal muscles.

Varicella Zoster

⇒ Communicable diseases (chickenpox), Herpesviruses and herpes.

Varicose Veins

⇒ Peripheral vascular diseases.

Vasoconstriction

⇒ Haemostasis.

Viruses

Viruses are a diverse group of micro-organisms that are visible using electron microscopy only. They contain either deoxyribonucleic acid (DNA) or ribonucleic acid (RNA), and can replicate within the host cell only. Viruses infect humans, animals, plants and other micro-organisms (bacteriophages). The families of viruses include adenoviruses, arboviruses, arenaviruses, coronaviruses, filoviruses, hepadnaviruses, herpesviruses, myxoviruses, papovaviruses, picornaviruses, poxviruses, reoviruses, retroviruses, rhabdoviruses and togaviruses. Diseases caused by viruses in humans include colds, rubella, influenza, measles, rabies, hepatitis, chickenpox, shingles, poliomyelitis and acquired immune deficiency syndrome (AIDS). There is increasing evidence to support the view that some viruses are carcinogenic and some are associated with cancer of the cervix, Burkitt's lymphoma and some types of leukaemia. ⇒ Asepsis, Disinfection, Herpesviruses and herpes, Human immunodeficiency virus, Human papilloma virus, Infection, Lymphatic system (lymphomas).

Vision

Sight is the faculty of seeing. The images focused on the retina are translated into electrical impulses that are transmitted via the visual pathway to the visual cortex of the cerebrum, where they are interpreted. To ensure that the images are seen as one, providing *binocular vision*, the nerve pathways follow a particular route. Those nerve fibres on the temporal (lateral) side of the retina of each eye continue on the same side, while the fibres on the nasal (medial) side cross over at the optic chiasma (*Fig. 185*). Damage, through disease or trauma, to any part of the visual pathway results in loss of part or all of the visual field, such as hemianopia (loss of half the visual field) after a stroke, or diplopia (double vision). ⇒ Eye.

VISUAL ACUITY AND TESTING

Visual acuity (VA) is a measure of the acuteness and fine detail of vision. Testing VA is one of the most important investigations for any patient who presents with reduced vision, ocular disease or trauma, and as a baseline measurement. The test most commonly used is the 'Snellen test type' (*Fig. 186A*), although others are available (see Practice application).

V

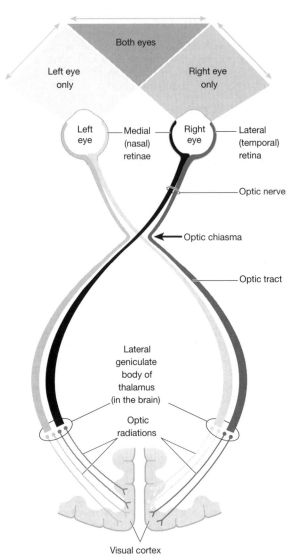

Fig 185 Visual pathways and visual fields

Practice application – testing visual acuity

The test chart should be located in a well-lit space that allows the patient's VA to be measured 6 metres from the chart.

The Snellen chart has a series of letters, numbers or tumbling Es arranged in lines of diminishing size. The largest single letter, number or E is on the top row and the smallest on the bottom row. All of the letters, numbers or Es, are of a particular shape and breadth and are black on a white background. As can be seen from *Figure 186*, as the image size reduces on each line, an additional letter, number or E is added. When the patient cannot read standard letters, understand what the letters represent or say the name of the letter, a number chart or the E type is used (*Fig. 186B*). These can be particularly helpful where language or learning disabilities are an issue. Patients look at the chart and show the position of the E with one they hold.

VA is usually expressed as a fraction. The first number, the numerator, represents the distance from the chart in metres. The second number, the denominator, is the distance at which a person who has average normal vision can read a particular line. For example, if a patient can read the second line from 6 metres, vision would be recorded as 6/36.

Vision should normally be tested at a distance of 6 metres, as at this distance accommodation is ruled out. Each eye must be tested separately. If patients normally wear glasses or contact lenses for distance, vision should be tested both with and without them and recorded as such.

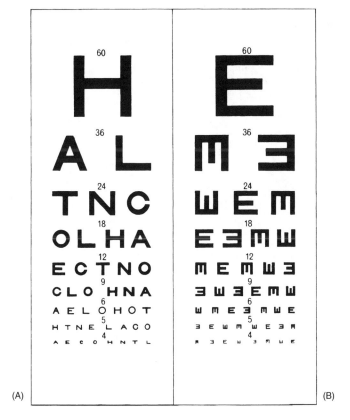

(A)

(B)

Fig 186 Visual acuity testing: (A) Snellen test type, (B) Snellen 'E' chart

VISUAL IMPAIRMENT

Visual impairment covers any problem with vision that affects the field of vision and/or the abilities to see near and distant objects clearly, to judge depth, to discriminate colour and to see one image at a time. ⇒ Colour vision.

Visual impairment may be a temporary phenomenon (e.g. soap that enters the eye causes watering and vision becomes blurred for a few moments). Cataracts, while having a major effect on vision, can in most cases be removed with a resultant improvement to vision. However, the visual impairment may also be permanent (e.g. trauma that results in the loss of an eye). In this instance, binocular vision and depth perception are lost.

The causes of visual impairment include:
- Congenital conditions (e.g. genetic abnormalities);
- Developmental anomalies [e.g. strabismus (squint)];
- Secondary to systemic disease (e.g. diabetic retinopathy);
- Primary disease of the eye itself (e.g. glaucoma, age-related macular degeneration);
- Trauma (e.g. penetrating injury);
- Damage to the visual pathway (e.g. after a stroke);
- Trachoma – caused by *Chlamydia trachomatis*;
- Vitamin A deficiency (xerophthalmia).

REFRACTIVE ERRORS

Many otherwise healthy adults do not see very well because of refractive errors such as myopia (image falls short of the retina – short-sightedness), hypermetropia (image falls behind the retina – long-sightedness) and astigmatism (defects in the curvature of the cornea). These visual anomalies are usually corrected with spectacles, contact lenses (*Fig. 187*) or laser surgery.

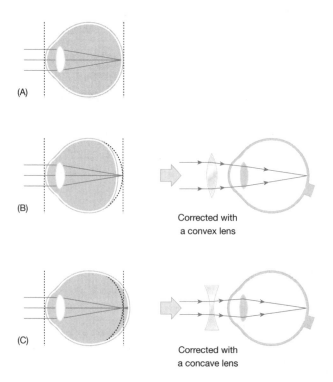

(A)

(B)

Corrected with
a convex lens

(C)

Corrected with
a concave lens

Fig 187 (A) Emmetropia (normal vision); (B) hypermetropia with correction; (C) myopia with correction

As we age (from the late 40s), the ability of the eye to accommodate to near objects, especially for reading, diminishes. People often compensate for this by holding books or newspapers further away. This condition (presbyopia) is normally corrected with reading glasses.

Further reading and resources

Brooker C and Nicol M (2003). *Nursing Adults. The Practice of Caring*, pp. 334–344. Edinburgh: Mosby.

Royal National Institute of the Blind – http://www.rnib.org.uk

VITAMINS

The vitamins are a group of organic compounds required in small amounts by the body. They are vital for many metabolic processes in which they act as co-enzymes. Most are obtained from dietary sources, but some can be synthesized in the body (e.g. vitamin K is made by commensal bacteria in the intestine and vitamin D is also synthesized in the skin). Vitamins are found in both plant and animal foods and are named alphabetically and by their structure. Vitamins may be fat-soluble (A, D, E and K) or water-soluble, as vitamin C and the B complex, which includes thiamin (vitamin B_1), riboflavin (vitamin B_2), niacin (nicotinamide and nicotinic acid), pyridoxine (vitamin B_6), folates, cobalamins (vitamin B_{12}), biotin and pantothenic acid. (Further details about vitamins can be found in the Further reading suggestions.)

Lack of vitamins in the diet and/or inability to absorb them can lead to deficiency diseases (e.g. scurvy, beri-beri, megaloblastic anaemia, xerophthalmia, etc.). However, severe toxicity can occur when some vitamins are taken in excess (hypervitaminosis).

Further reading

Barker H (2002). *Nutrition/Dietetics for Healthcare*, Tenth Edition. Edinburgh: Churchill Livingstone.

Brooker C and Nicol M (2003). *Nursing Adults. The Practice of Caring*, pp. 205–209. Edinburgh: Mosby.

VOMITING

Vomiting is the disagreeable experience that occurs when stomach contents are reflexly expelled through the mouth – it is often accompanied by feelings of nausea (unpleasant sensation felt in the upper abdomen and throat, sweating, pallor, etc.). Vomiting may be effortless, associated with abdominal pain or projectile, such as with pyloric stenosis. The causes of vomiting include gastroenteritis, intestinal obstruction, infection, coughing, radiotherapy, hypercalcaemia, toxins, drugs (e.g. as used in chemotherapy and opioids), motion sickness, pregnancy, unpleasant sights and/or smells, pain, etc. ⇒ Early pregnancy problems (nausea and vomiting, hyperemesis gravidarum).

VOMITING REFLEX

Vomiting is initiated and co-ordinated by two centres in the brain (medulla) – the *vomiting (emetic) centre*, which has overall control, and the *chemoreceptor trigger zone* (CTZ). The vomiting centre and the CTZ respond to various stimuli.

The neurotransmitters involved in vomiting include histamine, dopamine, 5-hydroxytryptamine (serotonin) and acetylcholine. The CTZ and vomiting centre contain receptors able to respond to different stimuli that arrive via receptors in other areas. A knowledge of the receptors is central to controlling nausea and vomiting because each type of antiemetic drug has a different site of action (see below).

ANTIEMETIC DRUGS

Antiemetic drugs exert their action in a variety of ways, so it is essential to target treatment appropriately. Types of antiemetics include (Rang *et al.* 1995):

- Histamine receptor (H_1) antagonists (e.g. cyclizine, which is used for motion sickness and after radiotherapy to the head or neck);
- Central dopamine (D_2) receptor antagonists (e.g. metoclopramide, domperidone) are used for gastrointestinal problems and the nausea and vomiting associated with radiotherapy, toxins and opioids;
- 5-Hydroxytryptamine receptor (5-HT_3) antagonists (e.g. ondansetron) are useful in the management of nausea and vomiting induced by chemotherapy and radiotherapy;
- Muscarinic receptor antagonists (AChM; e.g. hyoscine) are used for motion sickness, and also dry secretions so may reduce nausea and retching if bronchial secretions are excessive;
- Synthetic cannabinoids (e.g. nabilone) are used where other antiemetics fail to control vomiting induced by cytotoxic drugs.

The route of administration of antiemetics is important, as oral drugs are only effective for preventing or treating mild nausea. Persistent nausea or vomiting causes gastric stasis and impedes the absorption of oral drugs. If this occurs, antiemetics should be given by suppository, injection or subcutaneous infusion.

> **Practice application – care of a person who is vomiting**
> The basic needs of a vomiting person include privacy and support, a suitable receptacle and a denture container if appropriate, facilities for teeth cleaning, a mouthwash and a wash and bedding and/or clothing change as appropriate. Postoperatively, people should be encouraged to support wounds with their hands to reduce stress on the incision. The vomit and type of vomiting (e.g. projectile) should be observed and accurate records of fluid balance kept. Apart from these simple measures, nurses should ensure that the most appropriate antiemetic drugs are administered as prescribed. Antiemetics should always be given in anticipation of expected vomiting, as for cancer chemotherapy with cytotoxic drugs.

VULVA

The vulva comprises the structures of the external genitalia (or pudendum; see *Fig. 155B*). The vulva is bounded by two fatty, skin-covered outer folds, the labia majora, which merge posteriorly with the perineal skin. Within the protective outer labia are two smaller folds called the labia minora, which enclose the vestibule. Anteriorly, the labia minora fuse to form the prepuce, which covers the clitoris, and posteriorly they form the fourchette. The clitoris contains erectile tissue and has an abundant nerve supply.

The vestibule contains the openings of the urethra and vagina and the vestibular glands – two tiny Skene's glands (lesser vestibular glands) and two larger Bartholin's glands (greater vestibular glands). Bartholin's glands produce mucus.

The area between the fourchette and the anal canal is called the perineum.

VULVAL DISORDERS

BARTHOLINITIS

Bartholinitis is inflammation of Bartholin's (greater vestibular) glands.

Pruritus vulvae

Pruritus vulvae is intense itching of the external genitalia. The causes include vaginitis from candidiasis and trichomoniasis, glycosuria, malignancy and psychogenic illness.

Vulval cancer

Vulval cancer is relatively uncommon and usually occurs in older women. It normally involves the labia and sometimes the clitoris, and spread is locally to adjoining tissue and lymph nodes.

Clinical presentation includes pruritus, ulcers or, in more advanced cases, a mass with soreness and slight bleeding.

Surgery is the most common form of management. However, radiotherapy may be indicated, but not usually as the sole treatment. Traditionally, surgery was nearly always radical in nature. However, surgery has been modified to reduce morbidity, but still achieve beneficial outcomes. Wide local excision of the cancer with bilateral inguinal node dissection, if necessary, is now undertaken, although if the cancer and tissue affected cover a large area, radical vulvectomy may be indicated. This involves dissecting away the invasive lesion, skin, subcutaneous fat, the vulva and inguinal and femoral nodes.

V

WEANING

Weaning describes the process whereby solid food is gradually added to the milk-only diet of infants. It should not commence before the infant is 17–18 weeks old. Breast milk (or formula milk) alone is considered to be the ideal diet for the first 6 months

The word 'weaning' is also used in the sense of helping to withdraw a person from something on which he or she is dependent (e.g. mechanical ventilation or drug dependency).

> **Practice application – first weaning foods**
> Suitable first weaning foods include:
> - Purées of vegetables and fruits (e.g. carrot, yam, potato, banana and apple), with no added sugar or salt;
> - Nonwheat cereals (e.g. sago, rice and maize) mixed with the baby's usual milk.

WEIL'S DISEASE

⇒ Leptospirosis.

WEST NILE FEVER

West Nile fever is caused by an arbovirus (one transmitted by arthropods) of the genus *Flavivirus*. The virus infects birds and mosquitoes mainly. However, the virus can be transmitted to humans by the bite of an infected mosquito. Although West Nile fever is not transmitted between people, there have been some cases of infection after blood transfusion.

West Nile fever is generally asymptomatic, but may cause a mild febrile illness, with headache and other aches and pains. Less than 1% of those infected develop meningoencephalitis (inflammation of the brain and spinal cord; Health Protection Agency 2003). Meningoencephalitis is characterized by severe frontal headache, pyrexia, neck stiffness, seizures, disorientation and changes in conscious level. Deaths have occurred, especially in those over 50 years of age.

WORLD HEALTH ORGANIZATION

World Health Organization (WHO) is a health organization that co-ordinates health activity and promotes public health worldwide. It was established through a 'declaration' during the United Nations Conference on International Organization held in San Francisco in 1945. A number of disparate health organizations were joined together under the aegis of the United Nations with a headquarters in Geneva, Switzerland.

WOUNDS AND WOUND CARE

Wounds may be acute (e.g. surgical incision or trauma) or chronic (e.g. leg or pressure ulcer). Wounds may also be classified as:
- *Clean* – certain surgical procedures (e.g. hysterectomy) in which aseptic technique is maintained;
- *Clean – contaminated* surgical operations that involve the respiratory or gastrointestinal tract;
- *Contaminated* – acutely inflamed without pus, or in which leakage from a hollow organ has occurred, or clean procedures in which aseptic techniques were breached or recent traumatic wound;

- *Dirty* – presence of pus, perforated internal organs and nonrecent traumatic wounds.
⇒ Burn injuries, Leg ulcers, Pressure ulcers, Tissue viability.

WOUND HEALING

Normal wound healing has three overlapping stages – inflammatory, proliferative and maturation, which may take many months (*Fig. 188*). The healing process may be prolonged by local factors (e.g. poor blood supply, drying of wound bed, mechanical stress, necrotic tissue and/or foreign body, etc.) or general factors that include ageing, nutritional state, dehydration, stress, drugs (e.g. corticosteroids and cytotoxic drugs), etc.

Wound healing may take place by:

- *Primary intention*, when the edges of a clean wound are accurately held together, there is minimal tissue loss and healing occurs with the minimum of scarring and deformity;
- *Secondary intention*, when the edges of a wound are not held together, there is significant tissue loss, the wound heals from the base and the gap is filled by granulation tissue before epithelium can grow over the wound (re-epithelialization);
- *Third intention*, when a wound is left open until infection has been treated or a foreign body removed, and then the wound edges are brought together.

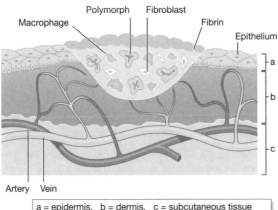

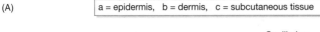

(A)

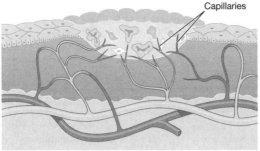

(B)

Fig 188 The stages of wound healing: (A) inflammatory stage, (B) proliferative stage – note the epithelial growth at the wound margins and extension of capillaries into the wound bed (*cont.*)

W

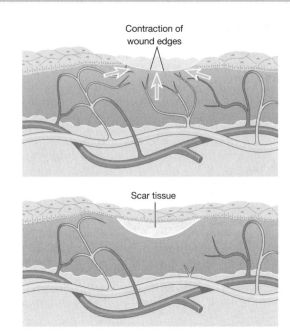

(C)

(D)

Fig 188 *(cont.)* The stages of wound healing: (C) maturation stage, (D) mature stage (early) – note the complete re-epithelialization of the wound surface

Some associated terms are defined in *Box 43*.

Box 43 Wound healing terms

Angiogenesis – formation of new blood vessels.

Debridement – removal of slough or necrotic tissue from wounds, which may be accomplished surgically. However, the three most common forms are:

- Enzymatic – with specialized dressings that contain proteolytic enzymes (streptodornase, streptokinase);
- Autolytic – facilitated by the provision of a moist wound environment using dressings such as hydrogels or hydrocolloids;
- Biosurgery – larval (maggot) therapy.

Dehiscence – the process of splitting or bursting open, as of a wound.

Epithelialization – the migration of epithelial cells over the raw area of a wound, which occurs during the proliferative stage.

Exudate – the serous fluid that is produced from the surface of a wound. It is a clear straw-coloured secretion that varies in consistency from very runny to thick and viscous.

Granulation and/or granulation tissue – the growth of new capillaries and supporting collagen in the base of a wound during the proliferative stage. Healthy granulation tissue is moist and red, and is fragile.

Keloid – elevated progressive scar formation without regression. The upper mantle of the body is most susceptible to keloid formation, as are those with dark skin.

Slough – cellular debris and bacteria that collect at the surface of a wound. It is viscous and can range in colour from creamy white to yellow.

WOUND DRESSINGS

Turner (1985) defined what is now widely accepted as the minimum criteria for the optimum dressing products (*Box 44*).

Box 44 The ideal dressing
The ideal dressing should:
- Maintain a high humidity at the wound/dressing interface (i.e. moist wound healing);
- Remove excess exudate and toxic components;
- Allow gaseous exchange;
- Provide thermal insulation;
- Be impermeable to bacteria;
- Be free from particulate and toxic contaminants;
- Allow removal without causing additional trauma.

Many proprietary dressing materials are available. The choice of dressing depends on the wound characteristics, the needs of the patients and the function required of the dressing. Types include alginates, deodorizing products, foams, hydrocolloids, hydrogels, semi-permeable films, silicone sheets (gels or wound contact layers), low adherent primary contact dressings (medicated) and polysaccharide bead dressings (see Further reading).

WOUND DRAINS

Wound drains are used most often in surgical wounds. They may be inserted as a therapeutic measure (e.g. to drain an abscess) or prophylactically (e.g. to prevent haematoma formation, or in case of the escape of bile). Drainage may be active if the drain is attached to a vacuum system or suction apparatus to produce a 'closed wound suction'.

Further reading

Brooker C and Nicol M (2003). *Nursing Adults. The Practice of Caring*, Ch 10. Edinburgh: Mosby.

REFERENCES

Abrams P, Cardozo L, Fall M, *et al.* (2002). The standardisation of terminology of lower uri-nary tract function: Report from the standardisation sub-committee of the International Continence Society. *Neurol Urodyn.* **21**:167–178.

Addison R (2000). How to administer enema and suppositories. *Nurs Times* **96** (6, Suppl.):3–4.

Aggleton P and Chambers H (2000). *Nursing Models and Nursing Practice*, Second Edition. Basingstoke: Macmillan.

American Psychiatric Association. *Diagnostic and Statistical Manual of Mental Disorders*, Fourth Edition (DSM-IV). Washington DC: American Psychiatric Association.

American Society of Anesthesiologists (1963). New classification of physical status. *Anaesthesiology* **24**:111.

Autar R (1996). Nursing assessment of clients at risk of deep vein thrombosis. The Autar DVT scale. *J Adv Nurs.* **23**(4):763–770.

Avorn J, Monane M, Gurwitz JH, *et al.* (1994). Reduction of bacteriuria and pyuria after ingestion of cranberry juice. *JAMA* **271**(10):751–754.

Ayliffe GAJ, Lowbury EJL, Geddes AM and Williams JD (1992). *Control of Hospital Infection: A Practical Handbook*, Third Edition. London: Chapman & Hall Medical.

Badger C (1987). Lymphoedema: Management of patients with advanced cancer. *Prof Nurse* **2**(4):100–102.

Bateman NT and Leach RM (1998). ABC of oxygen: Acute oxygen therapy. *Br Med J.* **317**:798–801.

Baylis V, Davies L, Gunner C, *et al.* (2001). *North Hampshire Bowel Care Pathway*. London: GI Education, Norgine Ltd.

Behrens H (1998). Ageism real or imagined? *Elderly Care* **10**(2):10–13.

Blair P, Bensley D, Smith I, *et al.* (1996). Smoking and sudden infant death syndrome: Results from 1993–5 case-control study for confidential enquiry into stillbirths and deaths in infancy. *Br Med J.* **313**:195–198.

Borbély A (Schneider D, trans) (1987). *Secrets of Sleep*. Harlow: Longman Scientific and Technical.

Boud D, Keogh R and Walker D (198). *Reflection: Turning Experience into Learning*. London: Kogan Page.

Braithwaite R (1992). *Violence: Understanding, Intervention and Prevention*. Oxford: Radcliffe Professional Series.

British Committee for Standards in Haematology (1999). The administration of blood and blood components and the management of transfused patients. *Transfusion Med.* **9**:227–238.

Brooker C and Nicol M (2003). *Nursing Adults: The Practice of Caring*. Edinburgh: Mosby.

Brugne JF (1994). Effects of night work on circadian rhythms and sleep. *Prof Nurse* **10**(1):25–28.

Butler G (2000). Emotion and the brain. *Psychologist* **13**(3):131–132.

Campbell S and Glasper EA (1995). *Whaley and Wong's Children's Nursing*. London: Mosby.

Cancer Research UK (2003). Online. Available at: http://www.cancerresearchuk.org

Cardozo L (1991). Urinary incontinence in women: Do we have anything new to offer? *Br Med J.* **303**(6815):1453–1457.

Cassano GB, Tundo A and Micheli C (1994). Bi-polar and psychotic depressions. *Curr Opin Psychiatry* **7**:5–8.

Cohen MR, Senders J and Davis NM (1994). Failure mode and effects analysis: A novel approach to avoiding dangerous medication errors and accidents. *Hospital Pharm.* **29**(4):319–330.

CRHP (2003). Council for the Regulation of Health Professionals – functions. Online. Available at: www.crhp.org.uk/functions.html 2003

Crouch R and Marrow J (1996). Towards a UK triage scale. *Emerg Nurse* **4**(3):4–5.

Davis N (1995). Potassium perils. *Am J Nurs.* **95**(3):14.

Department of Health (1991a). *Report on Health and Social Subjects 41. Dietary Reference Values for Food Energy and Nutrients for the United Kingdom*. London: HMSO.

Department of Health (1991b). *The Patient's Charter*. London: HMSO.

Department of Health (1994). *Working in Partnership: A Collaborative Approach to Care (Butterworth Report)*. London: HMSO.

Department of Health (1996). *Breastfeeding: Good Practice Guidance to the NHS*. London: HMSO.

Department of Health (1997). *The New NHS: Modern, Dependable*. London: Department of Health.

Department of Health (1998a). *A First Class Service: Improving Quality in the NHS*. London: The Stationery Office.

Department of Health (1998b). *Guidance for Clinical Health Care Workers: Protection against Blood-Borne Viruses*. London: HMSO.

Department of Health (1999a). *Making a Difference: Strengthening the Nursing, Midwifery and Health Visiting Contribution to Health and Health Care*. London: The Stationery Office.

Department of Health (1999b). *Saving Lives: Our Healthier Nation*. London: The Stationery Office.

Department of Health (2000a). *The NHS Plan*. HMSO.

Department of Health (2000b). *National Service Framework for Coronary Heart Disease. Modern Standards and Service Models*. London: Department of Health.

Department of Health (2001). *Good Practice in Consent Implementation Guide: Consent to Examination or Treatment*. London: Department of Health.

Department of Health (2003). *Death Rates by Selected Causes*. Online. Available at: www.dh.gov.uk

Dimond B (2001). *Legal Aspects of Nursing*. Harlow: Pearson Higher Education.

Eisenberg N, Fabes RA, Guthrie IK and Reiser M (2000). Dispositional emotionality and regulation: The role in predicting quality of social functioning. *J Pers Soc Psychol*. **78**(1):136–157.

Engel GL (1964). Grief and grieving. *Am J Nurs*. **64**:93–98.

European Pressure Ulcer Advisory Panel (1999a). *Pressure Ulcer Treatment Guidelines*. Oxford: European Pressure Ulcer Advisory Panel (EPUAP).

European Pressure Ulcer Advisory Panel (1999b). *Pressure Ulcer Prevention Guidelines*. Oxford: European Pressure Ulcer Advisory Panel (EPUAP).

Folstein MF, Folstein SE and McHugh PR (1975). Mini mental state: A practical method for grading the cognitive state of patients for the clinician. *J Psychiatr Res*. **12**(3):189–198.

Getliffe K (1993). Informed choices for long term benefits, the management of catheters in continence care. *Prof Nurs*. **9**(2):122–126.

Gibbs G (1988). *Learning by Doing: A Guide to Teaching and Learning Methods*. Oxford: Further Education Unit, Oxford Brookes University.

Gibson CH (1991). A concept of empowerment. *J Adv Nurs*. **16**:354–356.

Gibson HB (1961). *The Gibson Spiral Maze*. Sevenoaks: Hodder and Stoughton.

Greenberg JS (1992). *Health Education: Learner-Centered Instructional Strategies*, Second Edition. Iowa: Brown.

Haward R (1999). *Improving Outcomes in Gynaecological Cancer*. London: NHS Executive.

Hawton K, Fagg J, Simkin S, *et al*. (1997). Trends in deliberate self-harm in Oxford, 1985–1995: Implications for clinical services and the prevention of suicide. *Br J Psychiatry* **171**:556–560.

Health Protection Agency, Communicable Disease Surveillance Centre (2003). *West Nile Virus, Q&A*. Online. Available at: http://www.hpa.org.uk

Henderson V (1966). *The Nature of Nursing: A Definition and its Implications for Practice, Research and Education*. New York: Macmillan.

Jefferson T, Demicheli V and Mugford M (2000). *Elementary Economic Evaluation in Health Care*, Second Edition. London: BMJ Books.

Johns C (1996). Using a reflective model of nursing and guided reflection. *Nurs Stand*. **11**(2):34–38.

Kempe R and Kempe C (1984). *The Common Secret: Sexual Abuse of Children and Adolescents*. New York: Freeman.

Leff J and Vaughn C (1985). *Expressed Emotion in Families*. New York: Guildford Press.

Lish JD, Dime-Meenan S, Whybrow, *et al*. (1994). The National Depressive and Manic-Depressive Association (DMDA) survey of bipolar members. *J Affective Disord*. **31**:281–294.

Macmillan (1996). *Professional Relationships: Influences on Health Care*. London: Macmillan.

Maslow AH (1974). *Motivation and Personality*, Second Edition. New York: Harper and Row.

McCaughan D (1999). Developing critical appraisal skills. *Prof Nurse* **14**:843–847.

Melzack R and Wall PD (1988). *The Challenge of Pain*, Second Edition. London: Penguin Books.

Metheny NM (1996). *Fluid and Electrolyte Balance*, Third Edition. Philadelphia: Lippincott.

Milsom I, Abrams P, Cardozo L, *et al.* (2001). How widespread are the symptoms of an overactive bladder and how are they managed? A population-based prevalence. *Br J Urol Int.* **87**:760–766.

Montazeri A, Gillis CR and McEwen J (1996). Measuring quality of life in oncology: Is it worthwhile? *Eur J Cancer Care* **5**:159–167.

Moppett S (2000). Which way is up for a suppository? *Nurs Times Plus* **96**(19):12–13.

Murthy P and McKerrow W (1995). Nasal septal surgery: Is routine follow-up necessary. *J Laryngol Otol.* **109**:320–323.

NANDA (2001). *Nursing Diagnosis: Definitions and Classification 2001–2002*. Philadelphia: NANDA International.

NICE (2001). *Alzheimer's Disease – Donepezil, Rivastigmine and Galantamine* (Guidance No 19). Online. Available at: http://www.nice.org.uk

NICE (2002). *Full Guidance on the Use of Drugs for Early Thrombolysis in the Treatment of Acute Myocardial Infarction* (Guidance No 52). Online. Available at: http://www.nice.org.uk

NICE (2003). Head Injury – *Triage, Assessment, Investigation and Early Management of Head Injury in Infants, Children and Adults*. Online. Available at: http://www.nice.org.uk

NBS (1999). *Preceptorship in Action: A Guide*. Edinburgh: National Board for Nursing, Midwifery and Health Visiting for Scotland.

NHS Executive (1999). *Agenda for Change*. National Health Service Executive: Leeds.

Nicol M, Bavin C, Bedford-Turner S, Cronin P and Rawlings-Anderson K (2000). *Essential Nursing Skills*. London: Mosby.

NMC (2002a). *The Code of Professional Conduct*. London: Nursing and Midwifery Council.

NMC (2002b). *Guidelines for Records and Record Keeping*, pp 7–10. London: Nursing and Midwifery Council.

NMC (2003). *NMC Begins Work on Higher Level Practice Standards*. Press statement 104/03 5 September 2003. London: Nursing and Midwifery Council.

O'Brien E and O'Malley K (1981). *Essentials of Blood Pressure Measurement*. Edinburgh: Churchill Livingstone.

O'Brien E, Beevers D and Marshall H (1995). *ABC of Hypertension*, Third Edition. London: BMJ Publishing Group.

Oliver M (1998). Theories of disability in health practice and research. *Br Med J.* **317**:1446–1449.

Oliver N and Kuipers E (1996). Stress and its relationship to expressed emotion in community care workers. *Int J Soc Psychiatry* **42**(2):150–159.

Parkes CM (1975). *Bereavement: Studies of Grief in Adult Life*. London: Penguin.

Pattie AH and Gilleard CJ (1979). *Manual of the Clifton Assessment Procedures for the Elderly (CAPE)*. London: Hodder and Stoughton.

Petticrew M, Watt I and Sheldon T (1998). Executive summary. *Systematic Review of the Effectiveness of Laxatives in the Elderly*, Vol. 13. NHS Research and Development, Health Technology Assessment Programme. London: HMSO.

Pilling S and Frank J (1994). Evaluation back-up. *Nursing Stand.* **8**(35):22–23.

Pilowsky I (1978). A general classification of abnormal illness behaviours. *Br J Med Psychol.* **51**:131–137.

Price B (1990). *Body Image: Nursing Concepts and Care*. London: Prentice Hall.

Rang HP, Dale MM and Ritter JM (1995). *Pharmacology*, Third Edition. Edinburgh: Churchill Livingstone.

Resuscitation Council (2000). *ALS Manual*, Fourth Edition. London: Resuscitation Council (UK).

Roberts J (2000). Developing an oral assessment and intervention tool for older people. 3. *Br J Nurs.* **9**(19):2073–2078.

Robins J and Mangan M (1999). Seen and not heard. *Nurs Times* **95**(37):30–32.

Rogers R, Salvage J and Cowell R (1998). *Nurses at Risk: A Guide to Health and Safety at Work*, Second Edition. London: Macmillan Press.

Roper N, Logan WW and Tierney AJ (1996). *The Elements of Nursing*, Fourth Edition. Edinburgh: Churchill Livingstone.

Royal College of Nursing (1998). *Clinical Practice Guidelines. The Management of Patients with Venous Leg Ulcers*. London: Royal College of Nursing (RCN).

Royal College of Surgeons (1992). *Commission on the Provision of Surgical Services. Guidelines for Day Case Surgery.* London: Royal College of Surgeons.

Sarafino EP (1994). *Health Psychology: Biophysical Interactions,* Second Edition. Chichester: John Wiley.

Selye H (1984). *The Stress of Life.* New York: McGraw-Hill.

Shekelle PG, Woolf SH, Eccles M and Grimshaw J (1999). Clinical guidelines: Developing guidelines. *Br Med J.* **318**:593–596.

Sims A and Owens D (1993). *Psychiatry,* Sixth Edition. London: Balliere Tindall.

Sobin LH and Wittekind C (1997). *TNM Classification of Malignant Tumours,* Fifth Edition. Chichester: John Wiley.

Strauss A (1976). *Chronic Illness and the Quality of Life.* St Louis: Mosby.

Sutherland VJ and Cooper CL (1990). *Understanding Stress. A Psychological Perspective for Health Professionals.* London: Chapman Hall.

Sylva K (1993). Play in hospital – when and why it's effective. *Curr Paediatr.* **3**:247–249.

Teasdale G and Jennett B (1974). Assessment of coma and impaired consciousness: A practical scale. *Lancet* **ii**:81–84.

Thompson GW, Creed F, Drossman AJ, *et al.* (1992). Functional bowel disease and functional abdominal pain. *Gastroenterol Int.* **5**:75–91.

Tolman E (1932). *Purposive Behaviour in Animals and Men.* New York: Appleton.

Turnbull S, Ward A, Treasure J, *et al.* (1996). The demand for eating disorder care: An epidemiological study using the general practice research data base. *Br J Psychiatry* **169**:705–712.

Turner TD (1985). Which dressing and why? In: Westerby S, Ed. *Wound Care.* London: Heinemann Medical Books.

UKCC (1999). *Fitness for Practice: The UKCC Commission for Nursing and Midwifery Education* (Chair: Sir Leonard Peach). London: United Kingdom Central Council for Nursing, Midwifery and Health Visiting.

Vieta E (1997). Differential features between bipolar I and bipolar II disorder. *Compr Psychiatry* **38**:98–101.

Von Schoenberg M, RobinsonP and Ryan P (1993). Nasal packing after nasal surgery – is it justified? *J Laryngol Otol.* **107**:902–905.

Vowden K, Goulding V and Vowden P (1996). Hand held Doppler assessment for peripheral arterial disease. *J Wound Care* **5**(3):125–128.

Wald A (1994). Constipation and faecal incontinence in the elderly. *Semin Gastrointes Dis.* **5**:179–188.

Waterlow JA (1985). A risk assessment card. *Nurs Times* **81**(48):49–55.

Watson R (1993). *Caring for Elderly People.* London: Balliere Tindall.

WHO (1980). *International Classification of Impairments, Disabilities and Handicaps.* Geneva: World Health Organisation.

WHO (1986). *Ottawa Charter for Health Promotion.* Geneva: World Health Organisation.

WHO (1990). *Cancer Pain Relief and Palliative Care.* Technical Report, Series 804. Geneva: World Health Organisation.

WHO (1992). *International Classification of Disease. ICD-10,* Tenth Edition. Geneva: World Health Organisation.

WHO (1998a). *The World Health Report. Life in the 21st Century A Vision for All.* Geneva: World Health Organisation.

WHO (1998b). *Obesity: Preventing and Managing the Global Epidemic.* Geneva: World Health Organisation.

WHO (2001). *International Classification of Functioning Disability and Health.* Geneva: World Health Organisation.

Woodward S (1997a). Neurological observations – 1. Glasgow coma scale. *Nurs Times* **93**(45, Suppl.):1–2.

Woodward S (1997b). Neurological observations – 2. Pupil response. *Nurs Times* **93**(46, Suppl.):1–2.

Worden WJ (1991). *Grief Counselling and Grief Therapy,* Second Edition. London: Routledge.

Workman B (1999). Safe injection techniques. *Nurs Stand.* **13**(39):47–53.

Zubin J and Spring B (1977). Vulnerability: a new view of schizophrenia. *J Abnorm Psychol.* **86**:260–266.

Sources

The editor would like to thank the authors and editors of the following books, all of which have been used as a source of text and artwork for *Churchill Livingstone's Mini Encyclopaedia of Nursing*.

Anderson DM, Anderson LE and Glanze WD (2002). *Mosby's Medical, Nursing and Allied Health Dictionary*, Sixth Edition. St Louis: Mosby.

Bale S and Jones V (1997). *Wound Care Nursing*. London: Balliere Tindall.

Brooker C (1998). *Human Structure and Function*, Second Edition. London: Mosby.

Brooker C (2002). *Churchill Livingstone's Dictionary of Nursing*, Eighteenth Edition. Edinburgh: Churchill Livingstone (Dictionary entries, Appendices 8, 9).

Brooker C (2002). *Mosby Nurse's Pocket Dictionary*. Edinburgh: Mosby.

Brooker C (2003). *Churchill Livingstone's Pocket Medical Dictionary*, Fifteenth Edition. Edinburgh: Churchill Livingstone (Dictionary of medical terms, Appendix 5).

Brooker C and Nicol M (2003). *Nursing Adults: The Practice of Caring*. Edinburgh: Mosby (Chapters 1–35).

Davis PS (1994). *Nursing the Orthopaedic Patient*. Edinburgh: Churchill Livingstone.

Fraser DM and Cooper MA (2003). *Myles Textbook for Midwives*, Fourteenth Edition. Edinburgh: Churchill Livingstone (Chapters 4, 16, 17, 20, 23).

Gamble C and Brennan G (2000). *Working with Serious Mental Health: A Manual for Clinical Practice*. Edinburgh: Churchill Livingstone (Chapters 7, 15).

Gangar EA (2001). *Gynaecological Nursing. A Practical Guide*. Edinburgh: Churchill Livingstone.

Gunn C (2001). *Using Maths in Health Science*. Edinburgh: Churchill Livingstone.

Haslett C, Chilvers ER, Hunter JAA and Boon NA (1999). *Davidson's Principles and Practice of Medicine*, Eighteenth Edition. Edinburgh: Churchill Livingstone (Chapters 2, 3).

Heath H (1995). *Potter and Perry's Foundations in Nursing Theory and Practice*. London: Mosby.

Hinchcliff S, Montague S and Watson R (1996). *Physiology for Nursing Practice*, Second Edition. London: Bailliere Tindall (Chapters 1.3, 3.1, 5.3, 6.3).

Huband S and Trigg E (2000). *Practices in Children's Nursing Guidelines for Hospital and Community*. Edinburgh: Churchill Livingstone (Chapters 20, 32, Appendix 1).

Jamieson E, McCall J and Whyte L (2002). *Clinical Nursing Practice*, Fourth Edition. Edinburgh: Churchill Livingstone.

Kanski JJ (1999). *Clinical Ophthalmology*, Fourth Edition. Oxford: Butterworth/Heinemann.

Kenworthy N, Snowley G and Gilling C (2002). *Common Foundation Studies in Nursing*, Third Edition. Edinburgh: Churchill Livingstone (Chapters 1, 3, 4, 7, 9, 10, 12, 14, 16).

MacConnachie AM, Hay J, Harris J and Nimmo S (2002). *Drugs in Nursing Practice: An A–Z Guide*. Edinburgh: Churchill Livingstone.

Maclean H (2002). *The Eye in Primary Care*. Oxford: Butterworth Heinemann.

Mallik M, Hall C and Howard D (1998). *Nursing Knowledge and Practice*. London: Bailliere Tindall (Chapters 1.2, 2.1, 2.5, 3.3, 3.4, 3.5,4.1, 4.2, 4.3, 4.5, 4.6).

Middleton S and Roberts A (2000). *Integrated Care Pathways: A Practical Approach to Implementation*. Oxford: Butterworth Heinemann (Chapter 1).

Newell R and Gournay K (2000). *Mental Health Nursing: An Evidence-Based Approach*. Edinburgh: Churchill Livingstone (Chapters 7, 9, 10, 11, 12, 13, 14, 15, 17).

Nicol M, Bavin C, Bedford-Turner S, Cronin P and Rawlings-Anderson K (2000). *Essential Nursing Skills*. Edinburgh: Mosby.

Niven N (2000). *Health Psychology for Health Care Professionals*, Third Edition. Edinburgh: Churchill Livingstone.

Parkinson J and Brooker C (2004). *Everyday English for International Nurses: a Guide to Working in the UK*. Edinburgh: Churchill Livingstone (Chapter 3).

Peattie PI and Walker S (1995). *Understanding Nursing Care*, Fourth Edition. Edinburgh: Churchill Livingstone (Chapter 6).

Prosser S, Worster B, MacGregor J, *et al*. (2000). *Applied Pharmacology*. Edinburgh: Mosby (Chapters 2, 3, 5, 12).

Pudner R (2000). *Nursing the Surgical Patient*. Edinburgh: Bailliere Tindall (Chapters 15, 16).

Rankin-Box D (2001). *The Nurse's Handbook of Complementary Therapies*, Second Edition. Edinburgh: Bailliere Tindall.

Robotham A and Sheldrake D (2000). Health *Visiting Specialist and Higher Level Practice*. Edinburgh: Churchill Livingstone (Chapters 7, 13).

Roper N, Logan W and Tierney A (1985). *The Elements of Nursing*, Second Edition. Edinburgh: Churchill Livingstone.

Rutishauser S (1994). *Physiology and Anatomy. A Basis for Nursing and Health Care*. Edinburgh: Churchill Livingstone.

Sheppard M and Wright M (2000). *Principles and Practice of High Dependency Nursing*. Edinburgh: Bailliere Tindall (Chapter 6).

Smith M (1999). *Rehabilitation in Adult Nursing Practice*. Edinburgh: Churchill Livingstone (Chapter 1).

Smith P (1997). *Research Mindedness for Practice. An Interactive Approach for Nursing and Health Care*. Edinburgh: Churchill Livingstone (Chapter 8).

Thompson IE, Melia KM and Boyd KM (2000). *Nursing Ethics*, Fourth Edition. Edinburgh: Churchill Livingstone.

Thompson T and Mathias P (2000). *Lyttle's Mental Health and Disorder*, Third Edition. Edinburgh: Bailliere Tindall (Chapters 1, 5, 6, 17).

Wallace M (2002). *Churchill Livingstone's A–Z Guide to Professional Healthcare*. Edinburgh: Churchill Livingstone.

Watson R (2000). *Anatomy and Physiology for Nurses*, Eleventh Edition. Edinburgh: Bailliere Tindall.

Waugh A and Grant A (2001). *Ross and Wilson Anatomy and Physiology*, Ninth Edition. Edinburgh: Churchill Livingstone.

Westwood O (1999). *The Scientific Basis for Health Care*. London: Mosby.

Wilson J (1995). *Infection Control in Clinical Practice*. London: Bailliere Tindall.

Wong D, Hockenberry-Eaton MJ, Wilson D, *et al.* (1999). *Whaley and Wong's Nursing Care of Infants and Children*, Sixth Edition. St Louis: Mosby.

INDEX

This index is of the sub-headings found within the main encyclopaedia entries, which are not in the index unless required for clarity (see the Preface). An arrow ⇒, either within or at the end of the entry, is used to indicate cross-references that contain related material.